Practice of Pediatric Orthopedics

Lynn T. Staheli, M.D.

Professor, Department of Orthopedics
University of Washington School of Medicine
Seattle, Washington

Editor, *Journal of Pediatric Orthopaedics*

Orthopedist,
Department of Orthopedics
Children's Hospital and Regional Medical Center
Seattle, Washington

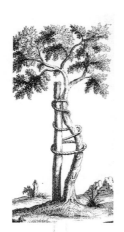

Contents

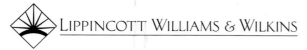

LIPPINCOTT WILLIAMS & WILKINS

i

Table of Contents

Consultants – find current e-mail addresses on Web site *www.childortho.com*

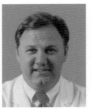

James Beaty, MD
Femur fracture
Memphis TN USA
Jbeaty@
campbellclinic.com

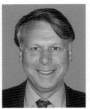

Michael Benson, FRSC
Developmental hip dys.
Oxford UK
michael.benson@
iname.com

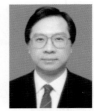

Jack Cheng, MD
Asian consultations
Hong Kong China
jackcheng@cuhk.edu.hk

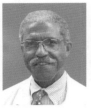

Alvin Crawford, MD
Spine chapter
Cincinnati OH USA
crawa0@chmcc.org

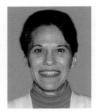

Sharon DeMuth, PhD
Physical and
occupational therapy
Los Angeles CA USA
demuth@hsc.usc.edu

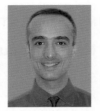

Mohammad Diab, MD
Syndrome chapter
Seattle WA USA
diab@chmc.org

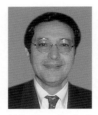

Alain Dimeglio, Prof.
Growth & clubfoot
Montpelier France
a-dimeglio@
chu-montpellier.fr

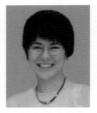

Marybeth Ezaki, MD
Upper extremity chapter
Dallas TX USA

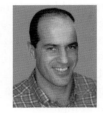

Edison Forlin, MD
South American
consultations
Curitiba Brazil
eforlin@cwb.matrix.com.br

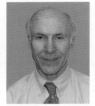

Anthony Herring, MD
Perthes
Dallas TX USA
johnher@ix.netcom.com

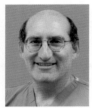

John Herzenberg, MD
Ponseti clubfoot treatment
Baltimore MD USA
frcsc@aol.com

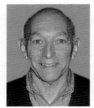

Mark Hoffer, MD
Brachial palsy
Los Angeles, CA, USA
sribas@laoh.ucla.edu

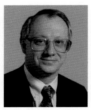

Randy Loder, MD
Slipped epiphysis
Minneapolis MN USA
rloder@shrinenet.org

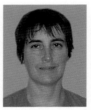

Anne Lynn, MD
Anesthesia
Seattle WA USA

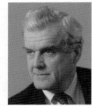

Dean MacEwen, MD
Risk management
Philadelphia PA USA
honsandtraps@webtv.net

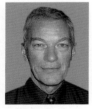

Colin Moseley, MD
Straightline chart
Leg length inequality
Los Angeles CA USA
cmoseley@ucla.edu

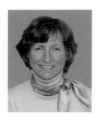

Carol Mowery, MD
PPO review
Seattle WA USA
cmow@
u.washington.edu

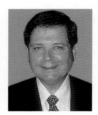

William Oppenheim, MD
Cerebral palsy
Los Angeles CA USA
woppenhe@ucla.edu

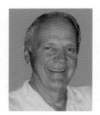

Ham Peterson, MD
Bridge resection – bunion
Rochester MN USA
peterson.hamlet@
mayo.edu

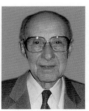

Ignacio Ponseti, MD
Clubfoot management
Iowa City IA USA
ignacio-ponseti@
uiowa.edu

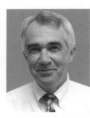

George Rab, MD
Tumor chapter
Sacramento CA USA
george.rab@
ucdmc.ucdavis.edu

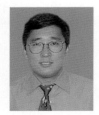

Kit Song, MD
**Infection & Spine
chapters**
Seattle WA USA
ksong@chmc.org

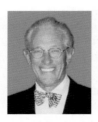

Carl Stanitski, MD
**Knee & Sports
chapters**
Charleston SC USA
stanitsc@musc.edu

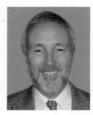

Peter Stevens, MD
Lower limb malalignment
Salt Lake City UT USA
peterstevens@
m.cc.utah.edu

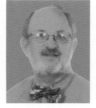

Michael Sussman, MD
**Neuromuscular
chapter**
Portland OR USA
msussman@
shrinenet.org

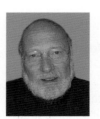

Hugh Watts, MD
Limb deficiency, polio,
& tuberculosis
Los Angeles CA USA
hwatts@ucla.edu

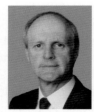

John Wedge, MD
Salter osteotomy
Toronto Canada
john.wedge@
sickkids.on.ca

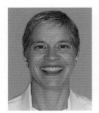

Jane Burns, MD
Antibiotic treatment
Seattle WA USA
jburns@chmc.org

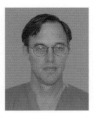

Chappie Conrad, MD
Tumors chapter
Seattle WA USA
chappiec@u.
washington.edu

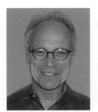

Richard Gross, MD
**Evaluation & Management
chapters**
Charleston SC USA
grossr@musc.edu

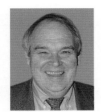

Robert Hensinger, MD
Cervical spine
Ann Arbor MI USA

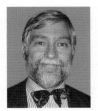

Freeman Miller, MD
Cerebral palsy
Wilmington DE USA
frmiller@nemours.org

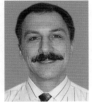

Vince Mosca, MD
Foot chapter
& myelodysplasia
Seattle WA USA
vmosca@chmc.org

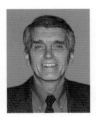

Perry Schoenecker, MD
Pseudoarthrosis tibia
St Louis MO USA
pschoenecker@
shrinenet.org

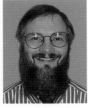

David Sherry, MD
Arthritis & RSD
Seattle WA USA
dsherry@chmc.org

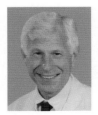

Stuart Weinstein, MD
Spine chapter
Iowa City IA USA
stuart-weinstein@uiowa.edu

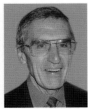

Kaye Wilkins, MD
Trauma chapter
San Antonio TX USA
drkwilkins@aol.com

Preface

The *Practice of Pediatric Orthopedics* (**PPO**) was designed to make learning children's orthopedics efficient and pleasant. This book provides core information, references, and e-mail access to experts. I designed, wrote, and illustrated PPO utilizing desktop publishing technology that made possible a full-color, extensively illustrated book that is affordable. To insure accuracy and clarity, each section was reviewed by at least two consultants. Consultants are acknowledged authorities. The general features of PPO are listed below. Please read – *Instructions to Readers*.

General Features

- Designed for general orthopedists and residents
- Provides core information on pediatric orthopedics
- 37 *consultants* edited content and may accept e-mail consultations
- Current references are provided
- Compact, efficient design, with over 400 pages & 2500 illustrations
- Practical, *how to* book details common problems
- Management recommendations are *whole child* oriented
- *Mainstream* approach to management – safe and proven
- Management recommendtions are current
- Trauma and procedures are presented in greatest detail
- Flowcharts are added to guide management

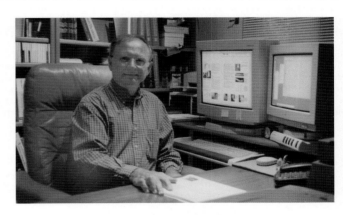

Lynn T. Staheli, M.D.
e-mail: staheli@u.washington.edu

Text editing: Sandra Rush
Reference editing: Christian Alexander
Communications: Gail Nealon
Section editor: Robert Hurley*
Executive vice president: Kathey Alexander*
* Lippincott, Williams & Wilkins

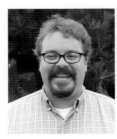

Jeff McCord
Design &
technical consultant
jeff@free-lancelot.com

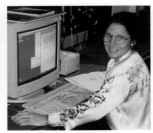

Lana Staheli, PhD
Consultant – advisor
Wife

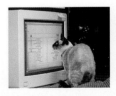

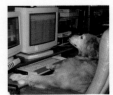

More help
Sabrina (upper)
Bear (lower)

Acquisitions Editor: Bob Hurley
Production Editor: Cassie Carey
Manufacturing Manager: Tim Reynolds

LIPPINCOTT WILLIAMS & WILKINS
530 Walnut Street
Philadelphia, PA 19106 USA
LWW.com

Library of Congress Cataloging-in-Publication Data

Staheli, Lynn T.
    Practice of pediatric orthopedics / Lynn T. Staheli ; consultants, Beaty, J. ... [et al.].
        p. ; cm.
    Includes bibliographical references and index.
    ISBN 0-7817-3142-9
    1. Pediatric orthopedics. I. Beaty, James H.
    [DNLM: 1. Musculoskeletal Diseases—therapy—Child. 2. Musculoskeletal
System—physiopathology. WS 270 S781p 2001]
    RD732.3.C48 S733 2001
    618.92′7—7—dc21   00-069011

Care has been taken to confirm the accuracy of the information presented and to describe generally accepted practices. However, the authors, and publisher are not responsible for errors or omissions or for any consequences from application of the information in this book and make no warranty, expressed or implied, with respect to the currency, completeness, or accuracy of the contents of the publication. Application of this information in a particular situation remains the professional responsibility of the practitioner.

The authors and publisher have exerted every effort to ensure that drug selection and dosage set forth in this text are in accordance with current recommendations and practice at the time of publication. However, in view of ongoing research, changes in government regulations, and the constant flow of information relating to drug therapy and drug reactions, the reader is urged to check the package insert for each drug for any change in indications and dosage and for added warnings and precautions. This is particularly important when the recommended agent is a new or infrequently employed drug.

Some drugs and medical devices presented in this publication have Food and Drug Administration (FDA) clearance for limited use in restricted research settings. It is the responsibility of the health care provider to ascertain the FDA status of each drug or device planned for use in their clinical practice.

10 9 8 7 6 5 4 3 2 1

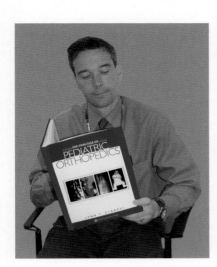

Instructions to Readers

Consultants

Consultants with e-mail addresses may accept e-mail questions from orthopedists. Questions should be non-urgent and general in nature. Find updated e-mail addresses on my web site at *www.ChildOrtho.com*

Abbreviations for journals

JPO Journal of Pediatric Orthopaedics

JBJS Journal of Bone and Joint Surgery

CO Clinical Orthopedics

OCNA Orthopedic Clinics of North America

Reference formats

Section reference citations are arranged by date. References in *Additional Reading* are listed by author. Syndromes references arranged chonologically to credit those making the original description.

Order of illustrations

The order of citing illustrations in the text is not always consecutive because of requirements for efficient page design.

Errors and suggestions

Please inform me of errors or make suggestions for the next edition by e-mail:
staheli@u.washington.edu

Dedication.....

To Letha Staheli, my mother and inspiration; Lana Staheli, my wife and best friend; and my children, Linda, Diane, and Todd

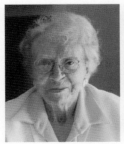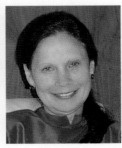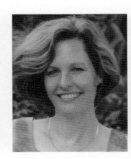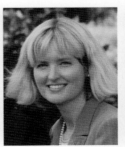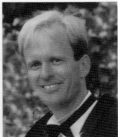

Chapter 1 – Growth

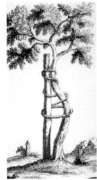

Fig. 1.1 Andry's Tree.

Pediatric orthopedics is a subspecialty of medicine that deals with the prevention and treatment of musculoskeletal disorders in children. In 1741, Nicholas Andry, professor of medicine at the University of Paris, published his treatise describing different methods of preventing and correcting deformities in children (Fig. 1.1). He combined two Greek words, *orthos*, or straight, and *paidios*, child, into one word, "orthopedics," which became the name of the speciality concerned with the preservation and restoration of the musculoskeletal system. Pediatric orthopedics is central to this specialty because of Andry's original focus on childhood problems, because of the large proportion of orthopedic problems that originate during the early period of growth, and finally, because pediatric orthopedics offers a dynamic and inherently interesting subspecialty.

A knowledge of normal and abnormal growth and development is vital to an understanding of pediatric orthopedics (Fig. 1.2). This knowledge increases our comprehension of the musculoskeletal system, improves our understanding of the causes of disease, and makes us better able to manage the varied orthopedic problems of childhood.

Dividing the period of growth into seven stages provides a convenient framework to review both normal and abnormal growth and development (Fig. 1.3). During the first stage, reproductive cells or gametes are formed.

Normal Growth

Gamete
Gamete is a collective term for ovum and sperm. During gametogenesis, meiotic division halves the chromosome number. Genetic material, which may include defective genes, is shuffled, and mature ova and sperm are formed (Fig. 1.4).

Early Embryo
This early embryonic phase encompasses the 2-week period from fertilization to the implantation of the embryo.

First week During the first week following fertilization, the zygote repeatedly divides as it moves through the fallopian tubes to the uterus. The zygote becomes a morula, then a blastocyst. The blastocyst implants itself on the posterior uterine wall.

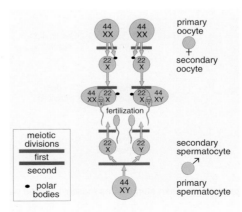

Fig. 1.2 Femoral torsion. Femoral torsion is often familial. Many common musculoskeletal problems have a genetic basis.

Category	Period
Gamete	Prior to fertilization
Early Embryo	0–2 weeks
Embryo	2–8 weeks
Fetus	8 weeks to birth
Infant	Birth to 2 years
Child	2 years to puberty
Adolescent	Transition to maturity

Fig. 1.3 Growth phases. The period of growth can be divided into seven phases.

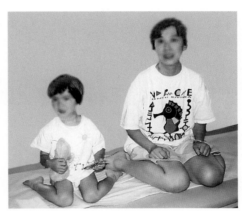

Fig. 1.4 Gametogenesis. The ovum and sperm are formed by two meiotic divisions that halve the chromosome number and shuffle genetic material. Fertilization combines the traits of both parents to create a unique individual.

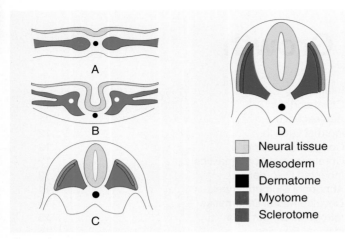

Fig. 1.5 Trilaminar Disc. The neural tube closes. The mesoderm differentiates into dermatome, myotome, and sclerotome.

Second week During this week, the amniotic cavity and trilaminar embryonic disc are formed (Fig. 1.5). The early embryo is usually aborted if a lethal or serious genetic defect is present. During these first two weeks, the early embryo is less susceptible to teratogens than during the following embryonic period.

Embryo

The organ systems of the body develop during the embryonic period. Differentiation to more specialized tissue occurs through complex mechanisms such as induction. *Induction* is the process by which cells act on other cells to produce entirely new cells or tissue.

Third week This is the first week of organogenesis. During this week, the trilaminar embryonic disc develops, somites begin to form, and the neural plate closes to form a neural tube.

Fourth week During this week, the limb buds become recognizable (Fig. 1.6). Somites differentiate into three segments. The dermatome becomes skin, the myotome becomes muscle, and the sclerotome becomes cartilage and bone. The apical ectodermal ridge develops in the distal end of each limb bud. The ridge has an inductive influence on limb mesenchyme, which promotes growth and development of the limb. Serious defects in limb development may originate at this time.

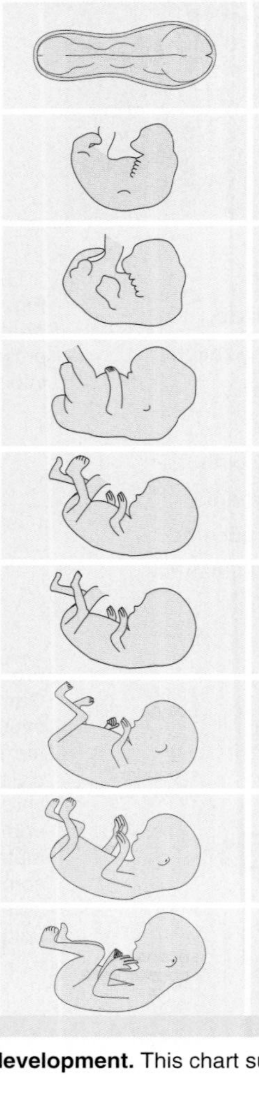

	AGE wks.	SIZE mm.	Shape	Form	Bones	Muscles	Nerves
Embryo				Trilaminar notochord			Neural plate
Embryo				Limb buds	Sclerotomes	Somites	Neural tube
Embryo				Hand plate	Mesenchyme condenses	Premuscle	
Embryo		12		Digits	Chondrification	Fusion myotomes	
Embryo		17		Limbs rotate	Early ossification	Differentiation	
Embryo		23		Fingers separate		Definite muscles	Cord equals vertebral length
Fetus	12	56		Sex determined	Ossification spreading		
Fetus	16	112		Face human	Joint cavities	Spontaneous activity	
Fetus	20 40	160-350		Body more proportional			Myelin sheath forms; cord ends L3

Fig. 1.6 Prenatal development. This chart summarizes musculoskeletal development during embryonic and fetal life.

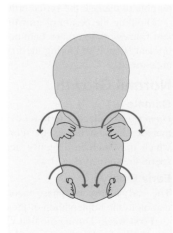

Fig. 1.7 Limb rotation. During the seventh week, the upper limb rotates laterally. The lower limb rotates medially to bring the great toes to the midline.

Fifth week The hand plate forms and mesenchymal condensations occur in the limbs.

Sixth week The rays of the digits become evident and chondrification of mesenchymal condensations occurs.

Seventh week The notches appear between the digit rays. Failure of the separation of rays results in syndactylism. During this week, the upper and lower limbs rotate in opposite directions (Fig. 1.7). The lower limb rotates medially to bring the great toes to the midline, whereas the upper limb rotates about 90° laterally to position the thumb on the lateral side of the limb.

Eighth week The fingers separate completely, the embryo assumes a human appearance, and the basic organ systems are completed.

Fetus

The fetal period is characterized by rapid growth and changes in body proportions.

Ninth to twelfth weeks The first bone, the clavicle, ossifies by a process of intramembranous deposition of calcium. The upper limbs become proportionate compared to the rest of the body, but the lower limbs remain short.

Thirteenth to twentieth weeks Growth continues to be rapid. The lower limbs become proportionate and most bones ossify. The fetal period is characterized by rapid growth and changes in body proportions.

Twentieth to fortieth weeks Growth continues and body proportions become more infant-like.

Connective Tissue

During early fetal life, the basic structure of connective tissue is formed largely of two families of macromolecules—collagens and proteoglycans.

Collagen Collagen is a family of proteins containing a triple helix of peptide chains (Fig. 1.8). Although at least ten different types of collagen are known, five types are most common (Fig. 1.9).

The biosynthesis of collagen starts in the endoplasmic reticulum, where the basic molecule is assembled. In the extracellular space, procollagen is formed. It is arranged into fibrils and reinforced by cross-linkages to become collagen. Collagen is the major component of connective tissue.

Disorders of collagen are common. They may be minor, producing only increased joint laxity (Fig. 1.10), or severe, causing considerable disability. The major collagen disorders are classified according to the site of the defect in the pathway of collagen biosynthesis.

Proteoglycans (mucopolysaccharides) Proteoglycans are macromolecules that form the intracellular matrix of hyaline cartilage and the other connective tissues. Polypeptides or proteins attach to glycosaminoglycan to become proteoglycans (Fig. 1.11). Proteoglycans attach to a hyaluronic acid by a link protein to become an aggregate with a molecular weight in excess of one million. Proteoglycans are highly hydrophilic, and in water, they combine with many times its weight of water to create an elastic matrix that is ideal for joint lining. Hyaline cartilage is composed of about equal amounts of proteoglycans and collagen, and it combines with about three times their weight of water. Defects in the formation of these complex molecules produce a variety of diseases.

Mucopolysaccharide (MPS) storage diseases result from a deficiency of specific lysosomal enzymes necessary for the degradation of glycosaminoglycans. These diseases are caused by intracellular accumulation of partially degraded molecules that result in cell dysfunction or death.

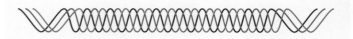

Fig. 1.8 Collagen helix. A triple helix of peptide chains form the basic collagen structure.

Location	Type	Comment
Interstitial	I	Ubiquitous, skin, tendons
	II	Cartilage and nucleus pulposus
	III	Like type I, but absent in bone
Segmentation	IV	Lens and kidney
	V	Minor component of bone

Fig. 1.9 Collagen types. Five basic collagen types in human connective tissue.

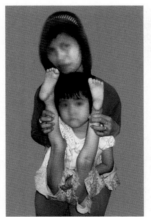

Fig. 1.10 Clinical manifestations of collagen types. Variations of collagen types are common in pediatric orthopedics. This child has developmental hip dysplasia with extreme joint laxity.

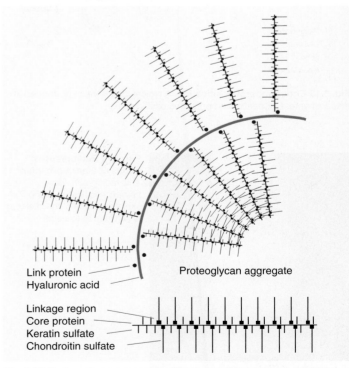

Link protein
Hyaluronic acid
Proteoglycan aggregate

Linkage region
Core protein
Keratin sulfate
Chondroitin sulfate

Fig. 1.11 Proteoglycan aggregate. These massive molecules combine with water to form a resilient matrix such as that of hyaline cartilage.

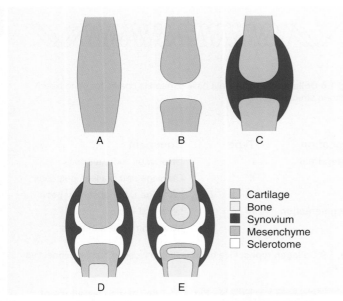

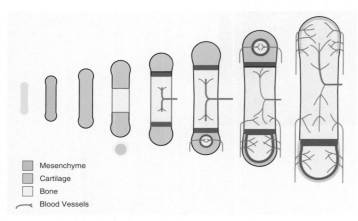

Cartilage
Bone
Synovium
Mesenchyme
Sclerotome

Fig. 1.12 Synovial joint formation. The synovial joints form first as condensations of mesenchyme. Cavitation, chondrification, synovial differentiation, and finally ossification complete the basic structure.

Mesenchyme
Cartilage
Bone
Blood Vessels

Fig. 1.13 Endochondral ossification. A typical long bone is preformed in mesenchyme. Chondrification precedes ossification.

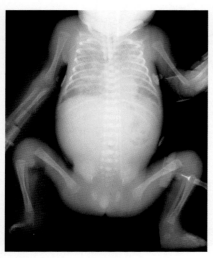

Fig. 1.14 Radiograph of bones of a newborn infant. This radiograph shows primary ossification of the skeleton. Much of the skeleton is cartilage at this age.

Synovial Joints

Synovial joints develop first as a cleft in the mesenchyme, which then chondrifies and cavitates (Fig. 1.12). Cavitation is completed by about the fourteenth week, with the inner mesenchyme becoming synovium and the outer mesenchyme becoming the joint capsule. Normal joint development requires motion, and motion requires a functioning neuromuscular system. Thus, defective joints are often seen in infants with neuromuscular disorders such as myelodysplasia or amyoplasia.

Bone Formation

Bones form in stages. First, mesenchymal cells condense to become models for future bones. The second stage, chondrification, is a time of rapid interstitial growth. Finally, cartilage is converted to bone by intramembranous and endochondral ossification.

Endochondral ossification takes place in most bones (Fig. 1.13). During the fetal period, primary ossification centers develop in long bones within the diaphysis. Ossification first occurs under the perichondrium. Within the cartilage, hypertrophied cells degenerate. Next, vascular ingrowth occurs, and then the core of the cartilage model is ossified to form the primary ossification center. Endochondral ossification proceeds at the cartilage–bone interphase. Later, secondary ossification centers develop at the ends of the bones, and the cartilage interposed between the primary and secondary ossification centers becomes the growth plate.

Primary ossification centers for long bones usually develop before birth (Fig. 1.14), whereas primary ossification centers for smaller bones, such as the patella and most carpal and tarsal bones, develop during infancy. Secondary ossification centers develop during infancy and early childhood. They fuse with the primary centers during late childhood, adolescence, and early adult life. Because osseous maturation continues throughout childhood and adolescence in a reasonably orderly fashion, the extent of ossification, as radiographically documented, has become the standard for assessing maturation.

Woven bone is formed during the fetal period. This bone has less structure, a relatively higher collagen content, and more flexibility than lamellar bone. This flexibility becomes essential during the transverse of the birth canal. Woven bone is gradually replaced by lamellar bone during infancy, and little remains in childhood.

Cortical thickness also increases throughout childhood. For example, the diameter of the diaphysis of the femur increases faster than the diameter of the medullary canal. This produces an increasing diaphyseal thickness with advancing age. This increasing thickness, lamellar structure, and proportion of calcium give mature bone great tensile strength but little flexibility. These changes are important factors in producing the varying patterns of skeletal injury seen during infancy, childhood, and adult life.

Growth Plate

The growth plate of long bones develops between the primary and secondary ossification centers. The function of the growth plate is to produce longitudinal growth (Fig. 1.15). This is accomplished by a complex process of proliferation and maturation of chondrocytes, matrix production, and mineralization, followed by endochondral ossification. Growth plates with more limited growth potential develop at other sites. These include the periphery of round bones, such as the tarsal bones or vertebral bodies, and the sites of muscle attachments, such as the margins of the ilium. Such sites are referred to as *apophyses*.

The typical long bone epiphysis is divided into zones that reflect morphological, metabolic, and functional differences.

The reserve zone (RZ) is adjacent to the secondary ossification centers and is a zone of relative inactivity. The RZ does not participate in the longitudinal growth of the bone, but it does provide some matrix production and storage functions.

The **proliferative zone (PZ)** is the zone of cartilage cell replication and growth. A high metabolic rate and abundant blood supply, oxygen, glycogen, ATP, and collagen make this rapid growth possible.

The **hypertrophic zone (HZ)** consists of three subzones: maturation, degeneration, and provisional calcification segments. In the HZ, the cartilage cells increase in size and the matrix is prepared for calcification. This is associated with a decline in blood supply, oxygenation, and glycogen stores and with a disintegration of aggregated mucopolysaccharides and chondrocytes. In the subzone of provisional calcification, a unique collagen X is synthesized that accepts calcium deposition.

The **metaphysis** is the site of vascularization, bone formation, and remodeling. The calcified matrix is removed, and fiber bone is formed and replaced by lamellar bone.

The **periphery** includes the growth plate and metaphysis, which are the primary sites for infections, neoplasms, fractures, and metabolic and endocrine disorders. Problems in the growth plate constitute a significant portion of diseases of the musculoskeletal system in childhood.

Bone Growth

The rate of growth may be retarded by many factors, such as injury, disease, and medical procedures. Brief periods of growth retardation may produce *growth arrest lines*. These lines may be visible on radiographs (Fig. 1.16).

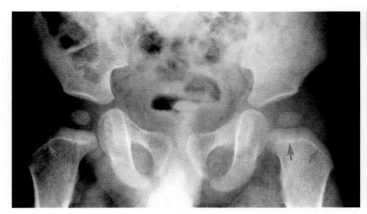

Fig. 1.16 Growth lines. Note the growth arrest lines (red arrows) in this child with developmental hip dysplasia. Presumably the anesthetic and closed reduction caused the arrest. Bone growth since the arrest is shown by the width of the new metaphyseal bone.

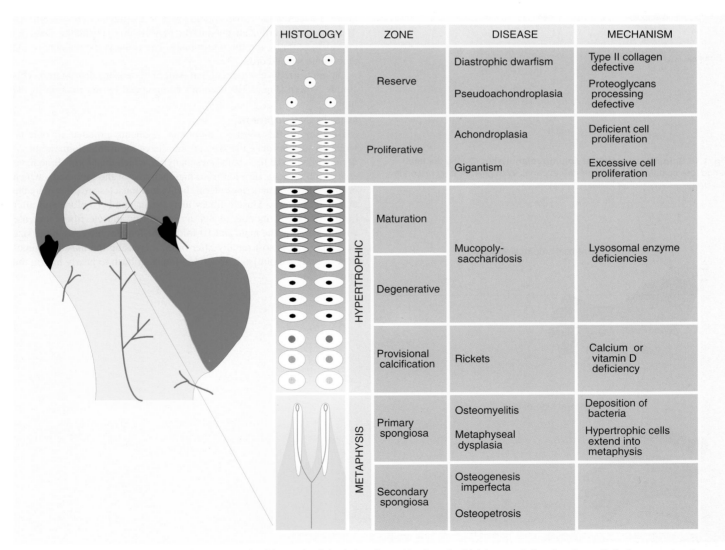

HISTOLOGY	ZONE		DISEASE	MECHANISM
	Reserve		Diastrophic dwarfism	Type II collagen defective
			Pseudoachondroplasia	Proteoglycans processing defective
	Proliferative		Achondroplasia	Deficient cell proliferation
			Gigantism	Excessive cell proliferation
	HYPERTROPHIC	Maturation	Mucopoly-saccharidosis	Lysosomal enzyme deficiencies
		Degenerative		
		Provisional calcification	Rickets	Calcium or vitamin D deficiency
	METAPHYSIS	Primary spongiosa	Osteomyelitis	Deposition of bacteria
			Metaphyseal dysplasia	Hypertrophic cells extend into metaphysis
		Secondary spongiosa	Osteogenesis imperfecta	
			Osteopetrosis	

Fig. 1.15 Growth plate. This section from the proximal femoral epiphysis is enlarged to show the histology and disordered growth that occurs at various levels of the growth plate.

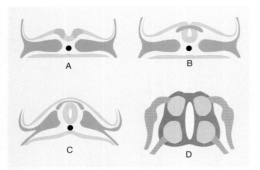

Fig. 1.17 Development of the nervous system. The nervous system is formed from the neural plate. (A) Infolding. (B) Neural crest. (C) Tube closure. (D) Dorsal and ventral root formation.

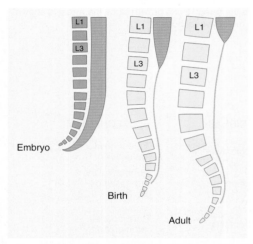

Fig. 1.18 Spinal cord vertebral column relationship. During the fetal period, the spinal cord fills the vertebral canal. With growth, the cord ends at a progressively higher level.

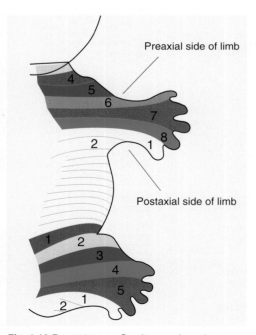

Fig. 1.19 Dermatomes. Somites produce dermatomes that are simple and well delineated. The simple pattern is altered by subsequent limb rotation.

Nervous System Development

During the third week of fetal life, the neural plate develops as a thickening of the dorsal portion of the ectoderm (Fig. 1.17). The neural plate then infolds to form the neural groove in the center, with neural folds on each side. During the fourth week, the neural groove closes to become the neural tube, and the neural crest separates and becomes interposed between the neural tube and surface ectoderm.

The neural crest becomes the dorsal root ganglia and the dorsal or sensory roots. The ventral or motor roots arise from the basal plates on the ventrolateral aspect of the neural tube. The combination produces the peripheral nerves.

Peripheral nerves grow into the forming limb buds of equivalent somites, penetrating the mesenchyme, and are distributed to the developing muscles. Cutaneous sensation is also provided in a segmental fashion.

Myelination of the spinal cord forms during the late fetal period and continues into early infancy.

Initially, the neural and bony elements of corresponding somites lie opposite each other. Thus, the caudal end of the spinal cord fills the spinal canal, and the spinal nerves pass through the corresponding intervertebral foramina. By the 24th fetal week, the cord ends at S1; at birth, at L3; and in the adult, at L1 (Fig. 1.18). This differential growth rate results in the formation of the caudal equina: the accumulation of the nerves traversing the subarachnoid space to the intervertebral foramina. The end of the cord is attached to the periosteum opposite the first coccygeal vertebra by the filum terminale. The filum is the residual of the embryonic spinal cord.

Somites produce a dermatomal pattern of sensory distribution. This simple pattern (Fig. 1.19) becomes complicated by the rotation of the limb.

Muscle Development

Mesoderm of the somites' myotome segments produce myoblasts, which in turn produce the skeletal muscle of the trunk. Somatic mesoderm produces the limb buds' mesenchyme, which then forms limb muscles. Limb muscles develop from mesenchyme of the limb buds, which originate from somatic mesoderm. Individual muscles are present by the eighth fetal week. Muscle fibers increase in number before and after birth. Between 2 months of age and maturity, muscle fibers increase about 15-fold in the male and 10-fold in the female. Increase in the size of fibers occurs most rapidly after birth, increasing the muscle component of body weight from about one-fourth at birth to nearly half in the adult.

Vertebral Column Development

The axial system develops during the embryonic period. During the fourth week, mesenchymal cells from the sclerotome grow around the notochord to become the vertebral body and around the neural tube to form the vertebral arches (Fig. 1.20). Cells from adjacent sclerotomes join to form the precursor of the vertebral body, an intersegmental structure. Between these bodies, the notochord develops into the intervertebral disc. Cells surround the neural tube to become the vertebral arches.

During the sixth fetal week, chondrification centers appear at three sites on each side of the mesenchymal vertebrae. The centrum is formed by the coalition of the two most anterior centers. Chondrification is complete before the ossification centers appear (Fig. 1.21). The centrum, together with an ossification center of each arch, make a total of three primary ossification centers for each vertebra.

During early childhood, the centers of each vertebral arch fuse and are joined to the vertebral body by a cartilaginous *neurocentral junction*. This junction allows growth to accommodate the enlarging spinal cord. Fusion of the neurocentral junction usually occurs between the third and sixth years. Anterior notching of the vertebrae is sometimes seen in the infant's or child's vertebrae and shows the site of somite fusion (Fig. 1.22).

Secondary ossification centers develop at the ends of the transverse and spinous processes and around the vertebral end plates at puberty. These fuse by age 25 years. Congenital defects are common in the axial system. Variations in the lumbar spine occur in about one-third of individuals. Spina bifida occulta is common. Hemivertebrae result from a failure of formation or segmentation. Such lesions are frequently associated with genitourinary abnormalities and less frequently with cardiac, anal, and limb defects and with tracheoesophageal fistula.

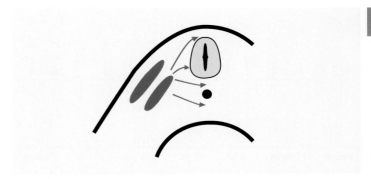

Fig. 1.20 Sclerotome growth. Cells from the sclerotome grow around the notochord and neural tube.

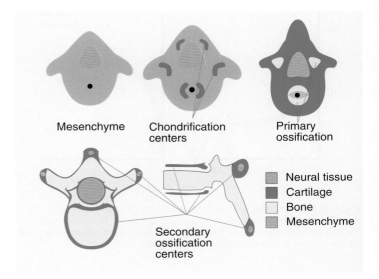

Mesenchyme — Chondrification centers — Primary ossification

Secondary ossification centers

Neural tissue
Cartilage
Bone
Mesenchyme

Fig. 1.21 Vertebral development. Vertebrae develop first as mesenchyme, then cartilage, and finally bone. Secondary ossification centers develop during childhood and fuse during adolescence or early adult life. From Moore (1988).

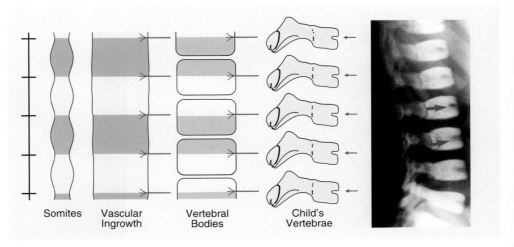

Somites — Vascular Ingrowth — Vertebral Bodies — Child's Vertebrae

Fig. 1.22 Vertebral intersegmental development. The vertebral bodies form as intersegmental structures. As blood vessels grow between somites, their final position is midvertebral. The site of blood vessel entry and somite fusion is sometimes seen radiographically as an anterior notch in the vertebral body of the child (red arrows).

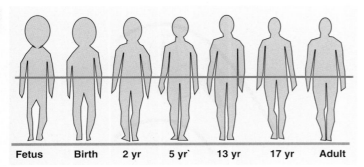

Fig. 1.23 Changes in body proportions with growth. At maturity, the position of the center of gravity (green line) is the level of the sacrum. From Palmer (1944).

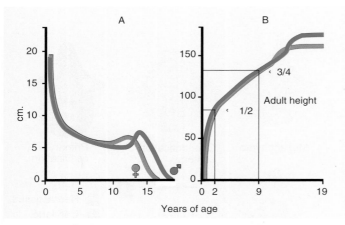

Fig. 1.24 Growth Rate. A. Growth rates for girls (red) and boys (blue) by age. The greatest rate of growth occurs during infancy. B. Growth rate as a fraction of adult height. About half of an individual's adult height is reached by age 2 years and three-fourths by age 9 years.

Infancy

Infancy extends from birth to 2 years of age. It encompasses the period of most rapid growth and development after birth.

Body proportions Growth of various body parts are different from one another. Upper limb growth occurs earlier than lower limb growth, and the foot grows earlier than the rest of the lower limb. In childhood, the trunk grows most rapidly; in adolescence, the lower limbs grow the fastest. Throughout growth, body proportions gradually assume adult form (Fig. 1.23).

Growth is greatest in early infancy, declines during childhood, and briefly increases again during the adolescent growth spurt. A child is about half his or her adult height at 2 years of age and about three-fourths by 9 years of age (Fig. 1.24).

Growth rates from various epiphyses varies. In the upper limb, growth is most rapid at the shoulder and wrist in contrast to the lower limb where most growth occurs just above and below the knee (Fig. 1.25).

The growth rate of tissues varies with age. Subcutaneous fat, which provides nutritional reserve and protection from cold and injury, develops during the first year. The fat also obscures the longitudinal arch of the foot, giving the infant a flatfooted appearance (Fig. 1.26). The percentage of muscle increases with age, but the percentage of neural tissue declines with advancing age.

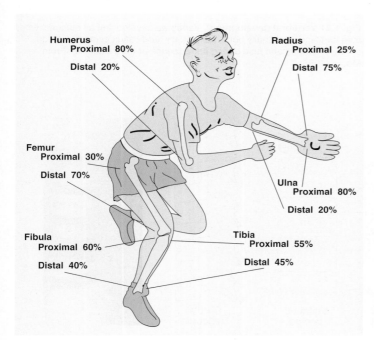

Fig. 1.25 Epiphyseal contribution of long bone growth. From Blount (1955).

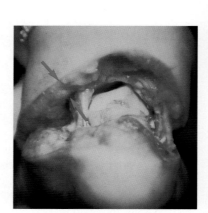

Fig. 1.26 Subcutaneous fat in infancy. Note the thickness in the subcutaneous fat (arrows) in this infant undergoing clubfoot correction.

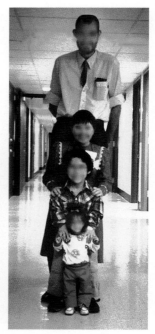

Fig. 1.27 Growth variations. These individuals show the wide variations in growth. Courtesy of Dr Judy Hall.

Growth control factors are systemic and local.

Systemic factors play a key role. Endocrine, nutritional, and metabolic disorders significantly alter growth (Figs. 1.27 and 1.28).

Local factors may retard or accelerate growth (Fig. 1.29). Procedures known to accelerate growth have been used in an attempt to lengthen the short limb due to poliomyelitis. Unfortunately, the gain in length is not predictable and is not enough to be clinically useful.

Compression of the physis retards growth in proportion to the load applied (Fig. 1.30). This has been studied in rats. Forelimb amputations result in upright walking. This bipedal walking causes significant anterior wedging of the lower lumbar vertebrae, presumably due to the greater loads applied to the anterior portion of the vertebral bodies.

Growth control factors are inherent in each growth plate. When juvenile limbs are transplanted onto adult rats, they continue to grow.

Gross motor development The standard for assessing motor development is the age of acquisition of gross motor skills. Such skills are easily measured and useful in assessing development (Fig. 1.31). Infants usually show head control by about 3 months, sit by 6 months, stand with support by 12 months, and walk unsupported by 15 months. These general guidelines are useful when screening.

Systemic Factors	Effects Growth
Osteochondral dystrophies	Retards
Neuromuscular disorders	Retards
Nutritional deficiencies	Retards
Most metabolic disorders	Retards
Pituitary tumors	Accelerates
Marfan syndrome	Accelerates

Fig. 1.28 Systemic factors affecting growth.

Local Factors	Effects Growth
Physeal compression	Retards
Denervation	Retards
Physeal ischemic injury	Retards
Sympathectomy	Accelerates
AV fistula	Accelerates
Periosteal division	Accelerates
Periosteal stripping	Accelerates
Diaphyseal fracture	Accelerates
Foreign body reaction	Accelerates
Chronic osteomyelitis	Accelerates

Fig. 1.29 Local factors affecting growth.

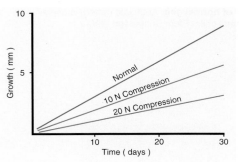

Fig. 1.30 Physeal compression effect on growth. Growth rate is reduced by compression (N = Newtons). From Bonnell (1983).

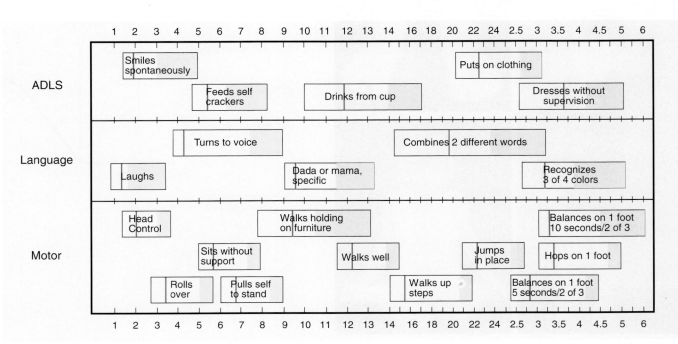

Fig. 1.31 Denver developmental screening test. From Frankenberg (1967).

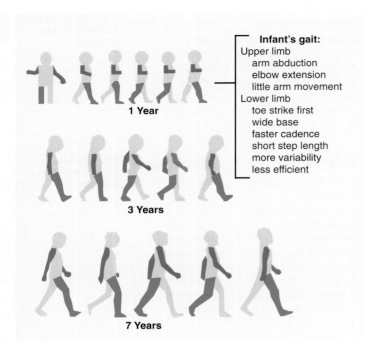

Infant's gait:
Upper limb
　arm abduction
　elbow extension
　little arm movement
Lower limb
　toe strike first
　wide base
　faster cadence
　short step length
　more variability
　less efficient

1 Year

3 Years

7 Years

Fig. 1.32 Development of normal gait. Adult gait pattern is achieved by about 7 years in the normal child. From Sutherland (1980).

Childhood

Childhood extends from the middle of the second year until adolescence. During this time, growth and development continue but at a slower rate than in infancy. Because childhood lasts so long, the majority of growth and development occurs during this period.

Gait during infancy is less stable and efficient than that of the child or adult (Fig. 1.32). Early gait is characterized by a wide-base irregular cadence, instability, and poor energy efficiency. The instability of gait in the infant is due to a high center of gravity, low muscle to body weight ratio, and immaturity of the nervous system and posture control mechanisms.

Developmental variations occur during infancy and childhood (Fig. 1.33). These variations are commonly mistaken for deformities. They include flatfeet, in-toeing, out-toeing, bowlegs, and knock-knees. These conditions resolve with time and seldom require any treatment. These conditions are covered in more detail in Chapters 4 and 5.

Prediction of adult height is valuable in managing certain deformities, particularly anisomelia (limb length inequality). A variety of methods for predicting adult height are available. A simple method involves establishing the percentile of height by plotting the child's height on the growth chart by bone age rather than by chronologic age. This percentile is projected out to skeletal maturity to provide an estimate of adult height (Fig. 1.34).

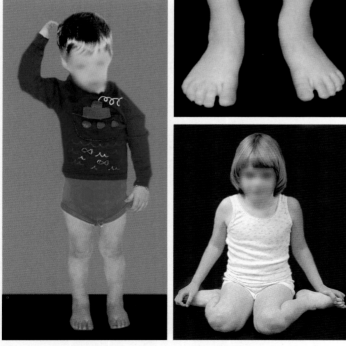

Fig. 1.33 Developmental variation in normal children. Common variations include knock-knees (left), flatfeet (top right), and femoral torsion (lower right).

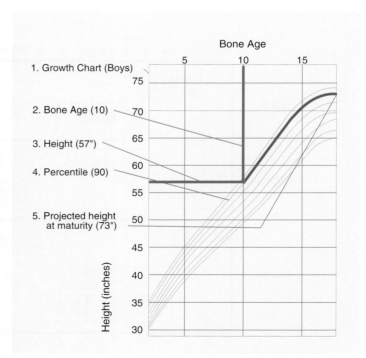

Fig. 1.34 Prediction of adult height. Predict adult height by plotting the child's bone age (vertical red line) against the current height (horizontal red line) to determine the percentile value (green). Follow the percentile (green line) to skeletal maturation to estimate final adult height.

Adolescence

Adolescence extends from the beginning of puberty until skeletal maturity. Certain diseases, such as scoliosis and slipped capital femoral epiphysis, develop during this time.

During adolescence, psychosocial factors receive a higher priority than in childhood. Physical appearance becomes increasingly important. Preexisting deformities or disabilities that may have caused little concern during childhood suddenly produce great distress. A boy with a small calf associated with a clubfoot deformity will request exercises to build up the limb size. A girl will become aware of old operative scars on her knee that before were ignored. A girl with an abductor lurch, present since infancy, may become concerned about it for the first time at age 13 years.

Obesity Obesity in children is becoming more common. The added weight is a factor in the development of several orthopedic problems. These include slipped capital femoral epiphysis and tibia vara (Fig. 1.35).

Determining maturation level Knowing the amount of growth remaining is important to the timing of physeal fusion and thus in correcting leg length inequality (Fig. 1.36) and in managing patients with scoliosis.

Hand–wrist radiographs Use the Greulich–Pyle atlas to estimate the bone age.

Tanner stages The level of maturation is based on the physical examination. Because this assessment requires an assessment of breast and genital development (Fig. 1.37) in a sensitive age group, its use is limited.

Risser sign is based on the extent of ossification of the iliac crest as assessed on the AP radiograph (Fig. 1.38). This sign has been commonly used in assessing maturity when managing scoliosis.

Other signs such as the velocity of height gain and the status of the triradiate cartilage (acetabulum) are becoming useful maturational indices.

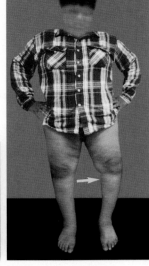

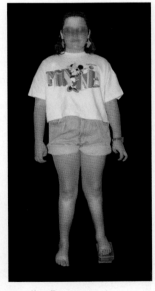

Fig. 1.35 Obesity and orthopedic problems. Two common serious orthopedic problems, slipping of the capital femoral epiphysis (red arrow) and tibia vara (yellow arrow), are commonly associated with obestiy.

Fig. 1.36 Leg length inequality. Bone age determination is helpful in planning correction by epiphysiodesis.

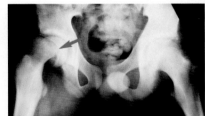

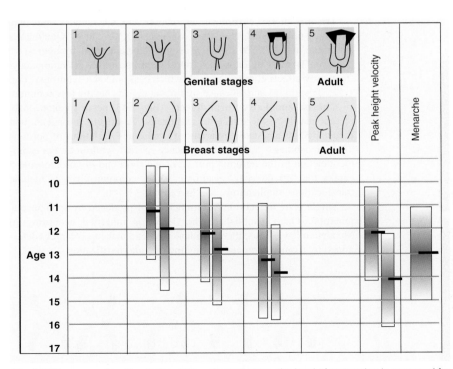

Fig. 1.37 Tanner maturation index. Using physical signs, the level of maturation is assessed for males (blue) and females (red). The columns show the 3–97% levels. Mean values are shown by the black bars.

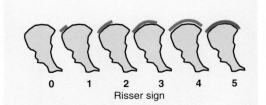

Fig. 1.38 Risser sign. The extent of ossification of the iliac apophysis is commonly used to assess the skeletal maturation of patients with scoliosis. Risser 0 = no iliac apophysis; Risser 5 = fusion of the apophysis with the ilium.

Disease	Prevalence estimated per 1000
Cerebral palsy	2.5
Trisomy 21	1.1
Developmental hip dysplasia	1.0
Clubfoot	1.0
Sickle cell disease	0.46
Muscular dystrophy	0.06

Fig. 1.39 Prevalence of orthopedic disorders.

Cause	Percentage
Chromosomal aberrations	6
Environmental factors	7
Monogenic or single gene	8
Multifactorial inheritance	25
Unknown	4

Fig. 1.40 Causes of congenital defects. From Moore (1988).

Chrom.	Disorder
1	Rh blood group, Gaucher's, CTM diseases
5	MPS VI, cri du chat syndrome
6	Histocompatibility complex
7	MPS VII, Ehlers–Danlos VII, some Marfan's
9	ABO typing, nail–patella syndrome
15	Prader–Willi syndrome
X	Duchenne dystrophy, chondrodysplasia

Fig. 1.41 Chromosome disorder location. Localization of musculoskeletal disorders to specific chromosomes.

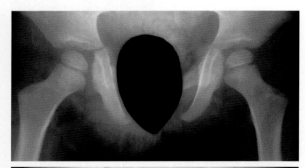
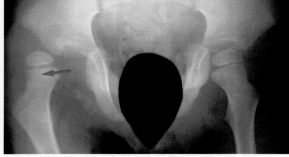

Fig. 1.42 Down syndrome hip instability. Due to the excessive joint laxity, recurrent dislocations (red arrow) may occur in these children.

Abnormal Growth

Disorders affecting the musculoskeletal system are relative common (Fig. 1.39). These and other conditions that cause limitation of activity in children have tripled during the past four decades because children with disabilities are more likely to survive today than in the past.

Congenital Defects

Multifactorial inheritance is the most common cause of congenital defects (Fig. 1.40). Of newborn infants, 3% show major defects and an additional 3% are discovered later during infancy. About 20% of perinatal deaths are attributable to congenital problems. Single minor defects are present in many newborns. Because infants with multiple minor defects have a higher incidence of major malformations, the finding of minor defects should prompt a careful search for more serious problems. Musculoskeletal problems account for about one-third of congenital defects. Hip dysplasia and clubfeet make up half of the primary musculoskeletal defects.

Although inherited disorders may manifest themselves during infancy, the majority of musculoskeletal problems of infancy are due to environmental factors, such as malnutrition, infection, and trauma.

Chromosomal Abnormalities

Chromosomes have been mapped to show the location of defective genes that create disorders often seen in orthopedic clinics (Fig. 1.41). The linkage of genes causing diseases with genes controlling distinguishable characteristics makes possible the identification of individuals at risk for certain diseases. For example, on chromosome 9, the gene carrying nail–patella syndrome is linked to the gene of ABO blood type. Offspring with the same ABO blood type as an affected parent will carry the syndrome.

Many chromosomal abnormalities are due to changes in number, structure, or content of chromosomes. Numerical changes in chromosomes are due to a failure of separation or nondisjunction during cell division. Nondisjunction results in monosomy or trisomy gametes. Monosomy of sex chromosomes produces the XO pattern of Turner's syndrome.

Trisomy of sex chromosomes causes 47XXX females who may have only mild mental retardation, whereas 47XXY causes Klinefelter's syndrome and 47XYY causes a disorder characterized by aggressive behavior. Trisomy of autosomes (nonsex chromosomes) is common and frequently affects chromosome 21, which causes Down syndrome (Fig. 1.42). Trisomy 13 and 18 cause significant defects but are less common.

Chromosomal structural defects (Fig. 1.43) occur spontaneously or secondarily to the effects of teratogens. Teratogens are agents that induce defects and cause a variety of syndromes. Deletions of portions of chromosomes 4, 5, 18, and 21 produce specific syndromes. For example, deletion of the terminal portion of the short end of chromosome 5 causes the "cri du chat" syndrome. Other common changes include translocations, duplications, and inversions.

Single gene defects may be inherited or produced by spontaneous mutation. Once established, the defect is inherited according to Mendelian laws. Thus, the individual's genetic makeup is largely determined by a random process during meiosis and fertilization.

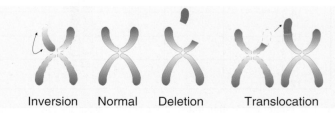

Fig. 1.43 Chromosome structural defects. Various structural defects include inversions, deletions, and translocations.

Inherited Disorders

Fertilization restores the diploid number of chromosomes and composites the traits of both parents. Fertilization may produce an abnormal zygote if the ovum or sperm carries defective genes. These conditions are transmitted by several mechanisms.

Dominant inheritance results in a disorder caused by a single abnormal gene (Fig. 1.44). Autosomal dominant conditions usually produce structural abnormalities (Figs. 1.48 and 1.49). Variable expressivity and incomplete penetrance suppress or minimize the expression of dominant inheritance.

Recessive inheritance is expressed only if both gene pairs are affected (Fig. 1.45). Metabolic or enzymatic defects that cause diseases such as the mucopolysaccharidoses are often inherited by autosomal recessive inheritance.

X-linked inheritance involves only the X chromosome (Fig. 1.46). In the male, the genetic inactivity of the Y chromosome allows even the recessive abnormal gene of the X chromosome to be manifested. A classic example of X-linked recessive inheritance is pseudohypertrophic muscular dystrophy. The female is the carrier, but only male offspring are affected. In recessive X-linked inheritance, the female is affected only in the rare situation in which both genes of the genetic pair are abnormal.

Polygenic inheritance (or multifactorial inheritance) involves multiple genes and an environmental "trigger" (Fig. 1.47). Such common conditions as hip dysplasia (Fig. 1.50) and clubfeet (Fig. 1.51) are transmitted by this mechanism.

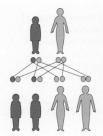

Achondroplasia
Brachydactyly
Cleidocranial
    dysostosis
Marfan syndrome
Multiple epiphyseal
    dysplasia
Nail-patella
    syndrome
Neurofibromatosis
Polydactyly

Fig. 1.44 Dominant inheritance. The dominant gene (red) causes structural defects in both parent and offspring. Musculoskeletal disorders transmitted by dominant inheritance are listed.

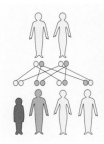

Congenital
    insensitivity to pain
Diastrophic dwarfism
Gaucher disease
Hurler syndrome
Morquio syndrome
Scheie syndrome
Hypophosphatasia

Fig. 1.45 Recessive inheritance. Carriers of the recessive genes (yellow) are expressed (red) only if both gene pairs are abnormal. Musculo-skeletal disorders transmitted by recessive inheritance are listed.

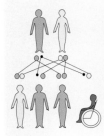

X-linked dominant
Vitamin D refractory
rickets

X-linked recessive
Hemophilia
Pseudohypertrophic
muscular dystrophy

Fig. 1.46 X-linked inheritance. X-linked defects (yellow) are carried by the female and expressed in the female if the gene is dominant. Most defects are recessive and are expressed only in the male (red).

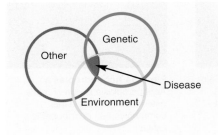

Fig. 1.47 Multifactorial inheritance. Many common orthopedic problems are transmitted by this mode. Genetic, environmental, and possibly other factors combine to cause the problems.

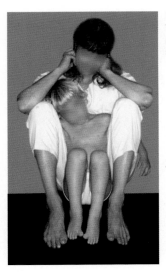

Fig. 1.48 Familial toe deformities. The mother and child have the same toe abnormalities. Toe and finger deformities are often familial.

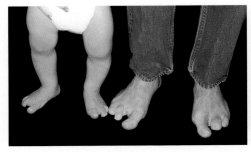

Fig. 1.49 Toe deformities. These toe deformities are exactly the same in the mother and child.

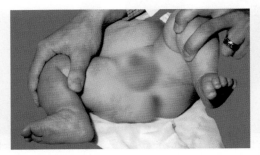

Fig. 1.50 Hip dysplasia. Developmental hip dysplasia is a common condition with a multifactorial etiology.

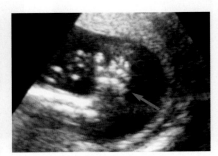

Fig. 1.51 Clubfoot *in utero*. High-resolution ultrasound shows a clubfoot deformity. Clubfeet are common deformities with a multifactorial etiology.

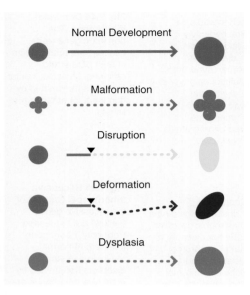

Fig. 1.52 Classification of abnormal morphogenesis. These categories provide a practical basis for understanding congenital defects. From Dunne (1986).

Abnormal Morphogenesis

Abnormal morphogenesis is classified into four categories (Fig. 1.52).

Malformations are defects that arise in the period of organogenesis and are of teratogenic or genetic origin. Phocomelia and congenital hypoplasia (Fig. 1.53) are examples.

Dysplasias result from altered growth that occurs before and after birth (Fig. 1.54).

Disruptions occur later in gestation when teratogenic, traumatic, or other physical assaults to the fetus interfere with growth. Ring constriction due to amniotic banding (Figs. 1.55 and 1.56) are examples.

Deformations occur at the end of gestation and are due to intrauterine crowding (Figs. 1.55 and 1.58). These deformities are milder and usually resolve spontaneously during early infancy.

Developmental Deformities

Metabolic disorders such as rickets cause osteopenia and a gradual bowing of long bones.

Inflammatory disorders may damage the growth plate or articular cartilage, causing shortening or angular deformity. Less commonly, chronic inflammation that does not affect the growth plate from conditions such as rheumatoid arthritis or chronic osteomyelitis may induce hyperemia and accelerate bone growth, thus causing bone lengthening.

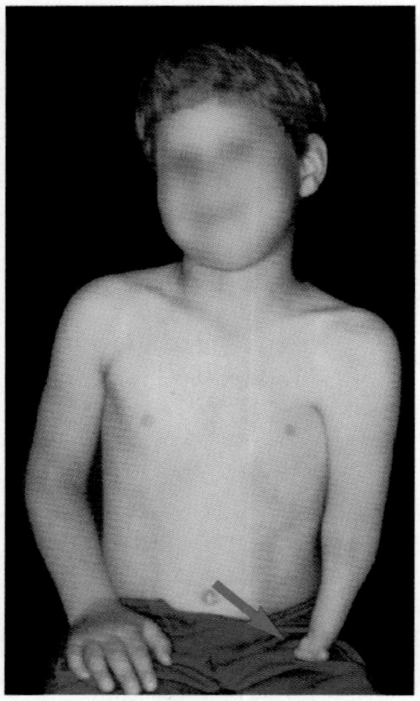

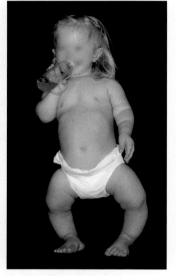

Fig. 1.53 Limb hypoplasia. Major limb defects are malformations arising from interruption of limb development.

Fig. 1.54 Achondroplasia. Achondroplasia is one of many osteochondral dysplasias commonly seen in orthopedic clinics.

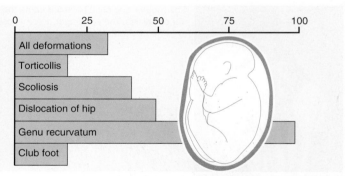

Fig. 1.55 Breech position. Common musculoskeletal defects associated with breech position. From Clarren (1977).

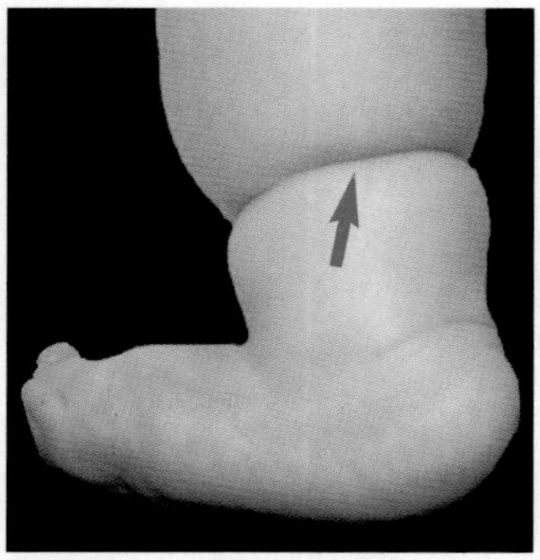

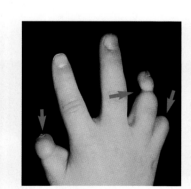

Fig. 1.56 Congenital constriction bands. Intrauterine adhesion caused this deep circumferential band.

Fig. 1.57 Constriction bands causing hand deformity. Amputation of the thumb and little finger and hypoplasia of the ring finger result from bands.

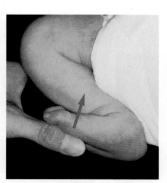

Fig. 1.58 Molding deformity. Intrauterine crowding caused this calcaneovalgus foot deformity.

Physical activity may alter bone growth. For example, long-term nonweight-bearing activity, as was once prescribed in treating Perthes disease, resulted in slight shortening of the involved leg. Similarly, professional tennis players who start their careers as children show relative overgrowth of the dominant upper limb.

Neuromuscular deformity may occur from muscle imbalance such as in the child with spasticity from cerebral palsy. Adductor spasm positions the head of the femur on the lateral acetabular rim causing deformity and erosion of the cartilage of the labrum, which in turn causes subluxation and eventual dislocation of the hip (Fig. 1.58). The combination of contractures, immobility, gravity, and time create the so-called windswept deformity common in spastic quadraplegia.

Trauma may cause deformity by malunion or growth plate damage (Fig. 1.59). If the growth plates are not damaged, growth contributes to the correction of residual malunion deformity through the process of *remodeling*.

Idiopathic disorders Sometimes the cause of the developmental deformity is not determined (Fig. 1.61).

Iatrogenic Deformities

The cradleboard, by positioning the infant's hip in extension, is a known cause of developmental hip dysplasia (Fig. 1.60). In some cultures, iatrogenic deformities are created in girls to enhance their beauty. Binding of the feet (Fig. 1.62) and placing rings around the neck (Fig. 1.63) of young girls has produced deformity and severe disability.

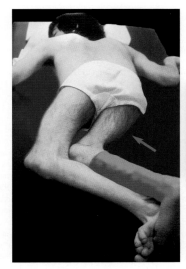
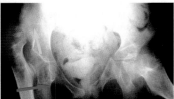

Fig. 1.58 Hip deformity in cerebral palsy. This boy with cerebral palsy (left) developed an adduction deformity (red arrows) and a secondary dislocation (yellow arrow) of the right hip.

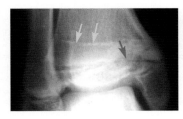

Fig. 1.59 Growth arrest lines. This post-traumatic physeal bridge (red arrow) caused asymmetrical growth of the distal tibia, as shown by the growth arrest line (yellow arrows).

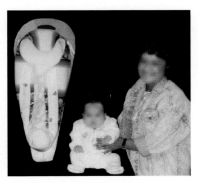

Fig. 1.60 Cradleboard. Cradleboards extend the infant's hips, causing an increased incidence of hip dysplasia.

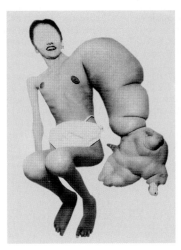

Fig. 1.61 Idiopathic growth acceleration. This girl pictured in the 1940s has massive overgrowth of the left upper extremity producing a grotesque disability. The girl died during the operation to remove the extremity.

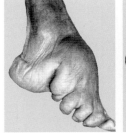
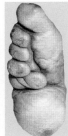

Fig. 1.62 Bound feet. A woman's feet show the effect of foot binding during childhood. The foot becomes triangular in shape (left and middle) and small in size so that it fits the shoe (right). The shoe is less than 6 inches in length.

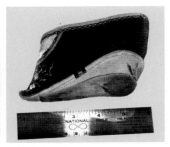
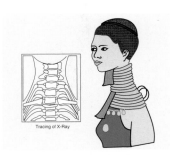

Fig. 1.63 Thoracic deformity. Rings placed around the neck in childhood produce constriction of the upper thorax in the adult woman (Padaung tribe, east Burma). From Roaff (1961).

Anderson M, Green WT, Messner MB. Growth and predictions of growth in the lower extremities. J Bone Joint Surg 1963; 45A:1-14.

Andry M. Orthopaedia: or the art of correcting and preventing deformities in children. London: A. Miller.

Blount, W. Fractures in Children, Williams & Wilkins Co., Baltimore, 1955

Bonnel F, et al. Effect of compression of growth plates in the rabbit. Acta Orthop Scand 1983; 54:730-3.

Brighton CT. The growth plate. Orthop Clin North Am 1984; 15:571-95.

Brighton CT. Longitudinal bone growth: the growth plate and its dysfunctions. AAOS Instruc Course Lect 1987; 34:3-25.

Brookes M, Wardle EN. Muscle action and the shape of the femur. J Bone Joint Surg 1962; 44B:398-411.

Buckwalter JA, Cooper RR. Bone structure and function. AAOS Instruc Course Lect 1987; 34:27-48.

Carvell JE. The relationship of the periosteum to angular deformities of long bones: experimental observations of rabbits. Clin Orthop 1983; 173:262-74.

Cassidy JD, Yong-Hing K, Kirkaldy-Willis WH. A study of the effects of bipedism and upright posture on the lumbosacral spine and paravertebral muscles of the rat. Spine 1988; 13:301-8.

Clarren SK, Smith DW. Congenital deformities. Ped Clin North Am 1977; 24:665-77.

Crossan JF, Wynne-Davies R. Research for genetic and environmental factors in orthopedic diseases. Clin Orthop 1986; 210:97-105.

Dietz FR. Effect of denervation on limb growth. J Orthop Res 1989; 7:292-303.

Dunne, KB, Clarren, S.K. The origin of prenatal and postnatal deformities. Ped Clin North Am 1986; 33:1277-1297.

Fuller DJ, Duthie RB. The timed appearance of some congenital malformations and orthopaedic abnormalities. AAOS Instruct Course Lect 1974; 23:53-61.

Greco F, de Palma L, Specchia N, Mannarini M. Growth plate cartilage metabolic response to mechanical stress. J Ped Orthop 1989; 9:520-4.

Greenfield GB. Radiology of bone diseases, 4th ed. Philadelphia: J.B. Lippincott, 1986.

Hansman CF. Appearance and fusion of ossification centers in the human skeleton. Am J Roentgen 1962; 88:476-82.

Haworth JB, Keillor GW. Use of transparencies in evaluating the width of the spinal canal of infants, children and adults. Radiology 1962; 79:109-114.

Hecht JT, Scott CI. Genetic study of an orthopedic referral center. J Ped Orthop 1984;4:208-23.

Hensinger RN. Standards in pediatric orthopedics: tables, charts, and graphs illustrating growth. New York: Raven Press, 1986.

Iannotti JP. Growth plate physiology and pathology. Orthop Clin North Am 1990; 21:1-17.

Izumi Y. The accuracy of Risser staging. Spine 1995;20:1868.

Keck SW, Kelly PJ. The effect of venous stasis on intraosseous pressure and longitudinal bone growth in the dog. J Bone Joint Surg 1965; 47A:539-44.

Khrouf N, Spang R, Podgorna T, Miled SB, Moussaoui M, Chibani M. Malformations in 10,000 consecutive births in Tunis. Acta Paediatr Scand 1986; 75:534-9.

Kline SC, Hotchkiss RN, Randolph MA, et al. Study of growth kinetics and morphology in limbs transplanted between animals of different ages. Plastic Reconstr Surg 1990; 85:273-80.

Leppig KA, Werler MM, Cann CI, Cook CA, Holmes LB. Predictive value of minor anomalies: I. association with major malformations. J Pediatrics 1987; 110:531-7.

Li JY, Specker BL, Ho ML, et al. Bone mineral content in black and white children 1 to 6 years of age: early appearance of race and sex differences. Am J Dis Child 1989; 143:1346-9.

Little DG, Sussman MD. The Risser sign: a critical analysis. JPOa 1994;14:569.

Lowrey GH. Growth and development of children, 6th ed. Chicago: Year Book Medical Publishers, 1973:77-93.

Marshall WA, Tanner JM. Variations in pattern of pubertal changes in boys. Arch Dis Child 1970;45:13-23.

Moore KL. The developing human: clinically oriented embryology, 4th ed. Philadelphia: W.B. Saunders, 1988.

Moseley CF. Growth. In: Lovell WW, Winter RB, ed. Pediatric Orthopaedics, 2nd ed. Philadelphia: J.B. Lippincott, 1986:27-39.

Netter FH. The CIBA collection of medical illustrations, volume 8: musculoskeletal system, part I: anatomy, physiology, and metabolic disorders. Summit, NJ: CIBA-Geigy, 1987.

Ogden JA. Development and maturation of the neuromusculoskeletal system. In: Morrissey RT, ed. Lovell and Winter's Pediatric Orthopaedics, 3rd ed. Philadelphia: J.B. Lippincott, 1990:1-33.

Palmer CE. Studies of the center of gravity in the human body. Child Dev 1944;15:99.

Pritchett JW. Growth and predictions of growth in the upper extremity. J Bone Joint Surg 1988; 70A:520-25.

Reed RB, Stuart HC. Patterns of growth in height and weight from birth to eighteen years of age. Pediatrics 1959; 24:904-21.

Risser JC. The iliac apophysis: an invaluable sign in the management of scoliosis. CO 1958;11:111.

Roaff F. Giraffe-necked women: a myth exploded. J Bone Joint Surg 1961; 43B:114-120.

Robertson WW. Newest knowledge of the growth plate. Clin Orth 1990;253:270-8.

Scoles PV, Salvagno R, Villalba K, Riew D. Relationship of iliac crest maturation to skeletal and chronologic age. J Pediat Orthop 1988; 8:639-44.

Skinner R. Unifactorial inheritance. In: Emery AE, Rimoin DL, eds. Principles and practice of medical genetics, vol 1. New York: Churchill Livingstone, 1983:65-74.

Smith DW. Recognizing patterns of human malformation: genetic, embryologic, and clinical aspects. Philadelphia: W.B. Saunders, 1970:324-55.

Specker BL, et al. Bone mineral content in children 1 to 6 years of age. Am J Dis Child 1987; 141:343-4.

Speer D. Collagenous architecture of the growth plate and perichondrial ossification groove. J Bone Joint Surg [Am] 1982; 64:399-407.

Sutherland D, Olshen R, Cooper L, Woo S. The development of mature gait. JBJSa 1980;62:336.

Tachdjian MO. Pediatric Orthopedics, 2nd ed. Philadelphia: W.B. Saunders, 1990.

Tanner JM, Whitehouse RH, Takaishi M. Standards from birth to maturity for height, weight, height velocity and weight velocity: British children, 1965. Part I. Arch Dis Child 1966; 41:454-71.

Trueta J. Studies of the development and decay of the human frame. Philadelphia: W.B. Saunders, 1968.

Van Regemorter N, Dodion J, Druart C, Hayez F, Vamos E, Flament-Durend J, Perlmutter-Cremer N, Rodesch F. Congenital malformations in 10,000 consecutive births in a university hospital: need for genetic counseling and prenatal diagnosis. J Pediatrics 1984; 104:386-90.

Wilson J, Rhinelander F, Stewart C. Microvascular and histologic effect of circumferential wire on appositional bone growth in immature dogs. J Orthop Res 1985; 3:412-17.

Wynne-Davies R. Acetabular dysplasia and familial joint laxity. JBJSb 1970;52:704.

Chapter 2—Evaluation

Evaluation leading to an accurate diagnosis (Fig. 2.1) is the first and most important step in optimal management. Every condition requires a diagnosis, but only some require active treatment. The evaluation of the child is often more difficult than that of the adult. The child is a poor historian, and examination of the child can be difficult. Dealing with the family may be challenging. The history given by the parents is often laced with emotion. Reporting is often complicated by varying gender and generational hierarchy. The physician often finds that managing the child's problem is easier than dealing with the family. Establishing rapport during the first visit is essential.

Establishing Rapport

The goal is to reduce the fear in the child and establish confidence with the parents and family (Fig. 2.2).

Dress

Studies have shown that casual dress promotes approachability and more formal dress enhances confidence. Dress in a way that suggests you have good judgment and are more appropriate for the situation. More formal dress may be more appropriate in a major referral center than elsewhere. Avoid making a statement by dress. This usually translates into selecting conservative clothing that promotes an image of good taste.

Initial Introduction

On entering the examination room, acknowledge everyone in the room. Consider the cultural background of the family and conform to gender order for introductions. Shake hands with everyone including the child. Determine the relationship of each person with the patient.

Be professional yet friendly. Establishing a good rapport with *everyone* in the family may be critical to properly managing the child. Later, when difficult management decisions must be made, having rapport with every member of the family is necessary to avoid pressure on the parents to seek additional opinions. Once started, serial consultations usually end with some unnecessary treatment of the child.

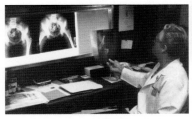

Fig. 2.1 Diagnosis. Evaluation requires integration of clinical, imaging, and laboratory findings.

Tips for the Physician

1. Knock on the door before entering to give anyone undressed a chance to cover-up before you go in.
2. Touch the patient either with a handshake or with a pat on the shoulder.
3. Introduce yourself and your colleagues to everyone in the examining room. Attempt to identify the cultural expectations to establish the order of introductions. Shake everyone's hand.
4. Establish the reason for the clinic visit.
5. Sit down in the room, preferably lower than the patient.
6. Show the family the x-ray, especially if it is normal.
7. Avoid technical terms.
8. Avoid leaving the room during consultation unless definitely necessary. Avoid looking at your watch.
9. Do not discuss other patients' treatment.
10. Avoid trying to impress patient with your credentials; the family has already selected you as their physician.
11. Discuss the problem, options, and recommendations.
12. Try to assess the family's reaction to the discussion. Continue discussion until the family's expectations are fulfilled.
13. Offer to provide follow-up if the family appears to need continued reassurance.

Fig. 2.2 Suggestions for establishing rapport.

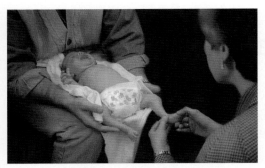

Fig. 2.3 Efficient, comfortable examination. Positioned on the parent's lap, the infant or child is most secure and quiet.

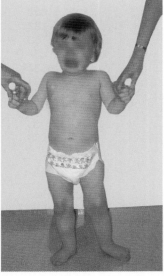

Fig. 2.4 When coaxing fails. Perform the examination without the cooperation of the child.

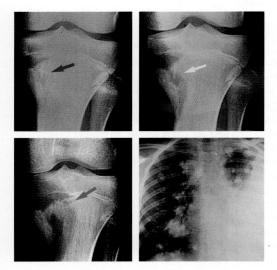

Fig. 2.5 Confusing trauma history. A 12-year-old boy gives a history of knee trauma and pain. The initial radiograph was considered normal, but a lesion is present (blue arrow). One month later, the lesion has enlarged (yellow arrow). A diagnosis of Osgood–Schlatter disease was made. A radiograph 2 months later showed further expansion of the lesion (red arrow). A radiograph of the chest just prior to death showed multiple pulmonary metastases from osteogenic sarcoma. Attributing this problem to "trauma" was disastrous.

Calming the Child

Reducing the child's fear is the next objective. Consider examining the infant or younger child on the parent's lap (Fig. 2.3). Ask the child on whose lap he or she wishes to sit. Children will often select the family member who they believe will offer the greatest safety.

Be friendly with the child. Suggest that this will be a *game*. Make some positive statements about the child, such as "Mary, you are such a nice child." Ask some child-oriented questions, such as "What is your pet's name?"

Start gently examining the child while taking the history from the family. This first step is to convince the child that the examination will not be painful. This is the time for the screening examination, starting with the area most removed from the problem. Being gentle often results in the child becoming less threatened and more cooperative.

Sometimes, these measures fail and the infant or young child remains aggravated and uncooperative. This is the time to move to strategy two—a firm approach (Fig. 2.4).

History

The child's complaints usually fall into the categories of deformity, altered function, or pain. Assessment of these complaints should take the patient's age into consideration. For example, the toddler usually manifests discitis (an intervertebral disc space infection) by altered function in the form of an unwillingness to walk. The child with discitis may primarily show a systemic illness, whereas the adolescent often complains of back pain.

A common pitfall in diagnosis is inappropriately attributing the child's problem to trauma. Although trauma is a common event in the life of a child, serious problems such as malignant tumors or infections may be mistakenly attributed to an injury (Fig. 2.5).

Deformity

Positional deformities such as rotational problems, flatfeet, and bowlegs are common concerns but seldom significant (Figs. 2.6 and 2.7). More significant problems, such as congenital or neuromuscular deformities, require careful evaluation. Inquire about the onset, progression, and previous management. Are there old photographs or radiographs that document the course of the deformity? Is there associated pain or disability? Does the deformity cause a cosmetic problem and embarrass the child? Is it noticeable to others? Finally, be cautious about relying solely on the family's estimation of the time of the deformity's onset. Often a deformity originates long before it is first noticed.

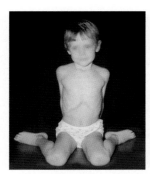

Fig. 2.6 Developmental variation. This child with femoral antetorsion shows the classic sitting posture.

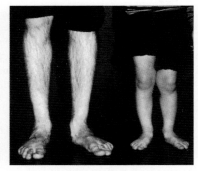

Fig. 2.7 Familial flatfeet. Since the father has flatfeet, it is more likely that the child's flatfeet will persist into adult life.

Altered Function

Function can be altered by deformity, weakness, or pain. Pain is a common cause of altered function in the infant and child; the most common example is a limp. A toddler's fracture of the tibia may be manifested by a limp or an unwillingness to walk. The young child with toxic synovitis may simply limp; the older child might complain of pain. The newborn whose clavicle is fractured during delivery shows a loss of arm movement on the affected side. This may be confused with a birth palsy. Altered function due to trauma, inflammation, or infection without neurologic damage is referred to as *pseudoparalysis*.

Pain

The expression of pain is age related. The infant may simply avoid moving the painful part, may fuss and cry, or cry continuously if the pain is severe. The child may show altered function, avoid moving the affected part, or complain of discomfort (Fig. 2.8). The adolescent usually complains of pain.

The perception and expression of pain differs widely among individuals, particularly as adolescents grow more adult-like in their responses. A young athlete might minimize his discomfort to improve his chances of participating in the next sporting event. Others might exaggerate the problem. Some adolescents minimize pain by pain-relieving positioning. A herniated disc or an osteoid osteoma may cause scoliosis. This scoliosis results from positioning the spine in a pain-relieving posture. This secondary deformity rather than the underlying condition may be the focus of the evaluation. Unless the underlying condition is identified by the physician, a serious diagnostic error can occur.

Past History

The past history is essential, not only for understanding the background and general health of the child but also for gaining insight into the current problem. Important aspects of past history include the following:

Birth history Were the pregnancy and delivery normal?

Development Have the developmental milestones been met at the appropriate age? When did the infant first sit and walk? About one-third of late walkers are pathologic. In children with conditions such as cerebral palsy, walking is always delayed and may be important in establishing whether or not the condition is progressive (Fig. 2.9).

Mother's intuition The mother's intuition is surprisingly accurate (Fig. 2.10). For example, the mother's sense that something is wrong with her infant is one of the most consistent findings in infants with cerebral palsy. Take the mother's concerns seriously.

Family history Do others have problems similar to those of the patient? If so, what disability is present? A surprisingly large number of orthopedic problems run in families, and knowledge of the disability, or absence of disability, provides information regarding the patient's prognosis.

References

1999 Malignancies in children who initially present with rheumatic complaints. Cabral DA, Tucker LB. J Pediatr 134:53

1998 Musculoskeletal pain in primary pediatric care: analysis of 1000 consecutive general pediatric clinic visits. de Inocencio J. Pediatrics 102:E63

1998 Self-reported bodily pain in schoolchildren. Smedbraten BK, et al. Scand J Rheumatol 27:273

1997 Prevalence of pain combinations and overall pain: a study of headache, stomach pain and back pain among school-children. Kristjansdottir G. Scand J Soc Med 25:58

1997 Outcome and predictive factors in children with chronic idiopathic musculoskeletal pain. Flato B, et al. Clin Exp Rheumatol 15:569

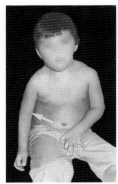
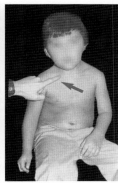

Fig. 2.8 Pseudoparalysis. Use of the arm (yellow arrow) is restricted because of pain. A painful lesion of the right clavicle (red arrow) was due to a leukemic infiltrate.

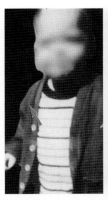
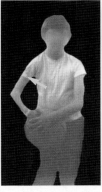
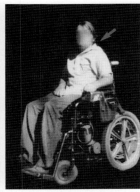

Fig. 2.9 Importance of medical history. This boy had normal function of his right arm (green arrow) as an infant. During early childhood, he developed weakness of the arm (yellow arrow), and a diagnosis of cerebral palsy was made. The weakness increased, and finally during adolescence, he was found to have a tumor involving the cervical spinal cord (red arrow). He became quadriplegic. The progressive nature of the condition is inconsistent with a diagnosis of cerebral palsy. A medical history of progression would have prompted an earlier diagnosis and may have prevented this disastrous outcome.

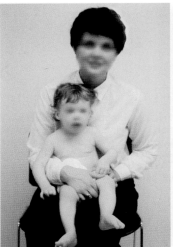
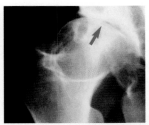
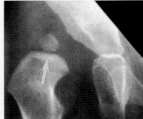

Fig 2.10 Mother's intuition. The mother with painful degenerative arthritis from developmental hip dysplasia (red arrow) sensed something was abnormal about her infant's hip. Her concern, based on intuition, was discounted by the primary physician, and the asymmetry present on examination was attributed to the child's mild hemiparesis. This resulted in a delay in diagnosis of developmental hip dysplasia until 18 months of age (yellow arrow).

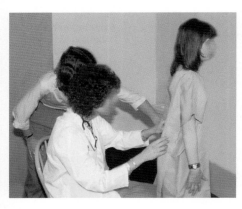

Fig. 2.11 Examination. Examine the adolescent in a gown.

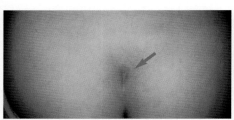

Fig. 2.12 Sacral dimple. A midline skin lesion such as a sacral dimple suggests the presence of a congenital spinal dysraphism.

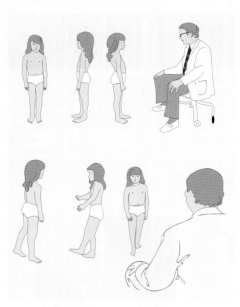

Fig. 2.13 Screening. Inspect from front, side, and back. Observe the child walking normally, then on heels and toes.

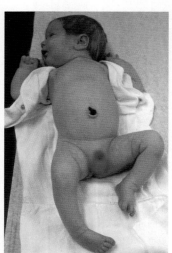

Fig. 2.14 Importance of observation. This infant shows reduced spontaneous movement of the left leg and an abducted position of the left hip. The infant has septic arthritis of the left hip.

Physical Examination

Examination of the musculoskeletal system should include two steps: (1) a screening examination and (2) a complete musculoskeletal evaluation performed to assess a specific complaint. The history and physical examination provide the diagnosis in most cases. It should be thorough and carefully performed. With the proper approach, it is usually possible to perform an adequate examination even without the cooperation of the infant or child.

Approach

Approach the child in a friendly and gentle fashion. Examining the child on the mother's lap is helpful. If the child is still nervous, keep your distance while obtaining the history. Reassure the child that all you plan to do is to watch her walk or move her legs. If the child is still nervous, examine the parent or sibling first. The child may find it reassuring for you to go through the examination with the parent first. If the child will not cooperate in walking, carry her to the opposite side of the room. The child will usually walk or run back to the parents. If the child has pain, always examine the painful site last.

Screening Evaluation

Examine the child in his underclothing. Examine the adolescent in a gown (Fig. 2.11) or, even better, in a swimsuit. It is essential to see the whole child to avoid missing important clues in diagnosis, such as the midline spinal skin dimple that may accompany an underlying spinal deformity (Fig. 2.12).

Perform the screening examination (Fig. 2.13) first before focusing on the principal complaint. This screening ensures that you do not miss any other orthopedic problems and will provide a general overview of the musculoskeletal system necessary to understand the specific problem. For example, knowledge of the degree of generalized joint laxity is valuable in assessing a flatfoot or a dysplastic hip. The examination of the back is an essential part of an evaluation of foot deformities. A cavus foot deformity is a common feature of diastematomyelia.

Infant screening Examine the infant on the mother's lap. First, observe the general body configuration. Next, observe the infant's spontaneous movement patterns for evidence of paralysis or pseudoparalysis (Fig. 2.14). Any reduction of spontaneous movements is an important finding. For example, the only consistent physical finding of the neonate with septic arthritis of the hip is a reduction in spontaneous movement of the affected limb. Finally, systematically examine the limbs and back for joint motion and deformity. Always perform a screening hip examination to rule out developmental hip dysplasia.

Examining the child and adolescent The examination requires several steps:

General inspection Does the child look sick (Fig. 2.15)? With the child standing in the anatomic position, observe her from the front, side, and back. Look at body configuration, symmetry, and proportions and for specific deformities.

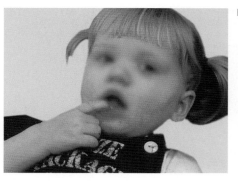

Fig. 2.15 Ill child.

Pelvis and back Place your hands on the iliac crests—are they level? A pelvic tilt usually results from a limb length difference. Next, ask the child to raise one leg at a time. A drop in the pelvis on the opposite side indicates a weakness of the hip abductors found in conditions such as hip dysplasia and cerebral palsy. With the child facing you, assess thoracic and lumbar symmetry for evidence of scoliosis by the forward-bending test. Observe the sagittal alignment of the spine (Fig. 2.16).

Assessing gait Ask the child to walk slowly across the room and back first with normal gait and then repeated on her toes and heels. Observe the gait for evidence of asymmetry, irregularity, or weakness. Any abnormal or questionable findings discovered during the screening examination should prompt a more complete evaluation of the problem. For example, a finding of in-toeing should prompt an assessment of the rotational profile.

Specific Evaluations

The history and findings of the screening examination serve as guides to more in-depth evaluation.

Joint laxity Joint mobility is greatest in infancy and gradually declines throughout life. Joint laxity, like other traits, varies widely among individuals and is usually genetically determined (Fig. 2.17). Extremes in joint laxity are seen in certain disorders, such as Ehlers–Danlos and Marfan syndromes.

Assess joint laxity by testing the mobility of the ankles, knees, elbows, thumbs, and fingers (Fig. 2.18). Excessive laxity in four or all of the five joints tested occurs in about 7% of children. Joint laxity is a contributing factor in the pathogenesis of hip dysplasia, dislocating patellae, and flatfeet, and it increases the risk of injuries such as sprains. In general, excessive joint laxity suggests the possibility of other problems.

Range of motion (ROM) The normal values of joint motion change with age. Generally, the arc of motion is greatest in infancy and declines with age. Specific joints are affected by intrauterine position. For example, lateral hip rotation is greatest in early infancy and declines during the first 2 or 3 years of growth. In assessing ROM, a knowledge of normal values is helpful. Make certain that the position of the pelvis is determined by palpation when assessing hip abduction (Fig. 2.19).

Contractures of diarthrodial muscles are common in children and sometimes require lengthening. For example, contracture of the gastrocnemius and gracilis occur in cerebral palsy. By proper positioning of the joints above and below the contracture, it is possible to differentiate contractures of these muscles from adjacent elements of the same muscle group.

Hip flexion motion is difficult to measure due to compensatory motion of the lumbar spine. Measurements can be made by the Thomas or prone extension tests. The prone extension test has been found to be more reliable. Most ROM measurements of most joints are reproducible within about ±4°.

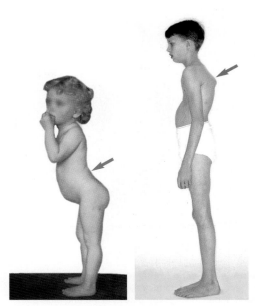

Fig. 2.16 Sagittal alignment. Note the increased lordosis (red arrow) and dorsal kyphosis (blue arrow).

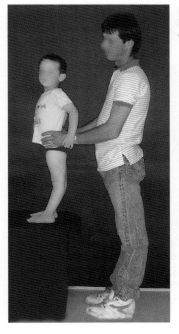

Fig. 2.17 Familial joint laxity. Note hyperextension of the knee in both the child and father.

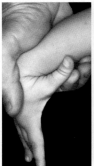
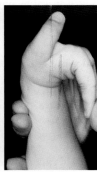

Fig. 2.18 Finger tests for joint laxity. The ability to approximate the thumb and the forearm and extend the fingers to a parallel relationship with the forearm suggests an excessive degree of joint laxity.

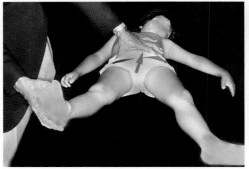

Fig. 2.19 Assessing hip abduction. Stabilize the pelvis with one hand (arrow) and abduct the hip with the other. Assess abduction using the anterior iliac spines as points of reference.

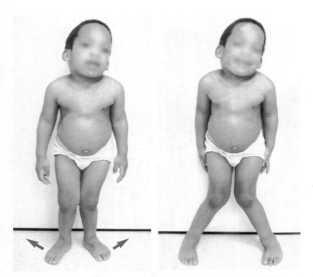

Fig. 2.20 Differentiate transverse and frontal plane deformity. This child compensates a severe genu valgum deformity by walking with the feet laterally rotated (red arrows). When the legs are placed in the anatomic position, the valgus deformity of the knees becomes apparent.

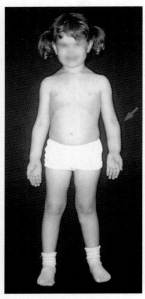

Fig. 2.21 Cubitus varus deformity. This deformity is secondary to a malunited fracture. The child is unaware of any problem.

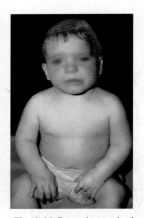

Fig. 2.22 Pseudoparalysis. This child has loss of spontaneous movement of the left arm from a "pulled elbow."

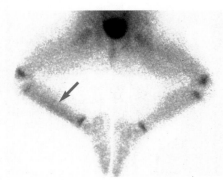

Fig. 2.23 Limp. This infant had an obscure limp. The bone scan demonstrated increased uptake over the tibia consistent with a toddler's fracture (arrow).

Deformity

Deformity is classified as either functional or structural. Functional deformity is secondary to muscle contracture or spasm-producing fixation of a joint in an abnormal position. For example, a fixed hip adductor contracture elevates the pelvis on the affected side, producing a functional shortening of the limb. This deformity is commonly seen in cerebral palsy and Perthes disease. In contrast, structural deformity originates within the limb. An example is the limb shortening associated with fibular hemimelia.

Assess deformity in reference to body planes with the body in the anatomic position (Fig. 2.21). Frontal or coronal plane deformity is most easily observed and creates the most significant cosmetic disability. Sagittal plane deformity produces problems in the plane of motion. Finally, transverse or horizontal plane deformity is most difficult to visualize and was often overlooked in the past. Currently, CT and MRI studies allow visualization and documentation of this plane and increased the appreciation of transverse plane problems. In assessing and documenting deformity, it is essential that each plane be separated clearly and described independently (Fig. 2.20). For example, in tibia vara, deformity occurs in both the frontal and transverse planes. Failure to clearly separate these planes may result in serious errors if operative correction is undertaken.

Altered Function

Function may be impaired by many mechanisms. The impairment is most obvious when the onset is acute and recent. The parents are aware when the pseudoparalysis is due to their child's "pulled" or "nursemaid's" elbow (Fig. 2.22). Conversely, long-standing changes in function may be overlooked or just considered as an unusual characteristic of the child. A child's bilateral abductor lurch from dislocated hips may go unappreciated for years. Limping of recent origin is usually obvious to the parents. Sometimes the examination is normal, and imaging studies are necessary to establish the diagnosis (Fig. 2.23).

Evaluate altered function of recent onset for evidence of trauma or infection. Look for deformity, swelling, or discoloration. Palpate to determine if tenderness is present. Finally, evaluate joint motion for stiffness or guarding. For example, inflammatory and traumatic hip disorders cause a loss of medial hip rotation and guarding of the joint. Evaluate chronic problems for evidence of deformity and an underlying disease. The chronic problem is much more likely to be serious and require a complete and thorough evaluation.

Functional disability is more significant than deformity. Deformity is static; function is dynamic. Deformity is most significant when it adversely affects function. This concept is becoming more universally accepted with time. In the past, handicapped children with conditions such as cerebral palsy were subjected to endless treatments to correct deformity. Often, deformity was corrected at the expense of function. The net effect was harmful.

Some alteration in function is subtle and not readily apparent. For example, a malunited bone forearm fracture may cause a permanent reduction of forearm rotation in the older child. The child compensates for the deformity by rotating the shoulder and may not be aware of any problem. This loss of motion can be detected by physical examination. Determine the degree of disability by functional tests that focus on activities requiring pronation and supination.

Pain

Pain in the child is usually significant. For example, the majority of adults experience back pain but rarely does it require active treatment. In contrast, back pain in children is much more likely to be organic. Pain in the adolescent is more likely to have a functional basis, as is so common in adults. The most common cause of pain in children is trauma. Trauma may result from acute injury or from the so-called microtrauma or overuse syndromes. Overuse syndromes account for the majority of sports medicine problems in children and adolescents.

Point of Maximum Tenderness

The most useful test in establishing the cause of pain is determining its anatomic origin by locating the *point of maximum tenderness (PMT)* (Fig. 2.24). Localization of the PMT, together with the history, often establishes the diagnosis. For example, a PMT over the tibial tubercle in a 13-year-old boy very likely means the boy has Osgood–Schlatter disease (Fig. 2.25). A PMT over the anterior aspect of the distal fibula (Fig. 2.26), together with a history of an ankle injury, probably points to an ankle sprain. A PMT over the tarsal navicular in a 12-year-old girl suggests the diagnosis of an accessory ossicle (Fig. 2.26).

The examination to establish the PMT should start distant from the problem. Palpate gently, moving progressively closer to the site of discomfort. Watch the child's face for signs of discomfort. Often a change in facial expression is more reliable than a verbal response. Be gentle. Ask the child to tell you where the tenderness is greatest. With gentleness, patience, and sensitivity, the PMT can usually be established accurately with minimal discomfort.

The PMT is a useful guide in ordering radiographs. A PMT over the tibial tubercle suggests the diagnosis of Osgood–Schlatter disease. If confirmation is necessary, order a lateral radiograph of the knee. Similarly, order oblique radiographs of the elbow if the PMT is over the lateral condyle and the AP and lateral views of the elbow are normal. Fracture of the lateral condyle may be demonstrated only on the oblique radiograph.

The PMT is helpful in evaluating the radiographs. For example, locating the PMT aids in differentiating an accessory ossification center from a fracture. Only a fracture will be tender. To determine if a subtle cortical irregularity in the contour of the distal radius represents a buckle fracture, locate the PMT. If the cortical irregularity represents a fracture, the PMT and the questionable radiographic change will coincide exactly in location.

Spondyloarthropathy Seronegative spondyloarthropathies in the incipient stage are associated with a PMT in specific locations. These are referred to as *enthesopathies*. Common sites include the metatarsal heads, plantar fascia, achilles tendon insertion, greater trochanter, and SI joints.

Muscle Testing

Muscle testing is done to determine the strength of muscle groups (Fig. 2.27). Testing is performed for neuromuscular problems such as poliomyelitis and muscular dystrophy. The grades can be further subdivided by a plus or minus designation.

Growing Pains

Growing pains are discomforts of unknown cause that occur in 15–30% of otherwise normal children. Headaches, stomachaches, and leg aches, in that order, are the common pains of childhood. Leg aches characteristically occur at night, are poorly localized, of long duration, and produce no limp or apparent disability. Spontaneous resolution occurs, without sequelae, over a period of several years.

Because the pain of leg aches is so diffuse and nondescript, the differential diagnosis includes most painful disorders of childhood. The conditions a physician must rule out include neoplastic disorders such as leukemia, hematologic problems such as sickle cell anemia, infections such as subacute osteomyelitis, and various inflammatory conditions. The diagnosis of growing pains is one of exclusion, relying primarily on the medical history and the physical examination. Rarely are a CBC and ESR or radiographs necessary. Evaluation and management of growing pains is discussed in greater detail in Chapter 3.

References

1992 Pain of musculoskeletal origin in children. Staheli LT. Curr Opin Rheumatol 4:748
1986 Screening for congenital dislocation of the hip, scoliosis, and other abnormalities affecting the musculoskeletal system. Asher MA. Pediatr Clin North Am 33:1335

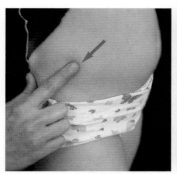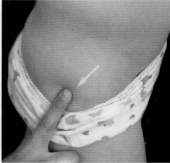

Fig. 2.24 PMT about the hip. The anterior iliac spine (red arrow) and the greater trochanter (yellow arrow) are useful landmarks for determining the PMT about the hip.

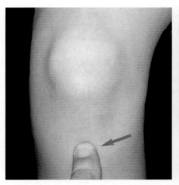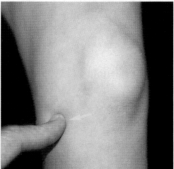

Fig. 2.25 PMT about the knee. The PMT is easily determined about the knee. The tibial tubercle (red arrow) is tender in Osgood–Schlatter disease. Medial joint line tenderness (yellow arrow) is found with meniscal injuries.

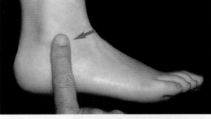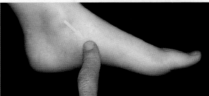

Fig. 2.26 PMT about the foot. Because bone and joints of the foot are subcutaneous, the PMT is very accurate and an especially valuable sign. The PMT over the lateral malleolus (red arrow) and over the navicular (yellow arrow) are readily localized.

Grade	Strength	Physical Finding
0	None	No contraction
1	Trace	Palpable contraction only
2	Poor	Moves joint without gravity
3	Fair	Moves joint against gravity
4	Good	Against gravity and resistance
5	Normal	Normal strength

Fig. 2.27 Muscle grading. Manual muscle testing is useful in documenting and classifying muscle strength into six categories.

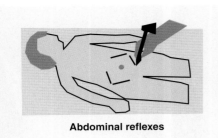

Abdominal reflexes

Fig. 2.28 Abdominal reflexes. The abdomen is stroked in all four quadrants. This stimulation causes the umbilicus to move toward the quadrant stimulated. The absence of this response is abnormal.

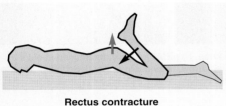

Tibial length
Ellis test

Femoral length
Galeazzi sign

Fig. 2.29 Assessing femoral and tibial lengths. Note the difference in tibial and femoral lengths as observed at the flexed knee. With the feet on the table, tibial length differences are apparent (red arrows). With the hips flexed and the feet free, note the differences in femoral lengths (blue arrows).

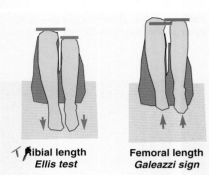

Rectus contracture
Ely test

Fig. 2.30 Rectus femoris contracture evaluation. With this contracture, flexion of the knee (black arrow) causes elevation of the pelvis (red arrow).

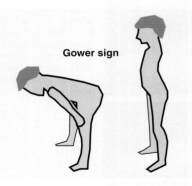

Gower sign

Fig. 2.31 Gower sign for generalized muscle weakness.

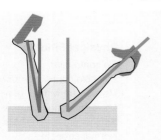

Hip rotation test

Fig. 2.32 Hip rotation test. This screens for traumatic or inflammatory hip problems. A reduction of medial rotation (red angle) is significant, as hip rotation is usually symmetrical in children.

Clinical Tests

Various tests are useful to supplement the general physical examination in children. Some of the more commonly used tests are described below, presented in alphabetical order.

Abdominal Reflex

Stimulate each quadrant of the abdomen (Fig. 2.28). Normally the umbilicus moves toward the side being stimulated. This test is commonly used to assess a neurologic basis for spinal deformity (see Chapter 8).

Anvil Test

This tests for the localization of discitis. Percussion on top of the head causes pain at the site of discitis.

Barlow Maneuver

This maneuver is a provocative test for hip instability in developmental hip dysplasia. See page 137.

Coleman Block Test

This tests for hindfoot flexibility. Ask the child to stand on a block positioned under the lateral side of the foot. With weight bearing, the failure of the heel to assume a valgus position is indicative of a fixed deformity.

Ellis Test

This test assesses the tibia–hindfoot length (Fig. 2.29). With the patient supine, flex the knees fully. The difference between the knee heights indicates the amount of shortening. This test can also be performed with the child prone. This allows the knees to be flexed to a full 90°.

Ely Test

The Ely test assesses for rectus contracture (Fig. 2.30). Place the child prone and flex the knee. If the rectus is spastic or contacted, the pelvis will rise.

Foot-Progression Angle

This test assesses the degree of in-toeing or out-toeing (see Chapter 4).

Forward Bend Test

This assesses the functional and structural stiffness and deformity of the back. While observing the patient from the back and again from the side, ask the patient to bend forward as far as possible. Note asymmetry and stiffness. The normal child should show symmetrical flexion and be able to extend the fingers to at least the knee. The spine should show an even flexion of the thoracic spine and reversal of the lumbar lordosis. The thorax should be symmetrical as viewed from the back and front. Spinal cord tumors, inflammatory lesions, spinal deformity, and hamstring contractures all cause abnormal findings.

Galeazzi Sign

This tests for shortening due to developmental hip dysplasia (Fig. 2.29). Flex both hips and knees to a right angle. Note any difference in apparent length of thighs.

Goldthwaite Test

This test detects lumbar spine inflammation as occurs with discitis. Position prone with hips extended and knees flexed. Moving the pelvis from side to side causes a synchondrous movement of the lumbar spine.

Gower Test

This tests for general muscle weakness (Fig. 2.31). Ask the patient to sit on the floor and then stand up without external supports. With trunk weakness, the child uses his hands to climb up his thighs for support.

Hip Rotation Test

The hip rotation test screens for inflammatory or traumatic hip problems (Fig. 2.32). Place child in prone position, knees flexed to 90°, and medially rotate both hips. A loss of medial rotation is a positive sign.

Nélaton's Line

This test is useful in clinical assessment of hip dislocation. The tip of the trochanter should fall below a line connecting the anterior iliac spine and the ischael tuberosity.

Ober Test

This tests for tensor fascia contracture (Fig. 2.33). Position the patient on one side with the lower knee and hip flexed to a right angle. Abduct and fully extend the upper hip. While maintaining the hip extended, allow the leg to fall into full adduction. An abduction contracture is present if the thigh fails to fall into adduction. The degree of contracture equals the abducted position above the neutral or horizontal position.

Ortoloni Maneuver

This maneuver tests for hip instability in DDH. See page 137.

Patellar Apprehension Sign

This test is for patellar instability. With the knee extended, gradually apply pressure to laterally displace the patella while observing the patient's facial expression. Apprehension indicates previous experience with patellar dislocation.

Patrick Test

This test detects sacroiliac (SI) inflammation (Fig. 2.34). Place the ipsilateral foot over the opposite knee. While holding down the opposite ilium, apply a downward force on the flexed knee. Pain at the SI joint is a positive finding.

Pelvic Obliquity Test

This differentiates suprapelvic from infrapelvic obliquity. Position the child prone with the pelvis on the edge of the examining table, allowing the lower limbs to flex. Windswept positioning of the legs brings the pelvis to neutral if the obliquity is infrapelvic in origin.

Phelps Gracilis Test

This test is a measure of gracilis spasticity or contracture. Position prone and abduct the hip with the knee flexed. Passive knee extension causes hip adduction if the gracilis is contracted.

Popliteal Angle Measure

This measures hamstring contracture (Fig. 2.35). With the patient supine, flex the hip to a right angle and the knee to a comfortable maximum. The contracture equals the degree of lack of full knee extension.

Prone Extension Test

This tests for hip flexion contracture (Fig. 2.36). Position the patient prone with the thigh over the edge of the examining table, with one hand on the pelvis and other holding on the leg. Extend the leg until the pelvis starts to elevate. The horizontal–thigh angle demonstrates the degree of contracture.

Thigh–Foot Angle

This is a measure of tibial and hindfoot rotation. See page 71.

Thomas Test

This tests for hip flexion contracture. Flex the contralateral hip fully. The ipsilateral horizontal–thigh angle equals the hip flexion contracture.

Transmalleolar Angle

This angle is a measure of tibial rotation. See page 71.

Trendelenburg Test

The Trendelenburg test assesses abductor strength (Fig. 2.37). While observing the pelvis from behind, ask the patient to raise one leg (without holding for support). A drop in the contralateral pelvis indicates weakness of the ipsilateral abductors.

A *delayed* Trendelenburg test is performed by determining the time necessary for the abductors to fatigue, allowing the pelvis to sag. If the elevation of the contralateral pelvis cannot be maintained for 60 seconds, the test is positive.

References

1977 The prone hip extension test. Staheli LT. CO 123:12

1977 A simple test for hindfoot flexibility in cavovarus foot. Coleman SS, Chesnut WJ. CO 123:60

1974 The natural history of torsion and other factors influencing gait in childhood. Engel GM, Staheli LT. CO 99:12

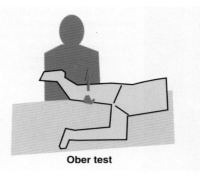

Ober test

Fig. 2.33 Ober test. This tests for tensor fascia contracture. Abduct and extend the leg, then allow it to fall. A failure of adduction is positive for a tensor contracture.

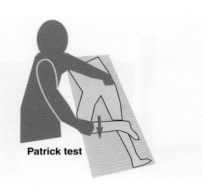

Patrick test

Fig. 2.34 Patrick test. This test is performed by positioning the leg across the other and applying downward pressure. This elicits pain in the ipsilateral sacraliliac joint region.

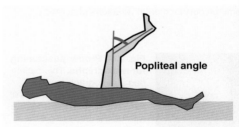

Popliteal angle

Fig. 2.35 Popliteal angle. With the hip flexed, extend the knee. The degrees short of full extension equal the popliteal angle (blue arc).

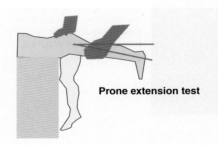

Prone extension test

Fig. 2.36 Prone extension test for assessing hip flexion contracture. With the contralateral hip flexed, extend the ipsilateral side to the degree that causes the pelvis to elevate. The degrees short of full extension equal the degrees of contracture.

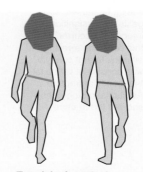

Trendelenburg test

Fig. 2.37 Trendelenburg test. Standing on the normal side elicits an elevation in the opposite side (green line). A drop in the opposite side (red line) indicates weakness of hip abduction.

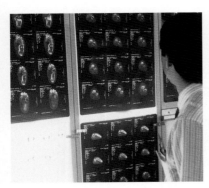

Fig. 2.38 Be cautious about over-reading. New imaging techniques often result in over-reading which sometimes results in over-treatment.

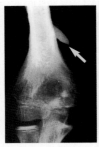
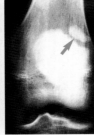
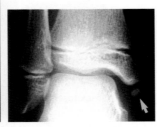

Fig. 2.39 Normal variation. The supracondyloid process of the humerus (yellow arrow), a bipartite patella (green arrow), and malleolar ossicles (orange arrow) are uncommon developmental variations of normal.

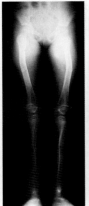
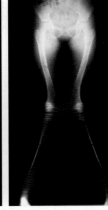

Fig. 2.40 Proper positioning for radiographs. This patient had a radiograph made for measuring mechanical axis of the lower limb. The technician rotated the limbs to get the radiograph on one film (left image). A second film was necessary (right image) in which the physician positioned the child in the anatomic position necessary for an accurate measurement.

Imaging

New imaging methods make musculoskeletal evaluation more rapid, precise, and complete. However, new images must be interpreted with caution (Fig. 2.38). Even after 100 years of experience reading conventional radiographs, we sometimes have difficulty separating disease from normal variability (Fig. 2.39). The lack of experience with new imaging methods makes interpretation even more difficult. Over-reading imaging, such as the MRI, poses risks and may lead to over-treatment. For example, MRI studies of discitis often show extensive soft tissue changes, which might prompt operative drainage if the nature of the disease is not appreciated.

Conventional Radiography

Conventional radiographs are still the mainstay of diagnostic imaging. They are the least expensive, most readily available, and the least apt to be misread. Radiographs show bone, water, fat, and air density well. Bone density must be reduced by 30–50% to show changes on radiographs. Proper positioning of the child is essential. Sometimes the physician needs to position the child. For example, to study genu varum or genu valgum, the child must be placed in the anatomic position with the patellae directed forward. The technician may try to rotate the limbs laterally to fit the legs on the film, creating a deceptive image (Fig. 2.40).

Limiting radiographs Try to limit radiation exposure by reducing the number of radiographs ordered. The risk of one chest x-ray is considered comparable to smoking 1.4 cigarettes or driving 30 miles. Although the risk is small, it is prudent to limit exposure when possible. Use the following principles to limit exposure to your patients:

1. Shield the gonads when possible except for the initial pelvic image.
2. When possible, order screening radiographs first. For example, if spondylolisthesis is suspected, a single lateral standing spot view of the lumbosacral junction may demonstrate the lesion. AP and oblique studies may not be necessary.
3. Single radiographs are often adequate. For example, a single AP view of the pelvis is usually adequate for evaluating hip dysplasia in the infant or child.
4. Lower extremity and spine radiographs should be taken in the upright position. These standardized views are less likely to be repeated if a referral is necessary.
5. Suggest to primary care physicians that if a consultation is necessary, have the consultant order the studies. Suggest that parents hand carry previous radiographs for consultation, as radiographs are often mysteriously lost in the mail.
6. Order follow-up radiographs only when the information is likely to alter management. For example, ordering a radiograph of a wrist fracture at 3 weeks is generally useless. It is too soon to discontinue immobilization and too late to change position.
7. Finally, the routine practice of ordering a comparative radiograph of the opposite side is often inappropriate.

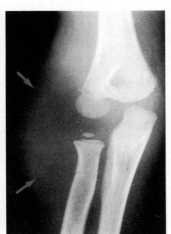

Fig. 2.41 Soft tissue swelling. Soft tissue swelling is an important finding because it suggests that a significant injury has occurred. In this case, the swelling over the lateral condyle was consistent with a lateral condylar fracture. Additional radiographs showed the fracture.

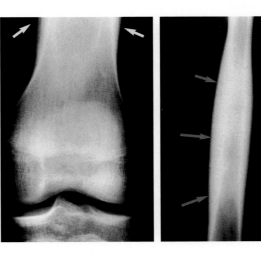

Fig. 2.42 Study the edge of the film. Initial radiograph of adolescent complaining of leg pain. The film was read as normal and a diagnosis made of a "conversion reaction." In a later review of the radiograph, periosteal reaction involving femoral distal diaphysis (yellow arrows) was appreciated. Additional radiographs of the whole femur showed extensive sclerosis of the diaphysis (red arrows) due to chronic sclerosing osteomyelitis.

Reading errors Here are some suggestions to avoid reading errors:
1. Study the radiographs in a standardized sequence, starting with the soft tissues (Fig. 2.41).
2. Study the edge of the film before concentrating on the presumed area of pathology (Fig. 2.42).
3. If the radiographic and physical findings are inconsistent, order additional views. For example, order oblique radiographs of the elbow if the child has unexplained swelling over the elbow (Fig. 2.41) and no evidence of a fracture on the initial AP and lateral views. The oblique views will often demonstrate a fracture.
4. Be aware that false negative studies occur in certain situations, such as in the early phase of osteomyelitis and in septic arthritis or developmental hip dysplasia in the newborn.
5. Finally, variations of ossification are often misleading. The accessory ossicles of the foot may be confused with fractures; irregular ossification on the lateral femoral condyle may be misinterpreted as osteochondritis dissecans.

Computerized Tomography Imaging

CT studies provide excellent bone and soft tissue detail (Fig. 2.43). The soft tissue images can be manipulated by computer to enhance tissue separations. This makes the method useful for assessing soft tissue lesions about the pelvis. CT studies can be combined with contrast material for special evaluations, such as CT myelography. Images are obtained in the transverse plane and can be reconstructed by computer with the frontal and sagittal planes or presented as 3-D images for a more graphic display (Fig. 2.44). These studies show relationships well, such as the concentricity of hip reduction and the detailing of dysplasia (Fig. 2.45). For complex deformity, plastic models can be fabricated based on the CT study (Fig. 2.46).

The disadvantages of CT imaging include the need for sedation in the infant and young child, greater radiation exposure, and greater cost than for conventional studies.

Arthrography

Arthrographic studies provide visualization of soft tissue structures of the joints (Fig. 2.47). The contrast is usually provided by air, nitrogen, carbon dioxide, or an iodinated contrast solution. The procedure can be combined with CT or tomography. Arthrography is most useful in evaluating the hip (Fig. 2.48) and knee. In septic arthritis, an arthrogram is helpful to confirm joint entry. Arthrography is useful for hip dysplasia and meniscal lesions and in identifying loose or foreign bodies in joints. Disadvantages include the need for sedating younger children and occasional reactions to the iodinated contrast material.

References
2000 Magnetic resonance arthrography in children with developmental hip dysplasia. Kawaguchi AT, et al. CO 235
1999 MR imaging of congenital anomalies of the pediatric spine. Egelhoff JC. Magn Reson Imaging Clin N Am 7:459
1999 Neuroimaging of scoliosis in childhood. Kim FM, Poussaint TY, and Barnes PD. Neuroimaging Clin N Am 9:195

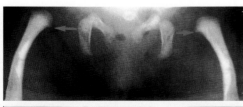
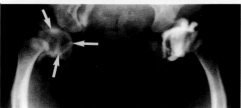

Fig. 2.47 Arthrography. Initial radiograph showed a lateral displacement of the upper femoral metaphysis (red arrows) suggesting the possibility of a hip dislocation or subluxation. The arthrogram shows the femoral head to be reduced (yellow arrows) and established the diagnosis of coxa vara.

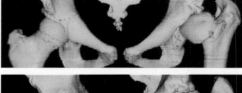

Uses for CT Scans
Bone detailing—when conventional radiographs are inadequate
Spine and pelvic lesions—inflammatory, neoplastic, traumatic
Complex hip deformity prior to reconstruction
DDH assessment of reduction in cast
Physeal bridge assessment
Complex fractures—such as triplane ankle fractures

Fig. 2.43 Uses of CT scans. These are some typical examples of the use of CT scans in assessing musculoskeletal problems in children.

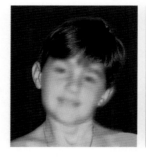
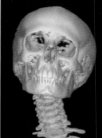

Fig. 2.44 Torticollis with plagiocephaly. Asymmetry of the face and skull are demonstrated by 3D CT reconstructions.

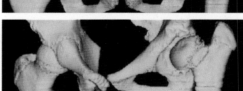

Fig. 2.45 3-D reconstruction in hip dysplasia. These reconstructions allow assessment of complex hip pathology and often facilitate operative planning.

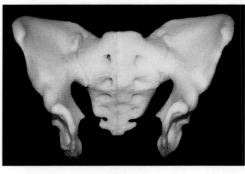

Fig. 2.46 Plastic model from CT reconstruction. Models in plastic can be created that allow preoperative planning and execution of operative correction.

Uses for Arthrography
DDH—initial evaluation and when management uncertain
Perthes disease—to assess shape of cartilagenous femoral head
Complex trauma—such as elbow injuries in the infant
Osteochondritis dissecans

Fig. 2.48 Arthrography uses. These are typical examples of the use of arthrograms for assessing musculoskeletal problems in children.

Uses for Bone Scans

Screening—for child abuse
Limp—localization of site of problem
Trauma—early stress fractures
Tumors—localizing lesions, lesion age, differentiating cyst types
Infections—localizing site or early osteomyelitis, discitis
Avascular necrosis—LCP disease, osteochondritis staging

Fig. 2.49 Uses of bone scans. These are some examples of the use of bone scans for assessing musculoskeletal problems in children.

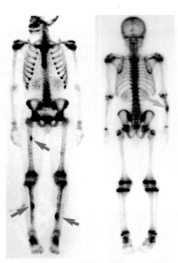

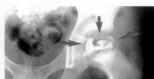

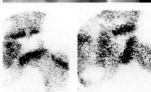

Fig. 2.50 Bone scans for screening. These screening bone scans demonstrated unsuspected multiple stress reactions in an athlete (red arrows). The other boy (right) has osteomyelitis that is localized to the left ulna (orange arrow).

Fig. 2.51 Pinhole collimated bone scan. Conventional radiograph shows avascular necrosis of the femoral head (red arrows). Pinhole collimated scans show reduced uptake in the avascular femoral head (orange arrows).

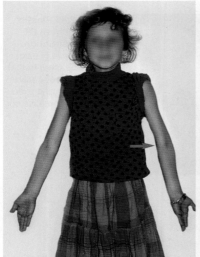

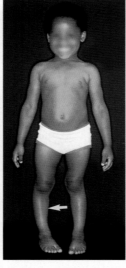

Fig. 2.52 Clinical photography. Note the cubitus varus deformity of the girls left arm (red arrow) and the bowing of the boy's right tibia (yellow arrow). The value of each photograph is enhance by the nondistracting backgrounds, careful positioning, and inclusion of both limbs for comparison. Both photographs document the deformity well and were useful for subsequent evaluation of the effect of growth on severity.

Scintography

Scans utilizing technetium-99m, gallium-67, and indium-111 provide imaging of a variety of tissues. Scintographies are more sensitive and show abnormal uptake much earlier than radiographic imaging (Fig. 2.49). In addition, bone scanning has a broad scope of applications, including the evaluation of obscure skeletal pain (Fig. 2.50). The radiation exposure is equivalent to a skeletal survey with conventional radiographs. Useful options in scanning include a variety of agents, collimator selection, timing of scans, and the use of special techniques.

Collimation "Pinhole" collimation increases the resolution of the image. This is particularly useful for assessing avascular necrosis of the femoral head. Order both AP and lateral views (Fig. 2.51).

Agents The vast majority of scans use technetium-99m. This agent has a half-life of 6 hours and, combined with phosphate, is bone seeking. It is highly sensitive, and the images usually become positive in 24–48 hours. Gallium-67 and indium-111 are used primarily for localization of infections. Indium is combined with a sample of the white blood cells from the patient.

Timing Phasic bone scans show the initial perfusion immediately. The soft tissue phase or pooling occurs at 10–20 minutes, and finally, the bone phase is shown after 3–4 hours. Bone scans are not affected by joint aspiration.

Photography

Medical photography provides an excellent means of documentation (Fig. 2.52). Photographs are inexpensive, safe, and accurate. They are useful in documentation and parent education. The documenting value of photographs is increased by taking certain steps:

Positioning Position for photographs as for a radiograph. Make anterior, lateral, or special views. Position the patient in the anatomic position.

Background Attempt to find a neutral, nondistracting background.

Distance Take photographs as close as possible while including enough of the body to orient the viewer.

Magnetic Resonance Imaging

MRI provides excellent images of soft tissue (Fig. 2.53) without exposure to ionizing radiation. However, it requires expensive, sophisticated equipment and sedation or anesthesia in the infant or younger child for necessary immobilization. Bone imaging is poor, but for soft tissues, MRI is excellent. The interpretation may be difficult because of limited experience, making over-reading a potential problem. Despite these problems, MRIs are proving useful for an increasingly wide variety of conditions (Figs. 2.54–2.56).

Uses for MRI Studies

Cartilage imaging—meniscal lesion, growth plate injuries
Avascular necrosis—LCP disease, AVN at hip, distal femur
Neural status—spinal cord lesions
Tumors—margins, staging
Infections—soft tissue lesions

Fig. 2.53 Uses for MRI. These studies are useful in imaging soft tissue lesions. The usefulness in infants and children is limited by the cost and the need for sedation or anesthesia for immobilization.

Ultrasound Imaging

Ultrasound applications for the musculoskeletal system are numerous, and the technique is underutilized (Fig. 2.57).

Prenatal ultrasound These studies (Fig. 2.58) have the potential of making dramatic changes in orthopedic practice. Here are some useful applications of prenatal ultrasound:

Pathogenesis Improving our understanding of disease in turn improves our ability to prevent or treat diseases.

Prenatal treatment Prenatal treatment, utilizing replacement, substitution therapies, or improving intrauterine environment may correct or improve the problem.

Family preparation Resources can be made available for early postnatal treatment as necessary and preparing families psychologically and educationally.

Pregnancy termination For serious conditions, ultrasound can help determine the need for termination based on the family's choice.

Musculoskeletal disorders The number of these disorders that can be diagnosed by prenatal ultrasound (Fig. 2.59) are increasing rapidly with higher resolution studies and greater user experience. False positive studies do occur, however, and may cause considerable unnecessary anxiety in the families.

Clinical uses These studies are highly dependent on operator skill and experience, and in North America, they are usually performed by the radiologist (Fig. 2.60). Ultrasound studies are probably underutilized and could become a practical extension of the physical examination. Ultrasound is safe, potentially inexpensive, versatile, and underutilized in North America.

References

1999 Prenatal sonographic diagnosis of musculoskeletal disorders. [editorial; comment]. Wientroub S, et al. JPO 19:1

1999 Prenatal sonographic diagnosis of clubfoot: implications for patient counseling. Treadwell MC, Stanitski CL, King M. JPO 19:8

1998 Musculoskeletal trauma in children. Jaramillo D, Shapiro F. Magn Reson Imaging Clin N Am 6:521

1998 The role of magnetic resonance imaging in the investigation of spinal dysraphism in the child with lower limb abnormality. Ward PJ, Clarke NM, Fairhurst JJ. JPO-b 7:141

1998 6-year experience of prenatal diagnosis in an unselected population in Oxford, UK [see comments]. Boyd PA, et al. Lancet 352:1577

1998 Pre-natal diagnosis of occult spinal dysraphism by ultrasonography and post-natal evaluation by MR scanning. Sattar TS, et al. Eur J Pediatr Surg 1:31

1997 Pediatric fracture without radiographic abnormality. Description and significance. Naranja RJ Jr, et al. CO 141

1996 Musculoskeletal ultrasound. Gibbon WW. Baillieres Clin Rheumatol 10:561

1995 Usefulness of magnetic resonance imaging for the diagnosis of acute musculoskeletal infections in children. Mazur JM, et al. JPO 15:144

1995 The use of ultrasound for the diagnosis of soft-tissue masses in children. Abi Ezzi SS, Miller LS. JPO 15:566

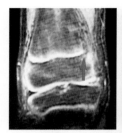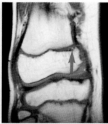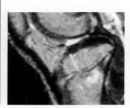

Fig. 2.54 MRI in physeal injury. Note the defect in the distal femoral physis (red arrows) and the proximal tibial growth plate (yellow arrow).

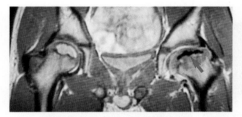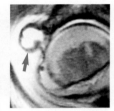

Fig. 2.55 MRI in Perthes disease. The avascular necrosis is clearly demonstrated (arrow).

Fig. 2.56 Synovial cyst hip. The cyst (arrow) is clearly seen on this MRI study.

Uses for Ultrasound—Postnatal

DDH—evaluation in the young infant
Infections—localization of abscess, joint effusions
Foreign bodies—of the foot
Tumors—especially cystic varieties
Trauma—cartilagenous injuries in young children
Research—measuring torsion, joint configuration

Fig. 2.57 Postnatal ultrasound diagnosis. These are typical examples of the use of ultrasound for assessing musculoskeletal problems in children.

Uses for Ultrasound—Prenatal

Clubfeet
Skeletal dysplasias
Limb deficiencies
Spina bifida
Arthrogryposis

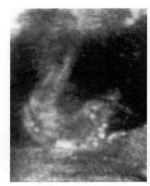

Fig. 2.58 Prenatal ultrasound diagnosis. These musculoskeletal problems can usually be diagnosed.

Fig. 2.59 Clubfoot. This clubfoot was identified at 16 weeks of gestation by ultrasound.

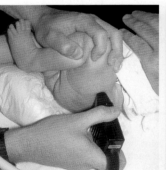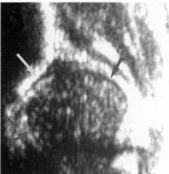

Fig. 2.60 Ultrasound hip evaluation. The ultrasound evaluation (left) of the hip allows effective imaging before ossification occurs. The ultrasound image clearly shows the acetabulum (yellow arrow) and the femoral head (red arrows).

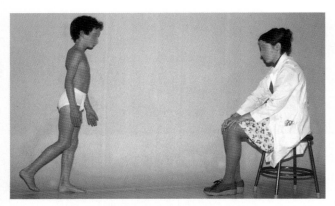

Fig. 2.61 Clinical observational gait examination. Evaluation of the child's gait is best performed in an open area.

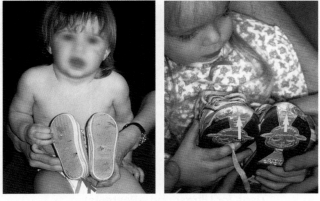

Fig. 2.62 Value of observing foot wear. The lack of heel wear (red arrow, left) is evidence of an equinus gait on the left side. Excessive wear on the toes of the shoes is indicative of a more severe degree of equinus (yellow arrows, right) in a child with spastic diplegia.

Gait Evaluation

Gait can be evaluated at three levels of sophistication.

Screening Examination

This is part of the standard screening examination and is usually performed in the hallway of the clinic (Fig. 2.61).

Clinical Observational Examination

This examination (Fig. 2.63) is indicated if (1) the family has reported that the child limps, (2) an abnormality is seen during the screening examination, or (3) the physical findings point to a disease likely to affect gait. In the hallway of the clinic, observe the child walking from the front, behind, and both sides if possible. Look at the child's shoes for evidence of abnormal wear (Fig. 2.62). An abnormal gait often falls into readily identifiable categories:

Antalgic gait Pain with weight bearing causes shortening of the stance phase on the affected side.

In-toeing and out-toeing gaits Assess the foot–progression angle for each side. Average the estimated values and express in degrees.

Equinus gait Toe strike replaces heel strike at the beginning of the stance phase.

Abductor lurch or Trendelenburg gait Abductor weakness causes the shoulders to sway to the opposite side.

Instrumented Gait Analysis

Gait can be assessed by using a video camera to record visual observations. More sophisticated techniques can also be used, including dynamic electromyography to assess muscle firing sequences, kinemetric techniques for assessing joint motion, force plate to measure ground reaction forces, and sequence and rate measurements (Fig. 2.64). These values are usually compared with normal values.

Currently, greater attention is being focused on the efficiency of gait by analyzing oxygen consumption and heart rate changes. Over time, we become more concerned about effective and efficient mobility and less about mechanical variations.

The role of the gait laboratory is still controversial. It is clearly an important research tool, but its practicality as a clinical tool remains uncertain.

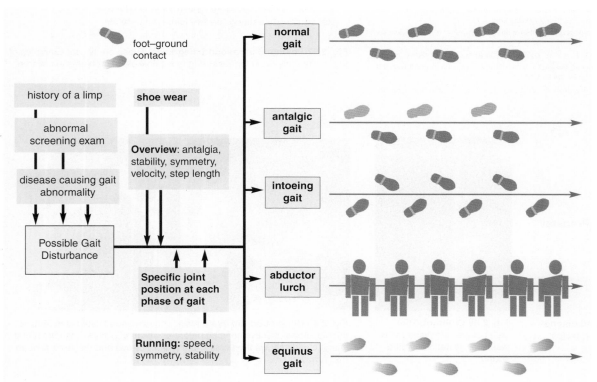

Fig. 2.63 Algorithm for gait assessment.

Laboratory Studies

Laboratory studies provide a limited but useful role in orthopedics. The studies can be combined to reduce the number of needle aspirations.

Hematology

Order a complete blood count (CBC) and erythrocyte sedimentation rate (ESR) and/or C reactive protein (CRP) as part of a screening evaluation to assess the general health of the patient (Fig. 2.65), or when infection, neoplasm, or hematologic conditions are suspected.

The ESR is valuable in differentiating infections from inflammation and traumatic conditions. The CRP elevates more rapidly and returns to normal sooner than the ESR. The upper range of value for the ESR is 20 mm/hr. Inflammatory conditions such as toxic synovitis may raise the ESR to the 20–30 mm/hr range, but ESRs above 30 mm/hr are usually due to infection, neoplasm, or significant trauma. Except in the neonate, the CRP and ESR are usually always elevated by infections such as septic arthritis and osteomyelitis. In contrast, a leukocytosis is a less consistent finding.

Chemistry

Serum studies of calcium metabolism are occasionally useful when the possibility of conditions such as rickets is suspected. The normal range of these values is age dependent.

Enzymes

Screen for muscular dystrophy by ordering a creatinine phosphokinase (CPK) determination. Order the test if the young child appears weak, shows a clumsy gait, and has tight heel cords.

Chromosomal Studies

Chromosome studies are indicated for evaluating syndromes with features suggestive of a genetic disorder. These features include multiple system congenital malformations; mental retardation of unknown cause; abnormal hands, feet, and ears; and skin creases.

Bone Mineral Content

Mineral content of bones can be quantitated using several techniques. Cortical measurements can be made by radiography. The second metacarpal is a common standard. Single and dual photon absorptiometry are other alternatives. These studies are indicated for metabolic diseases, idiopathic osteopenia, and similar disorders.

Joint Fluid

Joint fluid should be visually examined (Fig. 2.66) and also sent to the lab for cell counts, chemistry, culturing, and staining (Fig. 2.67). The joint sugar is usually about 90% serum level and is reduced in infection. In about one-third of cases of septic arthritis, cultures are negative.

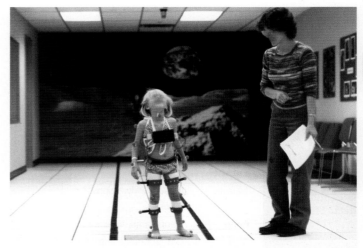

Fig. 2.64 Gait laboratory. The modern gait lab has sophisticated measuring devices to analyze gait.

Condition	Indication for CBC, ESR, and/or CRP
Growing pain	Suspicious features, rule out leukemia
Bone pain	Rule out sickle cell anemia
Stress fracture	Rule out infection
Hip pain	Separate septic arthritis and toxic synovitis
Back pain	Evaluate for discitis
Infection	Follow course of infection

Fig. 2.65 Indications for CBC, ESR, and/or CRP. These screening tests are helpful in evaluating a variety of clinical problems.

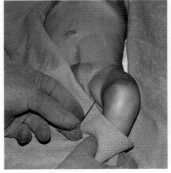

Fig. 2.66 Joint aspiration. The hip joint in the infant is readily aspirated by the medial approach. Visually examine the joint fluid.

Fig. 2.67 Joint fluid evaluation. Joint fluid differences can be seen among common causes of joint effusions.

Examination	Normal	Septic arthritis	JRA	Traumatic arthritis
Appearance	Straw colored	Grayish	Straw colored	Bloody
Clarity	Clear	Turbid	Slightly cloudy	Bloody
Viscosity	Normal	Decreased	Decreased	Decreased
Total WBC	0–200	50,000–100,000	20,000–50,000	RBCs
PMNS	90+%	Mostly PMNS	Predominate	
Bacteria	None	Seen in about half	None	None
Culture	Negative	Positive 2/3	Negative	Negative
Protein	1.8 g/100 mL	4 g/100 mL	3–4 g/100 mL	Normal
Glucose	20 mg/100,ml below serum	30–50 mg/100 mL below serum	Normal	Normal
Inspection				Fat in aspirate

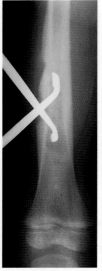

Tissue	Indication
Muscle	Muscular dystrophy
	Myositis
Bone	Neoplasms, infections
Skin	Osteogenesis imperfecta
Nerve	Neuropathy

Fig. 2.68 Common indications for biopsy. Tissue from bone (left) or other tissues is useful to establish the diagnosis.

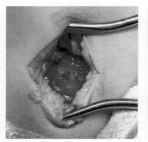
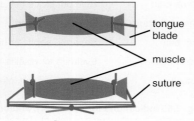

tongue blade

muscle

suture

Fig. 2.69 Technique of muscle biopsy. Remove a segment of muscle for biopsy (left). Secure the specimen to a segment of a tongue blade with sutures (blue lines, right) to maintain length and orientation during transport and initial fixation.

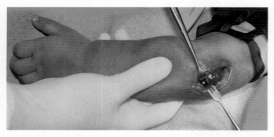

Fig. 2.70 Biopsy of bone. Biopsies are important procedures that require planning, careful technique, and competent pathologic evaluation.

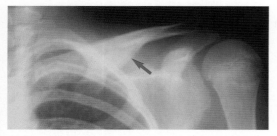

Fig. 2.71 Osteomyelitis of the clavicle. This lesion is often confused with a tumor. Be certain to obtain biopsy cultures.

Diagnostic Procedures

Other studies are sometimes helpful.

Electromyography

Electromyography (EMG) is done using either surface or deep electrodes. Surface electrode studies are limited because of artifacts and poor muscle selectivity. The placement of deep electrodes is painful and thus poorly tolerated in children. Furthermore, EMG studies do not show the strength of contraction, only the electrical activity.

EMG is useful in evaluating peripheral nerve injuries, anterior horn cell degeneration, and diseases such as myotonia and myelitis. In peripheral nerve injuries, denervation causes fibrillation potentials 1–2 weeks after injury. During regeneration, the EMG will show polyphasic wave forms. In anterior horn cell degeneration, fasciculations appear.

Nerve Conduction Velocity

Nerve conduction velocity is measured by the time difference shown between the point of stimulation and the recording by EMG. Normal values change with age, from about 25 m/sec at birth to 45 m/sec at age 3 years to about 45–65 m/sec in mid-childhood. The peroneal, posterior tibial, ulnar, median, and facial nerves are usually studied. In children, perform these studies in evaluating peripheral and hereditary neuropathies.

Diagnostic Blocks

Diagnostic blocks are most useful in children for evaluating incisional neuroma and for pain of unknown cause around the foot. By this means, it is possible to localize the site of pain precisely.

Biopsy

The biopsy is an important diagnostic procedure (Fig. 2.68) and is not always a simple process. It is preferable for the same surgeon to perform both the biopsy and any reconstructive or ablative procedures. Planning is important. Generally, open biopsy is routine, with needle biopsy performed for lesions in inaccessible sites such as vertebral bodies. Plan ahead with the lab to coordinate tissue removal (Figs. 2.69 and 2.70), transfer solutions, frozen sections, and electron microscopic studies. Culture the lesion if there is even the remotest possibility of an infectious etiology (Fig. 2.71).

Arthrocentesis

Joint aspiration is diagnostic (Fig. 2.72) and sometimes therapeutic. These studies are indicated whenever an infectious etiology is possible. See pages 379 and 380.

References

1996 Biopsy: complicated and risky [editorial; comment] [see comments]. Springfield DS, Rosenberg A. JBJS 78A:639

1996 The effect of arthrocentesis in transient synovitis of the hip in the child: a longitudinal sonographic study. Kesteris U, et al. JPO 16:24

1995 Normal values of nerve conduction in children and adolescents. Hyllienmark L, et al. Electroencephalogr Clin Neurophysiol 97:208

1994 Biopsy of bone and soft-tissue lesions. Simon MA, Biermann JS. Instr Course Lect 43:521

1994 Single-incision combination biopsy (muscle and nerve) in the diagnosis of neuromuscular disease in children. Hurley ME, et al. JPO 14:740

1985 Evolution of nerve conduction velocity in later childhood and adolescence. Lang HA, et al. Muscle Nerve 8:38

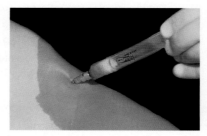

Fig. 2.72 Arthrocentesis. Pus is aspirated from this septic hip.

Time Line

The effect of time and growth on a disorder is called the *time line.* This is also referred to as the *natural history,* or what would happen without treatment. The natural history of many conditions is well known. For instance, we know that nearly all rotational problems resolve with time. Unfortunately, variability from child to child makes the best predictions only estimates. In less common conditions, the course is unknown and the time line is of even greater importance. Sometimes the time line is established by chance (Fig. 2.73), but it is usually established by serial radiographs (Figs. 2.74– 2.76) or photographs (Fig. 2.77). To establish a time line, the status of the disorder is documented at intervals. During the first visit, obtain baseline studies. The studies are repeated at intervals depending on the disease.

A classic example is in physeal bridge management. If a child sustains a medial malleolar Salter type III or IV injury, it is useful to obtain a baseline full-length radiograph of both tibiae on one film. The same study is made at 3-month intervals. A change in relative lengths of the tibia or a tilting of the articular surface of the ankle is early evidence of a physeal bridge.

Chapter consultant Richard Gross, e-mail: grossr@musc.edu

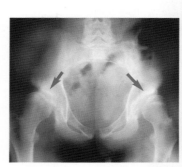
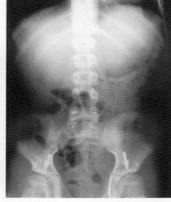

Fig. 2.73 Chance "time line." This 15-year-old boy was seen for bilateral hip pain. Radiographs demonstrated severe hip dysplasia with subluxation (red arrows). By chance in his old x-ray folder, a KUB was found that was taken when he was 12 years old. His hips showed only mild dysplasia (yellow arrows) at that age.

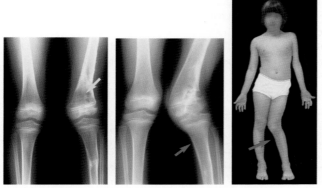

Fig. 2.74 Effect of growth. These radiographs show the effect of time and growth when a physeal bridge is present (yellow arrow). Two years later, this 12-year-old boy shows a dramatic increase in valgus deformity of the knee (red arrows).

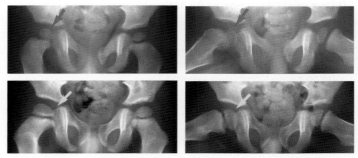

Fig. 2.75 Remodeling. Childhood remodeling of fracture deformity is one of the most graphic demonstrations of the effect of time and growth. This infant sustained a physeal fracture with malunion at 12 months (red arrows). Note the extensive remodeling of the deformity by age 24 months (yellow arrows).

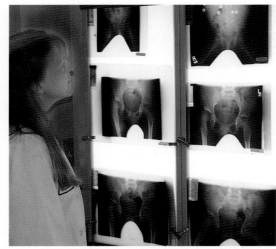

Fig. 2.76 Time line using radiographs. Comparing a sequence of radiographs is a very practical method of assessing the effect of time on deformity.

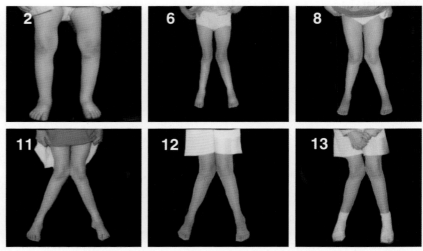

Fig. 2.77 Time line using photographs. In this child with vitamin D-resistant rickets, the progression of the genu valgum deformities at ages 2, 6, 8, 11, 12, and 13 years is illustrated. The family and patient elected to delay correction until 14 years of age to avoid recurrence.

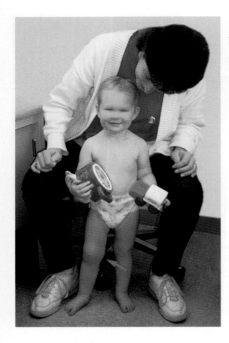

Fig. 2.78 Pauciarticular juvenile rhematoid arthritis. This young girl has little discomfort. Note the swollen right knee.

Joint Swelling

Joint inflammation is termed *arthritis* (Fig. 2.78), whereas joint pain without signs of inflammation is referred to as *arthralgia*. Rheumatologists call pain at ligament and tendon insertions *endthesopathy*. Arthritis occurs in about 2 in 1000 children. The causes of swollen joints in children are numerous (Fig. 2.79). In most cases, the diagnosis (Fig. 2.80) is established through the approach outlined below.

Approach

History Ask the patient and family about systemic symptoms, night pain, morning stiffness, other illnesses, family history, duration, severity, and general health.

Examination Perform a careful screening examination. Is the child systemically ill? Carefully examine all extremities to determine if any other large or small joints are involved. Note the degree of inflammation, localization of tenderness, joint range of motion, and any fixed deformities.

Laboratory studies If one suspects juvenile rheumatoid arthritis (JRA), order a CBC, ESR, CRP, ANA, RF, and urinalysis. Order other studies to help separate your short-list differential diagnosis.

Imaging Start with conventional radiographs and add other studies as appropriate.

Joint aspiration Joint aspiration is indicated if an infectious etiology is included in the differential diagnosis.

Clinical Types

Polyarticualar JRA occurs in two clinical patterns (Fig. 2.81): young girls and those in adolescence with multiple small and large joint involvement.

Differential Diagnosis of Arthritis

Primary

Traumatic
Direct injury—dislocation, fracture
Slipped capital femoral epiphysis
Introduction—foreign body synovitis

Infection
Bacterial
Lyme disease
Tubculosis

Juvenile rheumatoid arthritis
Systemic JRA
Polyarticular JRA
Pauciarticular JRA
Spondyloarthopathy

Tumors
Intraarticular hemangiomata
Pigmented villonodular synovitis

Vascular
Legg-Calvé-Perthes disease
Osteochondritis dissecans

Idiopathic
Toxic synovitis hip

Secondary

Adjacent inflammation
Osteomyelitis
Osteoid osteoma

Systemic disorders
Leukemia
Acute rheumatic fever
Hemophilia with joint effusion
Acute rheumatic fever
Systemic lupus erythematosis
Henoch–Schönlein purpura
Sarcoidosis
Postinfectious disorders
Reflex sympathetic dystrophy

Fig. 2.79 Differential diagnosis of joint swelling and pain.

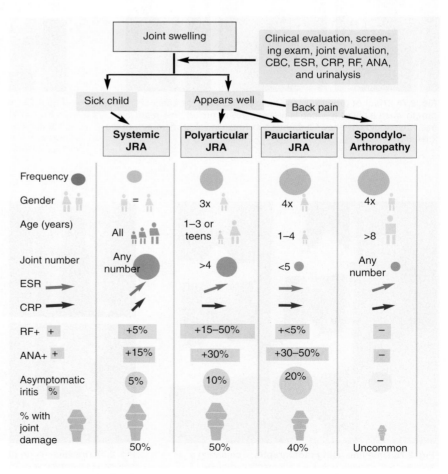

Fig. 2.80 Differential diagnosis of JRA

Pauciarticular arthritis is the most common form of juvenile arthritis. The patient is most likely a 1 to 4 year old girl (Fig. 2.80). About a quarter have no pain but are seen because of a swollen joint such as the knee, ankle, and fingers. ANA is positive in 70%, RF negative. About 20% have iritis (Fig. 2.85). Early referral of these patients to an ophthamologist is essential.

Systemic JRA occurs in boys and girls usually between 3 and 10 years (Fig. 2.80). These children are febrile, toxic, have severe myalgias, enlarged nodes, liver, and spleen, and sometimes pericarditis, myocarditis, disseminated intravascular coagulation, and polyarthritis (Fig. 2.82). The course of the disease is variable. Some cases resolve in months, others persist causing joint destruction and disability.

Seronegative spondyloarthropathies Seronegativity is an absence of rheumatoid factor. These disorders include ankylosing spondylitis, reactive synovitis, Reiter syndrome, and those associated with inflammatory bowel disease and psoriasis. These patients are frequently HLA-B27 positive and are usually adolescent boys. These patients may have low-grade systemic signs of fever, weight loss, and malaise.

Ankylosing spondylitis This condition is most common in adults but does occur in older children. Inflammation involves the spine, SI, and large joints. Back pain and morning stiffness are common complaints. Stiffness on forward bend test is found. Laboratory findings usually include a mildly elevated ESR, CRP, a positive HLA-B27, and negative ANA and RF. Radiographic changes are late.

Reiter syndrome The triad of arthritis, urethritis, and conjunctivitis are usually found. Painful photophobic iritis can occur. The disease usually follows dysentery or sexually transmitted disease.

Management

Intraarticular triamcinolone hexacetonide (steroid) injections are effective in reducing synovitis and sometimes preventing joint destruction (Fig. 2.83).

Systemic agents include ibuprofen, and methotrexate and etanercept. These drugs are best administered by a pediatric rheumatologist.

Joint damage occurs in most types of JRA (Fig. 2.84). Pauciarticular arthritis causes damage but the interval between onset and damage is longer.

Pitfalls

Confused with trauma A swollen joint is frequently thought to be secondary to an injury. As injuries are a daily occurrence in the life of a child, a history of an injury is common. Swollen joints are seldom the result of an injury. They require evaluation and an accurate diagnosis.

Iritis can accompany pauciarticular and some polyarticular forms of JRA (Fig. 2.85). The iritis is usually asymptomatic and can lead to blindness. Children with these forms of arthritis should be referred to an ophthalmologist for evaluation. The risk of iritis makes an early diagnosis of arthritis of great importance.

Missing septic etiology Permanent joint damage is most likely to occur quickly from septic arthritis. Septic arthritis of the hip is most difficult to differentiate. Monarticular arthritis of the hip is seldom due to JRA.

Missing leukemia Bone and joint complaints are the initial symptoms in 20% of children with leukemia. Leukemia causes bone pain, systemic illness, high ESR, and anemia.

Consultant David Sherry, e-mail: dsherry@u.washington.edu

References

2000 What's new in diagnosis and treatment of juvenile rheumatoid arthritis, Editorial. Sherry DD. JPO 20:419

1998 Intraarticular corticosteroid injection in the management of children with chronic arthritis. Padeh S, Passwell JH. Arthritis Rheum 41:1210

1997 Isolated digital swelling as the initial presentation of juvenile rheumatoid arthritis. Naidu SH, et al. J. Hand Surg. 22A:653

Feature	Early	Late
Age	1–4 years	Adolescence
Sex	Girls	Girls
Joint involvement	Varied and sym.	Large and small, sym.
ANA	Positive	Few
RF	Negative	Half positive
Iritis	Uncommon	Rare

Fig. 2.81 Types of polyarticular JRA. This shows two types of presentation of polyarticular JRA. From Sherry (1998).

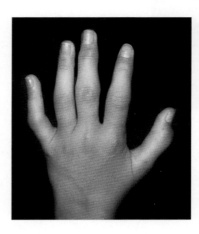

Fig. 2.82 Hand involvement in systemic JRA. Note the swelling of multiple joints.

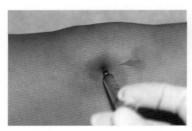

Fig. 2.83 Joint injections with steroids. Injections in JRA-affected joints dramatically reduce the synovitis and joint destruction.

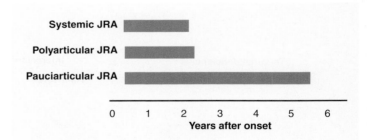

Systemic JRA

Polyarticular JRA

Pauciarticular JRA

0 1 2 3 4 5 6
Years after onset

Fig. 2.84 Time between onset and joint damage. Mean time between onset of different types of JRA and onset of joint damage.

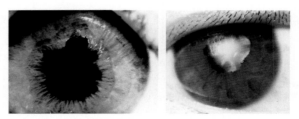

Fig. 2.85 Features of iritis. These photographs show irregularity of the pupil. These are late findings that result from adhesions between the iris and lens. Courtesy DD Sherry.

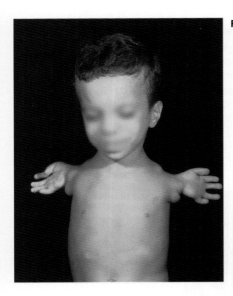

Fig. 2.86 Phocomelia.

Limb Deficiencies

Congenital limb deficiencies occur in about 0.1 to 0.2 in 1000 children, or about one-tenth the frequency of clubfeet or DDH.

Causes

Most deficiencies occur in children who are otherwise normal and have no genetic basis. Thalidomide is known to cause multi-limb deficiencies (Fig. 2.86). Most limb deficiencies are sporadic (Fig. 2.87 and 2.90). Tibial hemimelia (Fig. 2.88) is transmitted as a dominant trait. In other cases, deficiencies are associated with various syndromes such as the radial aplasia–thrombocytopenia syndrome. Acquired amputations result from trauma or treatment of malignant tumors.

Nomenclature

The most widely accepted nomenclature is that of Frantz and O'Rahilly, which divides limb deficiencies into intercalary and terminal types (Fig. 2.89). Every type of deficiency is usually classified (Figs. 2.91–2.96). These classifications aid in defining severity and indicating treatment methods (see Chapters 4 and 9 for details of treatment).

Prevalence

Males outnumber females 3:2, and lower extremities are twice as affected as upper. In 80% of cases, single limbs are involved. Congenital causes are three to four times more frequent than acquired amputations.

Evaluation

Most deficiencies are associated with limb shortening. Order comparative radiographs if a reduction deformity is suspected. Classify the deformity according to the radiographic appearance. Classification is more difficult early on because of lack of ossification. Consider possible associated problems, especially in children with radial deficiencies.

Refer most patients to a limb deficiency clinic. Such clinics provide several important resources for the family: (1) geneticists to evaluate for possible associations and provide family genetic counseling, (2) families to provide support groups, (3) prosthetics to provide often complex fitting problems, and (4) orthopedic surgeons to provide overall management.

Consultant Hugh Watts, e-mail: hwatts@ucla.edu

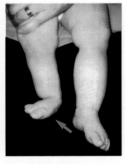

Fig. 2.87 Fibular deficiency. Note the shortening, ankle valgus, and hypoplasia of the foot.

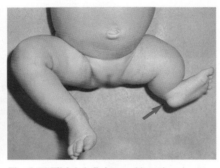

Fig. 2.88 Tibial deficiency. Note the short leg with a normal foot.

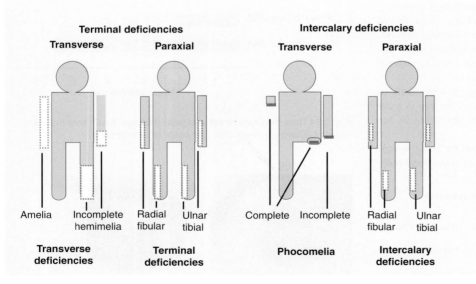

Terminal deficiencies
Transverse   Paraxial

Intercalary deficiencies
Transverse   Paraxial

Amelia   Incomplete   Radial   Ulnar   Complete   Incomplete   Radial   Ulnar
hemimelia   fibular   tibial   fibular   tibial

Transverse deficiencies   **Terminal deficiencies**   **Phocomelia**   **Intercalary deficiencies**

Fig. 2.89 Frantz–O'Rahilly classfication of congenital limb deficiencies.

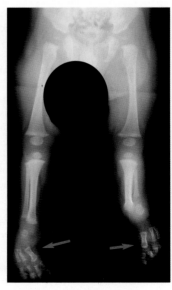

Fig. 2.90 Fibular deficiency with bilateral three-rayed feet.

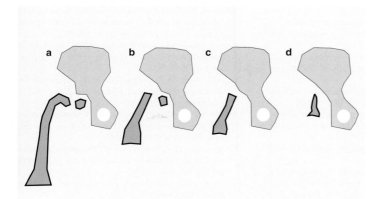

Fig. 2.91 Proximal focal femoral deficiency. (a) Good acetabulum, varus deformity of femur. (b) Fair acetabulum, delayed ossification of femur. (c) Poor acetabulum, femoral head absent, femur very short. (d) No acetabulum, femur nearly absent. Based on Aitken (1968).

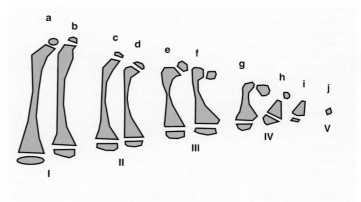

Fig. 2.92 Spectrum of the congenitally short femur. This figure shows the wide variation in deformities included in this classification. Based on Hamanishi, JBJS 62B:569 (1980).

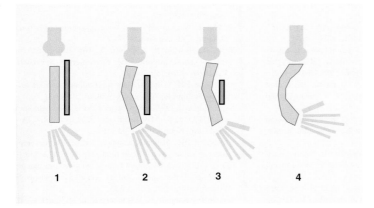

Fig. 2.93 Heikel classification of radial deficiencies. (1) Hypoplasia of distal radius. (2) Distal and proximal shortening and ulnar bowing. (3) Varied ulnar shortening with carpal deviation. (4) Radial aplasia. From Heikel, AOS Suppl 39:1 (1959).

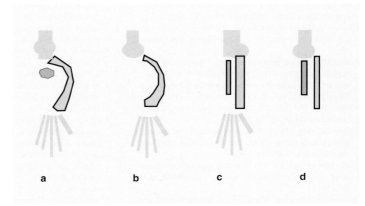

Fig. 2.94 Swanson classification of ulnar deficiencies. (a) Hypoplasia of the ulna. (b) Absence of the ulna. (c) Fusion of the humerus and radius with hypoplasia of the ulna. (d) Hypoplasia of the ulna with absence of the hand. From Swanson et al., J Hand Surg 9A:658 (1984).

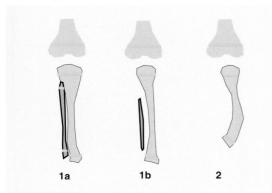

Fig. 2.95 Fibular defeciency classification. Type I includes all cases in which some fibula is present. In type 1a, the fibula is short with the proximal fibular physes below that of the tibia and the distal physis above the ankle. In type 1b, the fibula is significantly shortened and not supporting the ankle. In type 2, no fibula is present. From Achterman and Kalamchi, JBJS 61B:133 (1979).

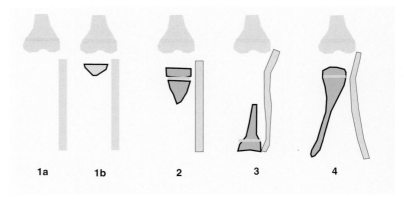

Fig. 2.96 Tibial deficiency classification. (1a) The tibia is not seen. (1b) Tibia seen on MRI or US. (2) Distal tibia not seen. (3) Proximal tibia not seen. (4) Diastasis. Based on Jones et al., JBJS 60B:31 (1978).

Aitken GT, Proximal femoral focal deficiency–definition, classification, and management. In: Symposium Washington DC June 13, 1968. pp 1-22, National Academy of Sciences, Washington DC.

Ashton BB, Pickles B, Roll JW. Reliability of goniometric measurements of hip motion in spastic cerebral palsy. Dev Med Child Neurol 1978;20:87.

Bartlett MD, Wolf LS, Shurtleff DB, et al. Hip flexion contractures: A comparison of measurement methods. Arch Phys Med Rehabil 1985;66:620-625.

Beck RJ, Andriacchi TP, Kuo KN, et al. Changes in gait patterns of growing children. J Bone Joint Surg 1981;63A:9.

Bettmann MA, Morris TW. Recent advances in contrast agents. Radiol Clin North Am 1986;24:347.

Bowker JH, Hall CB. Normal human gait in atlas of orthotics, biomechanical principles and application. American Academy of Orthopaedic Surgeons. St. Louis: CV Mosby, 1975:133.

Burnett CN, Johnson EW. Development of gait in childhood. Part I. Dev Med Child Neurol 1971;13:196.

Callanan D. Causes of refusal to walk in childhood. South Med J 1982;75:20-22.

Canale ST, Harkness RM, Thomas PA, et al. Does aspiration of bones and joints affect results of later bone scanning? J Pediatr Orthop 1985;5:23.

Cann CE. Quantitative CT for determination of bone mineral density:A review. Radiology 1988;166-509.

Choban S, Killian JT. Evaluation of acute gait abnormalities in preschool children. J Pediatr Orthop 1990;10:74-78.

Cohen MD. Clinical utility of magnetic resonance imaging in pediatrics. Am J Dis Child 1986;140:947.

Coleman SS, Chesnut WJ. A simple test for hindfoot flexibility in cavovarus foot. CO 123:60 1977.

Collier BD, Hellman RS, Krasnow AZ. Bone SPECT. Semin Nucl Med 1987;17:247.

Covey DC, Albright JA. Clinical significance of the erythrocyte sedimentation rate in orthopedic surgery. J Bone Joint Surg 1987;69A:148-151.

Engel GM, Staheli LT. The natural history of torsion and other factors influencing gait in childhood. CO 1974;99:12.

Engfeldt B, Hjerpe A, Mengarelli S. Morphological and biochemical analysis of biopsy specimens in disorders of skeletal development. Acta Paediatr Scand 1982;71:353-363.

Erlich MG, Zaleske DJ. Pediatric orthopedic pain of unknown origin. J Pediatr Orthop 1986;460-468.

Fisher MR, Hernandez RJ, Dias LS, et al. Computed tomography in the evaluation of the gluteal region. J Pediatr Orthop 1983;3:516-522.

Fornage BD. Achilles tendon: US examination. Radiology 1986;159:759.

Fornage BD, Schernberg FL. Sonographic diagnosis of foreign bodies of the distal extremities. AJR 1986;147:567.

Gilsanz V, Gibbens DT, Roe TF, et al. Vertebral bone density in children: Effect of puberty. Radiology 1988;166:847.

Graham CB. Assessment of bone maturation—methods and pitfalls. Radiol Clin North Am 1972;10:185.

Greulich WW, Pyle SI. Radiographic atlas of skeletal development of the hand and wrist. 2nd ed. Stanford, CA, Stanford University Press, 1959:50.

Hall FM. Arthography: Past, present and future. AJR 1987;149:561.

Hankin FM, Braunstein EM. Intraoperative radiographs: A modified technique. J Pediatr Orthop 1985;5:107-108.

Harcke HT, Grissom LE, Finkelstein MS. Evaluation of the musculoskeletal system with sonography. AJR 1988;150:1253.

Heckmatt JZ et al. Diagnostic needle muscle biopsy. A practical and reliable alternative to open biopsy. Arch Dis Child 1984;59:528-532.

Hernandez RJ. Visualization of small sequestra by computerized tomography. Report of six cases. Pediatr Radiol 1985;15:238.

Herndon WA, Alexieva BT, Schwindt ML, et al. Nuclear imaging for musculoskeletal infections in children. J Pediatr Orthop 1985;5:343-347.

Jones ET. Use of computed axial tomography in pediatric orthopedics. J Pediatr Orthop 1981;1:329-338.

Kozlowski K et al. Unilateral mid-femoral periosteal new-bone of varying aetiology in children. Radiographic analysis of 25 cases. Pediatr Radiol 1986;16:475-482.

Lancaster SJ, Cummings RJ. Hip aspiration: verification of needle position by air arthography. J Pediatr Orthop 1987;7:91-92.

Lang HA, Puusa A, Hynninen P, et al. Evolution of nerve conduction velocity in later childhood and adolescence. Muscle Nerve 1985;8:38-43.

Mayerson NH, Milano RA. Goniometric measurement reliability in physical medicine. Arch Phys Med Rehabil 1984;65:92-94.

McCoy JR, Morrissy RT, Seibert J. Clinical experience with the technetium-99m scan in children. Clin Orthop 1981;154:175.

Menkveld SR, Knipstein EA, Quinn JR. Analysis of gait patterns in normal school-aged children. J Pediatr Orthop 1988;8:263-267.

Merten DF, Radkowski MA, Leonidas JC. The abused child: a radiological reappraisal. Radiology 1983;146:377.

Miller JH, Ettinger LJ. Gallium citrate (67Ga) scintigraphic detection of chronic osteomyelitis in children with leukemia. Am J Dis Child 1986;140:230-232.

Perry J. Pre-op and post-op dynamic EMG as an aid in planning tendon transfers in children with CP. J Bone Joint Surg 1977;59A:531.

Rab GT, Wyatt M, Sutherland DH, et al. A technique for determining femoral head containment during gait. J Pediatr Orthop 1985;5:8-12.

Rothstein JM, Miller PJ, Roettger RF. Goniometric reliability in a clinical setting. Elbow and knee measurements. Phys Ther 1983;63:1611.

Shapiro A, Susak Z, Malkin C, et al. Preoperative and postoperative gait evaluation in cerebral palsy. Arch Phys Med Rehabil 1990;71:236.

Siffert RS, Katz JF. Growth recovery zones. J Pediatr Orthop 1983;3:196-201.

Sorenson JA. Perception of radiation hazards. Semin Nucl Med 1986;16:158.

Staheli LT. The prone hip extension test: a method of measuring hip flexion deformity. CO 1977;123:12-15.

Staheli LT. Strontium 87m scanning. Early diagnosis of bone and joint infections in children. JAMA 1972;221:1159.

Staheli LT. Fever following trauma in childhood. JAMA 1967;199:503-504.

Staheli LT. A clamp for isometric muscle biopsies. Surgery 1966;59:1154-1155.

Statham L, Murray MP. Early walking patterns of normal children. Clin Orthop 1971;79:8.

Strife JL, Towbin R, Crawford A. Hip arthography in infants and children: the inferomedial approach. Radiology 1984;152:536.

Sutherland DH. Gait disorders in childhood and adolescence. Baltimore: Williams & Wilkins, 1984:631.

Sutherland DH, Olshen R, Cooper L, et al. The pathomechanics of gait in Duchenne muscular dystrophy. Dev Med Child Neurol 1982;23:3.

Sutherland DH, Olshen R, Cooper L, et al. The development of mature gait. J Bone Joint Surg 1980;62A:336.

Szalay EA, Roach JW, Smith H, et al. Magnetic resonance imaging of the spinal cord in spinal dysraphisms. J Pediatr Orthop 1987;7:541-545.

Todd FN, Lamoreux LW, Skinner SR, et al. Variations in the gait of normal children. A graph applicable to the documentation of abnormalities. J Bone Joint Surg 1989;71:196-216.

Yokochi K, Aiba K, Horie M, et al. Magnetic resonance imaging in children with spastic diplegia: Correlation with the severity of their motor and mental abnormality. Dev Med Child Neurol 1991;33:18-25.

Chapter 3 – Management

This chapter covers principles of management. Details are provided in later chapters.

Managing the Family

Skill in dealing with the parents and family is essential in providing optimum care for the child. This requires professional competence, patience, and empathy for child and family. Dealing with parents is often the area of greatest difficulty for the orthopedic resident. Developing appreciation, sensitivity, and skill in communicating with parents and the ability to calm their anxieties are essential skills in dealing effectively with the child's problem.

Child

The child's overall well-being is the primary objective of management (Fig. 3.1). Doing what is best for the child requires respect for the inherent value of childhood as an important time of life (Fig. 3.2). Childhood is more than just a preparatory period of life; it has intrinsic value. Moreover, unnecessary interference with the child's life deprives the child of important life experiences. This concept is especially important in pediatric orthopedics, where the physician often deals with chronic disease; "medicalization" of childhood is a serious risk. We may create what is referred to as the vulnerable child syndrome. These children are often harmed by unnecessary restrictions. Some philosophical and practical guidelines are given here:

1. Resist the pressure to treat the child simply to satisfy the parents or just to "do something." This is harmful to the child, disruptive to the family, expensive for society, and poor medical practice.

2. Order treatment only when intervention is both necessary and effective. In the past, treatment was commonly prescribed for conditions that resolve spontaneously, such as in-toeing, flexible flatfeet, and physiological bowlegs. Observational management, a policy of monitoring the child's condition with minimum intervention, provides optimum care for a large percentage of pediatric orthopedic problems. It is least disruptive to the child's and family's life and generates a reputation of honesty and competence for the physician.

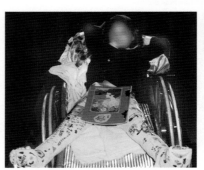

Fig. 3.1 Management. Managing children's problems is usually enjoyable and satisfying.

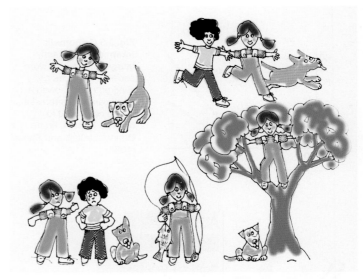

Fig. 3.2 Play is the occupation of the child. Childhood is the time for varied experiences and has intrinsic value. From Staheli (1986).

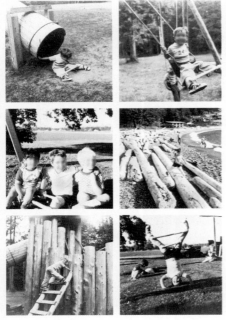

Fig. 3.3 Integrate treatment with play. Encourage families to have their child participate in physically active play during treatment. These pictures were taken by a mother who achieved this goal.

3. Limit the child's activity only after thoughtful consideration Play is the primary occupation of the child. Unnecessary restriction denies the child play experiences vital to enjoying childhood and developing critical skills. In some situations the physician may need to curb the parents' tendency to overprotect the child. It may be in the child's best interest to risk injury rather than to have long-term constraints on natural activity (Fig. 3.3).

4. Avoid medicalization of the handicapped child Overtreatment can further limit the child and overwhelm the family. Excessive numbers of physician's visits, operations, therapies, braces, and other treatment will result in a large share of the child's life being expended on treatment that may provide little or no benefit.

5. Before considering any treatment, consider the child as a whole Treatment methods readily prescribed for children would never be accepted by an adult (Fig. 3.4). Orthopedic treatment can be damaging to the individual's self-image (Fig. 3.5) and be uncomfortable or embarrassing for the child (Fig 3.6). Make certain that the anticipated benefits of treatment exceed the harmful psychological, social, and physical effects on the child.

6. Care of the child requires the highest medical standard The results of treating a child, whether good or bad, may remain with the patient for 70 years or more.

Parents

Dealing with parents is an essential part of a pediatric practice (Fig. 3.7). Each family has certain rights, such as privacy, that must be respected, as well as differing needs and values.

Family coping ability should be respected. Respect the family's resources concerning time, energy, and money. A handicapped child adds stress and complexity for any family. Balance the treatment plan and the family's resources. Consider the well-being of the other children and the health of the marriage; if these are marginal, it may be prudent to order only essential treatment. At different times during management, encourage questions and discuss progress with the family. Being sensitive to the coping ability of the family is part of the physician's responsibility. Demanding more than the family can handle results in noncompliance that may be more the fault of the physician than the family.

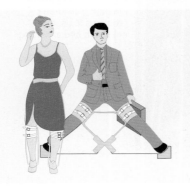

Fig. 3.4 Child's treatment unacceptable for adults. Treatment that has been commonly prescribed for children such as twister cables for intoeing girls or Perthes disease braces for boys, would never be accepted by an adult patient.

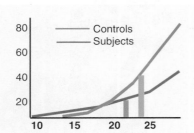

Fig. 3.5 Orthopedic treatments and self-image. Adults who wore corrective devices as children (red) showed a significantly lowered self-image compared to controls (green). From Driano, Staheli, and Staheli (1988).

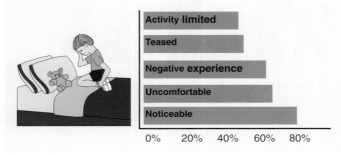

Fig. 3.6 Recollections. Percentage of adults recalling experience about wearing orthopedic devices during childhood. From Driano, Staheli, and Staheli (1998).

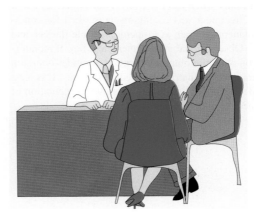

Fig. 3.7 Parent discussions. Take the families' concerns seriously. Allow enough time to explain the disease and treatment options thoroughly.

Informed consent should be part of all management, whether surgical or not. The family has the right to know the pros and cons of the management alternatives. The physician's influence is greater with adults as parents than as patients. Most parents are very sensitive to the possibility that the child's current condition may cause some disability in adult life. Certain words such as "arthritis," "crippled," and "pain" have a powerful effect on parents and should be used with caution. For example, in the past, many rotational osteotomies were performed to correct femoral antetorsion under the assumption that the procedure would prevent arthritis of the hip. Although the prophylactic value of the procedure was uncertain, parents readily gave their consent under the presumed threat of arthritis (Fig. 3.8). Several recent studies have shown no relationship between femoral antetorsion and arthritis.

Support and reassurance should be provided for patients and parents. In managing common resolving problems such as intoeing (3.9), reassurance is the main treatment. With more serious problems, reassurance may take the form of providing information that dispels the parents' fears about the future. In critical conditions, reassurance consists of assuring the family that you will support them throughout the disease. The process of providing effective support and reassurance involves several steps:

1. Make certain that you understand the family's concerns and take these concerns seriously.

2. Conduct a thorough evaluation of the child. Pay attention to the family's specific concerns. For example, if they are anxious about the way the child runs, be certain that you observe the child running in the hallway.

3. Provide information about the condition, especially the natural history. Make copies of appropriate page of *what families should know* on pages 413–417 to take home and show other family members.

4. Offer to follow the problem in the future. Not all positional deformities resolve with time. Offer to see the child again if the family has additional concerns. If the family is obviously apprehensive, or there is someone in the family who is the major source of concerns, such as the grandmother, it may be necessary to provide reassurance repeatedly. Suggest that the grandmother accompany the child during the next visit.

5. If the family is still unconvinced, suggest a consultation. An offer to refer the child usually increases the family's confidence in the physician. Be certain to communicate to the consultant the family's need for reassurance and not that you are recommending some treatment.

6. Avoid submitting to family pressure for treatment that is not medically indicated. Performing unnecessary or ineffective procedures because of family pressure is never appropriate.

Procedures are a source of family stress. Whether or not the family should be present during procedures, such as joint aspiration, should be managed individually. Some parents prefer not to be present; others insist on being with the child. Whenever possible, give the family a choice. Be aware that if the parents are present, one of them (usually the father) may feel ill or dizzy and need to lie down. More often, a parent can help calm the child (Fig. 3.10). Moreover, the presence of parents helps to prevent feelings of abandonment in the child (Fig. 3.11). In summary, even though the parents' presence may add a complicating factor for the physician, it may be of benefit to the child.

Litigious problems are fortunately less common in pediatrics compared with other orthopedic subspecialties. However, the legal exposure period for the physician is much longer, because the statute of limitations usually starts at the age of majority. Medical competence, attention to detail, and good rapport with the family are the best protective measures. Additional measures include complete records, generous use of consultants, and avoidance of nonstandard treatments. If an unusual or tragic incident occurs, document the circumstances honestly and thoroughly. Be especially attentive to the family at this time and respond quickly to their concerns.

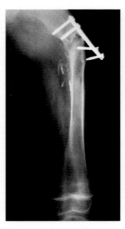

Fig. 3.8 Complications of rotational osteotomy. This patient underwent an osteotomy for correction of femoral antetorsion. He developed a streptococcal wound infection. This was further complicated by failure of the fixation, nonunion, osteomyelitis, and limb shortening. He had 13 operations to manage complications.

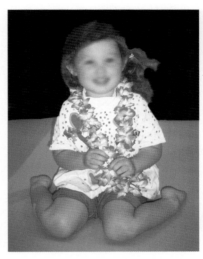

Fig. 3.9 Femoral antetorsion improves with growth. This is considered a variation of normal that requires no treatment.

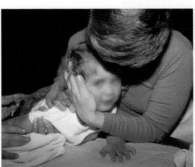

Fig. 3.10 Procedures are less stressful in a supportive environment. Often the mother is best able to comfort the child.

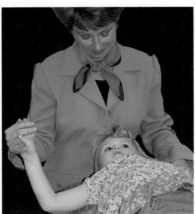

Fig. 3.11 Supportive measures during casting. Ongoing support of the child during simple procedures calms and quiets the child.

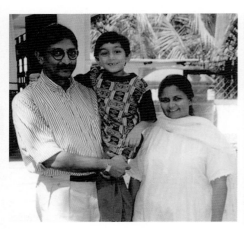

Fig. 3.12 Religious beliefs. Respect the family's right to make or at least influence medical decisions that do not compromise the child's treatment.

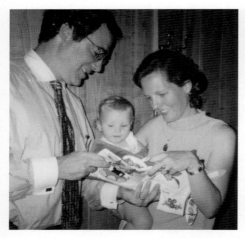

Fig. 3.13 Families values. Incorporate these values in planning management.

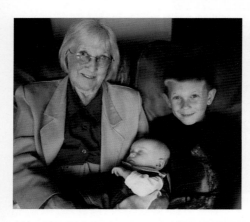

Fig. 3.14 Grandparents in clinic. This grandmother is very well informed and an asset in helping the parents deal with their children's problems.

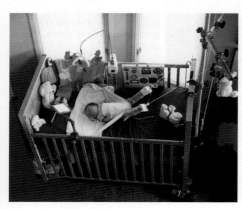

Fig. 3.15 Home traction. Home treatment programs provide cost-effective and convenient management.

Religious beliefs may affect the physician's management. Religious beliefs should be respected to the extent that they do not compromise the child's treatment (Fig. 3.12). Discuss the parents' beliefs and concerns openly. Issues regarding blood replacement are common. Alternatives are possible, so do not victimize the child by taking a rigid position against the family. With planning, careful technique, hypotensive anesthesia, and staging if necessary, nearly all orthopedic procedures can be managed without blood replacement. Some families will want a period of time for prayer before giving consent for an operative procedure. Unless time is critical, a negotiated delay is appropriate. Establish a time limit and determine some objective outcome measures in advance.

Family values should be incorporated into the management plan. For some medical conditions, management indications are unclear or controversial. Inform the family of the situation and discuss the choices openly so that the management is consistent with the family's values (Fig. 3.13). Family feelings about operative procedures, bracing, therapy, and other treatment methods vary considerably. The family's feelings and values should be respected but should not supersede the delivery of optimal medical care. Performing an operation that is medically not indicated because of an insisting family is not appropriate.

Difficult families may tax the physician's ability to deal with the parents' reaction to their child's illness. The parents may become overprotective or, conversely, may abandon the child. Some parents become abusive toward the physician and staff. Be sure that the parents' behavior does not adversely affect your management of the child. Be understanding but firm, and when appropriate, support abused staff members. Write a note in the chart summarizing the parents' behavior.

Grandparents often accompany the child to clinic (Fig. 3.14). Grandmothers are often concerned about infants' flatfeet, intoeing, or bowlegs. In the grandmother's child-rearing era, positional problems were poorly understood and routinely treated. Overcoming such misconceptions requires a willingness to respectfully explain the reasons for current management.

Unorthodox methods of care by nonphysician practitioners are often considered by parents. Such practitioners usually prescribe treatment, and the treatment often continues over a long period of time. By current standards, such treatments are generally unnecessary and ineffective. Moreover, the treatment may delay necessary treatment. Avoid criticism when discussing these "treatments" with the family; instead, focus on parent education. This is much more effective than criticism. If the parents insist on unorthodox treatment, suggest an objective outcome measure and reevaluate the child later. If appropriate management cannot wait, use a more aggressive approach. Start with the basic facts, obtaining consultations for reinforcement if necessary.

Society

The physician's responsibility to society is seldom addressed. Physicians do have the responsibility to keep health care costs to a minimum by avoiding inappropriate management. We can also choose the least expensive alternatives among equivalent management methods (Fig. 3.15).

Consultant Dean MacEwen, e-mail: honsandtraps@webtv.net

References
1986 Philosophy of care. Staheli LT. Pediatr Clin North Am 33:1269
1998 Psychosocial development and corrective shoewear use in childhood. Driano AN, Staheli L, Staheli LT. JPO 18:346

Shoes

For a long time, shoe modifications were a traditional treatment of infants and children for a wide variety of pathological and physiological problems. Because shoe modifications were usually prescribed for spontaneously resolving conditions, resolution was falsely attributed to the shoe. This led to the concept of the "corrective shoe." Recently, data-based studies have consistently shown that natural history, rather than shoe modifications, was responsible for the improvement (Fig. 3.16). We now know that the term "corrective shoe" is a misnomer. Barefooted people have been shown to have feet that are stronger, more flexible, and less deformed than those wearing shoes (Figs 3.17 and 3.18). The feet of infants and children do not require support and do best with freedom of movement without shoes.

Shoe Selection

The selection of shoes should be the same as for other clothing. The shoe should protect the foot from injury and cold and be acceptable in appearance. The best shoes are those that interfere least with function and simulate the barefoot state (Fig 3.19). High-top shoes are necessary in the toddler to keep the shoes on the feet. Proper fit is desirable, not to promote support but to avoid falls and compression of the toes. Falls are more common if the shoes are too long or have sole material that is slippery or sticky.

Useful modifications

Shock-absorbing footwear may be helpful for the adolescent in reducing the incidence of overuse syndromes (3.21). Some shoe modifications are helpful (Fig. 3.20). These are not for correction but to improve function or provide comfort. Shoe lifts may be useful if leg length difference exceeds 2.5 cm. Orthotics are effective in evenly distributing loading of the sole of the foot.

References

1999 Comparison of gait with and without shoes in children. Oeffinger D, B Brauch, S Cranfill, C Hisle, C Wynn, R Hicks and S Augsburger. Gait Posture 9:95

1992 The influence of footwear on the prevalence of flat foot. A survey of 2300 children. Rao UB, Joseph B. JBJS 74B:525

1991 Shoes for children: a review. Staheli LT Pediatrics 88:371

1989 Corrective shoes and inserts as treatment for flexible flatfoot in infants and children. Wenger DR, et al. JBJS 71A:800

1958 A comparison of foot forms among the non-shoe and shoe wearing Chinese population. Simfook L, and Hodgson A. JBJS 40:1058

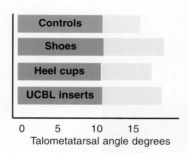

Fig. 3.16 Effect of shoe modifications in flatfeet. This prospective, controlled study compared arch development with various treatments. No difference was found. Talarmetatsal angles before (light shade) and after treatment (dark shade). From Wenger et al. (1989).

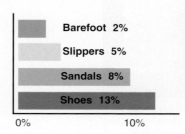

Fig. 3.17 Effect of shoe wearing on incidence of flatfoot in adults. In a survey of adults, the percentage with flatfeet was related to shoewear during childhood. Note that flatfeet were least common among barefoot children. From Roe and Joseph (1992).

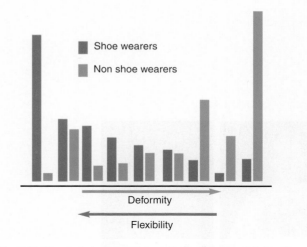

Fig. 3.18 Effect of shoe wearing on the incidence of deformity and flexibility in adults. In a survey of Chinese adults, those who wore shoes had more deformity and less flexibility than nonshoe wearers. From Simfook and Hodgson (1958).

Feature	Purpose
Flexible	Improve mobility and strength
Flat	Distributes weight evenly
Foot Shaped	Noncompressive
Friction	Prevents slipping & sticking
Appearance	Acceptable for the child
Cost	Acceptable for the parent

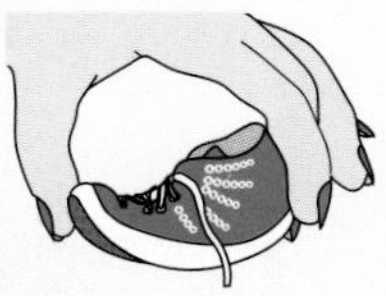

Fig. 13.19 Characteristics of a good shoe. The best shoes are those that allow normal function of the foot.

Problem	Modification
Short Leg	Shoe lift for differences >1"
Rigid Deformity	Orthotic to equalize loading
Heel Pain	Elevate heel
Overuse Syn.	Shock absorbing features
Bunions	Stretch shoe over bunion

Fig. 3.20 Useful shoe modifications. This modifications are useful to improve the mechanics of load bearing.

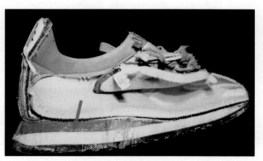

Fig. 3.21 Cushioned shoes. Shoes have cushioned heels and soles (arrow) that may reduce the incidence of overuse syndromes.

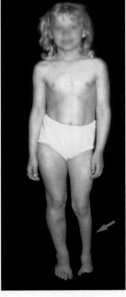

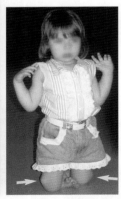

Fig. 3.22 Limb deficiencies. Fibular hemimelia (red arrow) causes moderate disability, whereas this child with bilateral tibial hemimelia (yellow arrows) is severely disabled.

Surgery

Operative Indications

Operative procedures are the most definitive mode of treatment in pediatric orthopedics. The outcome of the procedure is largely determined by the judgment and skill of the surgeon. Children have both greater healing potential and fewer complications than adult patients, increasing the chances for a successful outcome.

Indications for operations include pain, limited function, unsatisfactory appearance, and as a means of preventing future disability. Prophylactic operations are appropriate only when the natural history is known and serious disability is relatively certain. In some, the need for surgery is well accepted (Fig. 3.22); in others, persisting deformity is unexpected (Fig. 3.23).

Management options Orthopedists can choose from among a wide range of treatment options. First, try a nonoperative treatment, if there is a reasonable chance of success. If the patient has a tarsal coalition and pain, immobilize the foot in a cast for several weeks as a trial. If the pain recurs, excise the bar. If the family is seeking multiple consultations, it is often wise to start with an nonoperative approach. If the family is uncertain, and waiting will not jeopardize the outcome, simply delay the needed operative correction until the family is ready to make a decision.

Conservative management Sometimes an operation is the most conservative of the treatment options. If so, proceed with this treatment first. This approach benefits both the family and child. There are a number of classic examples where delays in operative correction harms the child. A 12-year-old girl with a 50-degree right thoracic scoliosis is given a trial of treatment with a brace and physical therapy for several years, only to have the 60-degree curve instrumented and fused at age 15. This unfortunate girl experienced the hardships of 3 years of unnecessary brace treatment. Long-term brace treatment is not a benign option; it is often a psychologically damaging experience. In another case, a child with cerebral palsy and a subluxation of the hip is managed by physical therapy. Subluxation progresses to dislocation. An early adductor lengthening or transfer would have been the conservative approach.

Cosmetic disability A cosmetic disability may justify operative correction. Unsightly genu varum or valgum may be corrected by a hemiepiphysiodesis. An abductor lurch may be corrected with a trochanteric transfer. A severe kyphotic deformity may justify instrumentation, correction, and fusion. Each treatment carries risks. Weighing the risks and benefits is often difficult.

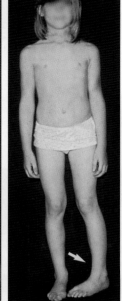

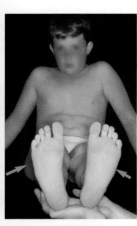

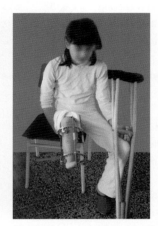

Fig. 3.23 Uncommon outcomes. Normal variability allows atypical outcomes. In these children the severe genu valgum (red arrow), tibial torsion (yellow arrow), and persisting forefoot adductus (green arrows) are rare outcomes of conditions that nearly always resolve spontaneously.

Fig. 3.24 Inappropriate lengthening. This child is undergoing a lengthening of the tibia without a functional foot. The child should have had a Syme type amputation and prosthetic fitting.

Families Role Provide factual information regarding risks and benefits of each alternative, and then allow the family to choose among the medically acceptable options. Be aware that issues concerning body image peak during early adolescence. What is bothersome at age 14 may become acceptable at age 17. Delay the correction of marginally disabling deformities until it is clear that the concern is lasting. Performing an unnecessary operation just because the parent wishes to do something is not appropriate (Fig. 3.24). First and foremost, the orthopedist is the advocate of the child.

Preoperative Planning
During the final preoperative evaluation, think through each step of the procedure to make certain that the preoperative planning is complete. Be certain that special tools or implants will be available.

Anticipate Possible Complications Look for problems that may complicate the procedure. The most common problems are respiratory infections and skin lesions. Check the temperature, evaluate the ears, throat, and lungs. Examine the skin about the operative site for inflammation. The decision regarding respiratory status is generally made by the anesthesiologist. It is usually wise to reschedule the procedure if the child has an unexplained fever, a respiratory infection, infected or inflamed skin lesions in the operative area, or documented exposure to a contagious disease, such as chickenpox or measles. Make certain the family understands the procedure and follow-up plans. Use a model or a skeleton to explain the operation to the family.

Discharge Plans Make discharge plans at this time. Arrange for adaptive equipment necessary for home care (Fig. 3.25). If the child will be using crutches or splints (Fig. 3.26) after the procedure, make fittings before the operation. Plan transportation home and anticipate special needs (Fig. 3.27). Plan for home teaching if the child will be away from school for more than 2 weeks. Make certain someone will be available to care for the child at all times.

Preparing the Child Prepare the child for the operation with a simple and honest explanation. Describe the procedures in terms appropriate to the child's or adolescent's age, and detail what he or she is likely to experience. Use the material in the reference section of this book and use models (Fig. 3.28). A teddy bear in a spica cast is a useful model for young patients. Let the child make choices wherever it is possible; for example, choosing the color of the cast. Arrange for the child to tour the hospital. All of these measures will help to reduce fear and to build a positive attitude toward the experience and the doctor.

Special Operative Needs Be certain fixation, bank bone graft, special tools, or implants will be available (Fig. 3.29.).

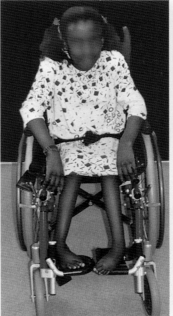
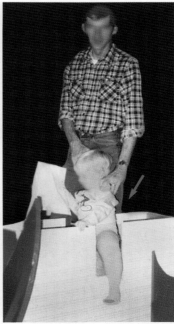

Fig. 3.25 Adaptive equipment. Order devices such as wheelchairs in advance. Devices to help in management of children with casts are created by the families and are very effective such as this support that provides stable seating for his daughter in a spica cast (red arrow).

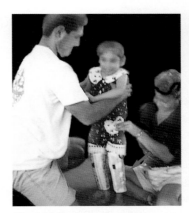
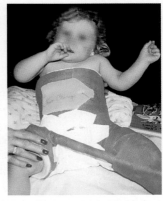

Fig. 3.26 Preoperative trials. Sometimes it is useful to try splints in advance to prepare the child for standing after surgery.

Fig. 3.27 Mobility home. This child will be traveling home by plane. Make arrangements for special seating in advance.

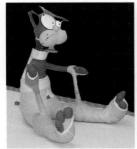
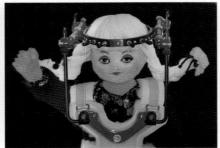

Fig. 3.28 Preparing the child. Dolls are very useful in preparing the child for various types of treatment.

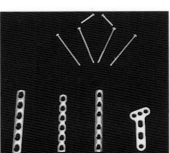
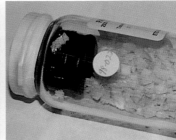

Fig. 3.29 Special operative needs. Special fixation devices are often needed for children. Order bone graft material well in advance.

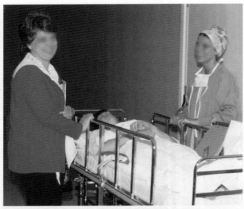

Fig. 3.30 Well-prepared girl. This girl and her mother were well prepared for surgery.

Disease	Anesthetic concerns
Achondroplasia	Limited cervical spine mobility, restrictive airway disease
Arthrogryposis	TM joint and C spine stiffness, GE reflex, postop airway obstruction, difficult IV access
Cerebral palsy	Gastroesophageal reflux, airway obst postop
Duchenne muscular dystrophy	Respiratory insufficiency, cardiomyopathy, malig. hyperthermia, hyperkalemia, hyperthermia, carditis, pulmonary dysfunction
JRA	TM joint ankylosis, cervical stiffness or instability

Fig. 3.31 Anesthetic problems by disease. Childhood disorders carry certain anesthetic risks that should be understood before surgery.

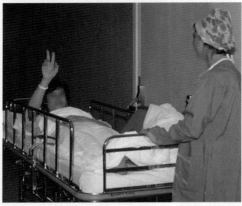

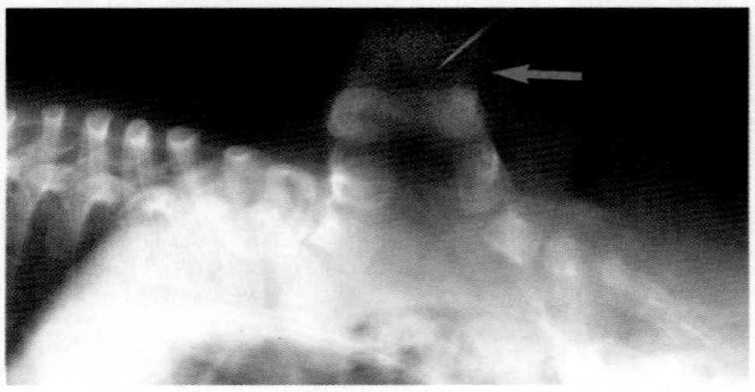

Fig. 3.32 Kyphosis in myelodysplasia. Correction is difficult technically and blood loss can be substantial.

Anesthesia

Anesthesia in children has advanced dramatically during the past two decades. Subspecialization, new techniques, a focus on pain management and preparing children psychologically (Fig. 3.30) provide improved care.

Preoperative Problems

Respiratory infections The average younger child has 4–5 upper respiratory infections per year. These infections complicate operative planning. Such infections pose operative hazards by increasing the risks of laryngospasm, bronchospasm, and coughing. Coughing during inductions increases the risks of regurgitation and aspiration. These problems can lead to a reduction in oxygen saturation during and after surgery.

Elective surgery If the child has an upper respiratory infection, cancel surgery if the infant is less than a year of age, if signs of viremia or bacteremia are found, if scheduled for a long or complicated procedure, or if findings suggest a lower respiratory component is present.

Reschedule Allow about 2 weeks after cessation of symptoms following a URI and 4–6 weeks after a lower respiratory infection.

Oral intake restrictions

Infants under 6 months Allow feeding breast milk or formula to 6 hours before surgery and clear liquids to 3 hours before surgery.

Older infants and children Allow feeding to 8 hours before surgery and clear liquids until 3 hours before surgery.

Perioperative Fluid Management

Fluids Management usually requires replacement and maintenance. Maintain using a balance salt solution (BSS) such as lactated Ringer's solution.

Fluid requirement Calculate fluid requirements on the basis of 4 ml/kg/hr for the first 10 kg of body weight, plus 2 ml/kg/hr for the next 10 kg and 1 ml/kg/hr above that.

Estimated blood volume for children Calculate the EBV in ml/kg at 90 for newborns, 80 for infants in first year, and 70 for older children.

Indications for intraoperative blood replacement In the healthy child replace acute volume losses of 25–30%. The most reliable signs of hypovolemic shock in children are a tachycardia, diminished pulse pressure, and prolonged capillary refill time. Generally, replacement is indicated if the hematocrit drops below 21–25%.

Special Anesthesia Problems

Certain diseases carry special risk requiring special consideration (Fig. 3.31).

Meningomyelocele Start blood replacement early (Fig. 3.32).

Myopathies This group of patients presents special risks. They should be referred to the anesthesiologist in advance of the procedure for an evaluation, which often includes an EKG, chest X-ray, and pulmonary function studies. These patients are prone to develop a malignant hyperthermia syndrome, cardiac rhythm dysfunction, and postoperative respiratory problems.

Cervical spine abnormalities Be concerned if the patient has disproportionate dwarfism, Down syndrome, Goldenhar syndrome, Klippel–Feil syndrome, systemic JRA, or neck trauma. These patients should have preoperative evaluation and require special precautions especially during induction.

JRA Children may have TM joint ankylosis, cervical spine stiffness, and/or instability.

Latex allergy Latex allergy includes a spectrum of dermatitis, rhinitis, asthma, urticaria, bronchospasm, laryngeal edema, anaphylaxis, and interoperative cardiovascular collapse.

High risk patients Include those with spina bifida, and those with repeated procedure and exposure to latex and who show varied allergic reactions.

Current status Suspect and send for preoperative anesthesia consultation. Plan a latex-free surgical environment during the operation.

Anesthetic Risks

Anesthesia is generally a greater risk than most orthopedic procedures. Still, the risk of anesthesia is small. Fatal complications of anesthesia occur in 3–4 per 100,000 procedures. Most complications can be prevented by close monitoring, maintaining adequate oxygenation, and careful control of the level of anesthesia. Greater sophistication and cooperation between the surgeon and anesthesiologist (Fig. 3.33) can reduce these risks. Complications include laryngeal and bronchospasm, aspiration, and cardiac arrhythmia and arrest.

General anesthesia is the standard for infants and children (Fig. 3.34). The induction technique is determined by the age of the child and the planned procedure. Rectal induction is used for some infants (over 6 months) and for simple procedures such as spica cast changes. Intervenous induction is appropriate for the adolescent when the IV is placed before the procedure. In children, induction is often provided by inhalation anesthesia. The IV is then started quietly, with the child asleep. The preferred sites are hand or foot, antecubital veins, scalp, or external jugular vein. Avoid the femoral vein. In infants with small veins and abundant subcutaneous fat, IV insertion can be very difficult.

Regional anesthesia Occasionally, local or regional anesthesia will be used for upper extremity fracture management. This may be achieved by a hematoma block, intravenous anesthesia, or axillary or peripheral nerve blocks.

Sedation Some procedures are planned with sedation only and anesthesia ready if needed. This is suitable for early spica cast application for femoral shaft fractures, dressing changes, or minimally painful procedures.

Blood Replacement

Order blood preoperatively if replacement is a reasonable possibility. Generally, major procedures done without a tourniquet may require replacement. Families are extremely concerned about the risks of AIDS when the possibility of transfusion is considered. The risk depends in part on the competence of the blood bank. Statistically, when transfused, the risk of receiving infected blood is roughly equivalent to the risk of receiving the anesthetic. Special situations may complicate blood replacement. Transfusions may be restricted by religious beliefs or the fear of AIDS. Minimizing blood loss may be necessary in difficult cases, such as spinal fusions and limb salvage procedures. Hypotensive anesthesia may be adequate. The mean blood pressure is maintained between 50 and 60 mm. Hypothermia is seldom indicated in orthopedics. Hemodilution is a technique by which blood is removed just prior to surgery and replaced at the end of the procedure. Finally, autologous blood donation and cell-saving techniques are becoming more widely available. Blood substitutes will be available in the future.

Postoperative Pain Management

Postoperative pain management can begin before the procedure with placement of an epidural catheter (Fig. 3.35). Epidural blocks are contraindicated when there is a need to monitor postoperative pain, as when a compartment syndrome is a possible postoperative problem. Problems with epidural blocks include itching and urinary retention (Fig. 3.36). Consider injecting marcaine into the wound edges at the end of the procedure to provide comfort in the early postoperative period. Patient-controlled analgesia (PCA) is a valuable technique for the child over 7 years of age. Morphine or meperidine are useful agents. Provide oral pain control by codeine or oxycodone.

Anesthesia Consultant Anne Lynn

References

1998 Anesthesia. Safavi FZ. Pediatric Orthopedic Secrets. Philadelphia, Hanley & Belfus.

1996 Intravenous regional anesthesia for management of children's extremity fractures in the emergency department. Blasier RD, White R. Pediatr Emerg Care 12:404

1995 Self-administered nitrous oxide and a hematoma block for analgesia in the outpatient reduction of fractures in children. Hennrikus WL, Shin AY, Klingelberger CE. JBJS 77A:335

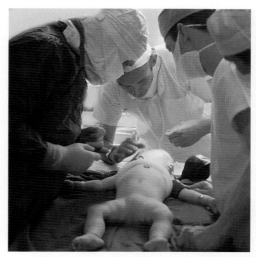

Fig. 3.33 Surgical team. Cooperation between the surgeon and anesthesiologist reduces risks.

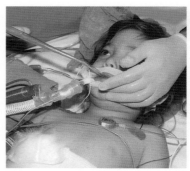
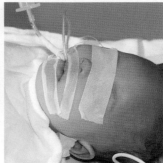

Fig. 3.34 General anesthesia. Provides excellent control of airway.

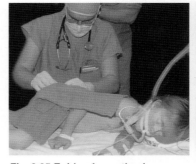
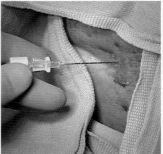

Fig. 3.35 Epidural anesthesia.

Epidural Anesthetic Complications

Nausea, emesis
Masking compartment syndrome
Pressure sore – heel ulcer
Urinary retention
Prolonged hospitalization
Itching

Fig. 3.36 Epidural anesthetic complications. Consider these problems when making the anesthetic choice and when following the child after surgery.

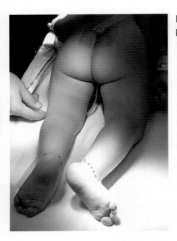

Fig. 3.37 Positioning. Thoughtful positioning facilitates surgery.

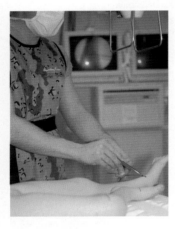

Fig. 3.38 Mark the operative sites before draping. Marking the exact surgical site sometimes allows for the shortest possible operative incision.

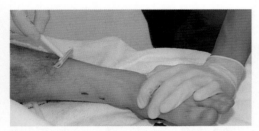

Fig. 3.39 Shaving. The need is minimal in children.

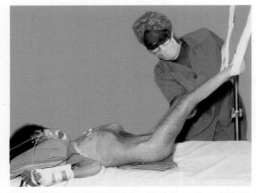

Fig. 3.40 Surgical prep with iodine solution. Mechanical support may simplify the surgical prep.

Surgical Preparation

Positioning

Position for ease of access (Fig. 3.37). Use prone position for clubfoot surgery and for release of knee flexion deformity. Positioning at the end of the table when possible allows greater freedom to maneuver around the patient during various stages of the procedure. Positioning on the child's side allows procedures to be done from the front and back of the child without the need for redraping. If an intraoperative image is planned, place the X-ray cassette under the patient before draping.

Mark Sites for Skin Incisions

To minimize incisional length, consider marking the exact sites for surgical procedures using the imaging intensifier (Fig. 3.38).

Skin Preparation

Shave if excessive hair is present (Fig. 3.39). Perform a surgical prep. 1% iodine in alcohol is effective and efficient, but has no commercial promoters, so its use is seldom appreciated (Fig. 3.40). We have used iodine successfully for thirty years. Apply one coat of the iodine solution and allow it to dry. This provides a sterile field and enhances the adhesion of the plastic film used for draping. For open wounds, a bacteriostatic soap solution is used. Shaving is usually not necessary in children. Shaving may cause superficial skin lacerations and irritation causing discomfort during the postoperative period.

Draping

Draping should provide adequate exposure for the surgical incision, a sterile barrier, and, if needed, free movement of the limb (Fig. 3.41). The margins, or the entire operative field, may be secured with an adhesive plastic film. Without clips, radiographs are less cluttered. Drape to provide wide exposure of the operative field. This allows the surgeon to extend the incision if more exposure is required.

For reconstructive procedures that require intraoperative alignment, drape one or both extremities free. This allows the surgeon to make certain the alignment is correct for lower limb alignment osteotomies, hip fusions, and similar procedures. Prep and drape both limbs, then use a sterile tourniquet.

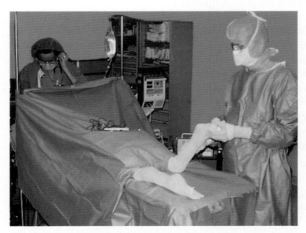

Fig. 3.41 Drape to allow full access. Plan for access well above and below the operative sites to allow intraoperative evaluation of joint motion.

Operative Scars

Plan the location and length of the incision as carefully as the fixation. The fixation is temporary, the scar permanent. Children are often embarrassed about their scars (Fig. 3.42) even when they become adults. Not infrequently, scars from orthopedic procedures cause children to avoid sports like swimming, running, or basketball that require clothing that exposes the scar. Make the scar as inconspicuous as possible by limiting its length and making the incision in the least noticeable location that allows adequate access for the procedure. Try to avoid incisions that are known to cause bad scars.

Minimizing Scars

Several techniques will be useful in reducing the disability from operative scars.

Shorten scars Make a short incision exactly over the site of the procedure. Before the skin prep, mark the position for the osteotomies using fluoroscopy.

Least conspicuous position Use the axillary approach for the upper humerus, the anterior approach for draining the hip, etc.

Avoid incision that cause wide scars For example, avoid making the vertical portion of the Smith–Peterson approach. To achieve the same exposure, extend the incision more medial in the *bikini line*. This provides adequate access with a much more cosmetic outcome. Likewise, avoid incisions over the clavicle. Make the approach below the clavicle even if a longer incision is necessary. Consider the anterior midline longitudinal incision for major knee procedures. The scar is more cosmetic, and if additional procedures are required later, the same approach can be used avoid multiple knee incisions.

Bilateral procedures Mark the position and scar length before preparing the skin (Fig. 3.43). Anticipate that the patient and family will compare the scars later. Asymmetrical scars for the same procedure creates doubt about the precision of the surgeon.

Short incision with mobilizing skin allows satisfactory exposure with minimal incision length (Fig. 3.44).

Skin Closure

Close the skin with subcutaneous absorbable sutures (3.45). Skin closure can be done quickly. Place a few subcutaneous sutures, and close the skin with subcuticular 3-0 absorbable suture. Supplement this closure with skin tape while approximating the skin edges by applying traction on both ends of the suture. The suture ends are cut off flush with the skin. This closure technique is rapid and definitive.

For incisions that are or will be under tension, close with 4-0 interrupted nylon sutures placed relatively close to the incision. Remove the sutures in 7 days. Avoid wide sutures to minimize the scar.

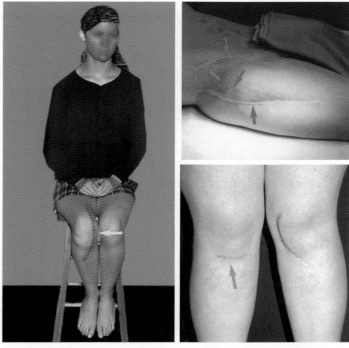

Fig. 3.42 Orthopedic scars. Operative scars may be unsightly and cause permanent embarrassment. Note the numerous scars on this boy's hip (red arrows). The improved appearance of the transverse scar on this girls knee (green arrow) and the disfiguring scar (yellow arrow) on the adolescent girl. Every day she planned her clothing in an attempt to hide this scar.

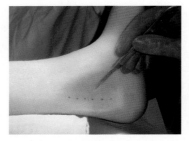

Fig. 3.43 Mark position for incisions. Make symmetrical incisions for bilateral procedures. Whenever possible avoid scars over prominences such as malleoli or heel-cords.

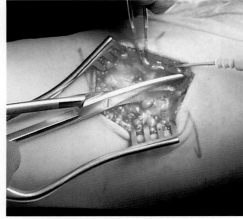

Fig. 3.44 Make minimal incision and mobilize. Often a short incision with subcutaneous skin mobilization will minimize the final scar length.

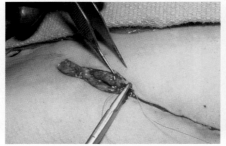
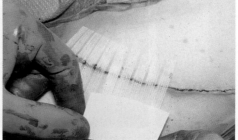

Fig. 3.45 Subcuticular closure. Close the skin with absorbable subcuticular sutures. Supplement with skin tapes if necessary.

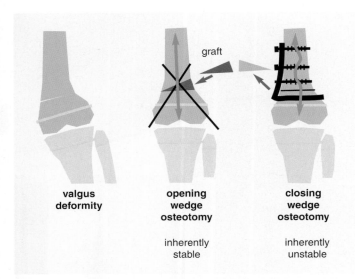

Fig. 3.46 Stability and osteotomy type. Opening wedge osteotomies are more stable and require less rigid fixation than closing wedge procedures.

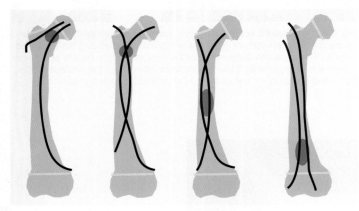

Fig. 3.47 Intramedullary fixation by level. The configuration of IM rods is in part determined by the level (red circle) of the lesion or fracture.

Fixation

Fixation of fractures or osteotomies in children take many forms (Fig. 3.48). The options of fixation in children are many. Take into consideration the child's age, location, inherent stability (Fig. 3.46), and the likely time for healing. Internal fixation is usually necessary for bony procedures. When fixation is supplemented with a cast, the internal fixation need not be rigid. Often minimal fixation supplemented with a cast is adequate for children.

Plates

Plates have a limited role in fixation in children. Plates have inherent disadvantages. They require broad exposure, produce stress risers through end screws, and their removal is a major procedure. Plate fixation is useful for such procedures as the repair of congenital pseudarthrosis of the clavicle.

Intramedullary Fixation

Intramedullary fixation (IM) has many advantages in children. Flexible, small diameter, IM fixation is adequate for children, making reaming and large nails unnecessary. Adequate fixation is provided by pins, Rush rods, or special purpose devices. Because of their length and shape, IM rods seldom migrate long distances. Make certain the fixation extends well above or below the site to be fixed (Fig. 3.47) and pins may traverse the growth plate. For tumors, plan to leave fixation until the lesion is healed. For conditions that permanently weaken bone, fixation is best left in place indefinitely. When pins remain for long periods, make certain the ends are deep enough to avoid skin irritation.

External Fixators

External fixators of a variety of types are suitable for children. Pins fixing bone may be stabilized externally with casts, frames, or special devices. They are used for stabilizing fractures and osteotomies, and for correcting deformities involving both bone and soft tissues. External fixators provide exceptional versatility, allowing changes in alignment, apposition, and length (Fig. 3.48). The disadvantages include the risk of pin tract infections, multiple scars, and the prolonged need for close medical attention.

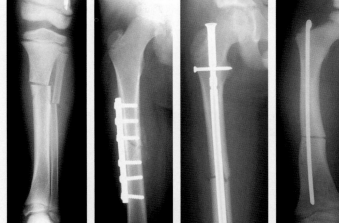
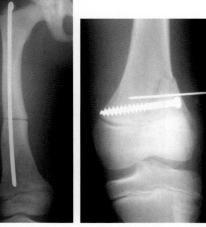
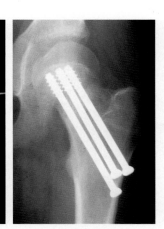

Fig. 3.48 Varied fixation in children orthopedics.

Pins

Pins can be for the orthopedist what nails are for the carpenter. Pins may be placed with varied configurations (Fig. 3.50). Pins are versatile, inexpensive, and rapidly applied and removed. Osteotomies fixed with crossed pins require small skin incisions (Fig. 3.52). Generally, smooth pins are most useful; they may traverse growth plates and are left outside the skin for removal in clinic. Threaded pins may be cut off just beyond the cortex, may not require removal, and should not be placed across the physis. Pins provide adequate fixation for bony procedures in nearly all infants, most children, and some adolescents. The absence of commercial promotion leaves the usefulness of pins often unappreciated.

Grafts

Tissue grafting involves autogenous and banked bone, fat, fascia, and cartilage (Fig. 3.51). Autologous organ transplants include bone, physeal plates, muscle, blood vessels, and nerves. Organ transfers require microsurgical techniques.

Autogenous Grafts

Bone Autografts are widely used, safe, rapidly incorporated, osteogenic, and readily available.

Local grafts Harvest bone from the site of the primary procedure when possible. Calcaneal bone for subtalar fusions, bone iliac bone for acetabular shelf procedure, cranial bone for upper C spine fusions, etc.

Iliac grafts Small amounts of bone can be removed percutaneously using a curette. Bicortical grafts in children are rapidly filled in.

Vascularized grafts Complexity and donar site problems limit the usefulness of vascularized grafts of bone joints or growth plates.

Soft tissue Free fat grafts are commonly used to replace defects in bone following physeal bridge resections.

Organ grafts Composite grafts are used to cover traumatic defects, for toe to finger transfers, etc.

Allografts

Bone Cadaver bone is convenient, carries a small risk of AIDS transmission, and incorporates more slowly than autogenous grafts. Such grafts are useful in procedures such as calcaneal lengthenings and bone replacement following resection of malignant tumors.

Osteochondral grafts are used for replacing joints for management of malignant tumors or trauma. The survival of cartilage is poor. Bone typing may improve results.

References

1998 Local bone-graft technique for subtalar extraarticular arthrodesis in cerebral palsy. Jeray KJ, Rentz J, Ferguson RL. JPO 18:75

1995 Iliac crest bone graft harvest donor site morbidity. A statistical evaluation. Banwart JC, Asher MA, Hassanein RS. Spine 20:1055

1995 The use of autologous skull bone grafts for posterior fusion of the upper cervical spine in children. Casey AT, et al. Spine 20:2217

1991 Autograft versus allograft for benign lesions in children. Glancy GL, et al. CO 262:28

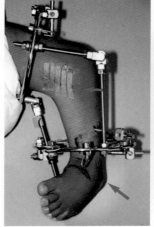
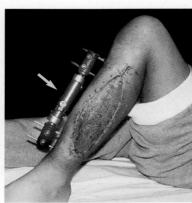

Fig. 3.49 External fixation. These fixators are useful for correcting deformities in arthrogryposis (red arrow) or for the tibia following a release for a compartment syndrome (yellow arrow).

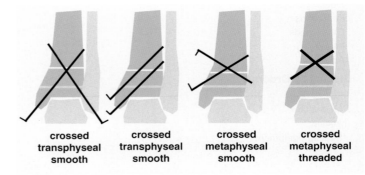

crossed transphyseal smooth   **crossed transphyseal smooth**   **crossed metaphyseal smooth**   **crossed metaphyseal threaded**

Fig. 3.50 Types of pin fixation. Varied uses of cross pins may be made based on the osteotomy level, age of patient, and indications for pin removal.

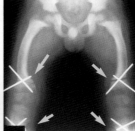
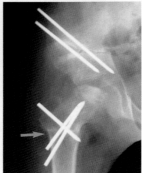
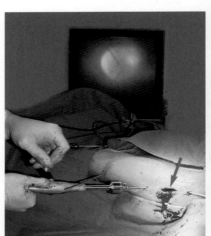

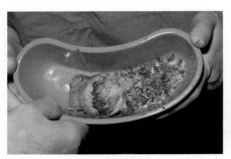
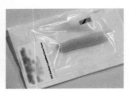

Fig. 3.51 Allografts. These may be from a femoral head (arrow) or packaged commercially.

Fig. 3.52 Cross pin fixation. Pins simplify fixation as a minimal incision is often adequate (red arrow) with the pins placed percutaneously. Usually crossed pin configuration is used as appropriate in rickets (yellow arrows) or for a double level osteotomy (green arrows) in Perthes disease.

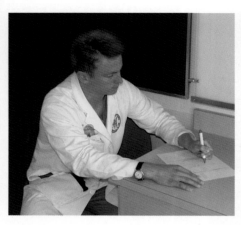

Fig 3.53 Postoperative care. Work out a plan that is comprehensive and includes follow-up and home care.

Physician Inpatient Orders

Position
Vital signs
Fluids
Pain meds
Other meds
Intake
Activity

Discharge Orders

Follow-up
Medication
Activity
Special equipment

Fig 3.54 Postoperative orders. Include these categories of needs.

Water (ml/kg/day) per body weight

First 10 kg	100
Second 10 kg	50
Each additional kg	20

Fig 3.55 Standard fluid maintenance for children.

Narcotic Medication	Usual Dosage
Acetaminophen + codeine elixir	Acetaminophen 15 mg/kg + Codeine 1 mg/kg/dose PO q 4–6 hrs
Acetaminophen + codeine tablets	1–2 tablets PO q 4–6 hrs prn
Morphine sulphate oral solution	0.3 mg/kg PO q 4 hrs prn
Acetaminophen (325 mg) + oxycodone (5 mg) *Percocet*	1–2 tablets PO q 4–6 hrs prn
Hydrocodone (5 mg) + acetaminophen (500 mg) *Vicodin*	1–2 tablets PO q 4–6 hrs prn

Anti-inflammatory Drugs

Ibuprofen *Motrin*	8 mg/kg PO q 6 hrs for 24–48 hrs

Fig. 3.56 Oral analgesic for children. From Ezaki (1998).

Postoperative Care

During the immediate postoperative period, the child is usually seen once or twice a day depending upon the magnitude of the procedure. Fortunately, most children have few postoperative problems and recovery is rapid.

Postoperative Orders

General orders include positioning, activity, vital signs circulation monitoring and other special considerations (Figs 3.53 and 3.54).

Fluid management A common error during and after surgery is prescribing too much fluid – especially dextrose in water. Most patients require little or no potassium because of tissue damage. Limit intake the first 24 hours after usual maintenance doses (Fig. 3.55).

Pain Management

IV analgesia Administer morphine 0.1–0.2 mg/kg as a loading dose and continuous infusion of 0.01-0.03mg/kg/hr as necessary to maintain comfort (Fig. 3.56). This is reduced by 10% every 12–24 hours.

Oral analgesia The patient is switched to oral analgesic when oral intake is allowed. Several agents are acceptable.

Patient controlled analgesia (PCA) In children older than about 5–6 years of age, this method is useful. Administer a loading dose of about 0.2 mg/kg. Allow doses of 0.02–0.03 mg/kg be given every 5–10 minutes with a maximum of 0.75–0.1 mg/kg per hour.

Epidural anesthesia This neuraxis analgesia is administered by the caudal route in children under years of age 6 or by lumbar route. Higher level administration may be necessary in selected cases.

Children with epidural pain management after surgery may be more comfortable, but be aware that epidural anesthesia may mask compartment syndromes.

Postoperative Problems

Fever Fever (temperature >38˚C) is seen in most children following surgery (Fig. 3.57). Be concerned if the fever is severe, the child looks more ill than expected, or if the child has positive physical findings suggesting a pulmonary or urinary problem.

Vomiting Nausea and vomiting following anesthesia are twice as common in children compared with adults. Causes of vomiting include agents such as nitrous oxide anesthesia and morphine. A history of motion sickness also increases the risk.

Special needs

Continuous passive motion (CPM) is a valuable technique in restoring motion (Fig. 3.58). The excursion is set at the range achieved by the interoperative releases. Continue the CPM for about 6 weeks.

Splints or braces may be fitted and completed during hospitalization (Fig. 3.59).

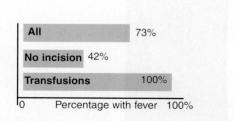

Fig. 3.57 Factors associated with fever following orthopedic procedures in children. Fever is common following orthopedic procedures. Fever is related to the duration and magnitude of the procedure. From Angel et al. (1994).

Time for Discharge

Observing the child's general appearance and behavior are valuable methods of monitoring recovery. Be concerned if the child is not becoming progressively better. As the child becomes comfortable and smiling, the parent's concerns diminish. At this point, the child is ready for discharge.

Scheduling Follow-up Visits

Order the follow-up clinic visits thoughtfully. Make certain each visit has a specific purpose. Plan the postoperative visits to approximate the time when the child is at risk for a complication or when some change in management is anticipated. Most operative complications, such as infections, loss of reduction, or position or pressure sores will occur within the first week.

Time follow-up visits to coincide with timing for orthotic, physical therapy, or other postoperative visits. Being thoughtful about the family's resources will be appreciated.

Activity Status

Compliance with orders to limit activity is poor. If necessary ensure compliance by immobilization in a cast. Avoid burdening the family with the duty to enforce activity restriction; it is an impossible task and an unfair assignment.

Physical Therapy

Crutch training is best done preoperatively. Mobilize the child (Fig. 3.60) when possible before discharge. Therapy is necessary for special situations such as for children with muscular dystrophy following contracture release procedures. Physical therapy is not necessary for routine postoperative care.

Hardware Removal

Generally smooth pins may be removed in the clinic. Often threaded pins and fixation hardware require removal under anesthesia. Most hardware removals are performed 3–9 months following surgery.

Indications In the past, removal of fixation devices was routine. As hardware requires an anesthetic, operative exposure, and sometimes added complications, routine removal is not appropriate. Indications for hardware removal include:

Prominent hardware Hardware that alters the body contour and may cause discomfort such as proximal femoral fixation for varus osteotomies.

Fixation complicating known future procedures Large fixation devices that are buried in bone about the hip may complicate total hip replacement.

Fixation causing stress risers in the femur may require removal.

Hardware that extends into a joint.

Metal reaction or infections are relative indications.

Contraindications of hardware removal include:

Fixation that reduces the risk of pathologic fracture should be permanent. This includes IM fixation of benign tumors, or fractures through osteopenic bone. This permanet fixation strengthens the bone and usually prevents refracture.

Fixation that is likely to be very difficult to remove The difficulty of hardware removal is classically unappreciated. Complication rates can be significant. Make certain the benefit is worth the risks.

References

1999 Complications of blade plate removal. Becker CE, Keeler KA, Kruse RW, and Shah SA. JPO 19:188

1998 Anesthesia. Safavi FZ. Pediatric Orthopedic Secrets. Philadelphia, Hanley & Belfus.

1997 Management of completely stiff pediatric knee. Cole PA, Ehrlich MG. JPO 17:67

1994 Posteoperative fever in pediatric orthopaedic patients. Angel JD, Blasier RD, Allison R. JPO 14:799

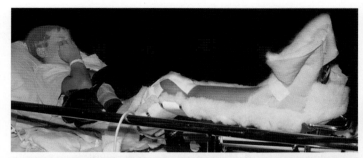

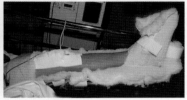

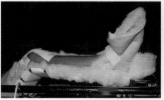

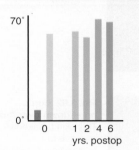

Fig. 3.58 Continuous passive motion for knee stiffness. CPM is effective in restoring knee motion in children. Children with stiff knees had operative release and postoperative CPM. Preoperative motion (red) showed substantial improvement (blue) with maintenance of motion over the next several years (green). From Cole and Ehrlich (1997).

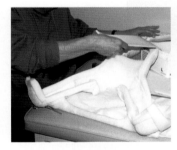

Fig 3.59 Making splints for postoperative care. The postoperative period in the hospital is an ideal time for fabrication of splints, orthotics, or adaptive equipment for home use.

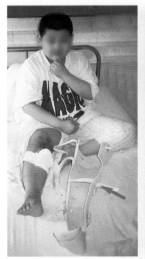

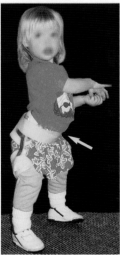

Fig. 3.60 Mobilizing the child following discharge. Make certain braces are constructed before the procedure (red arrow). Sometimes the child can be mobilized in the brace (yellow arrow) or with support.

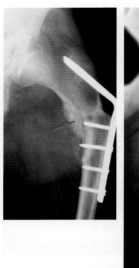

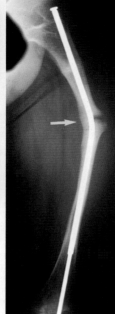

Fig. 3.61 Fractures around fixation. Sometimes the problem is preventable, as in this osteotomy, which was performed too low (red arrow). In others, the problem is not preventable, as in this bent rod in a child with osteogenesis imperfecta (yellow arrow).

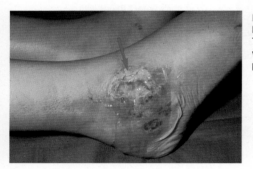

Fig. 3.62 Skin breakdown over foot. This skin breakdown was due to postoperative swelling.

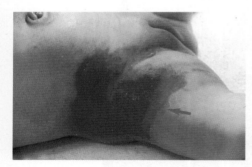

Fig. 3.63 Skin irritation under a spica cast. This severe irritation is due to poor home care.

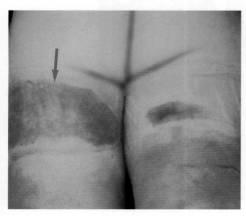

Fig. 3.64 Tourniquet burns. This skin breakdown occurred under a tourniquet.

Complications

Avoiding complications is a major operative objective. Orthopedists have been divided into *risk avoiders* and *risk acceptors*. Be a *risk avoider* when managing children. Complications are fewer in the pediatric age group because the child is more physiologically resilient. For example, thrombophlebitis and cardiopulmonary problems are uncommon in children. Complications sometimes cannot be prevented whereas others are secondary to poor technique (Fig. 3.61). Others are due to technical problems, such as inadequate correction, loss of position or fixation, or pressure sores from a tight cast.

It is usually possible to avoid complications if the risks are identified prior to the treatment and preventive measures to taken in advance. For example, when planning a proximal tibial osteotomiy be aware that the procedure is associated with peroneal nerve palsies and compartment syndromes. These complications can often be prevented by (1) altering the level of osteotomy, performing rotational osteotomies in the distal rather than proximal level; (2) performing a prophylactic fasciotomy; (3) splitting the cast and, (4) careful postoperative monitoring.

As another example, when pinning a slipped capital femoral epiphysis, be aware of the risks of joint penetration and postfixation fracture. Fixing with a single central pin reduces the risk of joint penetration. Making the entry point proximal reduces the risk of postop fractures. Entry points at or below the lessor trochanter are associated with a risk of fracture through the site of pin penetration of the lateral cortex.

Other high-risk procedures include procedures using external fixation, or major procedures such as spine operations, extension osteotomies of the distal femur, unstable slipped capital epiphysis cases, procedures on myelodysplasic or poorly nourished children, etc.

Wound Infections

Wound infections are less common in children than adults. The risk of infection is greatest in operations of long duration; infections are most serious if the procedures involve bones and joints.

Prophylactic antibiotics can often prevent infection and should be administered intravenously at the beginning of the operative procedure. The single dose is adequate unless the procedure is prolonged.

Clinical signs of wound infections develop as early as 24 hours in streptococcal infections. The more common staphylococcal infections appear after 3-4 days. The child with a wound infection often shows systemic signs of fever and malaise, and the wound becomes more swollen, warm, and erythematous. The fever from infection must be differentiated from the common benign postoperative fever that commonly occurs after most procedures. Such fever resolves in a day or two. Be concerned if a secondary temperature elevation occurs. It should be considered a sign of an infection until proven otherwise.

If the child shows systemic signs of infection, search for the cause. Examine the ears and throat. Listen to the lungs. Window the cast and examine the wound. Perform a urinalysis. Culture the urine, blood, and wound. If the child is ill, start antibiotic therapy while the cultures are incubating. If the wound is infected, it should be opened, cultured, and drained under sterile conditions in the operating room. Close the wound after the infection is controlled.

Skin Problems

Skin problems may be due to irritation under the cast (Fig. 3.62) and is common in infants immobilized for hip dyplasia (Fig. 3.63). Prevent skin problems by keeping casts as dry as possible. The inflammation resolves once the cast is removed.

Tourniquet Irritation

Tourniquet "burns" (Fig. 3.64) can usually be prevented by avoiding prep solution from seeping under the tourniquet. Treat as a burn.

Pressure Sores

Pressure sores are most common in children with neuromuscular problems. Anesthetic skin and the child's difficulty in communicating are major contributing factors. Take added precautions in patients with myelodysplasia and cerebral palsy. Pressure sores occur in characteristic locations: the heels (Fig. 3.65), trochanters, sacrum, and other bony prominences (Fig. 3.66). They can usually be prevented by careful casting technique. Apply thick padding, avoid a snug cast, and window the cast over the heels if necessary. During the postoperative period, rotate the patient frequently, and inspect areas at risk, such as the sacrum, often. In communicative patients with intact sensation, ask about localized pain, such as over the lateral malleolus. Cast pressure pain is often described as a burning pain. Detecting pressure sores is sometimes difficult. Be concerned if a foul odor is present. The stench of devitalized tissue is different from the usual fecal-urine odor. *Sniffing* the cast or wound is a simple and effective test. Operative related pressure sores will heal if the wound is kept clean and protected from pressure (Fig. 3.67) or abrasion. Identify pressure sores early so they can be healed by the time the cast is removed.

Stiffness

Joint stiffness as an operative complication is uncommon in children. Simple postoperative stiffness is temporary and resolves as the child resumes activity. This makes physical therapy unnecessary. Persistent stiffness usually results from joint damage due to compression, ischemia, or infection. Manage joint stiffness by active range-of-motion exercises and observation. If improvement plateaus and the stiffness produces disability, consider performing an arthrolysis and employing continuous passive motion or special splints to maintain the correction gained. Generally expect to retain about half of the range of motion obtained intraoperatively.

Pin Migration

Smooth pins may migrate long distances in the body. They have been found in the mediastinum and in the heart. Migration is best prevented by bending the end of the pin. Bend the protruding end of the pin to a right angle and cut the pin off about 1 cm from the bend.

Pin Tract Infections

Pin tract infections are usually due to motion around the pin, or tension on the adjacent soft tissue (Fig. 3.68), producing necrosis. Both of these problems are usually preventable. After placing the pin, if the skin is tented, incise the skin to relieve the tension. Stabilize the pin-skin junction. Immobilize the limb in a cast. Pin tract infections should be cultured and treated with antibiotics. Open drainage is seldom necessary.

Cast Syndrome

The cast syndrome, or superior mesenteric artery syndrome refers to a spectrum of disorders caused by compression of the second portion of the duodenum between the superior mesenteric artery and aorta. This is sometimes referred to as the "nutcracker effect." The clinical manifestations vary from partial duodenal obstruction to bowel infarction. Predisposing factors include hyperextension of the trunk, supine positioning, and poor nutritional status. Each tends to increase the nutcracker-like squeeze of the artery and aorta on the duodenum. This syndrome may develop in a hyperextended body cast or prolonged supine positioning. Treat by removing the cast, prone positioning, and increased caloric intake.

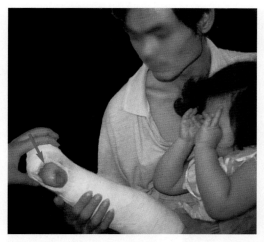

Fig. 3.65 Heel ulcer. This ulcer is due to excessive pressure from the cast.

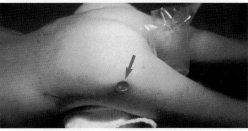

Fig. 3.66 Skin breakdown in cerebral palsy. These are common sites of skin breakdown under the spica cast in a child with cerebral palsy.

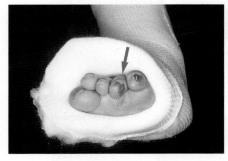

Fig. 3.67 Skin breakdown in myelodysplasia. The heavily padded cast protects the skin and allows healing.

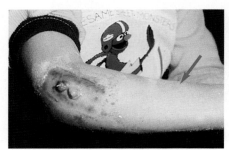

Fig 3.68 Pin tract infection. This infection around a percutaneous pin was due to excessive tension on the skin.

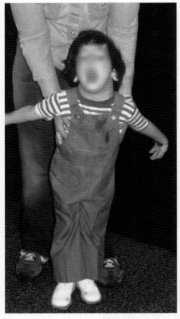

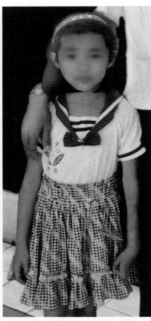

Fig 3.69 Motor regression. This child lost the ability to walk following surgery. Recovery took many months.

Fig 3.70 Volkmann ischaemic contracture. This complication resulted from management of supracondylar fracture of the humerus.

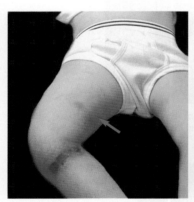

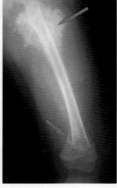

Fig 3.71 Pathological fractures in myelodysplasia. These fractures causes extensive soft tissue swelling and callus formation.

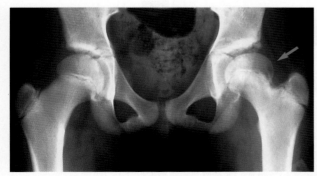

Fig 7.72 Partial AVN complicating DDH management. This type 2 AVN causes a deformity of the upper femur.

Motor Regression

Most children experience some temporary motor regression following immobilization after operative procedures. In children with neuromuscular disorders, the regression is much more profound (Fig. 3.69). In severely disabled adolescents, recovery may be incomplete, and full return to the preoperative motor level never achieved. For example, the adolescent with cerebral palsy who is a marginal walker preoperatively may not return to walking after a long recovery from a triple arthrodesis, hip, or spine procedure. Regression can be minimized by upright positioning, an active exercise program, and shortening the period of immobility.

Compartment Syndromes

Compartment syndromes, or ischemia from tight casts (Fig. 3.70) should be promptly diagnosed. Following any major procedure distal to the elbow or knee, the cast should be prophylactically bivalved and spread. Perform a prophylactic anterior and lateral compartment release whenever a proximal tibial osteotomy is performed.

Pathological Fractures

Postoperative pathologic fractures are most common in children with reduced sensitivity and flaccid paralysis. The risks are greatest in the child with myelodysplasia (Fig. 3.71). Fractures occur most commonly at the distal femoral level following cast removal. These fractures are difficult to prevent. Minimize the period of immobilization, load the limb by standing the child in the cast, and use special caution in applying physical therapy after cast removal.

Deep Vein Thrombosis

Deep vein thrombosis is most common in spinal surgery, spinal trauma with paralysis, and in children with predispositions such as those with protein C deficiency, vascular malformations, etc. External compression devices on limbs during surgery reduce the risk.

Toxic Shock Syndrome

Toxic shock syndrome (TSS) is a rare but catastrophic complication that occurs usually 2–3 weeks following surgery. TSS is a reaction to toxins from staphloccal and streptococcus infections. About half occur in menstruating girls. Sudden onset of fever, vomiting, diarrhea, rash, and hypotension are common. Multisystem organ failure may occur. Fatality rates in orthopedic patients are about 25%.

Hypertension

Hypertension is common following certain orthopedic procedures that cause stretching or lengthening of extremities. In these procedures monitor the child's blood pressure.

Avascular necrosis

Avascular necrosis (AVN) is a serious complication that may follow treatment of DDH (Fig. 3.72), acute slips, traumatic dislocated hips, displaced transcervical femoral fractures, lateral condylar fractures, radial neck fractures, and other problems. With this known risk, warn the parents and document in the chart an awareness of the risk and measures to avoid AVN before undertaking management. In many cases no effective prevention is available. In others, such as for lateral condylar fractures, careful operative technique avoiding excessive soft tissue dissection may prevent the complication.

Arterial Injury

Injuries to veins and small arteries can usually be controlled by pressure and time. In contrast, major arterial injuries may be limb-threatening. Unless you are skilled in vascular repair, ask a colleague with this expertise for assistance. If excessive pulsatile bleeding occurs, control by local pressure, pack the wound, and wait several minutes. While waiting, improve exposure, optimize the lighting, and have suction ready. If bleeding continues, the injured vessel can usually be found and ligated. For more severe injuries, proximal control and arterial repair may be necessary. Arteriography may delay the repair. Less common are aneurysms following operative procedures (Fig. 3.73). Aneurysms may become evident weeks or months postoperatively.

Bad Scars

Ugly scars are far too common following procedures in children (Figs. 3.74 and 3.75). Poorly placed, excessively long and sloppily closed operative scars last a lifetime. Bad scars embarrass children, limit their selection of clothing and restrict activities. Most are preventable.

Lack of Compliance

Children often exceed limits placed on postoperative activities. Families may not return for scheduled clinic visits. Often the child or family is blamed for the complication; however, it may be due to poor medical care (Fig. 3.77). Take precautions based on the assumption that the child will do whatever is possible. Be creative. Use fixation unlikely to cause problems with removal. Make casts excessively strong or activity-inhibiting by design. Employ a *tickler system* to automatically generate recall action if families miss appointments.

References

2000 Infectious complications in critically injured children. Patel JC, Mollitt DL, Tepas JJ, 3rd. J Pediatr Surg 35:1174

1998 Normal postoperative febrile response in the pediatric orthopaedic population. Merjanian RB, et al. JPO 18:497

1997 Surgical risk for elective excision of benign exostoses. Wirganowicz PZ, Watts HG. JPO 17:455

1995 Toxic shock syndrome as a complication of orthopaedic surgery. Grimes J, Carpenter C, Reinker K. JPO 15:666

1995 Complications in proximal tibial osteotomies in children with presentation of technique. Pinkowski JL, Weiner D. JPO 15:307

1994 Postoperative fever in pediatric orthopaedic patients. Angel JD, Blasier RD, Allison R. JPO 14:799

1994 Subtrochanteric fracture after fixation of slipped capital femoral epiphysis: a complication of unused drill holes. Canale ST, et al. JPO 14:623

1994 Peroneal nerve injury as a complication of pediatric tibial osteotomies: a review of 255 osteotomies. Slawski DP, Schoenecker PL, Rich MM. JPO 14:166

1994 Pulmonary embolism in pediatric trauma patients. McBride WJ, et al. J Trauma 37:913

1993 Refracture of adolescent femoral shaft fractures: a complication of external fixation. A report of two cases. Probe R, et al. JPO 13:102

1993 Supracondylar femoral extension osteotomy: its complications. Asirvatham R, et al. JPO 13:642

1993 Hypertension following orthopaedic surgery in children. Helal A, et al. JPO 13:773

1993 Complications of use of the Ilizarov technique in the correction of limb deformities in children. Velazquez RJ, et al. JBJS 75A:1148

1991 Metal removal in a pediatric population: benign procedure or necessary evil? Schmalzried TP, et al. JPO 11:72

1991 Protein C deficiency as a cause of pulmonary embolism in the perioperative period. Sternberg TL, et al. Anesthesiology 74:364

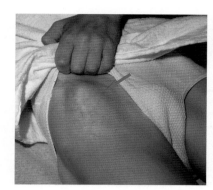
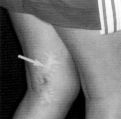

Fig. 3.73 Aneurysm of femoral artery. The artery was injured during an operative procedure.

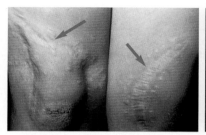

Fig. 3.74 Ugly scar about the knee. Note the bad scars in front of the knee from patellar realignment (red arrows) and behind the knee (yellow arrow) from a hamstring lengthening procedure.

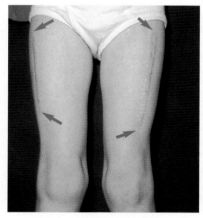

Fig. 3.75 Note the unnecessarily long scars from femoral osteotomies.

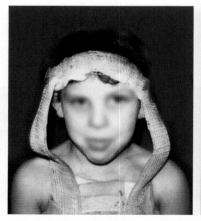
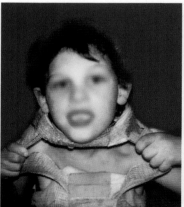
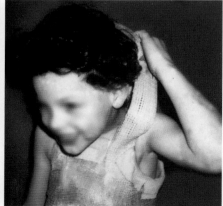

Fig. 3.76 Flimsy casts are no match for children. This cast was applied to hold the head in a neutral position following torticollis surgery. It was inadequate and quickly broke down. The child was not *noncompliant*, he was simply behaving like a normal child.

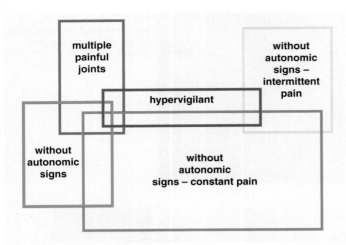

Fig. 3.77 Overlap of pain amplification syndromes. Note the varied patterns. From Sherry (2000).

Common Features of Amplified Pain Syndrome

Most common in preadolescent or adolescent girls
Increasing pain after minimal or no trauma
Significant disability
Crawls around house or on stairs
Discomfort with light touch – clothing, bed sheets, etc.
Autonomic changes – cold, color, clammy, edema
Worse or not better with cast immobilization
Unsuccessful previous treatment
High-level athletes or dancers
Personality features – mature, excels at school, perfectionistic, etc.
Recent major life change – move, school, friends, divorce, etc.
Mother speaks for the child
Incongruent affect for degree of pain or disability
La belle indifference about pain
Compliant when asked to use the limb
Autonomic signs especially after use
Pain not restricted to dermatome or peripheral nerve distribution
Negative neurological examination

Fig. 3.78 Common features of amplified pain syndrome. Based on Sherry (2000).

Amplified Musculoskeletal Pain Syndromes

Included in this category of syndromes include reflex sympathetic dystrophy (RSD) or reflex neurovascular dystrophy (RND), idiopathic pain syndrome, and fibromyalgia.

Scope

These pain syndromes are varied and may be associated with autonomic signs (Fig. 3.77). The patients typically present features of disability out of proportion to the trauma history or clinical findings. These patients are often seen first by the orthopedist because the pain is musculoskeletal and frequently follows minor injury.

Diagnosis

The patients present with a wide variety of clinical features (Fig. 3.78). The findings may show considerable variations from autonomic features (Fig. 3.79) to dynamic or fixed deformity (Fig. 3.80). Usually the evaluation elicits a sense of disparity. The pain or disability is exaggerated beyond any signs of underlying disease.

Management

These patients are difficult to manage. The psychological or functional underlying problem is often clear, but the family will often be offended if that possibility is presented as the primary problem.

Referral When available, consider referring the child to a pediatric rheumatologist to manage care.

Active treatment is usually successful. Order functional aerobic training using the involved limbs such as drills, running, play activities and swimming for a period of 5 hours daily. Desensitize skin with towel rubbing. Refer for psychological evaluation and provide psychotherapy as appropriate. This intensive treatment may require inpatient care with a follow-up home program for another month.

Outcome 80% cured, 15% improved, 5% unimproved; relapse 15%; 90% doing well at 5 years.

Consultant Sherry DD, e-mail: dsherry@u.washington.edu.

References
2000 An overview of amplified musculoskeletal pain syndrome. Sherry DD. J. Rheumatol Suppl 58:44

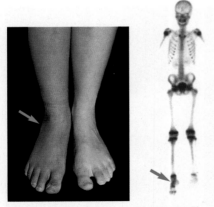

Fig. 3.79 Autonomic features of right foot. Note the discoloration and swelling of the leg and foot (red arrow) and increased uptake on bone scan (blue arrow).

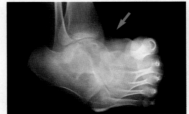
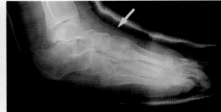

Fig. 3.80 Severe fixed deformity from RSD. This 15-year-old girl developed a fixed equinovarus deformity of the foot (red arrow) over a period of many months. Correction requires soft tissue releases and casting (yellow arrow).

Traction

Traction still has a role in management. Although less than in the past, specific indications have replaced standard management.

Common Indications for Traction

Temporary stabilization Skin traction is commonly used for femoral shaft fractures before cast immobilization or operative fixation and for preoperative management of unstable proximal femoral epiphyseal slips.

Home traction Home traction programs have been used for preliminary traction in DDH management (Fig 3.81) and in home management of femoral shaft fractures in young children.

Fracture management The common uses of traction include supracondylar humeral fractures, femoral shaft (Fig. 3.82) and subtrochanteric fractures.

Overcoming contracture Traction is sometimes used to improve motion in Perthe's disease or chondrolysis of the hip. Whether the improvement is due to the traction or simply the enforced bed rest and immobilization is unclear.

Spine problems Complex spine problems such as congenital and neuromuscular deformities are sometimes managed by a combination of traction and surgery.

Traction Cautions

Inflammatory hip disorders Avoid traction in inflammatory hip disorders such as toxic synovitis or septic arthritis. Traction often positions the limb in less flexion, external rotation, and abduction, resulting in increased intraarticular pressure and possible avascular necrosis.

Overhead leg position Avoid Bryant traction in patients weighing more than 25 pounds as the vertical positioning may result in limb ischaemia. This traction is seldom used today. It is preferable to reduce the flexion of the hips from 90° to about 45° to reduce the risk of ischaemia.

Proximal tibial pin traction Avoid proximal tibial skeletal traction as distal femoral traction (Fig. 3.82) provides greater safety. Reports of recurvatum deformity and knee ligamentous laxity make this treatment risky.

Complications of Traction

Skin irritation This is common under skin traction (Fig. 3.83). Prevent this problem by avoiding excessive traction or compression. Frequent inspection of the skin reduces this risk.

Nerve compression This most commonly involves the peroneal nerve (Fig 3.84) from skin traction. Avoid excessive pressure over the upper fibula.

Vascular compromise This complication is most commonly associated with overhead traction for femoral fractures in infants over 25 lbs.

Physeal damage from pins This complication has been most common from upper tibial pin traction.

Cranial penetration of halo pins The thin calvarium in children makes inadvertent penetration a risk (Fig. 3.85). The risks are reduced by using more pins with less compression. Preapplication CT studies may be helpful in determining proper sites for pin placement.

Superior mesenteric artery syndrome This serious complication may result from long periods of supine positioning in poorly nourished individuals.

Hypertension The mechanism is unknown.

Procedures

Traction procedures are detailed on pages 368 and 369.

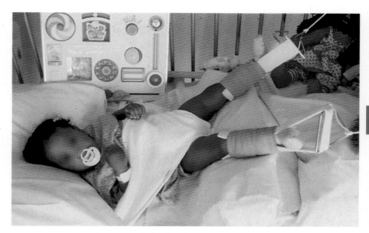

Fig. 3.81 Skin traction for DDH. Sometimes prereduction skin traction is used to overcome contractures to facilitate reduction and possibly reduce the risk of AVN.

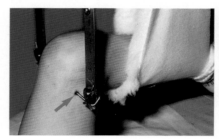

Fig. 3.82 Distal femoral traction. This is the preferable site for traction when treating femoral shaft fractures.

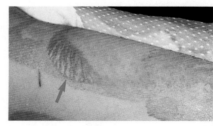

Fig. 3.83 Skin irritation under traction tapes. This skin blister is due to excessive pressure and traction.

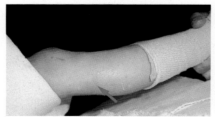

Fig. 3.84 Peroneal nerve palsy. The excessive pressure resulted in a loss of function.

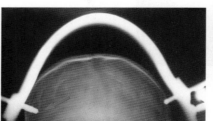

Fig. 3.85 Halo pin penetration. This is prevented by using multiple pins and limiting penetration pressure during application.

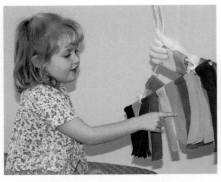
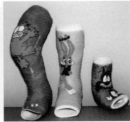

Fig. 3.86 Colorful casts. Allowing the child to choose the color makes the experience less threatening. Casts can be decorated.

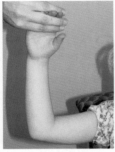
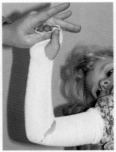
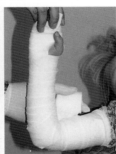

Fig 3.87 Padding. Hold the desired postion the same throughout the casting process. Apply the stockinette then the padding.

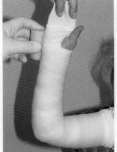
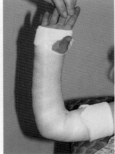
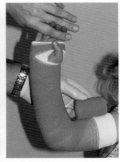

Fig 3.88 Cast application. Apply the first layers, turn the stockinette back for trim. Apply the final layer to trim the cast and add the desired color.

Casting

Casting is useful for immobilization, control of position, correction of deformity, and sometimes to ensure compliance with treatment. Cast treatment is relatively safe, inexpensive, and well tolerated by children. Casts may be made of plaster or fiberglass. Plaster casts are least expensive and readily molded. Fiberglass casts are expensive, lightweight, water-resistant, radiographically transparent, and less messy and provide many color and decorating options (Fig. 3.86). Sometimes the materials are combined in treating deformities such as clubfeet.

Categories of Casts

Casts are remarkably versatile and take many forms. They may be circumferential or applied as splints.

Cast Problems for Children

When applying casts for children, keep in mind the unique problems that may be encountered.

Compliance Children are less compliant than adults. They may not hold still for cast application, may allow their cast to become wet, or damage their cast in play.

Communication Infants or young children may not be able to communicate the pain that precedes the development of pressure sores over bony prominences.

Sensation The child with myelodysplasia or cerebral palsy has poor sensation and is at risk for pressure sores.

Cast Application

Positioning First, make certain the child is comfortable and the limb is held in the position desired after the cast is completed. For cylinder casts or body jackets, the child should be standing. For long-leg casts, it is helpful to apply the short-leg section first; after it has hardened, extend it to the thigh. Include the toes in children's casts to provide protection. Apply the cast only when the patient is comfortable and the limb immobile. Make certain the assistant holding the limb maintains the proper position until the cast has hardened.

Padding Apply at least two layers of padding (Fig. 3.87). The first is the tubular stockinette that allows a neat trim for the cast edges. The material is usually cotton or dacron. The second layer is the padding. Apply extra padding over bony prominences, if the child is likely to move during cast application, or if the child is at risk for pressure sores.

In applying the cast (Fig. 3.88), start at one end and proceed in an orderly fashion to the other end of the cast. Apply with a 50% overlap by rolling rather than pulling on the material. The techniques for application of plaster versus fiberglass are different. Tucks are taken in plaster casts to make a neat application.

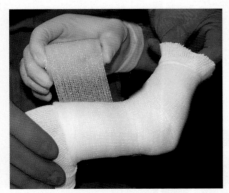

Fig. 3.89 Cast technique with fiberglass. Unroll a length and then lay the material down without tension.

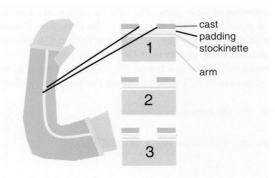

Fig. 3.90 Stages of cast splitting. Casts can be split to different levels. Note that in cross-section only the cast is divided (1); cast and padding are divided (2); or all layers are divided (3).

Fiberglass application Fiberglass rolls must be guided to maintain control of direction. *When applying fiberglass, free a segment of material from the roll, the apply it smoothly and without tension* (Fig. 3.89). Plaster has a definite time of crystallization and hardens rather abruptly. Fiberglass hardens slowly. The ideal thickness of most casts is three layers. Apply extra layers over sites of greater stress, such as the hip in spica casts or the knee and ankle in long-leg casts.

Early Cast Care

Bivalving Bivalving or splinting casts may be by degree (Fig. 3.90). Be aware that padding is often not elastic and may create as much compression as cast material. For complete relief of pressure, it is necessary to divide all layers of the cast on both sides.

Pressure relief If sensation is poor or communication limited, consider relieving pressure over bony prominences. Cut a rectangle of cast or cut a *X* over the site for relief. Elevate the cast edges and leave the padding intact. To make the child in a spica cast more comfortable, consider flaring the thoracic edges and creating a *stomach hole* (Fig. 3.91).

Trim cast edges To save operative room time, consider trimming the cast in the recovery room or on the ward. Provide a generous amount of space around the perineum.

Cast Care

When the child bathes or plays in the rain, cover the cast with a plastic bag to keep it dry. Even fiberglass casts are uncomfortable when wet. In infants, spica casts pose a special problem. Instruct staff and parents to change the infant's diapers frequently and to avoid tucking the diaper under the cast. Skin irritation is best managed by exposure to air and light. Avoid criticizing the child for the appearance of the cast. Often a worn cast is evidence of success in incorporating the treatment in the play activity of the child (Fig. 3.92).

Cast Removal

Cast removal is often the most risky phase of cast treatment (Fig. 3.93). Cast saws can cut the skin if the contact is made under pressure. Cast saw lacerations are most likely over bony prominences such as the malleoli. Plaster casts may be soaked off by the parents prior to clinic. The crying, struggling child is at special risk. Try to reassure the child by placing the moving blade gently against your arm to show that it only vibrates and normally does not cut skin. Compare the saw noise to an airplane. Have the mother comfort the child as well.

Avoid dragging the saw; use consecutive in-and-out movements to cut the cast. Try to avoid cutting directly over the bony prominences. Insist that the inexperienced assistant learn to remove casts on adolescents or adults and not infants or children.

Hair grows more rapidly under casts. The adolescent girl is often shocked by the amount of hair on her leg following cast removal. Reassure her that in a month or so the hair growth will return to normal.

Chapter Consultant Richard Gross, e-mail: grossr@musc.edu

References

1996 Parent satisfaction comparing two bandage materials used during serial casting in infants. Coss HS, Hennrikus WL. Foot Ankle Int 17:483

1992 Peroneal nerve palsy after early cast application for femoral fractures in children. Weiss AP, et al. JPO 12:25

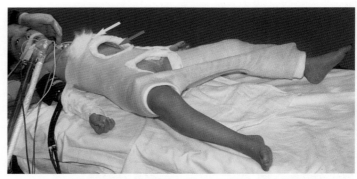

Fig. 3.91 Spica cast. Note the large abdominal window (red arrow) and extra space around the thorax (yellow arrow).

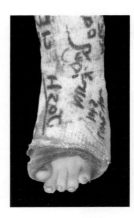

Fig. 3.92 "Well-used" cast. Ideally the child will be very active in the cast.

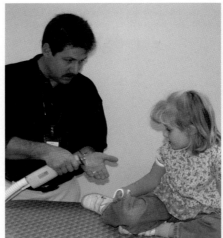
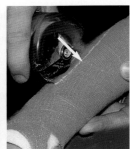
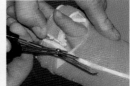
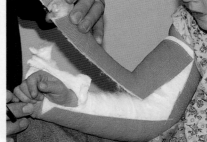
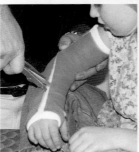

Fig 3.93 Cast removal. Reassure the child by applying the moving blade to the hand (upper left). Cut the cast with in and out movements (upper right). Cut both sides of the cast, spread the cut edges, and divide the padding with a sissors. This allows the cast to be removed.

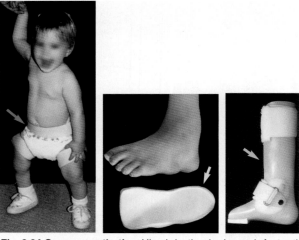

Fig. 3.94 Common orthotics. Hip abduction (red arrow), foot orthosis (yellow arrow), and ankle-foot orthosis (orange arrow) are most common braces.

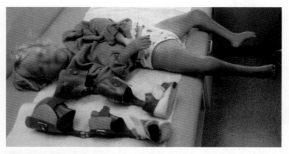

Fig. 3.95 Functional bracing. This child with arthrogryposis has special braces that incorporate light weight, heel elevations, knee flexion, and internal rotation components.

Prescribing Orthoses

Length
 AFO
 KFO
 HKFO
Material
 Molded
 Leather
 Polyprolene
Hinges
 Free
 Right angle stop
 Spring loaded
Upright
 Single – Double
 Steel – Aluminum
Closures
 Velcro
 Buckles
Special Features
 Stress – valgus or varus
 Pads – location

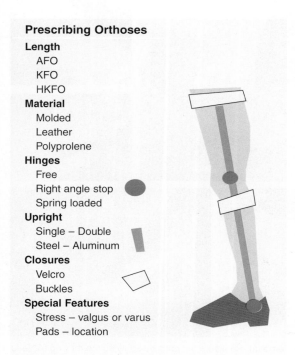

Fig. 3.96 Orthosis prescription. Specify each element of the brace.

Orthotics

Orthoses are used to control alignment, facilitate function, and provide protection. They include braces and splints (fig 3.94). Often the distinction between braces and splints is poorly defined.

Splints provide static support or positioning and often encompass only half of the limb. They are often worn only part-time.

Braces are usually more elaborate and worn while the child is active (Fig. 3.95). Braces are sometimes divided into passive and active types.

Passive braces are those that simply provide support such as some scoliosis braces in children with neuromuscular disorders.

Active Braces are those that facilitate function. Such braces may promote active correction as seen in scoliosis braces that incorporate pads.

Goals

Be realistic about the goals of bracing. Bracing will not correct static deformity or scoliosis. At best, braces prevent progression. Orthotics do not correct physiologic flatfeet or torsional deformity. Although radiographs taken with the orthotics in place may show improvement, this correction is not maintained after the brace is removed. Unbraced radiographs can be made to assess real correction.

Naming Orthoses

The name of the device is determined by which joints are involved. An AFO includes the ankle and foot; a KFO adds the knee; a HKFO includes the hip, knee, and ankle. Special braces are often named by city of origin.

Ordering Orthoses

The prescription should include several components: the extent, material, joint characteristics, and closure types (Fig. 3.96). Order orthoses thoughtfully as any orthoses is a burden for the child.

Minimizing the Orthotic Burden

Attempt to reduce the burden to the child.

Effective? Many orthoses are ineffective and should not be used. Examples include all orthoses for developmental deformities that occur in normal children. These include orthoses for flatfeet, twister cables for torsional problems, or wedges for bowlegs.

Perform *the child test* For children with neuromuscular problems, orthoses such as AFOs are frequently ordered to improve function. If the brace truly improves function, the child will usually prefer to use the brace. If the braces causes more trouble than benefit, the child will prefer to go without. Make certain the brace is comfortable and fitting properly. If the child prefers to go without a comfortable, well-fitting orthoses, it generally means that the brace is a functional liability. In most cases the unwanted brace should be discontinued.

Minimum duration Duration of bracing is critical to success and acceptance. The effectiveness of bracing to arrest progression of a deformity depends upon two factors: the amount of corrective force applied and the duration this force is applied (based on a 24-hour day). The effectiveness of bracing increases with duration. The psychological and physiological costs also increase with duration. Balancing the benefit and cost is a challenge. Nighttime bracing is least "costly" for the patient because bracing does not interfere with play, is convenient to use, and causes little effect on the child's self-image. The duration of bracing can vary from full-time (allow an hour free), to nighttime, or part-time. Part-time bracing is commonly ordered for 4-, 8-, or 12-hour periods per day. Negotiate with the child to make certain that the precious free hours coincide with the child's priorities, such as school or specific athletic or social activities. This will improve compliance.

Minimal length The longer the brace the greater the disability. Extending braces to the pelvis is seldom necessary. Likewise shoe lifts for leg length inequality may be prescribed that are less that needed to completely level the pelvis. Usually allowing up to 2 cm undercorrection is acceptable to reduce the weight, instability, and unsightly appearance of a higher lift.

Prosthetics

Prosthesis are artificial substitutes for body parts. Most prostheses in children are designed to replace limb deficiencies secondary to congenital, traumatic, or neoplastic problems.

Naming Prostheses

Name the prosthesis based on the level of the deficiency or type of amputation (Fig. 3.97).

Prescribing Prosthesis

Detail each element of the limb (Fig. 3.98).

Special Needs of Children

Children have special prosthetic needs. Children grow, making prosthetic adjustments necessary 3–4 times a year. The prosthesis must be rugged and simple in design. Because multiple limb deficiencies occur in up to 30% of congenital losses and 15% of acquired losses, customized prosthetic management is often necessary.

Age for Fitting

Lower limb Fit lower limb prosthetics when the child first pulls up to stand, about 10 months. Initially the knee may be omitted to keep the limb simple, light, and stable (Fig. 3.99). Delay bilateral amputee fitting a few months.

Upper limb Fitting upper limb deficiencies is controversial. Some fit at about 6 months of age. Others prefer to wait until a need is recognized by the child, which usually occurs in mid-childhood.

Acceptance

Lower limb prostheses are well accepted as they clearly enhance function and appearance (Fig. 3.100). Stability and symmetry required for walking are readily provided by the prosthesis.

Upper limb prostheses are less well accepted. Some find the artificial limb to be a burden without sufficient compensation in improved function to justify the trouble. The lack of sensibility limits function. Children learn to function well with one hand. Children seldom use the prehensile function of upper limb terminal devices. Cosmetic hands are useful in adolescence.

Myoelectric Power

Powered limbs have the advantage of slightly improving appearance but the disadvantages of being more complex, heavier, and slower. The results are mixed.

Consultant Hugh Watts, e-mail: hwatts@ucla.edu

References

1993 Performance comparison among children fitted with myoelectric and body-powered hands. Edelstein JE, Berger N. Arch Phys Med Rehabil 74:376

1993 Myoelectric and body-powered prostheses. Kruger LM, Fishman S. JPO 13:68

1992 Gait analysis in pediatric lower extremity amputees. Ashley RK, Vallier GT, Skinner SR. Orthop Rev 21:745

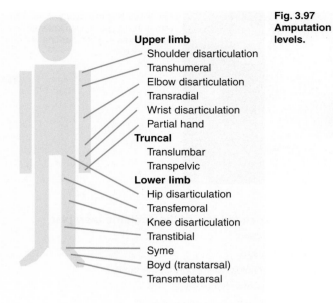

Fig. 3.97 Amputation levels.

Upper limb
- Shoulder disarticulation
- Transhumeral
- Elbow disarticulation
- Transradial
- Wrist disarticulation
- Partial hand

Truncal
- Translumbar
- Transpelvic

Lower limb
- Hip disarticulation
- Transfemoral
- Knee disarticulation
- Transtibial
- Syme
- Boyd (transtarsal)
- Transmetatarsal

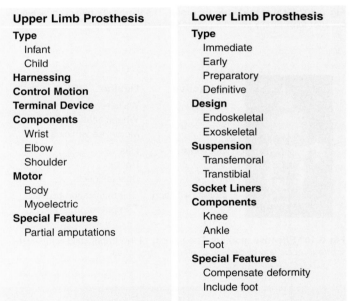

Upper Limb Prosthesis	Lower Limb Prosthesis
Type	**Type**
Infant	Immediate
Child	Early
Harnessing	Preparatory
Control Motion	Definitive
Terminal Device	**Design**
Components	Endoskeletal
Wrist	Exoskeletal
Elbow	**Suspension**
Shoulder	Transfemoral
Motor	Transtibial
Body	**Socket Liners**
Myoelectric	**Components**
Special Features	Knee
Partial amputations	Ankle
	Foot
	Special Features
	Compensate deformity
	Include foot

Fig. 3.98 Prostheses prescription. When ordering prostheses describe each of these features.

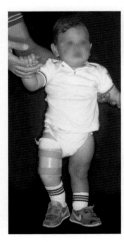

Fig. 3.99 Toddler with nonarticulated prosthesis. First prosthesis.

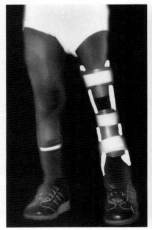

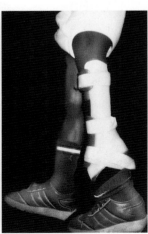

Fig. 3.100 High below knee prosthesis. This boy with tibial deficiency has a short stump with strong quads. He is fully active in sports.

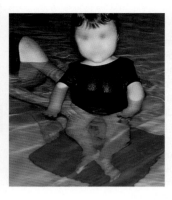

Fig. 3.101 Hydrotherapy. This child with arthrogryposis with knee flexion contractures is given her first walking experience.

Expanded role of the pediatric therapist

Assesses function

Educates family

Provides psychological support for the family

Explores uses of adaptive equipment

Documents management and research

Fig. 3.102 Role of pediatric therapist. The therapist's role is considerably broader than simply providing exercises and manipulation.

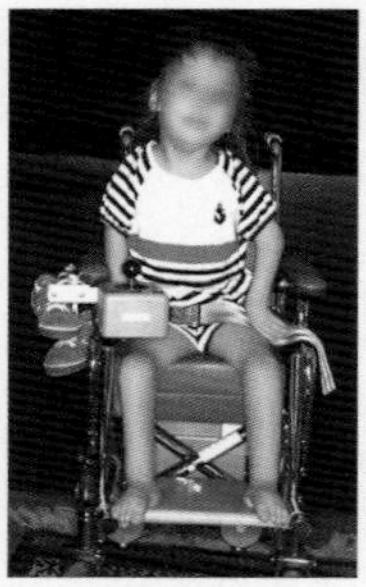

Objective	Device
Mobility	Walkers
	Wheelchairs
	Motorized vehicles
Self-Care	Lifts
	Ramps
	Special toilets
Communication	Communication boards
	Computers

Fig. 3.103 Effective mobility. The mobility of this bright child with severe arthrogryposis is provided by an electric wheelchair.

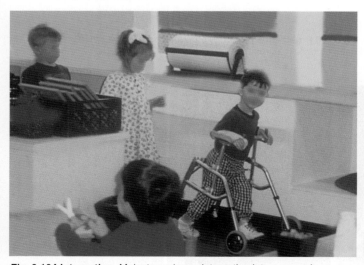

Fig. 3.104 Integration. Mainstreaming or integration into a normal environment is very helpful for social development.

Therapy

Therapy utilizes the treatment methods of physical medicine, including manipulations, exercises (Fig. 3.101), positioning, stimulation, massage, and application of cold and heat. The role of the pediatric therapist is much broader than that of the general therapist, requiring knowledge of growth and development (Fig. 3.102).

The current emphasis on function has improved the effectiveness of therapy programs. Emphasis on effective mobility, independence skills, and communication focuses therapeutic energy and resources on an outcome that optimizes the child's quality of life.

Physical Therapy

In pediatric orthopedics, the primary focus of physical therapy is on lower limb function and mobility.

Effective mobility A child needs independent and efficient mobility (Fig. 3.103). Without this capability, the child's psychosocial and educational experiences are significantly limited. The level of mobility should be appropriate to the child's mental age. The method of mobility is not critical.

Whether mobility is provided by walking or by the use of adaptive equipment (Fig. 3.104), the method of mobility should be manageable by the child himself, conserve the child's energy, and be functionally practical. Options range from the use of an electric wheelchair (Fig. 3.105) to unassisted walking. The objective of management is to provide effective mobility by whatever means necessary while helping the child progress toward a realistic mobility objective. The objective should be an optimistic target within a realistic range. The therapist's accurate appraisal of the child, knowledge of mobility potential for the disease, and periodic assessments of progress help protect the child from disappointment, frustration, and wasted efforts. With time, objectives may change, depending upon the rate of progress.

A major objective of therapy is support and education of the family. Often the family has unrealistic expectations that create an additional burden for the child. The family's major concern is often "Will my child walk?" A better objective would be "Will my child be independent and happy?" Assisting the family and guiding their concepts and expectations is an important role for the therapist.

Infant stimulation programs Helping the parents to interact positively with the child is a vital role of therapy. Parents may be uncomfortable with the infant, and this strained relationship further limits the child. Interactive play therapy, taught to the parents (Fig. 3.106) by the therapist, provides the positive physical contact infants need for optimal emotional and intellectual growth. Infant stimulation programs are effective in promoting cognitive, motor, language, emotional development.

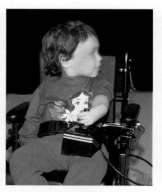

Fig. 3.105 Effective mobility. This electric wheelchair allows this child self determined mobility.

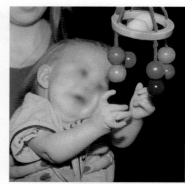

Fig. 3.106 Infant stimulation. This infant is provided play experience which is necessary for intellectual development

Neurodevelopmental therapy Neurodevelopment therapy (NDT) focuses on motor development. NDT is more effective than the original passive treatment methods but is being replaced by therapy with a broader focus.

Accepting disability Accepting the disability and working around it, using adaptive equipment, is often the most effective management strategy for the child. Usually the physician or therapist cannot cure the disease, but can minimize the disability.

Adaptive equipment is useful to help the child become more independent and functional. Adaptive equipment is useful for the child's mobility, self-care skills, and communication, and often enhances care of the child by the caregiver.

Exercises are not very useful for the young child because the child lacks the interest and discipline to perform the exercises. Fortunately, children have little need for exercises, as muscle strength and function usually recover spontaneously. Moreover, assistive or stretching exercises can be harmful. In posttraumatic stiffness, stretching often increases stiffness by adding new injury and scarring. Exercise should not be painful. Exercises take on a variety of forms (Fig. 3.107). Chronic passive motion is a new technique for maintaining joint motion following operative release or injury. The joint is moved slowly and continuously through a range of motion during healing.

Stretching is a traditional treatment for contracture (3.108). Flaccid contractures respond best to stretching. The prolonged effects of spasticity, as in cerebral palsy, cannot be controlled by intermittent stretching. To prevent contracture, the elongated or stretched position must be maintained for about 4 hours in each 24-hour day. This requires bracing or splinting. Stretching beyond the child's pain threshold is not advisable; overstretching causes further injury and scar formation.

Therapy at home, with a parent acting as therapist and the therapist as a consultant, is effective and practical when the family is willing and able. Home therapy programs reduce stress on the family by making the treatment more convenient and less expensive. The therapy can often be incorporated into the daily routines, increasing frequency and improving outcomes. Home therapy may also have a bonding effect on the family. This requires parent education and periodic visits to the therapist to assess technique and progress.

Treatments of doubtful value include massage, thermotherapy, injections, and diathermy. These "treatments" are not helpful in pediatric orthopedics.

Occupational Therapy

Occupational therapy focuses on upper extremity function (Fig. 3.109) and activities of daily living (Fig. 3.110), including independence skills and correction of deformity (Fig. 3.111). This aspect of therapy plays a broad role in managing childhood disabilities because modern management places greater emphasis on assessment and self-care skills. Physical and occupational therapists often work together, especially for children with long-term disabilities, as part of a management team.

Self-care skills are taught to increase independence in feeding, dressing, and toileting. Self-care can be achieved by learning special techniques from the therapist, using adaptive equipment, or making the environment more easily livable for the child. Independence learned in childhood enhances the individual's self-respect and happiness and reduces the burden for the family and the costs for society.

Consultant Sharon DeMuth, e-mail: demuth@hsc.usc.edu

References

1998 Physical and occupational therapy. Watts HG, DeMuth SK. Pediatric orthopedic Secrets. Philadelphia, Hanley & Belfus

1997 A comparison of intensive neurodevelopmental therapy plus casting and a regular occupational therapy program for children with cerebral palsy. Law M, et al. Dev Med Child Neurol 39:664

Form	Indication
Isotonic	Contraction through an arc
Isometric	Static contraction
Active Range of Motion	Maximum range of motion by patient unassisted
Assistive Range	Therapist-assisted maximum range of motion

Fig. 3.107 Forms of exercises for children. Several forms of exercise are available. Passive exercise that causes pain is contraindicated in children, as it often increases stiffness by injuring the joint.

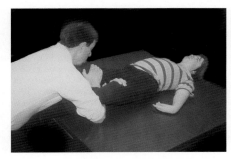

Fig. 3.108 Stretching. Stretching exercises should be done carefully to avoid fractures and causing pain.

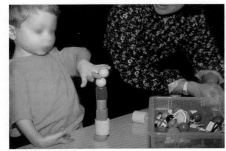

Fig. 3.109 Occupational therapy. Teaching families how to provide play activities for each child is essential for development.

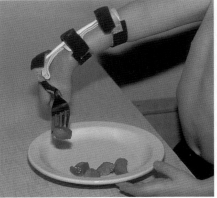

Fig. 3.110 Adaptive equipment. Selection or development of special devices to facilitate activities of daily living is very valuable in developing independence.

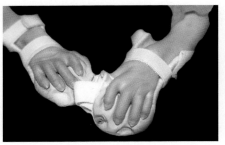

Fig. 3.111 Hand splints. These resting splints are invaluable in preventing recurrence of deformity in children with muscle imbalance, burns, or following surgery.

Abraham E. Remodeling potential of long bones following angular osteotomies. J Pediatr Orthop 1989;9:37-43.

American Academy of Orthopaedic Surgeons. Sports and recreational programs for the child and young adult with physical disability. Proceedings of the Winter Park Seminar, Winter Park, CO, April 11-13 1983, pp 883-993.

American Academy of Pediatrics. The Dorman-Delacato treatment of neurologically handicapped children: Policy statement. Pediatrics 1982;70:810-812.

Angel JD, Blasier RD, Allison R. Postoperative fever in pediatric orthopaedic patients. JPOa 1994;14:799.

Armstrong PF, Brighton CT. Failure of the rabbit tibial growth plate to respond to long-term application of a capacitively coupled electrical field. J Orthop Res 1986;4:446.

Bailey R, Dubow H. Evolution of the concept of an extensible nail accommodating to normal longitudinal bone growth: Clinical considerations and implications. Clin Orthop 1981; 159:157-171.

Birmingham PK, RM Dsida, JJ Grayhack, J Han, M Wheeler, JA Pongracic, CJ Cote and SC Hall Do latex precautions in children with myelodysplasia reduce intraoperative allergic reactions? J Pediatr Orthop 1996; 16:799-802.

Bleck EE. Severe orthopedic disability in childhood: Solutions provided by rehabilitation engineering. Orthop Clin North Am 1978; 9:509-28.

Breed A, Ibler I. The motorized wheelchair: New freedom, new responsibility and new problems. Dev Med Child Neurol 1982;24:366-371.

Brodke DS, Skinner SR, Lamoreux LW, et al. Effects of ankle-foot orthoses on the gait of children. J Pediatr Orthop 1989;9:702-708.

Brown K ,et al. Epiphysial growth after free fibular transfer with and without microvascular anastomosis. Experimental study in the dog. J Bone Joint Surg [Br] 1983;65:493.

Bull MJ, Weber K, DeRosa GP, et al. Transporting children in body casts. J Pediatr Orthop 1989;9:280-284.

Butler C, Okamoto GA, McKay TM. Motorized wheelchair driving by disabled children. Arch Phys Med Rehabil 1984;65:95.

Butler P, et al. Physiological cost index of walking for normal children and its use as an indicator of physical handicap. Dev Med Child Neurol 1984;26:607.

Carlson JM, Winter R. The "Gillette" sitting support orthosis. Orthotics Prosthetics 1978;32(4):35-45.

Chicarilli ZN. Pediatric microsurgery: Revascularization and replantation. J Pediatr Surg 1986;21:706.

Cole PA, Ehrlich MG. Management of completely stiff pediatric knee. JPOa 1997;17:67.

Connolly JF, et al. Epiphyseal traction to correct acquired growth deformities. Clin Orthop 1986;302:258.

DeCurtis M, et al. Gangrene of the buttock: A devastating complication of the infusion of hyperosmolar solutions in the umbilical artery at birth. Eur J Pediatr 1985;144:261.

Dietz FR, Weinstein SL. Spike osteotomy for angular deformities of the long bones in children. J Bone Joint Surg 1988;70:848.

Driano AN, Staheli LR, Staheli LT. Psychosocial development and corrective shoewear use in children. J. Pediatr Ortho 1998; 18:346.

Fischer AQ, Strasburger J. Footdrop in the neonate secondary to use of footboards. J Pediatr Orthop 1982;101:1033.

Forster RS, Fu FH. Reflex sympathetic dystrophy in children. A case report and review of literature. Orthopedics 1985;8:475.

Foulk DA; Boakes J; Rab GT; Schulman S The use of caudal epidural anesthesia in clubfoot surgery. J Pediatr Orthop 1995 Sep-Oct; 15 (5):604-7

Frimodt-Moller N, Riegels-Nielson P. Antibiotic penetration into the infected knee: A rabbit experiment. Acta Orthop Scand 1987;58:256.

Gould N. Shoes versus sneakers in toddler ambulation. Foot Ankle 1985;6:105.

Greene WB. Use of continuous passive slow motion in the postoperative rehabilitation of difficult pediatric knee and elbow problems. J Pediatr Orthop 1983;3:419-423.

Guidera KJ, Hontas R, Ogden JA. Use of continuous passive motion in pediatric orthopedics. J Pediatr Orthop 1990;10:120-123.

Hamdan JA, Taleb YA, Ahmed MS. Traction-induced hypertension in children. Clin Orthop 1984;185:87.

Hoffer MM, Feiwell E, Perry LR, et al. Functional ambulation in patients with myelomeningocele. J Bone Joint Surg 1973;55A:137-148.

Hoffer MM, Koffman M. Cerebral palsy: The first three years. Clin Orthop 1980;151:222-227.

Holzman RS Clinical management of latex-allergic children. Anesth Analg 1997; 85:529-33.

Jones KL, Robinson LK. An approach to the child with structural defects. J Pediatr Orthop 1983;3:238-244.

Kanda T, Yuge M, Yamori Y, et al. Early physiotherapy in the treatment of spastic diplegia. Dev Med Child Neurol 1984;26:438-444.

Knittel G, Staheli LT. The effectiveness of shoe modifications for intoeing. Orthop Clin North Am 1976;7:1019-1025.

Kokki H; Hendolin H Comparison of spinal anaesthesia with epidural anaesthesia in paediatric surgery. Acta Anaesthesiol Scand 1995 Oct; 39 (7): p896-900

Leslie I et al. A prospective study of deep vein thrombosis of the leg in children on halo-femoral traction. J Bone Joint Surg [Br] 1981;63:168-170.

Lynn AM et al. Systemic responses to tourniquet release in children. Anesth Analg 1986;65:865.

Maisami M, Freeman JM. Conversion reactions in children as body language: A combined child psychiatry/neurology team approach to the management of functional neurologic disorders in children. Pediatrics 1987;80:46.

McCall RE, Schmidt WT. Clinical experience with the reciprocal gait orthosis in myelodysplasia. J Pediatr Orthop 1986;6:157-161.

McGill SM, Dainty DA. Computer analysis of energy transfers in children walking with crutches. Arch Phys Med Rehabil 1984;65:115.

McGrath PJ, et al. Assistive devices: Utilization by children. Arch Phys Med Rehabil 1985;66:430.

Meyer S, Gordon RL, Robin GC. The pathogenesis of neurovascular complications following penicillin injection. J Pediatr Orthop 1981;1:215-218.

Nather A, Balasubramaniam P, Bose K. A comparative study of different methods of tendon lengthening: An experimental study in rabbits. J Pediatr Orthop 1986;6:456-459.

O'Hara M, McGrath PJ, D'Astous J, et al. Oral morphine versus injected meperidine (Demerol) for pain relief in children after orthopedic surgery. J Pediatr Orthop 1987;7:78-82.

Palmer FB, Shapiro BK, Wachtel RC, et al. The effects of physical therapy on cerebral palsy: A controlled trial in infants with spastic diplegia. N Engl J Med 1988;318:803-808.

Parette HP Jr, Houcade JJ. A review of therapeutic intervention research on gross and fine motor progress in young children with cerebral palsy. Am J Occup Ther 1984;38:462-468.

Rang M, Douglas G, Bennet GC, et al. Seating for children with cerebral palsy. J Pediatr Orthop 1981;1:279-287.

Respet PJ, Kleinman PG, Meinhard BP. Pin tract infections: A canine model. J Orthop Res 1987;5:600.

Rose GK, Sankarankutty M, Stallar J. A clinical review of the orthotic treatment of myelomeningocele patients. J Bone Joint Surg 1983;65B:242-246.

Rose J, Gamble JG, Medeiros J, et al. Energy cost of walking in normal children and in those with cerebral palsy: Comparison of heart rate and oxygen uptake. J Pediatr Orthop 1989;71A:276-279.

Rose J, Medeiros JM, Parker R. Energy cost index as an estimate of energy expenditure of cerebral-palsied children during assisted ambulation. Dev Med Child Neurol 1985;27:485-490.

Rosenthal RK. The use of orthotics in foot and ankle problems in cerebral palsy. Foot Ankle 1984;4:195-200.

Salter RB. The biologic concept of continuous passive motion of synovial joints. The first 18 years of basic research and its clinical application. Clin Orthop 1989;242:12.

Salter RB et al. Clinical application of basic research on continuous passive motion for disorders and injuries of synovial joints: A preliminary report of a feasibility study. J Orthop Res 1984;1:325.

Safavi FZ. Chapter 14 Anesthesia in Pediatric Orthopedic Secrets 1998 Hanley & Belfus, Staheli LT, editor.

Seibert JJ, et al. Acquired bone dysplasia secondary to catheter-related complications in the neonate. Pediatr Radiol 1986:16:43.

Short DL, Schade JK, Herring JA. Parent involvement in physical therapy: A controversial issue. J Pediatr Orthop 1989;9:444-446.

Simmons DJ, et al. The effect of protracted tetracycline treatment on bone growth and maturation. Clin Orthop 1983;180:253.

Spencer GE Jr, Vignos PJ Jr. Bracing for ambulation in childhood progressive muscular dystrophy. J Bone Joint Surg 1962;44A:234-242.

Staheli LT. Shoes for children: A review. Pediatrics 1991;88:371-375.

Staheli LT. Lower positional deformity in infants and children: A review. J Pediatr Orthop 1990;10:559-563.

Staheli LT. Philosophy of care. Pediatr Clin North Am 1986;33:1269-1275.

Stefanini M. Disseminated intravascular coagulation. How to recognize an insidious culprit. Modern Medicine; Feb 18, 1974: p.31.

Strain JD, et al. Intravenously administered pentobarbital sodium for sedation in pediatric CT. Radiology 1986;161:105.

Tardieu C, Lespargot A, Tabary C, et al. For how long must the soleus muscle be stretched each day to prevent contracture? Dev Med Child Neurol 1988;30:3.

Taylor D. Counseling the parents of handicapped children. Br Med J 1982;284:1027-1028.

Timberlake RW, Cook SD, Thomas KA, et al. Effects of anticonvulsant drug therapy on bone mineral density in a pediatric population. J Pediatr Orthop 1988;8:467-470.

Todd FN, Lamoreux LW, Skinner SR, et al. Variations in the gait of normal children: A graph applicable to the documentation of abnormalities. J Bone Joint Surg 1989;71A:196-204.

Chapter 4 – Lower Limb

This chapter covers problems of one or more lower limb segments and includes some of the most common problems in children's orthopedics (Figs. 4.1 and 4.2).

Leg Aches

Leg aches or growing pains, are idiopathic, benign discomfort of extremities, which occur in 15–30% of children. The pains are most common in girls, usually occur at night, and primarily affect the lower limbs. The condition produces no functional disability or objective signs and resolves spontaneously without residual. The cause is unknown. Undocumented speculation on cause includes genetic, functional, or structural (hypermobility) etiology. Leg aches follow headaches and stomach aches as the most common sites of pain during childhood.

Clinical Features

The differential diagnosis of leg aches includes most of the painful conditions involving the musculoskeletal system in children. The diagnosis is made by exclusion (Fig. 4.3).

    History The pain from leg aches is typically vague, poorly localized, bilateral, nocturnal, and seldom alters activity. This condition does not affect gait or general health. A history of long duration is most consistent with the diagnosis of leg aches. This long duration is helpful in separating out more serious problems, which over a period of time will usually produce objective findings.

    Screening examination Does the child appear systemically ill? Is deformity or stiffness present? Does the child limp?

    Tenderness Systematically palpate the limbs and trunk for tenderness.

    Joint motion Is joint motion guarded or restricted? Check for symmetry of medial rotation of hips.

Differential Diagnosis

Night pain may also be due to a tumor, such as ostoid osteoma, osteogenic, or Ewing sarcomas. Tumor pain is more localized, often associated with a soft tissue mass, progressive, and usually occurs later in childhood than growing pains.

Management

If the history is atypical for leg aches or signs are found on examination, imaging and laboratory studies are required. If the findings are negative, a presumptive diagnosis of growing pains or leg aches is made. Provide symptomatic treatment with heat and an analgesic. Reassure the family about the benign, self-limited course of the condition, but advise them that if the clinical features change, the child should be reevaluated.

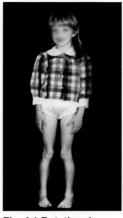

Fig. 4.1 Rotational deformity. This girl has medial femoral torsion. Note the medial rotation of the patellae.

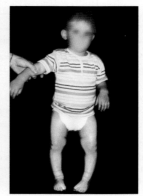

Fig. 4.2 Physiologic bowing. This symmetrical bowing is typical of this benign form of bowing.

Feature	Growing Pain	Serious Problem
History		
Long duration	Often	Usually not
Pain localized	No	Often
Pain bilateral	Often	Unusual
Alters activity	No	Often
Causes limp	No	Sometimes
General health	Good	May be ill
Physical Examination		
Tenderness	No	May show
Guarding	No	May show
Reduced range of motion	No	May show
Laboratory		
CBC	Normal	± Abnormal
ESR	Normal	± Abnormal

Fig. 4.3 Differentiating growing pains from more serious problems. The features of growing pains are usually so characteristic that special studies are seldom required.

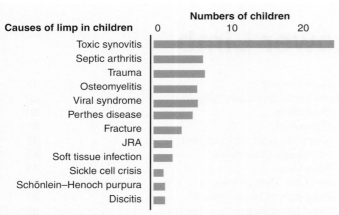

Causes of limp in children

Numbers of children

| | 0 | 10 | 20 |

- Toxic synovitis
- Septic arthritis
- Trauma
- Osteomyelitis
- Viral syndrome
- Perthes disease
- Fracture
- JRA
- Soft tissue infection
- Sickle cell crisis
- Schönlein–Henoch purpura
- Discitis

Fig. 4.4 Causes of limp in 60 young children. Data from Choban and Killian (1990).

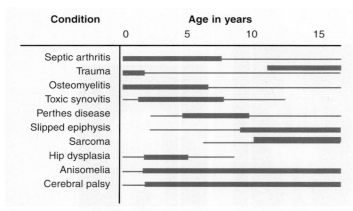

Fig. 4.5 Causes of limp by age. The causes of limp are related to the age of the child. The fine red lines show the range and the heavy lines the most common age range of involvement.

Limp

A limp is an abnormal gait that is commonly due to pain, weakness, or deformity. A limp is a significant finding and the cause should be established (Fig. 4.4).

Evaluation

A presumptive diagnosis can usually be made by the history and physical examination. Age is an important factor to consider during evaluation.

History First inquire about the onset (Fig. 4.5). When was the limp first noted? Was the onset associated with an injury or illness? Was it gradual or abrupt? If the limp has been present since infancy, inquire about developmental history, because children with neuromuscular disorders have delayed motor development.

Observation The type of limp can usually be determined by observation. Remove outer clothing to allow the full view of the legs. Watch the child walk in the hallway of the clinic (Fig. 4.6). Observe in three phases: (1) Overview. Look for obvious abnormalities. Which side seems abnormal? Is the stance phase on each side equal in duration? Is lateral shoulder sway present? Is circumduction seen? (2) Study each leg *individually*. Look for more subtle changes. Is the normal heel-to-toe gait pattern present? Does the knee approach full extension during stance phase? How is the hand carried? Elevation of the arm is seen in hemiplegia. (3) Make a presumptive diagnosis, and then make a final observation to be certain that this diagnosis is consistent with the characteristics of the limp.

Types of Limps

The common types of limping may be classified into four groups (Fig. 4.7). The hip is the most common site for the problem (4.8).

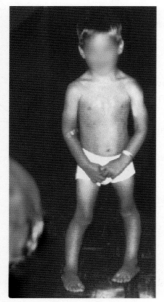

Fig. 4.6 Hallway observation. Evaluate the limp by studying the child's gait while the child walks in the clinic hallway.

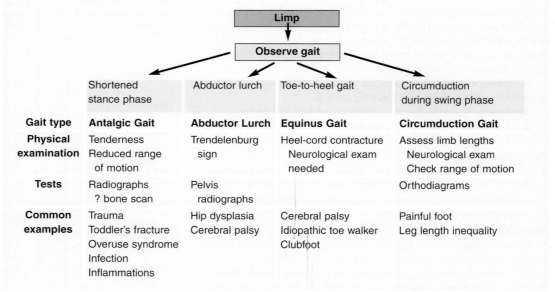

	Limp			
	Observe gait			
	Shortened stance phase	Abductor lurch	Toe-to-heel gait	Circumduction during swing phase
Gait type	**Antalgic Gait**	**Abductor Lurch**	**Equinus Gait**	**Circumduction Gait**
Physical examination	Tenderness Reduced range of motion	Trendelenburg sign	Heel-cord contracture Neurological exam needed	Assess limb lengths Neurological exam Check range of motion
Tests	Radiographs ? bone scan	Pelvis radiographs		Orthodiagrams
Common examples	Trauma Toddler's fracture Overuse syndrome Infection Inflammations	Hip dysplasia Cerebral palsy	Cerebral palsy Idiopathic toe walker Clubfoot	Painful foot Leg length inequality

Fig. 4.7 Algorithm for evaluation of limping. The major causes of limping are shown. A general categorization is first possible by observation. The exact causes are established by the physical examination and laboratory studies.

Antalgic limp This is a painful limp. The most prominent feature is a shortened stance phase on the affected side. To minimize discomfort, the time of weight bearing on the affected side is shortened. The child is said to "favor" one side or the other. The term "favor" is ambiguous because it may be used to describe either the affected or unaffected side. Find the anatomic location of the problem by determining the site of tenderness, joint guarding, or limitation of motion. Follow-up with radiographs. Often a CBC and ESR or CRP are helpful. If the radiographs are negative, order a bone scan to localize the problem (Figs. 4.9 and 4.10).

Equinus gait An equinus gait is due to a heel-cord contracture, which is usually due to cerebral palsy, residual clubfoot deformity, or idiopathic heel-cord tightness. Regardless of the etiology, the contracture causes a "toe-to-heel" sequence during stance phase on the affected side. In the young child, equinus is often associated with a "back knee" or recurvatum deformity of the knee that occurs during stance phase. Document the deformity by evaluating the range of dorsiflexion of the ankle with the knee extended. The ankle should dorsiflex more than 10°. If an equinus deformity is present, a thorough neurological examination is required.

Abductor lurch results from weakness of the abductor muscles, usually due to hip dysplasia or a neuromuscular disorder. An abductor lurch is characterized by lateral shoulder sway toward the affected side or sides. In normal gait, the abductor muscles contract during stance phase to maintain a level pelvis and a linear progression of the center of gravity of the body. If the abductors are weak, during stance, the pelvis tilts and falls on the unsupported side. To maintain the center of gravity over the foot, the shoulder shifts toward the weak side. This shift is referred to as an *abductor lurch* or a *Trendelenburg gait*. Weakness of the abductors is demonstrated by the Trendelenburg test or sign. The test is positive if the pelvis drops on the unsupported side during single leg standing. The cause of the abductor lurch is usually established by a standing radiograph of the pelvis and a neurological examination.

Circumduction allows a functionally longer limb to progress forward during swing phase. Circumduction is often due to a painful condition about the foot or ankle because circumduction requires less ankle movement, making walking more comfortable.

Management

The limp may be caused by something as simple as a stone in the shoe, or by something as serious as leukemia or osteogenic sarcoma. Thus, generalizations regarding management cannot be made. Sometimes the cause of the limp cannot be determined. Should the diagnosis be unclear, reevaluate the child weekly until the problem resolves or a diagnosis is established.

References

2000 Transient synovitis as a cause of painful limps in children. Do TT. Curr Opin Pediatr 12:48

1999 The limping child: epidemiology, assessment and outcome. Fischer SU, Beattie TF. JBJS 81B:1029

1999 Are growing pains a myth? Manners P. Aust Fam Physician 28:124

1998 Assessing the limping child with skeletal scintigraphy. Connolly LP, Treves ST. J Nucl Med 39:1056

1998 The limping child. Lawrence LL. Emerg Med Clin North Am 16:911

1996 Variability in physicians' reported ordering and perceived reassurance value of diagnostic tests in children with "growing pains." Macarthur C, et al. Arch Pediatr Adolesc Med 150:1072

1996 Occult fracture of the calcaneus in toddlers. Schindler A, et al. JPO 16:201

1995 Fracture of the cuboid in children. A source of leg symptoms. Simonian PT, et al. JBJS 77B:104

1992 Efficiency of the bone scan for occult limping toddlers. Aronson J, et al. JPO 12:38

1990 Evaluation of acute gait abnormalities in preschool children. Choban S, Killian JT. JPO 10:74

1985 The cause of gait disturbance in 425 pediatric patients. Singer JI. Pediatr Emerg Care 1:7

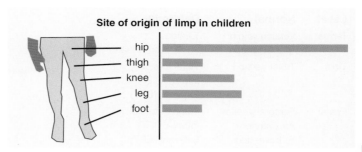

Site of origin of limp in children

Fig. 4.8 Origin of limp in 60 young children. Data from Choban and Killian (1990).

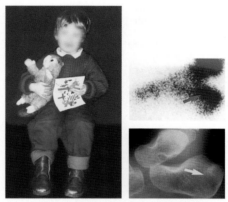

Fig. 4.9 Role of bone scan in limp evaluation. This child had an antalgic limp with a negative physical examination, radiographs, and ESR. The bone scan showed increased uptake over the calcaneus (red arrow). This suggested a stress injury to the calcaneus. This was confirmed by a radiograph 2 weeks later showing evidence of a stress fracture (yellow arrow). The child had been stressed by being taken on long walks in a shopping mall.

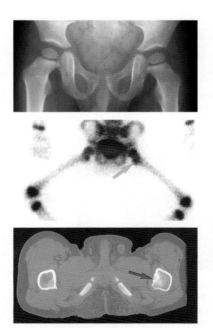

Fig. 4.10 Obscure limp from osteomyelitis. This 2-year-old complained of night pain and showed a subtle limp during the day. Radiographs were negative, the bone scan showed slight increased uptake in the upper femur (orange arrow). CT scan demonstrated an intracortical defect (red arrow). The differentiation from ostoid osteomy was made by a resolution with antibiotic treatment.

Level	Normal	Deformity
Terms	Version within ± 2 SD mean	Torsion >2 SD from mean
Tibia	Tibial version	Tibial torsion Internal (ITT) External (ETT)
Femur	Femoral version Anteversion Retroversion	Femoral torsion Internal (IFT) External (EFT)

Fig. 4.11 Terminology of rotational variations. Normal variations and deformity are described by different terms.

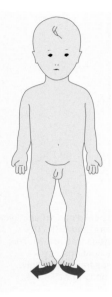

Fig. 4.12 Lower limb laterally rotates with age (left). Both the femur and tibia laterally rotate with growth. Femoral anteversion declines and tibial version becomes more lateral.

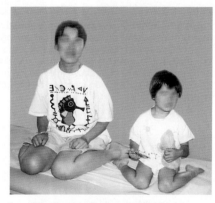

Fig. 4.13 Internal femoral torsion affecting mother and child (right). Often evaluation of the parent reveals a rotational pattern similar to that present in the child.

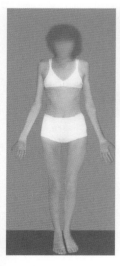

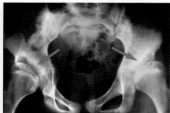

Fig. 4.14 Asymmetrical hip rotation requires further evaluation. This 12-year-old girl was seen for in-toeing. The rotational profile was abnormal, showing asymmetry of hip rotation. A radiograph of the pelvis showed severe bilateral hip dysplasia (arrows). Operative correction of the hip dysplasia was performed.

Torsion

Torsional problems, in-toeing, and out-toeing often concern parents and frequently prompt a variety of treatments for the child. Management of torsional problems is facilitated by clear terminology, an accurate diagnosis, a knowledge of the natural history of torsional deformity, and an understanding of the effectiveness of management options.

Terminology

Version describes normal variations in limb rotation (Fig. 4.11). Tibial version is the angular difference between the axis of the knee and the transmalleolar axis. The normal tibia is laterally rotated. Femoral version is the angular difference between the transcervical and transcondylar axes. The normal femur is anteverted.

Torsion describes version beyond ± 2 standard deviations (SD) from the mean and is considered abnormal and described as a "deformity." Internal femoral torsion (IFT) or antetorsion and external femoral torsion, (EFT) or retrotorsion describe abnormal femoral rotation. Internal tibial torsion (ITT) and external tibial torsion (ETT) describe abnormal tibial rotation.

Torsional deformity may be simple, involving one level, or complex, involving multiple segments. Complex deformities may be additive or compensating. Thus, internal tibial torsion and internal femoral torsion are additive. External tibial torsion and internal femoral torsion are compensatory.

Normal Development

The lower limb rotates medially during the seventh fetal week to bring the great toe to the midline. With growth, femoral anteversion declines from about 30° at birth and to about 10° at maturity (Fig. 4.12). Values for anteversion are higher in the female and in some families (Fig. 4.13). With growth, the tibia laterally rotates from about 5° at birth to a mean of 15° at maturity. Because growth is associated with lateral rotation in both the femoral and tibial segments, medial tibial torsion and femoral antetorsion in children improve with time. In contrast, lateral tibial torsion usually worsens with growth.

Evaluation

While the diagnosis of torsional deformities can be made by the physical examination, the history is helpful in excluding other problems and assessing extent of disability.

History Inquire about the onset, severity, disability, and previous treatment of the problem. Obtain a developmental history. A delay in walking may suggest a neuromuscular disorder. Is there a family history of a rotational problem? Often rotational problems are inherited and the status of the parent foretells the child's future.

Screening examination Screen to rule out hip dysplasia and neurological problems such as cerebral palsy.

Rotational profile The rotational profile provides the information necessary to establish the level and severity of any torsional problem. See the larger charts on page 419. Record the values in degrees for both right and left sides. Evaluate in four steps:

1. Observe the child walking and running. Estimate the *foot progression angle (FPA)* during walking (Fig. 4.15). This is the angular difference between the axis of the foot and the line of progression. This value is usually estimated by observing the child walking in the clinic hallway. The average degree of in-toeing or out-toeing is estimated. A minus value is assigned to an in-toeing gait. In-toeing of –5° to –10° is mild, –10° to –15° moderate, and more than –15° severe (Fig. 4.13). Ask the child to run. The child with femoral antetorsion may show an "eggbeater" running pattern with the legs flipping laterally during swing phase.

2. Assess femoral version by measuring hip rotation (Fig. 4.16). Measure external (ER) and internal rotation (IR) with the child prone, the knees flexed to a right angle and the pelvis level. Assess both sides at the same time. Internal rotation is normally less than 60°–70°. If hip rotation is asymmetrical, evaluate with a radiograph (Fig. 4.14).

3. Quantitate tibial version by assessing the *thigh-foot angle* (Fig. 4.18). With the child prone and the knee flexed to a right angle, the TFA is the angular difference between the axis of the foot and the axis of the thigh. The TFA measures the tibial and hindfoot rotational status. The TMA is the angular difference between the transmalleolar axis and the axis of the thigh. This is a measure of tibial rotation. The difference between the TMA and the TFA is a measure of hindfoot rotation. The normal range of both the TFA and TMA is broad, and the mean values increase with advancing age. For these measurements, positioning of the foot is critical. Allow the foot to fall into a natural position. Avoid manual positioning of the foot as this is likely to cause errors in assessment.

4. Assess the foot for forefoot adductus. The lateral border of the foot is normally straight. Convexity of the lateral border and forefoot adduction are features of metatarsus adductus. An everted foot or flat-foot may contribute to out-toeing. Include both in the rotational profile.

From the screening examination and rotational profile establish the cause of the torsional deformity (Fig. 4.17).

Special Studies

Order special imaging studies if hip rotation is asymmetrical or if the rotational problem is so severe that operative correction is being considered. In general, special imaging to document rotational problems is not very useful. Before operative correction, image severe antetorsion to rule out hip dysplasia and to measure the degree of femoral antetorsion. Measurements can be made by CT scans or biplane radiographs. Usually antetorsion exceeds 50° in children whose condition is severe enough to require operative correction.

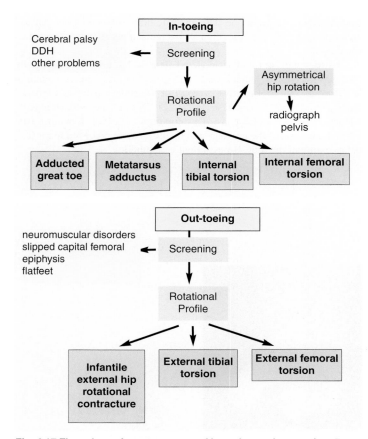

Fig. 4.17 Flow-charts for assessment of in-toeing and out-toeing. By the screening examination and the rotational profile, the diagnosis can usually be readily established.

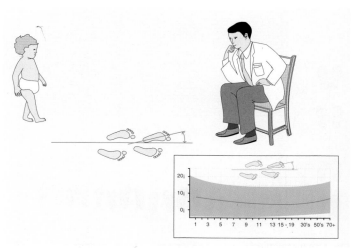

Fig. 4.15 Foot progression angle. Foot progression angle is estimated by observing the child walking. The normal range is shown in green.

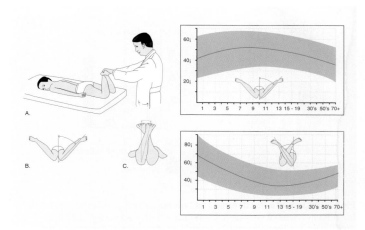

Fig. 4.16 Hip rotation. (A) Hip rotation is assessed with the child prone. **(B)** Internal rotation and **(C)** external rotation are measured. Normal ranges are shown in green.

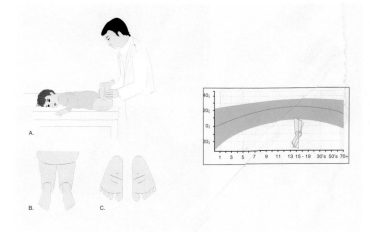

Fig. 4.18 Assessing rotational status of tibia and foot. The rotational status of the tibia and foot are best assessed by evaluating the child in the prone position (A) allowing the foot to fall into a natural resting position. (B) The thigh-foot axis and (C) shape of the foot are readily determined. The range of normal is shown in green.

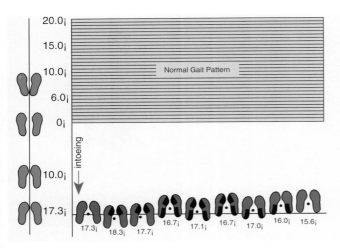

Fig. 4.19 Ineffectiveness of shoe wedges. Various wedges were placed (shown in black). Mean values for intoeing for each wedge are shown compared with the unwedged controls. Redrawn from Knittle and Staheli (1976).

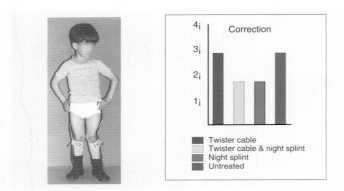

Fig. 4.20 Lack of effectiveness of twister cables. The chart compares the effectiveness of various "treatments" and the untreated child with antetorsion. These interventions made no difference in the measured femoral anteversion before and after treatment. From Fabry et al. (1973).

Management Principles

The first step is establishing a correct diagnosis. In managing rotational problems, the most common management challenge is dealing effectively with the family. Because the lower limbs laterally rotate with time, in-toeing spontaneously corrects in the vast majority of children. Thus, simply waiting to allow this spontaneous resolution is best for the child. Attempting to control the child's walking, sitting, or sleeping positions is impossible. Such attempts only create frustration and conflict between the child and parent.

Shoe wedges or inserts are ineffective (Fig. 4.19). Likewise, daytime bracing with twister cables only limits the child's walking and running activities (Fig. 4.20). Night splints that laterally rotate the feet are better tolerated and do not interfere with the child's play, but probably have no long-term benefit.

Thus, observational management is best. The family needs to be convinced that only observation is appropriate. This requires careful evaluation, education, reassurance, and follow-up. The family should be informed that only rarely does a torsional problem persist. Less than 1% of femoral and tibial torsional deformities fail to resolve and may require operative correction in late childhood. The need for rotational osteotomy is rare and the procedure is effective.

Infant

Out-toeing may be due to flatfeet with heel valgus or more commonly due to a lateral rotation contracture of the hips. In-toeing may be due to an adducted great toe, forefoot adductus, or internal tibial torsion.

Lateral hip rotational contracture Because the hips are laterally rotated *in utero*, lateral hip rotation is normal. When the infant is positioned upright, the feet may turn out (Fig. 4.21). This may worry the parents. Often only one foot turns out, usually the right. The turned out foot is the more normal one. The opposite limb, the one that is considered normal by the parents, often shows metatarsus adductus or medial tibial torsion.

Adducted great toe The adducted great toe has been described both as a spastic abductor hallucis and as a "searching toe." This is a dynamic deformity due to a relative overpull of the abductor hallucis muscle that occurs during stance phase (Fig. 4.22). This may be associated with adduction of the metatarsals. The condition resolves spontaneously when maturation of the nervous system allows more precision in muscle balance around the foot. No treatment is required.

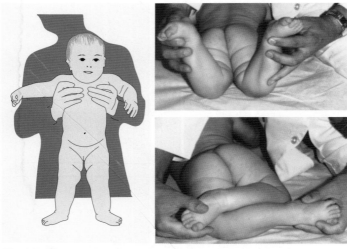

Fig. 4.21 Physiologic infantile out-toeing. Out-toeing in early infancy is usually due to a lateral rotation contracture of the hips. In this infant, medial rotation is limited to about 30° (upper photograph), whereas lateral rotation is about 80° (lower photograph). This results in a lateral rotation of the limb (drawing), which resolves spontaneously.

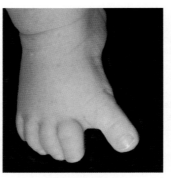

Fig. 4.22 Searching toe. This is a dynamic deformity due to overactivity of the abductor hallucis muscle.

Forefoot adductus describes a spectrum of foot deformities characterized by a medial deviation of the forefoot of different degrees (Fig. 4.23). The prognosis is clearly related to stiffness. The condition is detailed in the next chapter.

Metatarsus adductus Flexible deformities are deformations that occur from intrauterine crowding. Like other deformations, they resolve spontaneously with time. Most resolve within the first year and the rest over childhood. Manage with observation and reassurance. If the deformity persists after the second year, resolution may be hastened with bracing that holds the foot abducted and the leg laterally rotated.

Metatarsus varus Rigid forefoot adductus tends to persist. The deformity is characterized by stiffness and a crease on the sole of the foot. The natural history is for incomplete spontaneous resolution. The deformity produces no functional disability and is not the cause of bunions. It produces a cosmetic problem, and when severe, a problem with shoe fitting. Be sure to distinguish the rare skewfoot. Recall that the skewfoot occurs in loose-jointed children and is characterized by marked forefoot adductus and hindfoot valgus. Most parents want the deformity corrected. As described on page 98, correct by long-leg braces or casts (Fig. 4.24).

Toddler

In-toeing is most common during the second year, usually noticed when the infant begins to walk. This in-toeing is due to internal tibial torsion, metatarsus adductus, or an adducted great toe.

Internal tibial torsion Internal tibial torsion (ITT) is the most common cause of in-toeing. ITT is often bilateral (Fig. 4.25). Unilateral ITT is most common on the left side (Fig. 4.26). Observational management is best. Fillauer or Denis Browne night splints are commonly prescribed, but probably have no long-term value with resolution occurring with or without treatment (Fig. 4.27). Avoid daytime bracing and shoe modifications because they can slow the child's running and may harm the child's self-image.

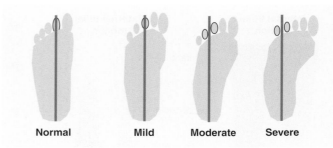

Fig. 4.23 Grading severity of forefoot adductus. Project a line that bisects the heel. **Normally** it falls on the 2nd toe. The projected line falls through the toe 3 in **mild**, between toes 3–4 in **moderate,** and between toes 4–5 in **severe** deformity. From Bleck (1983).

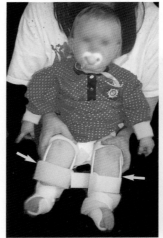
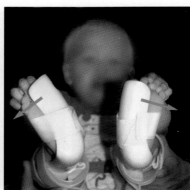

Fig. 4.24 Metatarsis varus. Stiff or persisting deformity can be corrected with long-leg splints (yellow arrows) that abduct the forefoot (red arrows).

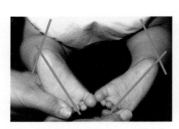

Fig. 4.28 Bilateral internal tibial torsion. The thigh-foot angled are negative (red lines) for both legs.

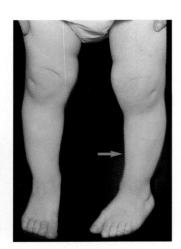

Fig. 4.29 Unilateral internal tibial torsion. Medial tibial torsion is often asymmetrical, usually worse on the left side (arrow).

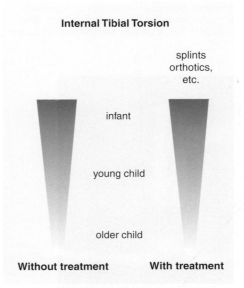

Internal Tibial Torsion

splints orthotics, etc.

infant

young child

older child

Without treatment   **With treatment**

Fig. 4.30 Management of internal tibial torsion. Management with or without intervention gives the same excellent results.

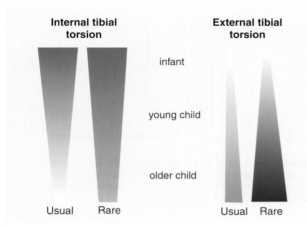

Fig. 4.28 Comparison of natural history of internal and external tibial torsion. As the tibia laterally rotates with growth, internal torsion improves and external torsion may worsen. Torsion severe enough to require tibial rotational osteotomy is more common with lateral torsional deformities.

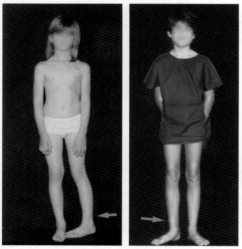

Fig. 4.29 Persisting tibial torsion. Rotational deformities do not always resolve with time. These girls show persisting tibial torsion (arrows), which caused enough disability to require tibial rotational osteotomy for correction.

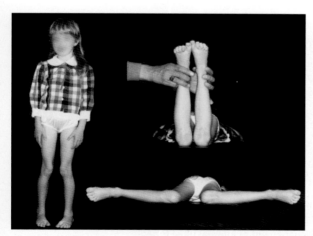

Fig. 4.30 Medial femoral torsion. This girl has medial femoral torsion. Her patella face inward on standing. Her lateral rotation is 0° (upper) and her internal rotation is 90° (lower).

Child

In-toeing in childhood is commonly due to femoral antetorsion and rarely to persisting internal tibial torsion. In late childhood, out-toeing may be due to external femoral torsion or external tibial torsion. The natural history is to externally rotate with growth, often correcting internal tibial torsion and making external tibial torsion worse (Fig. 4.28).

Internal tibial torsion is less common than external tibial torsion in the older child. ITT may also require operative correction if the deformity persists and produces a significant functional disability and cosmetic deformity in the child over 8 years of age (Fig. 4.29). Operative correction may be indicated if the thigh-foot angle is internally rotated more than 10°.

External tibial torsion Because the tibia normally rotates laterally with growth, ITT usually improves but ETT becomes worse with time (Figs. 4.29 right and 4.32). ETT may be associated with knee pain. This pain arises in the patellofemoral joint and is presumably due to malalignment of the knee and the line of progression. This malalignment is most pronounced when ETT is combined with IFT. The knee is internally rotated and the ankle externally rotated, both out of alignment with the line of progression, producing a "malalignment syndrome." This condition produces an inefficient gait and patellofemoral joint pain.

Femoral antetorsion or internal femoral torsion is usually first seen in the 3–5 year age groups and is more common in girls (Fig. 4.30). Mild residual deformity is often seen in the parents of affected children. The child with MFT sits in the "W" position, stands with the knees medially rotated ("kissing patella"), and runs awkwardly ("egg-beater"). Internal hip rotation is increased beyond 70°. IFT is mild if the internal hip rotation is 70°–80°, moderate if 80°–90°, and severe if 90+°. External hip rotation is reduced correspondingly, as the total arch of rotation is usually about 90°–100°.

Femoral antetorsion usually is most severe between 4 and 6 years of age and then resolves (Fig. 4.31). This resolution results from a decrease in femoral anteversion and from a lateral rotation of the tibia. In the adult, Femoral antetorsion does not cause degenerative arthritis and rarely causes any disability.

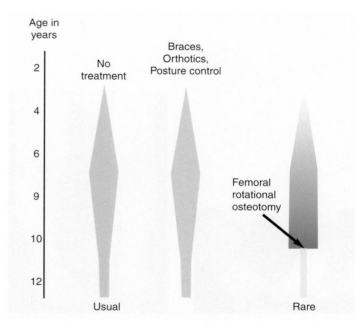

Fig. 4.31 Clinical course of femoral antetorsion. Femoral antetorsion becomes more clinically apparent during infancy and early childhood. The deformity is usually most severe between about 4 and 6 years of age. Resolution occurs regardless of common treatments. Rarely, the deformity is severe and fails to improve and requires rotational osteotomy for correction.

Femoral antetorsion is unaffected by nonoperative treatment. Persistence of severe deformity after the age of 8 years may necessitate correction by a femoral rotational osteotomy.

Femoral retrotorsion may be of greater significance than commonly appreciated. Retrotorsion is more common in patients with slipped capital femoral epiphysis. Presumably the shear force on the physis is increased. Retrotorsion is associated with increased degenerative arthritis and an out-toeing gait. The gait problem is not sufficiently severe to warrant operative correction.

Operative Correction

Rotational osteotomy is effective in correcting torsional deformities of the tibia or femur (Fig. 4.36). Osteotomy is indicated only in the older child, over age 8–10 years, who has a significant cosmetic and functional deformity, and with a single deformity 3 SD above the mean or combined deformity 2 SD above the mean. The child's problem should be sufficiently severe to justify the risks of the procedure. These procedures should not be considered "prophylactic."

Femoral correction Femoral rotational osteotomy is best performed at the intertrochanteric level. At this level healing is rapid, fixation most severe, scaring least obvious and should malunion occur, least noticeable. Usually rotational correction of about 50° is required. See page 401.

Tibial correction Tibial rotational osteotomy is best performed at the supramalleolar level (Fig. 4.33). Correct rotation to bring the thigh-foot angle to about 15°. See page 394.

Rotational Malalignment Syndrome

This syndrome usually includes external tibial and internal femoral torsion. The axis of flexion of the knee is not in the line of progression. Patellofemoral problems of pain and, rarely, dislocation follow.

Manage most conservatively. Very rarely operative correction is necessary. Correction is a major undertaking as it usually requires a 4 level procedure (both femoral and tibia). The site of the tibial osteotomy may be distal (most safe) or proximal. Proximal osteotomy just above the tibial tubercle has been reported.

Rarely, rotational malalignment is associated with severe patellofemoral disorders such as congenital dislocations (Fig. 4.34). Correction is complex and may require both osteotomy and soft tissue reconstructions.

Prognosis

The effects of adults with internal femoral torsion show little or no functional disability. Mild internal tibial torsion may facilitate sprinting by improving push-off. Degenerative arthritis of the knee has been associated with femoral antetorsion and of the hip with femoral retrotorsion.

Consultant Lynn Staheli, e-mail: staheli@u.washington.edu

References

1998 Distal tibial/fibular derotation osteotomy for correction of tibial torsion: review of technique and results in 63 cases. Dodgin DA et al. JPO 18:95

1996 Treatment of severe torsional malalignment syndrome. Delgado ED, et al. JPO 16:484

1996 Sprinting and intoeing. Fuchs R, Staheli LT. JPO 16:489

1994 Normal and abnormal torsional development in children. Fabry G, Cheng LX, Molenaers G. CO p. 22

1992 Tibial rotational osteotomy for idiopathic torsion. A comparison of the proximal and distal osteotomy levels. Krengel WF 3d, Staheli LT. CO 283:285

1991 Effects of lateral rotation splinting on lower extremity bone growth: an in vivo study in rabbits. Barlow DW, Staheli LT. JPO 11:583

1990 Lower positional deformity in infants and children: a review. Staheli LT. JPO 10:559

1985 Lower-extremity rotational problems in children. Normal values to guide management. Staheli LT, et al. JBJS 67A:39

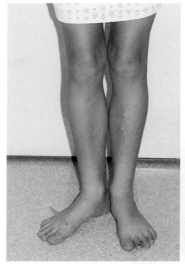
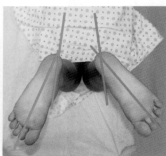

Fig. 4.32 External tibial torsion. External tibial torsion is often unilateral. When asymmetrical it is usually worse on the right side (red arrow). Note that the thight-foot angle is more external on the right (red lines).

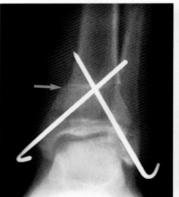
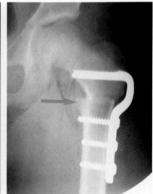

Fig. 4.33 Rotational osteotomy. Rotational osteotomies are usually performed at the supramalleolar tibial or intertrochanteric femoral levels (red arrows). Fix tibial osteotomies with crossed transcutaneous pins and a long leg cast. Fix femoral osteotomy with pins and a cast or a nail-plate.

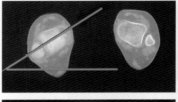
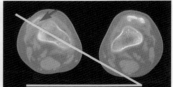
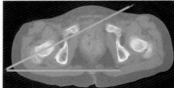

Fig. 4.34 Rotational malalignment with patellar dislocations. This CT study of a child with a dislocated patella (red arrow) shows torsional malalignment. Note the 40° lateral tibial torsion (blue lines), the 40° medial rotation of the axis of the knee (yellow lines), and 30° femoral anteversion (orange lines).

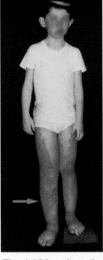
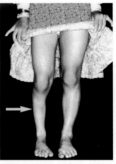

Fig. 4.35 Leg length differences. The boy has overgrowth of the right leg (red arrow) due to Klippel-Trenaunay syndrome.This girl has a short right leg due to weakness secondary to poliomyelitis (yellow arrow).

Category	Shortening	Lengthening
Congenital	Aplasia Hypoplasia Hip dysplasia Clubfoot	Hyperplasia
Neurogenic	Paralysis Disuse	Sympathectomy
Vascular	Ischemia Perthes disease	AV fistular
Infection	Physeal injury	Stimulation
Tumors	Physeal involvement	Vascular lesions
Trauma	Physeal injury Malunion	Fracture stimulation Distraction

Fig. 4.36 Causes of limb length discrepancy. The common causes of limb shortening and lengthening are shown.

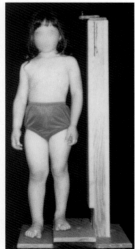
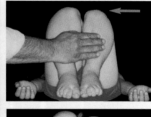
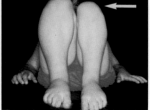

Fig. 4.37 Leg length inequality. In this child the right lower leg is hypertrophied. Note that the tibia is longer and the diameter greater. The left leg is more proportional in size to the rest of the body. The left limb is shorter both in the femur (red arrow) and tibia (yellow arrow).

Leg Length Inequality

Leg length inequality or *anisomelia* may be structural (Fig. 4.35) or functional. Functional anisomelia is secondary to joint contractures producing an apparent discrepancy in length. Structural discrepancies may occur at any site in the limb or pelvis. Often only discrepancies of the tibia or femur are measured. The height of the foot and pelvis should be included in calculating the total disparity. Discrepancies of 1 cm or more are considered significant.

Etiology

The causes of anisomelia are numerous (Fig. 4.36). Minor discrepancies are seen in clubfeet, hip dysplasia, and Perthes disease. Major differences are seen in tibial or femoral agenesis.

Natural History

The course of anisomelia is determined by the cause. The inhibition or acceleration that causes progressive forms of anisomelia varies according to the etiology. Growth inhibition from congenital defects is usually constant and makes predicting the final disparity feasible. Inhibition or acceleration from vascular, infectious, or neoplastic disorders are variable. For example, growth acceleration may be associated with chronic diaphyseal osteomyelitis. The acceleration occurs only when the infection is active.

Gait

The effect on gait depends on the magnitude of the discrepancy and the age of the patient. Children compensate for discrepancies by flexing the knee on the long side or by standing in equinus on the shortened limb. These compensations level the pelvis. Discrepancies are compensated by altered function. The long limb may be circumducted during swing phase or by "vaulting" over the long limb during stance phase. This vaulting results in a rise and fall of the body and consumes more energy than normal gait.

Adverse Effects

The adverse effects of anisomelia have been overstated. Limb length difference in childhood does not lead to an increased risk of structural scoliosis or back pain in adults.

Evaluation

During the evaluation, calculate the projected height of the patient and the degree of shortening at skeletal maturity if untreated. This evaluation requires a screening examination, a search for the cause, clinical and radiographic assessment of severity, and a determination of bone age. Serial evaluations are necessary during growth to improve the accuracy of the evaluation. From the history, determine if the child has been injured or experienced any musculoskeletal diseases.

Screening examination Note any asymmetry and alterations in body proportions. Does the asymmetry involve only the lower limbs? Is the long side the normal or abnormal side? Sometimes overgrowth makes the long side the abnormal one. Is it a hemihypertrophy or hemihypoplasia? Hemihypertrophy (Fig. 4.35) is important to recognize because it is sometimes associated with Wilm's tumor. The finding of hemihypertrophy should prompt an abdominal ultrasound evaluation. Hemihypoplasia is usually due to hemiparesis from cerebral palsy. Often these underlying problems are more significant than the length discrepancy itself. Observe the child walking. Is equinus, vaulting, circumduction, or abductor lurch present? Assess the abnormal limb to determine the site or sites of the discrepancy. Are the feet of equal length? Are the tibial and femoral segments equal? Are the forearms of equal length? Are any associated abnormalities present? Is joint motion symmetrical? Assess to determine whether the difference is in the femur, tibia, or combined (Fig. 4.37).

Clinical measures of discrepancy The limbs can be measured from the medial malleolus to the anterior iliac spine with a tape measure. This is usually accurate within about 1 cm. A more practical method uses blocks. Blocks of known thickness are placed under the short side until the pelvis is level. The patient will often sense when symmetry is established. By this method, all segments including foot and pelvis are assessed.

Imaging methods Image to measure discrepancies and determine any associated bone or joint deformities. Radiographic measures include the teleroentgenogram with a single exposure or orthodiagrams requiring multiple exposures on the same film. The orthodiagrams may be full length on a 36-inch film or telescoped on a 17-inch film (Fig. 4.38). For the infant and young child, order a teleroentgenogram because it provides an excellent screen for other problems such as hip dysplasia, it requires only one exposure, and it does not require patient cooperation. Enough serial studies should be made to provide adequate documentation to time the epiphysiodesis. These need not be done yearly. If the discrepancy is detected in the infant, obtain the baseline study early and repeat at about 3, 6, and 9 years of age.

Bone age Bone age is the most inaccurate of the measurements. Often measurements are given with a ±2 year qualification. The standard for assessment is the Gruelich and Pyle atlas. It is wise to sample bone ages over a period of several years and average any differences from the chronological age to improve reliability.

Body height at skeletal maturation The projected height at skeletal maturation is sometimes useful in planning correction of anisomelia. Shortening is more feasible for the tall individual, whereas lengthening may be more acceptable for those of short stature. The estimation can be made by comparing the child's height with the bone age to determine a percentile. This percentile is projected to maturity as an estimate of adult height.

Calculating discrepancy at maturation The discrepancy at maturation is the sum of the current discrepancy and the discrepancy accumulated during the period of remaining growth. The current discrepancy is assessed by clinical and radiographic measures. The discrepancy created by remaining growth must be calculated based on the percentage of growth retardation (or acceleration).

Minimal acceptable height (MAH) The MAH is the shortest stature that would be acceptable to the family. This will be based on racial, social, cultural, individual, and family differences. As a starting point for discussion, set the MAH at 2 SD below the mean value or about 65 inches for men and 59 inches for women (Fig. 4.39). Establishing the MAH involves an integration of complex issues such as the value the family gives to preservation of height and balancing this with the increased risks of lengthening over shortening.

Management Principles

The objective of management is to level the pelvis by equalizing extremity length without imposing excessive risk, morbidity, or height reduction. The severity of the discrepancy determines the general approach to management.

Severity Degrees of shortening can be categorized to aid in planning management. These values are influenced by the minimal acceptable height as determined during evaluation. In general, correct the discrepancy by shortening down to the MAH, then lengthen the limb as required to achieve the MAH.

Lifts Lifts may be useful in discrepancies greater than 2–3 cm (Fig. 4.40). Lifts cause problems for the child. They make the shoe heavier and less stable and are usually a source of embarrassment. Lifts make a clear statement, "I have a disability," which may be harmful to the child's self-image and status among piers. Because no immediate or late harmful effect of uncompensated anisomelia has been shown, the lift should improve function enough to compensate for inherent problems of wearing a lift. Walking without the lift will not damage the child. Lifts may be applied inside the shoe or on the heel. Make the lift as inconspicuous and lightweight as possible. More in-shoe correction can be placed in a high-top shoe. Consider placing 1 cm inside and another cm on the heel. Order tapered lifts when possible as the less bulk means a lighter, more stable and less conspicuous lift. To further reduce the lift size, order a lift that will leave the correction about 2 cm less than the disparity.

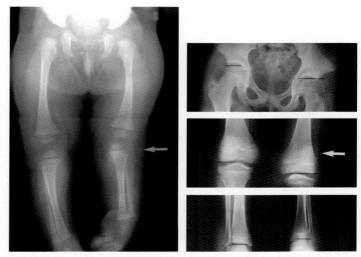

Fig. 4.38 Radiographic measures. The long radiograph (red arrow) is best for young children. The orthodiagam is more accurate for older children (yellow arrow).

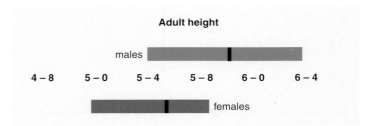

Fig. 4.39 Distribution of normal adult height. The mean value is shown in black with the range of ±2 SD shown in blue for men and red for women.

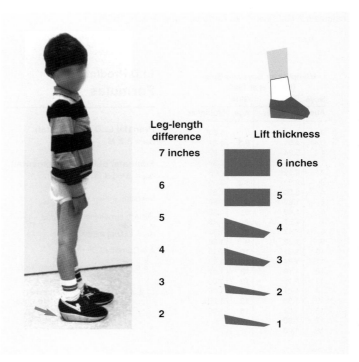

Fig. 4.40 Shoe lifts. Attempt to use wedges to minimize size and weight. For large discrepancies block lifts are necessary. Maintain correction below the actual discrepancy to minimize disability.

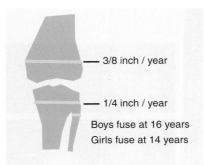

Fig. 4.41 Arithmetic method of predicting effect of epiphysiodesis. The growth rate per year for the lower femur and upper tibia are shown.

— 3/8 inch / year

— 1/4 inch / year

Boys fuse at 16 years
Girls fuse at 14 years

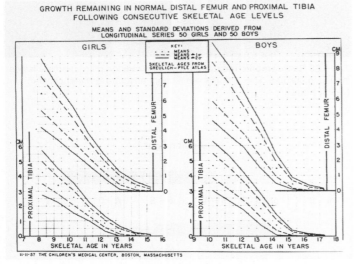

Fig. 4.45 Growth-remaining charts for girls and boys. The growth-remaining charts for girls and boys are different. Actual correction is based on growth of the short limb. To use it correctly, the discrepancy at maturity and the percentage of growth retardation of the short limb should be calculated. Redrawn from Anderson and Green (1963).

Timing of Correction

The usual objective of management is to correct the leg length discrepancy to within 1 cm of the opposite side. Because of its simplicity, effectiveness, and safety, epiphysiodesis remains the most effective means of correcting discrepancies between 2 and 5 cm.

The timing of epiphysiodesis determines the degree of correction, and 5 methods of timing are commonly used.

The simplistic method is useful for giving a rough estimate of the discrepancy at maturation from discrepancies of congenital origin. This is based on the assumption that the growth retardation is consistent. For example, a child with a congenital discrepancy of 3 cm at age 2 years has reached roughly half of his adult height. Thus, at skeletal maturation, the discrepancy is likely to be about 6 cm.

The arithmetic method is based on average growth rates and chronological age. On average, the distal femur contributes 3/8 inch of growth per year and the proximal tibia contributes 1/4 inch per year (Fig. 4.41). Girls complete growth at 14 and boys at 16 years of age. Use this method for long-term planning.

The growth-remaining method for timing of epiphysiodesis was the standard for many decades (Fig. 4.42).

The Paley multiplier method allows prediction of eventual discrepancy by simply multiplying the disparity with an age-adjusted factor (Fig. 4.43) to establish the disparity at maturation.

Straight line graph method requires a special graph for each patient (Fig. 4.44). The method is graphic and has the advantage of averaging the bone ages. This method has become the standard method of timing. The timing and procedure are detailed on page 398.

Correction

Plan management based on age of diagnosis, severity, projected height at maturity and any other special factors (Fig. 4.49).

Techniques of Correction

Bone shortening is a relatively safe and effective method of correcting discrepancies in the patient beyond the age when correction by epiphysiodesis is possible. Closed shortening procedures are now the standard (Fig. 4.48).

Multiplier for Boys and Girls (Paley, et al 1999)			
Boys		**Girls**	
Age	Multiplier	Age	Multiplier
0	5.08	0	4.63
0.4	4.01	0.3	4.01
1	3.24	1	2.97
1.3	2.99	2	2.39
2	2.59	3	2.05
3	2.23	3.3	2.00
4	2.00	4	1.83
5	1.83	5	1.66
6	1.68	6	1.53
7	1.57	7	1.43
8	1.47	8	1.33
9	1.38	9	1.26
10	1.31	10	1.19
11	1.24	11	1.13
12	1.18	12	1.07
13	1.12	13	1.03
14	1.07	14	1.00
15	1.03	15	1.00
16	1.01	16	1.00
17	1.00		
18	1.00		

LLD Prediction
Formulas

Prenatal LLD (Congenital)
$$\Delta_m = \Delta \times M$$

Postnatal LLD (Developmental)
$$\Delta_m = \Delta + I \times G$$

Inhibition $= I = 1 - \dfrac{S - S'}{L - L'}$

Growth remaining $= G = L(M - 1)$

Δ_m = LLD at maturity

Δ = Current LLD

L & S = Current length of long and short leg

L' & S' = Length of long and short leg at any other date since LLD began

Fig. 4.46 Paley multiplier. From the Maryland Center for Limb Lengthening and Reconstruction. This is a simple method of determining the leg length difference at maturation. This is applicable for shortening conditions in which growth retardation is consistent. From Paley et al (2000).

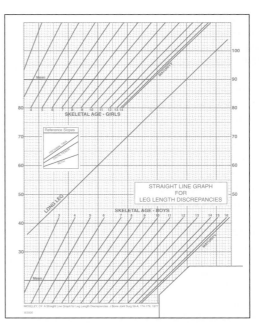

Fig. 4.47 Moseley straight line graph. This method utilizes graphic presentation of data to calculate the age for epiphysiodesis. See page 412 for full-size graph.

Stapling as a means of achieving an epiphysiodesis is appropriate only when calculating the appropriate timing for an epiphysiodesis is not possible due to difficulties in reading bone age and plotting growth.

Epiphysiodesis is the best method to correct most discrepancies between 2 and 5 cm. The traditional method leaves a long scar. Newer percutaneous methods use either a curette (Fig. 4.50) or a drill to remove the growth plate.

Lengthening as a means of correcting anisomelia has been practiced for 70 years. During the past two decades, new techniques have reduced the risks and made the procedure more effective (Fig. 4.51). This increased effectiveness is primarily due to the improved osteogenesis achieved by applying biological principles established through research.

Consultant Colin Moseley, e-mail: cmoseley@ucla.edu

References

2000 Multiplier method for predicting limb-length discrepancy. Paley D et al. JBJS 82A:1432

2000 The psychological and social functioning of 14 children and 12 adolescents after Ilizarov leg lengthening. Ramaker RR et al. Acta Orthop Scand 71:55

1999 Improvement in gait parameters after lengthening for the treatment of limb-length discrepancy. Bhave A, Paley D, Herzenberg JE. JBJS 81A:529

1997 The effect of limb-length discrepancy on gait. Song KM, Halliday SE, Little DG. JBJS 79A:1690

1991 Leg-length inequality in people of working age. The association between mild inequality and low-back pain is questionable. Soukka A et al. Spine 16:429

1988 Leg length inequality. A prospective study of young men during their military service. Hellsing AL. Ups J Med Sci 93:245

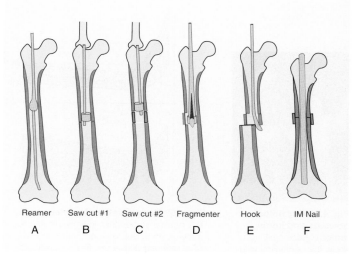

Fig. 4.48 Closed femoral shortening. A segment of femur is removed by a saw placed down the medullary canal from above. A segment is divided, split, displaced, then fixed with an intramedullary nail. From Winquist (1986).

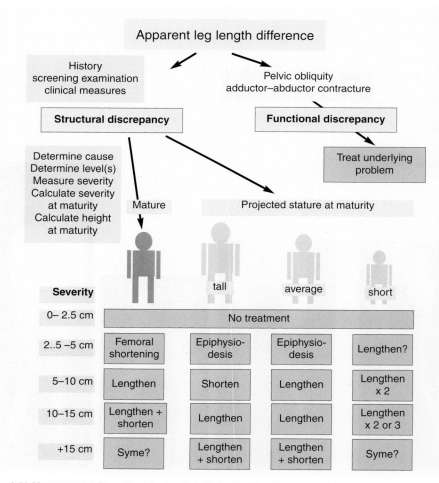

Fig. 4.49 Management flow-chart for leg length inequality. Management is based on the age of diagnosis, severity, and projected height at skeletal maturity.

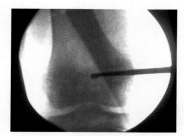

Fig. 4.50 Epiphysiodesis. The growth plate is being removed by curettage. This causes bony fusion across the growth plate and arrests growth.

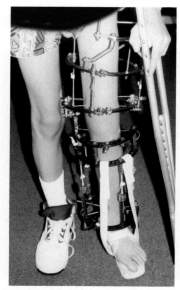

Fig. 4.51 Ilizarov lengthening.

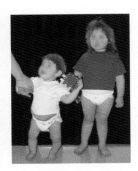

Fig. 4.52 Physiological bowlegs and knock-knees. These siblings show the sequence with the toddler with bowlegs and the older sister with mild knock-knees.

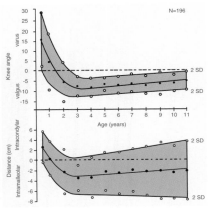

Fig. 4.53 Normal values for knee angle. The normal values for the knee angle are shown both in degrees and intracondylar or intramalleolar distances. From Heath and Staheli (1993).

Genu Varum and Genu Valgum

Genu varum and genu valgum are frontal plane deformities of the knee angle that fall outside the normal range, ±2 SD of the mean. Knee angle variations that fall within the normal range are referred to as *bowlegs* or *knock-knees* or physiologic variations (Fig. 4.52). The range of normal for knee angle changes with age (Fig. 4.53). Lateral bowing of the tibia is common during the first year, bowlegs are common during the second year (Fig. 4.54), and knock-knees are most prominent between 3 and 4 years (Fig. 4.55). Varus or valgus deformities are classified as either "focal" as seen in tibia vara or "generalized" as occurs in rickets.

Evaluation

History Inquire about the onset. Was there an injury or illness? Is the deformity progressing? Are old photographs or radiographs available for review? Is the child's general health good? Does the family provide a normal diet? Are other family members affected?

Physical examination Start with a screening evaluation. Does the child have normal height and body proportions? Short stature is common in rickets and various syndromes. Are other deformities present? Is the deformity symmetrical? Is the deformity localized or generalized? Are the limb lengths equal? Shortening and knee angle deformity may be due to epiphyseal injuries or some developmental problems such as fibular hemimelia. Measure the rotational profile. Often frontal and transverse plane deformities coexist; make a clear separation. Measure the deformity. With the patella directly forward, measure the knee angle with a goniometer. Measure the intramalleolar or intracondylar distance. Does the deformity increase when the child stands? If the collateral ligaments are lax, such as in achondroplasia, the varus deformity is worse in the upright position.

Laboratory If the child has a generalized deformity, order a metabolic screen including calcium, phosphorus, alkaline phosphatase, and creatinine, plus a hematocrit.

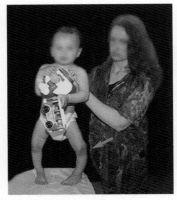

Fig. 4.54 Physiologic bowlegs. This 18-month-old infant has moderate bowing.

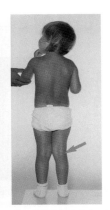

Fig. 4.55 Physiologic knock-knees. This 3-year-old girl has mild physiologic knock-knees.

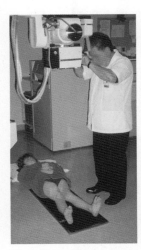

Fig. 4.56 Positioning for radiographs. This girl is being carefully positioned to assure an accurate study.

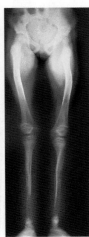

Fig. 4.57 Poor and well positioned radiographs. Patient positioned to get legs on radiographs (left). Properly positioned study shows deformity (right).

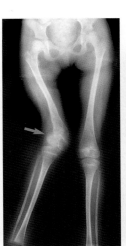

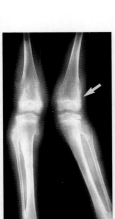

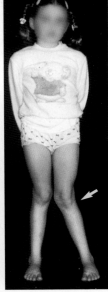

Fig. 4.58 Pathological genu valgum. Deformity due to physeal arrest from trauma (red arrow), and to osteochondromatosis (yellow arrows) are shown.

Imaging If findings suggest the possibility of a pathological basis for the deformity, order a single AP radiograph of the lower limbs (Fig. 4.56). If knee ligaments are loose, make the radiograph with the infant or child standing. Position the child with the patella directly forward (Fig. 4.57). Use a film large enough to include the full length of femora and tibiae. A 36-inch film is often required. Study the radiograph for evidence of rickets, tibia vara, or other problems. Measure the metaphyseal-diaphyseal angle of the upper tibia (page 84). Values above 11° are consistent with tibia vara. Measure the hip-knee-ankle angle. Complete the evaluation with other imaging studies if necessary. For knee deformities, a lateral radiograph is useful. Early tibia vara can be assessed with a bone scan. Uptake is increased in the medial portion of the proximal tibial epiphysis. CT or MRI studies may be useful in identifying and measuring a physeal bridge. Document the deformity by photography. A sequence of photographs provides a graphic record of the effect of time.

Diagnosis

Follow a plan (Figs. 4.61 and 4.62). First make the differentiation between physiologic and pathologic forms (Figs. 4.58 and 4.59). If a pathologic form is present, consider the various categories of causes (Fig. 4.60). Causes are varied and usually the diagnosis is not difficult.

Feature	Physiologic	Pathologic
Frequency	Common	Rare
Family hx	Usually negative	May occur in family
Diet	Normal	May be abnormal
Health	Good	Other MS abnormalities
Onset	Second year for bowing Third year knock-knees	Out of normal sequence Often progressive
Sequence	Normal sequence	Variable
Height	Normal	Less than 5th percentile
Symmetry	Symmetrical	Symmetrical or asym
Severity	Mild to moderate	Often beyond ±2 SD

Fig. 4.59 Differentiating physiologic and pathologic genu varum.

Cause	Genu Valgum	Genu Varum
Congenital	Fibular hemimelia	
Dysplasia	Osteochondrodysplasias	Osteochondrodysplasias
Developmental	Knock-knee >2 SD	Bowing >2 SD Tibia vara
Trauma	Overgrowth Partial physeal arrest	Partial physeal arrest
Metabolic	Rickets	Rickets
Osteopenic	Osteogenesis imperfecta	
Infection	Growth plate injury	Growth plate injury
Arthritis	Rheumatoid arthritis knee	

Fig. 4.60 Classification of pathologic knee angle. Causes of genu varum and genu valgum are listed.

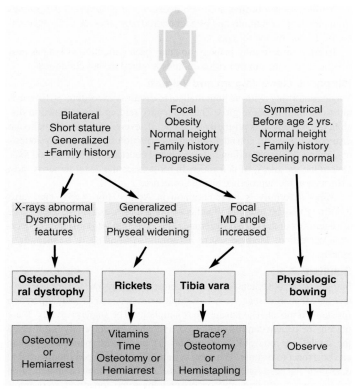

Fig. 4.61 Evaluation of genu varum or bowlegs. This flowchart shows the differentiation of the common causes of change in knee angle.

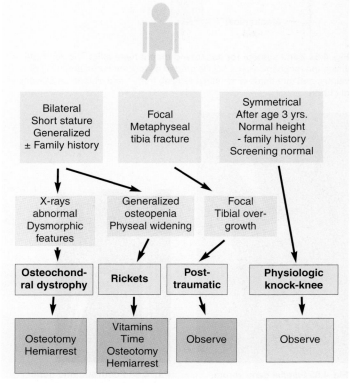

Fig. 4.62 Evaluation of genu valgum or knock-knees. This flowchart shows the differentiation of the common causes of change in knee angle.

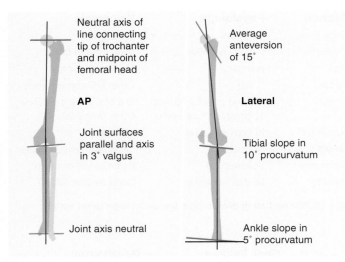

Fig. 4.63 Normal mechanical axis of lower limbs. These are average values. Based on Paley and Tetsworth (1992).

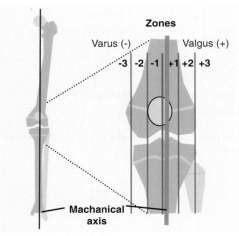

Fig. 4.64 Zone system for assessing mechanical axis. The zone into which the mechanical axis falls is graded as a (-) for varus and a (+) of valgus, and into thirds with values ranging from 1 to 3. Based on Stevens et al (1999).

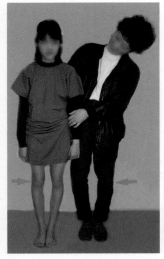

Fig. 4.65 Familial genu varum. Asians tend to have more varus than other groups.

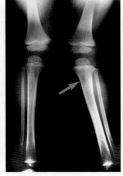

Fig. 4.66 Posttraumatic genu valgum. This deformity is due to overgrowth of the tibia following proximal tibial metaphyseal fracture.

Management

The vast majority of children have bowlegs or knock-knees that will resolve spontaneously. Document these physiological variations with a photograph and see the child again in 3–6 months for follow-up. No radiographs are necessary. If the problem is pathological, establish the cause. Treatment options are then considered.

Nonoperative treatment with shoe wedges is not effective and should be avoided. Long-leg bracing may be used for early tibia vara, but its effectiveness is uncertain. Avoid long-term bracing for conditions such as vitamin D–resistant rickets because the effectiveness of bracing is unclear and considerable disability results from brace treatment.

Operative correction options include osteotomy, or hemiarrest procedures either by hemiepiphysiodesis or unilateral physeal stapling. The objectives of operative treatment are to (1) correct knee angle, (2) place the articular surfaces of the knee and ankle in a horizontal position, (3) maintain limb length equality, and (4) correct any coexisting deformities. To achieve these directions, preoperative planning is required.

Mechanical axis Obtain a long, standing radiograph of the lower limbs. Be certain the child is positioned with the patella directly anterior when the exposure is made. Draw the axis of the femur and tibia connecting the center of the femoral head to the center of the distal femoral epiphysis (Fig. 4.63). Construct a second line between the midpoint of the upper and lower tibial epiphysis. Mark the articular surfaces. Measure the degree of valgus or varus.

Zone system On a full-length radiograph, draw a line between the femoral head and ankle. Note the position of the knee relative to this axis (Fig. 4.64).

Make cutouts Before undertaking any osteotomy, make tracings of the bone and perform the intended osteotomy on the paper. This allows previsualizing the outcome and making necessary modifications.

Make corrective osteotomies as close to the site of deformity as practical.

Translation of the osteotomy may be necessary to position the joint within the mechanical axis.

Mulilevel osteotomies are often necessary in generalized deformities from metabolic conditions and osteochondrodystrophies. Balance the number of osteotomies with risks.

Recurrent deformity is likely, so delay each correction as long as possible to reduce the number of procedures required during childhood.

Idiopathic Genu Valgum and Valgum

Valgus deformity with an intramalleolar distance exceeding 8–10 cm is most common in obese girls. This deformity seldom causes function disability; the problem is primarily cosmetic. If severe, with an intramalleolar distance of >15 cm, consider operative correction by hemiepiphysiodesis or stapling. Make a standing radiograph and construct the mechanical axis. Determine the site(s) of deformity. In most cases the distal femur is most deformed at the appropriate site of correction.

Varus deformity is most common in Asians (Fig. 4.65). The varus deformity may be familial. Whether or not it increases the risk of degenerative arthritis of the knee is uncertain. This deformity seldom requires operative correction. Manage severe deformity by stapling or hemiepiphysiodesis.

Stapling

Stapling is a convenient method of correction (Fig. 4.67). The disadvantages are the larger scar, the risk of staple extrusion, and a second operation for staple removal. The advantage is simplicity. The staples (usually 2) are placed, the patient carefully followed, and when the deformity is corrected the staples are removed. If the staples are placed extraperiosteal, growth can be expect to resume. The zone system (Fig. 4.64) is commonly used to determine the need for correction. A *zone 3* deformity may be an indication for stapling. A rebound often occurs undoing some correction, so overcorrect slightly in anticipation of this common problem, especially in the children <12 years. See page 397.

Hemiepiphysiodesis

With accurate timing, hemiepiphysiodesis has several advantages. The scar is short and the procedure simple and definitive. Bowen has developed a table to aid in timing (Fig. 4.68). Careful follow-up is essential because if the deformity appears to be destined for overcorrection, arresting the entire epiphysis becomes necessary.

Pathologic Deformities

Posttraumatic genu valgum Posttraumatic genu valgum results from overgrowth following fracture of the proximal tibial metaphysis in early childhood (Fig. 4.66). Valgus may also be due to malunion or soft tissue interposition.

Natural history The deformity develops during the first 12 to 18 months due to tibial overgrowth following the fracture. This is followed by a very gradual reduction of the valgus over a period of years. In the majority, this correction is adequate and no operative procedure is necessary.

Management Manage proximal tibial fractures by correcting any malalignment and immobilize with a long-leg cast applied with gentle varus molding. Document reduction and position with a long film that includes the entire tibia. Advise the family of the potential of this fracture to cause a secondary deformity, which cannot be prevented. Avoid early osteotomy because recurrence is frequent and the deformity usually resolves spontaneously with time. Reassure the family that the knee will not be damaged by the deformity. Should the deformity persist, correct by osteotomy or by hemiepiphysiodesis or stapling near the end of growth.

Rickets

Suspect rickets in a child with increasing genu valgum, short stature, and a history of an atypical diet or similar deformities in other family members. Rickets produces a generalized genu valgum with bowing of the diaphysis and rarefaction of the epiphysis. Low calcium and phosphorus and a high alkaline phosphatase are confirming laboratory findings. Document severity with a 36-inch radiograph of the entire femur and tibia. Measure the hip-knee-ankle angle and mechanical axis zone.

Manage by first referring the child to an endocrinologist to optimize the medical management of the rickets. Despite optimal medical management, the deformities often persist in vitamin D–resistant forms of rickets.

Bracing The role of bracing is controversial as long-term bracing imposes a major added burden on the child and the value of bracing has not been shown.

Surgery If possible, delay correction until late childhood for stapling or adolescence for osteotomy. Correction at the end of growth reduces the risk of recurrence. If deformity is severe, correction may be necessary in childhood (Fig. 4.69). Plan osteotomy as discussed earlier with long films and cutouts. Drape the entire limb free to visualize adequacy of correction. Correct at one or more levels on each bony segment following the preoperative plan. Immobilize for about 10 weeks as healing may be slightly slower than normal.

If operative correction is performed before the end of growth, recurrence is common. Recurrence is most rapid in the younger child.

Consultant Peter Stevens, e-mail: peter.stevens@mcc.utah.edu

References

1999 Physeal stapling for idiopathic genu valgum. Stevens PM, et al. JPO 19:645

1996 Hemiepiphyseal stapling for knee deformities in children younger than 10 years: a preliminary report. Mielke CH, Stevens PM. JPO 16:423

1995 Medial physeal stapling for primary and secondary genu valgum in late childhood and adolescence. Fraser RK, Dickens DR, Cole WG. JBJS 77B:733

1993 Normal limits of knee angle in white children--genu varum and genu valgum. Heath CH, Staheli LT. JPO 13 13:259

1992 Mechanical axis deviation of the lower limbs. Paley D, Tetsworth K. CO p 65

1985 Partial epiphysiodesis at the knee to correct angular deformity. Bowen JR, et al. CO 198:184.

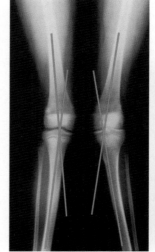
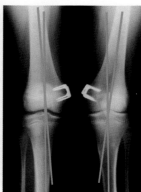

Fig. 4.67 Correction of excessive physiologic knock-knee by stapling. This 13-year-old girl had distal medial femoral stapling to correct this deformity. Note the knee angle before and after stapling.

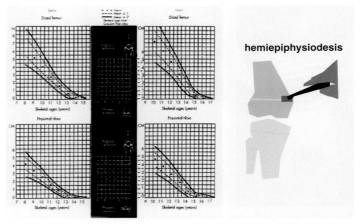

Fig. 4.68 Chart for timing hemiepiphysiodesis. This chart was created to time correction of angulatory deformities. From Bowen (1985).

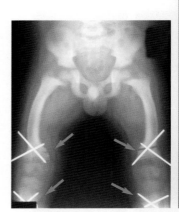
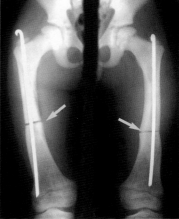

Fig. 4.69 Operative correction of richetic deformity. Multilevel correction is often necessary (red arrows). In some, intramedullary fixation can be used (yellow arrows).

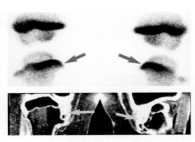

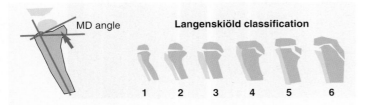

Fig. 4.70 Tibia vara. Bone scans early show increased uptake on the medial aspect of the proximal tibial epiphysis (red arrows). MR imaging of advanced disease shows cartilagenous replacement of the upper metaphysis (yellow arrows).

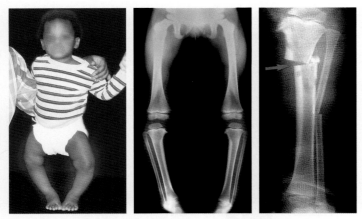

Fig. 4.71 Common measures for tibia vara. The metaphyseal–diaphyseal angle (red arrow) and the Langenskiöld classification are commonly used.

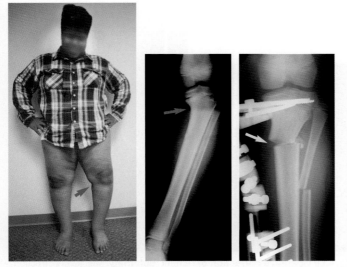

Fig. 4.72 Infantile tibia vara. This disease is usually bilateral and may cause cause deformity that requires correction by osteotomy (red arrow).

Fig. 4.73 Adolescent tibia vara. This form is often unilateral (red arrows) and usually requires operative correction. External fixation is often an excellent choice in operative correction (yellow arrow).

Tibia Vara

Tibia vara or Blount disease, is a growth disorder involving the medial portion of the proximal tibial growth plate that produces a localized varus deformity (Fig. 4.70). The incidence is greater if the child is black, obese, has an affected family, and resides in certain geographical locations such as the southeastern part of United States. The cause is unknown but it has been theorized that in susceptible individuals mechanical stress damages the proximal medial growth plate, thus converting physiologic bow legs into tibia vara.

Evaluation

Two clinical patterns of tibia vara are seen. Radiographs in early infantile tibia vara may be difficult to differentiate from physiologic bowing. The metaphyseal–diaphyseal angle is often used. This angle (Fig. 4.71) shows considerable overlap between physiologic and tibia vara cases. If the angle exceeds 15°, tibia vara is likely. Differentiation is made by following radiographs made every 3–6 months. Usually physiologic varus improves after the child's 2nd birthday. Tibia vara progresses and shows diagnostic metaphyseal changes.

Management

Treatment is based on the stage of the disease (Fig. 4.71) and the age of the child.

Bracing As mild deformities may resolve without treatment, the beneficial effect of the brace is often uncertain. Often braces are used to treat stage 1 and 2 disease. If treatment is elected, order a long-leg brace with a fixed-knee that incorporates valgus loading. The brace should be worn during active play and at nighttime.

Osteotomy in the child If the disease progresses or is first seen in stages 3 and 4, osteotomy is indicated. Perform the osteotomy before age 4 years if possible (Fig. 4.72). Deformities of stages 5 and 6 are more complex and may require a double-level osteotomy to correct both the genu varum and the articular incongruity. Also assess the shape of the distal femur as varus or valgus deformity may contribute to the deformity. Medial tibial torsion is also a common associated deformity. Correct the varus and torsion by a simple closing wedge with rotation or by an oblique osteotomy. Correct the thigh-foot angle to about +10 degrees and overcorrect the varus to about 10 degrees of valgus. Use a sterile tourniquet so the entire limb can be seen to ensure appropriate correction. Release the anterior compartment fascia to reduce the risk of a compartment syndrome. Fix the osteotomy with crossed pins and supplement the fixation with a long-leg cast.

Hemistapling may be an alternative to osteotomy for stage 2 or 3 deformities.

Physeal bridge resection Rarely a physeal bridge is suspected in unilateral involvement in mid to late childhood. CT or MRI studies confirm the presence of the bridge. Resect the bridge, fill the defect with fat, and correct the tibial deformity by osteotomy.

Surgery in the adolescent Operative correction in the older child or adolescent is usually complicated by obesity. Stabilize the osteotomy with an external fixator. External fixation provides adequate immobilization without need for a cast and allows the option to adjust alignment during the postoperative period (Fig. 4.73).

Prognosis

The prognosis depends upon severity, stage, and treatment. Recurrence of varus and increasing shortening are common during childhood. Persisting articular deformity often leads to degenerative arthritis in adult life.

References

1999 Tibia vara in adolescents. Apropos of 19 cases. Catonne Y, et al. Rev Chir Orthop Reparatrice Appar Mot 85:434
1998 Orthotic treatment of infantile tibia vara. Raney EM, et al. JPO 18:670
1998 Brace treatment of early infantile tibia vara. Zionts LE, CJ Shean. JPO 18:102
1997 Management of late-onset tibia vara in the obese patient by using circular external fixation. Stanitski DF, et al. JPO 17:691

Lower Limb Deficiencies

Lower limb deficiencies are rare deformities. The diagnosis and evaluation were covered in Chapter 2. Management of lower limb deficiencies is complex, requiring correcting length equalization, stabilizing unstable joints, and correcting angular and rotational deformity. Prudent management requires a balanced approach, balancing cosmetic and functional outcomes against risks and costs of surgery.

Principles of Management

1. Establish an accurate diagnosis. Refer to a children's limb deficiency clinic when available. Refer to a geneticist. Consider other problems.

2. Deal with the family's shock and guilt. Be positive. Most children can have a relatively normal childhood and can become independent and productive adults.

3. Plan a management strategy that is tailored to the unique deformities of the child and social and cultural values of the family.

4. Be prepared to deal with the family's preference to lengthening over amputation, even for deformities best managed by conversion and prosthetic fitting. Be prepared for the impact of the Internet, support groups and input from other parents on decision making.

5. Encourage the family to discuss management with others in support groups and medical centers.

6. Be prepared for the effect of growth.

7. Children rarely have phantom pain.

8. Amputations are well-tolerated in children, but peer and family issues often complicate management.

9. Children impose greater physical demands on prosthetics.

Dealing with Deformity

1. Preserve length and growth plates.

2. Stabilize the proximal joints when possible.

3. Save the knee joint if possible.

4. Be prepared to deal with problems other than limb deficiency, as deformities are often complex.

5. Estimate roughly the anticipated magnitude of shortening at maturity to plan management (Fig. 4.74).

6. Limit lengthening to roughly 15% of the bone length.

Surgical Principles

1. Perform disarticulations rather than transosseous amputations when possible to prevent diaphyseal overgrowth (Fig. 4.75).

2. The most commonly used procedures include: Syme amputation–disarticulation of ankle (Fig. 4.76); Boyd amputation (midtarsal amputation); knee disarticulation; modified Van Nes rotationalplasty (Fig. 4.77); Brown procedure–centralization of the fibula and ankle fusion.

3. Coordinate operative and prosthetic management thoughtfully.

Tibial Deficiency

Tibial deficiency is a congenital hypoplasia or aplasia of the tibia. Classify the deformity based on the extent of loss (Fig. 4.78). This deficiency may be genetic. Refer to a geneticist for a consultation and counseling. Management is based on the adequacy of the upper tibial segment.

Adequate upper tibial segment Centralize the fibula under the tibia and disarticulate the ankle at about one year of age. Fit the child with a Syme prosthesis.

Inadequate upper tibial segment Usually management includes disarticulation of the knee and prosthetic fitting in late infancy or early childhood.

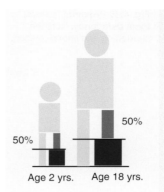

Fig. 4.74 Growth in congenital deficiencies. Note that the percentage shortening of the limb remains constant throughout growth for congenital deficiencies.

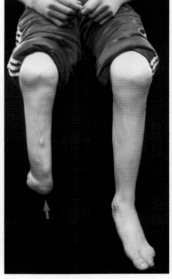

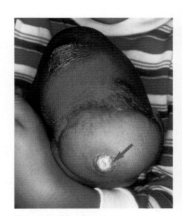

Fig. 4.75 Diaphyseal overgrowth. This causes "penciling" or penetration of the sharp end through the skin (arrow).

Fig. 4.76 Syme amputation. This child had this conversion for fibular deficiency. This stump is endbearing.

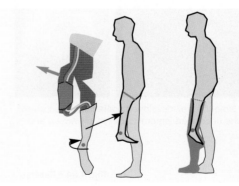

Fig. 4.77 Van Nes rotationalplasty. Thigh resection was required for tumor eradication. Note that ankle (blue dot) is rotated 180° and becomes the knee within the prosthesis. Based on Krajbich (1998).

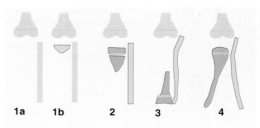

1a 1b 2 3 4

Fig. 2.78 Tibial deficiency classification. Based on Jones, Barnes, and Lloyd-Roberts (1978).

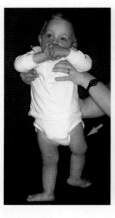
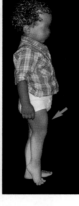

Fig. 4.80 Proximal femoral focal deficiency. Note the shortening and lateral rotation.

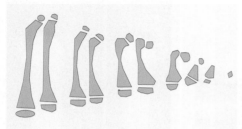

Fig. 2.81 Hamanishi's spectrum of the congenitally short femur. This figure shows the wide variation in deformities included in this classification. Based on Hamanishi (1980).

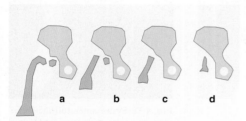

Fig. 4.82 Aiken's classification of proximal femoral focal deficiency.

a   b   c   d

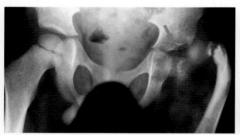
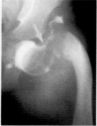

Fig. 4.83 PFFD type b. Note the well-developed acetabulum (red arrow). The arthrogram shows the unossified femoral neck (yellow arrow) and severe varus.

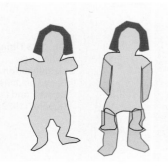

Fig. 4.84 Bilateral PFFD prosthetic fitting. Prosthetic fitting allows for increasing height and accommodates lateral limb positioning. Based on Krajbich (1998).

Proximal Femoral Focal Deficiency

Proximal femoral focal deficiency or PFFD (Fig. 4.80) includes a spectrum of deformities that may be associated with fibular deficiency. Differentiate PFFD from the congenitally short femur (Fig. 4.81), which involves the shaft rather than the proximal part of the femur. Management of these conditions is different as lengthening is often appropriate for managing the congenitally short femur and rarely appropriate for PFFD.

Natural History

The normal and abnormal sides remain proportionately the same throughout growth. The limb length inequality is the most obvious source of problems. Less obvious but often significant is hip joint instability. Less significant is an external rotation deformity of the femur.

Evaluation

Study the shape of the acetabulum, the shape of the proximal ossification of the femur, and the length of the femur. Classify the deformity traditionally (Fig. 4.82) or as simply *short* or *too short*.

Deformity

As PFFD causes a combination of deformities, consider each as part of general management.

Length Length is a major problem. Calculate the estimated discrepancy at maturity to guide management. Base the management decision on severity.

Hip joint Predict hip status based on the volume of the acetabulum. A poor acetabulum suggests that the hip will be unstable. Only mild degrees of dysplasia are correctable. Be aware that an unstable hip joint jeopardizes the success of femoral lengthening.

Proximal femur A bulbous shape of the upper femur suggests that the proximal femur is complete, but with a varus deformity and slow ossification. In contrast a pointed and sclerotic upper femur suggests a more severe deformity. Perform arthrography early to determine the pathology (Fig. 4.83). Correct the varus early to enhance ossification.

Timing of Correction

Correct proximal femoral deformity during the first year. Fit with temporary prosthesis by age 2. Staged lengthenings may be started as early as the second year. Rotationalplasties are best delayed until about age 4 years.

Procedures

Hip fusion is controversial. It provides stability for walking or lengthening procedures. It may make prosthetic fitting more difficult than the unfused mobile but unstable hip.

Subtrochanteric osteotomy is indicated for correction of varus. When associated with delayed ossification of the proximal femur, fusion and correction are more difficult.

Rotationalplasty includes excision of the knee joint and rotation the extremity 180° allowing the child's ankle to become the knee joint of the prosthesis. The procedure improves function but degrades appearance and is more suitable for males because clothing better hides the deformity.

Syme or Boyd amputation is indicated to allow prosthetic fitting with a knee disarticulation type of prosthesis. It is simple, cosmetic, easy prosthetic fit but at the sacrifice of efficiency.

Knee fusion is usually combined with Syme amputation to provide stability and to position the Syme stump just above the level of the opposite knee joint to facilitate prosthetic fitting.

Femoral lengthening may be considered for a congenital short femur expected to be less than 10–20 cm at the end of growth. With increasing length gained, complications and risk of joint damage increase. Rapidly changing technology will undoubtedly increase feasibility of greater lengthening in the future.

Alternatives

Special situations such as bilateral deformity may make prosthetic management without conversion an option (Fig. 4.84).

Fibular Deficiency

This deformity (Fig. 4.85) is the most common of lower limb deficiency. It occurs sporadically and seldom has a genetic basis.

Pathology

There is partial or complete absence of the fibula (Fig. 4.86). A fibrous analogue may replace osseous fibula. Fibular shortening causes lateral ankle instability. Tibial deformities may include shortening, anterior bowing, and valgus deformity. Foot deformities include absence of lateral portions of the foot (Fig. 4.80), talocalcaneal fusions, and ankle equinus.

Natural History

Shortening is progressive but remains proportionally shortened to the opposite normal side. Ankle instability results in deformity and pain in the second decade. Knee valgus may cause disability. Disability from shortening is proportional to severity.

Management

Classify type of deformity. Calculate roughly the expected shortening at skeletal maturation. Operative management is largely determined by the extent of foot deficiencies and ankle instability (Figs. 4.87 and 4.88). Managing the deformity is often less difficult than effectively dealing with the family.

Dealing with the family Families often have difficulty accepting Syme amputation and prosthetic management even for severe deformities. Families often wish to delay a decision in hope of new technology that will make amputation unnecessary or delay the decision until the child can participate in the decision. Families often use electronic communication with other families and may elect to visit centers where complex reconstructive procedures are offered. If the family cannot make a decision, provide a special prosthesis that can incorporate the foot while the decision is being made.

Operative management Plan amputation late in the first year just before the infant would normally stand and walk. Perform a Syme or Boyd procedure. The value of resection of the fibular analogue is controversial. Correct significant tibia vara to facilitate prosthetic fitting and walking. Lengthening is best delayed until midchildhood. A shoe lift may be necessary before lengthening. Make the lift light, least intrusive, and about one inch less in height than is necessary to level the pelvis.

Consultant Hugh Watts, e-mail: hwatts@ucla.edu

References

1999 Syme amputation for the treatment of fibular deficiency. Birch J et al. JBJS 81A:1511

1998 Severe progressive deformities after limb lengthening in type-II fibular hemimelia. Cheng JC, Cheung KW, Ng BK. JBJS 80B:772

1998 Lower-limb deficiencies and amputations in children. Krajbich JI. J Am Acad Orthop Surg 6:358

1997 Radiological study of severe proximal femoral focal deficiency. Court C, Carlioz H. JPO 17:520

1997 Management of fibular hemimelia: amputation or limb lengthening. Naudie D, et al. JBJS 79B:1040

1996 Management of forme fruste fibular hemimelia. Maffulli N, Fixsen JA. JPO 5B:17

1995 Proximal femoral focal deficiency: results of rotationplasty and Syme amputation. Alman BA, Krajbich JI, Hubbard S. JBJS 77A:1876

1992 Screening for behavioral and emotional problems in children and adolescents with congenital or acquired limb deficiencies. Varni JW, Setoguchi Y. Am J Dis Child 146:103

1980 Congenital short femur. Clinical, genetic and epidemiological comparison of the naturally occurring condition with that caused by thalidomide. Hamanishi C. JBJS 62B:307

1979 Congenital deficiency of the fibula. Achterman C, Kalamchi A. JBJS 61B:133

1978 Congenital aplasia and dysplasia of the tibia with intact fibula. Classification and management. Jones D, Barnes J, Lloyd-Roberts GC. JBJS 60B:31

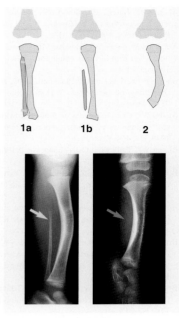

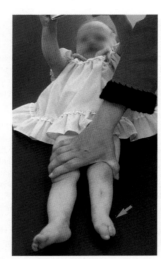

Fig. 4.85 Foot deformity with fibular deficiency. The foot deformity cannot be corrected.

Fig. 4.86 Fibular deficiency classification. Clinical examples of type 1b (yellow arrow) and type 2 (red arrow). From Achterman and Kalamchi (1979).

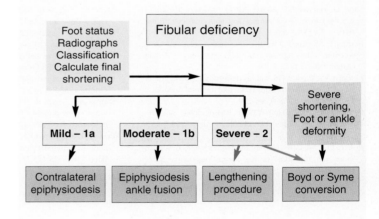

Fig. 4.87 Flowchart for managing fibular deficiencies.

	Amputation	**Lengthening**
Advantages	Definitive Few complications Resolves length and ankle problems	Attractive to family Restores body image

Disadvantages	Requires prosthesis
	Difficult to accept
		Many complications
		Complex procedure
		Sometimes:
		  retards tibial growth
		  damages knee and ankle

Fig. 4.88 Factors in making decision to lengthen or amputate. The choice between amputation for types 1b and 2 deformities and lengthening is often difficult. Consider these factors.

Altongy JF, Harcke HT, Bowen JR. Measurement of leg length inequalities by micro-dose digital radiographs. J Pediatr Orthop 1987;7:311-316.

Anderson M, Green WT, Messner MB. Growth and predictions of growth in lower extremities. J Bone Joint Surg 1963;45A:1-4.

Blair VP III, Schoenecker PL, Sheridan JJ, et al. Closed shortening of the femur. J Bone Joint Surg 1989; 71A:1440-1447.

Blount WP, Clark GR. Control of bone growth by epiphyseal stapling: A preliminary report. J Bone Joint Surg 1949;31A:464-478.

Blount WP. Tibia vara: Osteochondrosis deformans tibiae. J Bone Joint Surg 1937;19:1-29.

Bowen JR, Leahey JL, Zhang ZH et al. Partial epiphysiodesis at the knee to correct angular deformity. Clin Orthop 1985;198:184-190.

Bower GD et al. Isotope bone scans in the assessment of children with hip pain or limp. Pediatr Radiol 1985; 15:319.

Broughton NS, Dickens DRV, Cole WG, et al. Epiphysiolysis for partial growth plate arrest: Results after four years or at maturity. J Bone Joint Surg 1989;71B: 13-16.

Brougton NS, Olney BW, Menelaus MB. Tibial shortening for leg length discrepancy. J Bone Joint Surg 1989; 71B:242-245.

Bylander B, Hansson LI, Selvik G. Pattern of growth retardation after Blount stapling. J Pediatr Orthop 1983;3:63.

Cook SD, Lavernia CJ, Burke SW, et al. A biomechanical analysis of the etiology of tibia vara. J Pediatr Orthop 1983;3:449-454.

Cundy P, Paterson D, Morris L, et al. Skeletal age estimation in leg length discrepancy. J Pediatr Orthop 1988;8:513-515.

Fabry G, Macwen GD, Shands AR Jr. Torsion of the femur-A followup study in normal and abnormal conditions. JBJS 1973;55A:1726.

Ferriter P, Shapiro F. Infantile tibia vara: Factors affecting outcome following proximal tibial osteotomy. J Pediatr Orthop 1987;7:1-7.

Fonseca AS, Bassett GS. Valgus deformity following derotation osteotomy to correct medial femoral torsion. J Pediatr Orthop 1988:8:295-299.

Foreman KA, Robertson WW Jr. Radiographic measurement of infantile tibia vara. J Pediatr Orthop 1985;5:452-455.

Friberg O. Clinical symptoms and biomechanics of lumbar spine and hip joint in leg length inequality. Spine 1983;8:643-651.

Gibson PH, Papaioannou T, Kenwright J. The influence on the spine of leg-length discrepancy after femoral fracture. JBJS;1983;65B:584-587.

Giles LG, Taylor JR. Lumbar spine structural changes associated with leg length inequality. Spine 1982;7:159-162.

Gillespie R, Torode IP. Classification and management of congenital abnormalities of the femur. J Bone Joint Surg 1983;65B:557-568.

Green WT, Wyatt GM, Anderson M. Orthoentgenography as a method of measuring the bones of the lower extremities. JBJS 1977;59A174-179.

Hofmann A, Jones RE, Herring JA. Blount's disease after skeletal maturity. J Bone Joint Surg 1982;64A:1004-1009.

Huurman WW, Jacobsen FS, Anderson JC, et al. Limb-length discrepancy measured with computerized axial tomographic equipment. JBJS 1987;69A:699.

Jones CB, Dewar ME, Aichroth PM, et al. Ephiphyseal distraction monitored by strain gauges: Results in seven children. JBJS 1989;71B:651-656.

Kling TF Jr, Hensinger RN. Angular and torsional deformities of the lower limbs in children. Clin Orthop 1983;176:136-147.

Knittel G, Staheli LT. The effectiveness of shoe modifications for intoeing. Orthop Clin North Am 1976;7:1019-1025.

Langenskiold A, Riska EB. Tibia vara (osteochondrosis deformans tibiae): A survey of seventy-one cases. J Bone Joint Surg 1964;46A:1405-1420.

Levine AM, Drennan JC. Physiological bowing and tibia vara: The metaphyseal-diaphyseal angle. J Bone Joint Surg 1982;64A:1158-1163.

Loder RT, Johnston CE II. Infantile tibia vara. J Pediatr Orthop 1987;7:639-646.

Moseley CF. A straight-line graph for leg-length discrepancies. J Bone Joint Surg 1977;59A:174-179.

Ogilvie JW. Epiphysiodesis: Evaluation of a new technique. J Pediatr Orthop 1986;6:147-149.

Paley D. Modern techniques in limb lengthening: Section I: Symposium. Clin Orthop 1990;250:2-159.

Paley D. Current techniques in limb lengthening. J Pediatr Orthop 1988;8:73-92.

Pappas AM, Anas P, Toczylowski HM Jr. Asymmetrical arrest of the proximal tibial physis and genu recurvatum deformity. JBJS1984;66A: 575-581.

Park HM, Rothschild PA, Kernek CB. Scintigraphic evaluation of extremity pain in children: its efficacy and pitfalls. AJR 1985;145:1079.

Phillips WA. The child with a limp. Orthop Clin North Am 1989;18:489.

Price CT. Metaphyseal and physeal lengthening in children. In Barr JS Jr (ed):AAOS Instruct Course Lect 1989;38:331-336.

Shapiro E. Longitudinal growth of the femur and tibia after diaphyseal lengthening. J Bone Joint Surgery 1987;69A:684-690.

Skak SV, Jensen TT, Pousen TD. Fracture of the proximal metaphysis of the tibia in children. Injury 1987;18:149-156.

Sommerville EW. Persistent fetal alignments. J Bone Joint Surg 1957;39B:106.

Staheli LT, Corbett M, Wyss C, et al. Lower-extremity rotational problems in children. Normal values to guide management. JBJS 1985;67A:39-47.

Staheli LT. Lower positional deformity in infants and children: A review. J Pediatr Orthop 1990;10:559-563.

Staheli LT. Rotational problems of the lower extremities. Orthop Clin North Am 1987;18:503.

Steel HH, Sandrow RE, Sullivan PD. Complications of tibial osteotomy in children for genu varum or valgum. J Bone Joint Surg 1971;53A:1629-1635.

Stephens DC, Herrick W, MacEwen GD. Epiphysiodesis for limb length inequality: Results and indications. Clin Orthop 1978;136:41-48.

Svennigsen S, Apalset K, Terjesen T, et al. Regression of femoral anteversion. A prospective study of intoeing children. AOS;1989;60:170.

Svennigsen S, Terjesen T, Auflem M, Berg V. Hip rotation and in-toeing gait. Clin Orthop RR 1990;251:177.

Thompson GH, Carter JR, Smith CW. Late-onset tibia vara: A comparative analysis. J Pediatr Orthop 1984;4:185-194.

Wagner H. Operative lengthening of the femur. Clin Orthop 1978;136:125-142.

Wenger DR, Mickelson M, Maynard JA. The evolution and histopathology of adolescent tibia vara. J Pediatr Orthop 1984;4:78-88.

Winquist RA. Closed intramedullary osteotomies of the femur. Clin Orthop 1986;212:155-164.

Zionts LE, MacEwen GD. Spontaneous improvement of post-traumatic tibia valga. J Bone Joint Surg 1986;68:680-687.

Zuege RC, Kempken TG, Blount WP. Epiphyseal stapling for angular deformity at the knee. J Bone Joint Surg 1979;61A:320-329.

Chapter 5—Foot

Introduction

Developmental variations of the foot are common. Thus, they are a frequent source of concern to the family and a common reason for referral to an orthopedist.

Growth

The lower limb bud forms by about 4 weeks of gestation, and the foot develops over the next 4 weeks (Fig. 5.1). The foot achieves its adult length earlier than the rest of the body. Half of the adult length of the foot is achieved between 12 and 18 months of age. By comparison, half of adult height is achieved at 2 years and half of the lower limb length by 3 to 4 years of age. Rapid foot growth requires shoe changes frequently in infancy and childhood (Fig. 5.2).

Arch Development

The longitudinal arch of the foot develops with advancing age (Fig. 5.3). The flatness of the infant's foot is due to a combination of abundant subcutaneous fat and joint laxity common in infants. This joint laxity allows flattening of the arch when the infant stands, and the fatty foot further obscures the longitudinal arch.

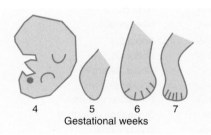

Fig. 5.1 Fetal foot development. The limb bud appears by about 4 weeks of gestation and the foot is well formed by about 7 weeks.

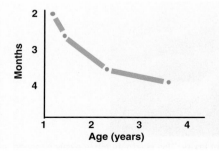

Fig. 5.2 Rapid foot growth. This graph shows the months required for a half size change in shoe size by year of age. From data by Gould et al. (1990).

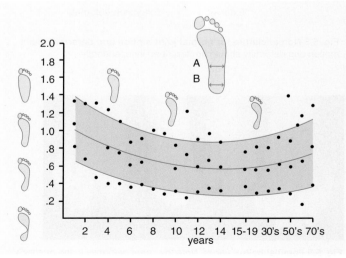

Fig. 5.3 Arch development. The longitudinal arch develops with growth in childhood. Note the wide range of normal. Flatfeet fall within the normal range. From Staheli et al. (1987).

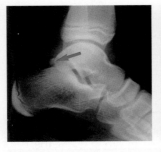
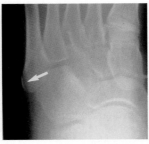

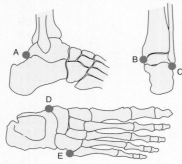

Fig. 5.4 Common accessory ossification centers about the foot. (A) Os trigonum (red arrow at top), (B) medial malleolar ossicle, (C) lateral malleolar ossicle, (D) accessory navicular (often painful), and (E) os vesalianum (yellow arrow at top).

Normal Variability

Accessory centers of ossification are common about the foot (Fig. 5.4). Most fuse with the primary center and become part of the parent ossicle. Others remain as separate ossicles, usually attached to the parent bone by cartilage or fibrous tissue. These ossicles are clinically important because they may be confused with a fracture, and they may become painful when the syndesmosis or synchondrosis is disrupted. Such disruptions commonly involve the accessory navicular and an ossicle inferior to the lateral malleolus.

Foot in Systemic Disorders

Evaluation of the foot is a useful aid in diagnosing constitutional disorders. For example, polydactylism is seen in chondroectodermal dysplasia. Dysplastic nails are found in the nail–patella syndrome.

Nomenclature

To clarify this discussion, terms describing joint motion versus those describing deformities are defined separately (Fig. 5.5). The anatomical position is considered neutral. Often deformity is designated simply by describing the motion and adding the term *deformity* behind it. Thus, the subtalar joint fixed in inversion is referred to as an *inversion deformity*. Note that the description of great toe position is inconsistent with standard terminology. The reference point is the center of the foot rather than the center of the body. Thus, the position of the great toe toward the midline of the body is referred to as *abduction*.

Both bones and joints may be deformed. For example, medial deviation of the neck of the talus occurs in clubfeet. This contributes to the adduction deformity. Joint deformity is usually due to stiffness with fixation in a nonfunctional position. Limit the use of the terms *varus* and *valgus* to describe deformities.

Evaluation

Family History

Foot shape often runs in families (Fig. 5.6). If the deformity is present in an adult, inquiry about disability may help in managing the child's problem.

Screening Examination

Perform a screening examination. Look at the back for evidence of a spinal dysraphism that may account for a cavus foot. Assess joint laxity (Fig. 5.7), as this may be a cause of a flexible flatfoot.

Site	Motion	Deformity
Ankle joint	Flexion	Equinus
	Extension	Calcaneus
Subtalar joint	Inversion	Heel varus
	Eversion	Heel valgus
Midtarsal joint	Adduction	Adductus
	Abduction	Abductus
	Flexion	Cavus deformity
	Extension	Rocker-bottom
	Pronation	Pronation deformity
	Supination	Supination deformity
Great toe	Abduction	Hallux varus
	Adduction	Hallux valgus
	Flexion	Flexion deformity
	Extension	Extension deformity
Toes	Flexion	Flexion deformity
	Extension	Extension deformity

Fig. 5.5 Nomenclature for normal joint motion and deformity. Joint motion and deformity should be described independently.

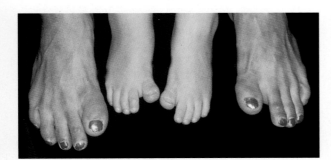

Fig. 5.6 Familial hallux varus. Note the same deformity in the mother's and daughter's feet.

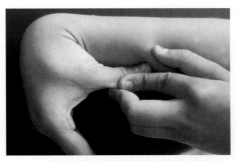

Fig. 5.7 Generalized joint laxity. This child's thumb is easily opposed to the forearm. The child also had a flexible flatfoot.

Foot Examination

The diagnosis of most foot disorders can be made by physical examination. Bones and joints of the foot have little overlying obscuring soft tissue, thus deformity and swelling are easily observed. Furthermore, localization of the point of maximum tenderness (PMT) is readily established.

Observation

Observe the skin on the sole of the feet for signs of excessive loading (Figs. 5.8 and 5.9). Excessive loading that causes calluses is not normal in children. Common sites of excessive loading include the metatarsal heads, the base of the fifth metatarsal, and under the head of the talus. The deformities that cause the calluses are likely to cause pain in adolescence.

Observe the foot with the child standing. Note any change in the alignment of the heel. Heel valgus is common. Note the height of the longitudinal arch. Next ask the child to toe stand. A longitudinal arch is established in children with a flexible flatfoot (Fig. 5.10). With the child seated and the foot unweighted, a longitudinal arch appears in the child with a flexible flatfoot.

Range of Motion

Estimate the range of motion of the toes and the subtalar and ankle joints. Estimate subtalar joint mobility by the range of inversion and eversion motion. Assess ankle motion both with the knee flexed and extended and with the subtalar joint in neutral alignment (Fig. 5.11). Dorsiflexion to at least 20° with the knee flexed and to 10° with the knee extended should be possible.

Palpation

By palpation, determine if any tenderness is present. Determining the PMT is especially helpful in the foot because much of the foot is subcutaneous. The PMT is often diagnostic or at least helpful in making decisions regarding imaging.

Imaging

Whenever possible, radiographs of the feet should be taken with the child standing (Fig. 5.12). If radiographs are indicated, order AP and lateral projections. If subtalar motion is limited, an oblique view of the foot is added to rule out a calcaneonavicular bar. The ankle can be evaluated by AP and lateral radiographs. Order a "mortise" view if a problem such as an osteochondritis of the talus is suspected. Other special views such as flexion–extension studies may be helpful. Compare the radiographs to published standards for children. The normal range is broad and changes with age (Fig. 5.13). CT scans are useful in evaluating the subtalar joint for evidence of a talocalcaneal bar. Bone scans are useful in confirming the diagnosis of osteochondrosis such as Freiberg disease. The scan will be abnormal before radiographic changes are present. MRI is useful for evaluating tumors.

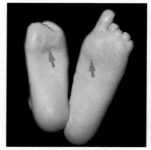

Fig. 5.8 Examine the sole for signs of excessive loading. Note the calluses under the metatarsal heads of both feet in this child with congenital toe deformities.

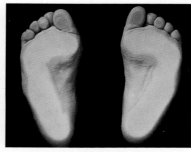

Fig. 5.9 Sole contact area. Note the broad even weight distribution on the soles of these normal feet. Child is standing on a mirrored glass surface.

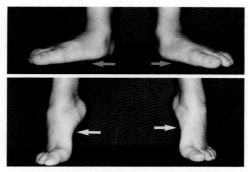

Fig. 5.10 Flexible flatfeet. The longitudinal arch absent on standing (red arrows) appears on toe standing (yellow arrows).

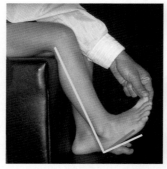
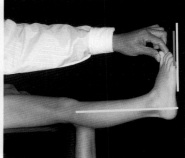

Fig. 5.11 Assessing ankle dorsiflexion. Right angle (yellow) is neutral position. Assess dorsiflexion (red lines) with the knee flexed and extended to determine site and severity of triceps contractures.

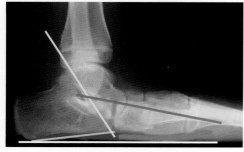

Fig. 5.12 Standing radiographs. Standing radiographs allow the most consistent evaluation. In the adolescent with a skewfoot deformity, the talar inclination (yellow line), metatarsal axis (red line), and calcaneal pitch (orange line) are readily measured.

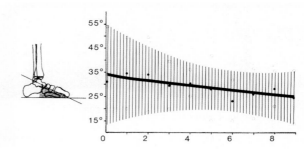

Fig. 5.13 Inclination of the talus by age. The shaded area represents two standard deviations above and below the mean (heavy line). Note that the values change with age and that the normal range is very broad. From Vander Wilde, et al. (1988).

Category	Disorder
Trauma	Fractures
	Sprains
	Soft tissue injuries
	Overuse syndromes
Infections	Osteomyelitis
	Septic arthritis
	Nail puncture wounds
	Ingrown toenail
Arthritis	Degenerative
	Juvenile rheumatoid
	Pauciarticular arthritis
Osteochondritis	Freiberg disease
	Köhler disease
Impingement pain	Os trigonum syndrome
	Anterior tarsal compression
Syndesmosis disruptions	Accessory navicular
	Lateral malleolar ossicle
	Medial malleolar ossicle
Idiopathic disorders	Osteochondritis dissecans
	Tarsal tunnel syndrome
	Reflex sympathetic dystrophy
Deformities	Bunions
	Bunionettes
	Tarsal coalitions
	Skewfoot
	Pathologic flatfeet

Fig. 5.14 Classification of foot pain. The causes of foot pain can be placed in categories for classification and diagnosis.

Foot Pain

Foot pain in children is common and varied (Figs. 5.14 and 5.15). During the first decade of life, foot pain is usually due to traumatic and inflammatory problems such as injuries and infections and is seldom due to deformity. During the second decade, foot pain is often secondary to deformity.

The cause of the foot pain can often be determined by the history and physical examination. Determining the PMT is especially useful about the foot because the structures are subcutaneous and easily examined (Fig. 5.16). This localization often allows a presumptive diagnosis.

Trauma

Stress–occult fractures Fractures without trauma history are not uncommon in infants and young children. They may be considered as part of the toddler fracture spectrum. Fractures of the cuboid, calcaneus, and metatarsal bones can be best identified by bone scans.

Tendonitis–fascitis Repetitive microtrauma is a common source of heel pain in children. This is most common about the os calcis either from the attachment of the heel-cord or the plantar fascia.

Infections

Infections of the foot are relatively common. Septic arthritis commonly affects the ankle and occasionally other joints of the foot. Osteomyelitis may occur in the calcaneus and other tarsal bones. Infection may be hematogenous or iatrogenic (heel sticks for blood sampling) or result from penetrating injuries.

Nail puncture wounds Nail puncture wounds are common injuries (Figs. 5.17 and 5.18) that may be complicated by osteomyelitis (Fig. 5.19). About 5% of nail penetrations become infected, but less than 1% develop osteomyelitis. Puncture wounds over the metatarsal are more likely to be infected with pseudomonas septic arthritis. Infections in the heel are commonly from staphlococcus or streptococcus.

Initial management Examine the foot and remove any protruding foreign material. Probing the wound will be noisy and unrewarding. Update tetanus immunization. Inform the family about the risk of infection and the need to return if signs of infection occur. Usually infections will show signs several days after the injury and include increasing discomfort, swelling on the dorsum of the foot, and fever.

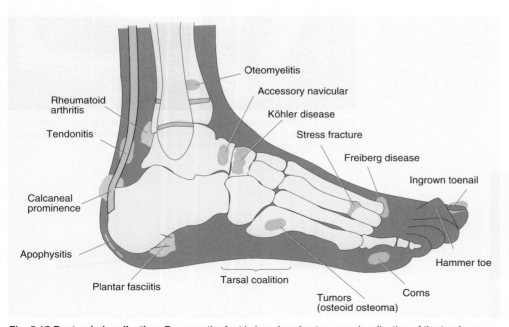

Fig. 5.15 Foot pain localization. Because the foot is largely subcutaneous, localization of the tenderness will often aid in establishing the diagnosis.

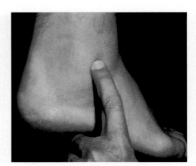

Fig. 5.16 Point of maximum tenderness. The ankle is swollen and tenderness is present just anterior to the distal fibula, typical of a sprain.

Management of infection Culture the wound and obtain an AP radiograph of the foot to serve as a baseline. The time of onset of signs of an infection suggests the infecting agent. If the interval between penetration and infection is 1 day, the organism is likely to be streptococcus. If the interval is 3–4 days, staphlococcus is most likely, and if a week, pseudomonas. Children with pseudomonas infections were usually wearing shoes at the time of the penetration. Operative debridement and drainage are indicated in all pseudomonas infections. Drainage is also indicated in all infections that fail to improve promptly with antibiotic treatment.

Ingrown Toenails Ingrown toenails (Fig. 5.20) are common infections resulting from a combination of anatomical predisposition, improper nail trimming, and trauma. Injury or constricting shoes or stockings may initiate the infection. In children prone to developing this problem, the nail is abnormal, often showing a greater lateral curvature of the nail into the nailbed.

Management of early infections Choose treatment based on the severity of the inflammation. Mild irritation requires only proper trimming of the nail and properly fitting shoes. Nails should be trimmed at right angles. Avoid trimming the nail to create a convex end. Instruct the family to trim the nail to create a concave end that leaves the nail edges extending beyond the skin to prevent recurrent ingrowth. Elevate the nail from the bed by packing cotton under the nail edge. Repeat this several times if necessary to lift the nail out of the inflamed nailbed. If inflammation is more severe, rest, elevation, protection from injury, soaking to clean and promote drainage, and antibiotics may be necessary.

Management of late infections Persistent severe lesions require operative management. The hypertrophic chronic granulation tissue is excised, and removal of the lateral portion of the nail together with a portion of the nail matrix may be necessary to prevent recurrence.

Pauciarticular Arthritis

Pauciarticular arthritis may present with foot pain in the infant or young child. A limp, limited ankle or subtalar motion and swelling for more than 6 weeks duration suggests this diagnosis (Fig. 5.21).

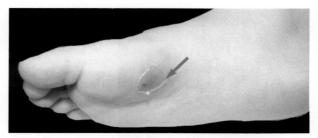

Fig. 5.17 Nail puncture wound. Erythema and a puncture wound (arrow) show the site of nail entry. Swelling is most prominent on the dorsum of the foot.

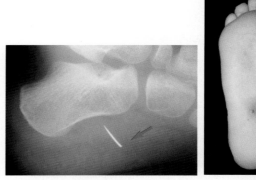

Fig. 5.18 Needle penetration into heel. Radiograph (left) shows broken needle. Photograph (right) shows site of entry of needle and surrounding inflammation.

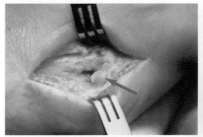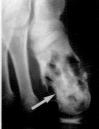

Fig. 5.19 Chronic osteomyelitis. A nail puncture wound through a shoe was followed by this infection that involved the bone and joint (red arrow). The joint was destroyed. Chronic osteomyelitis of the first metatarsal (yellow arrow) is evident in the radiograph.

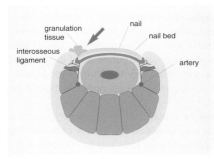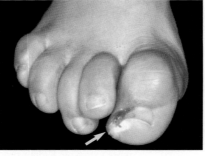

Fig. 5.20 Ingrown toenails. Granulation tissue grows over the site of nail penetration (red arrow). Photograph shows typical clinical appearance (yellow arrow).

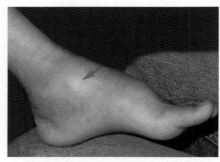

Fig. 5.21 Arthritis of the ankle. This child has pauciarticular arthritis of the ankle.

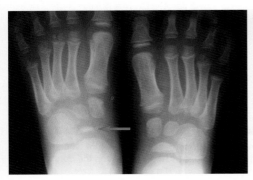

Fig. 5.22 Köhler disease in a 5-year-old boy. The tarsal navicular of the left foot is sclerotic (arrow) and the site of tenderness.

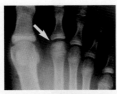
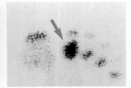

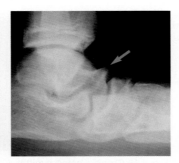

Fig. 5.23 Freiberg disease. Tenderness over the head of the second metatarsal is usually present in Freiberg disease. Minimal changes are present in the radiograph (yellow arrow), and the bone scan shows increased uptake over the second metatarsal head (red arrow). The photograph shows the point of maximum tenderness (blue arrow).

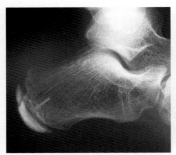
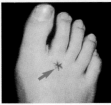

Fig. 5.24 Calcaneal apophysis. This apophysis often shows a sclerotic pattern in the normal child.

Fig. 5.25 Impingement. This is talar beaking associated with a tight heel-cord and impingement.

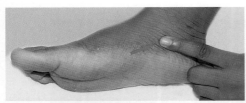

Fig. 5.26 Accessory navicular. The accessory navicular is located on the medial aspect of the foot (arrows). It often produces a prominence and is sometimes painful.

Osteochondritis

Köhler disease Tarsal navicular osteochondritis, also known as Köhler disease, is an avascular necrosis most common in boys between 3 and 5 years of age (Fig. 5.22). It also occurs uncommonly in girls 2 to 4 years of age. The disease produces inflammation, localized tenderness, and a limp. Radiographic changes depend on the stage of the disease. The navicular first shows collapse and increased density. Patchy deossification follows. Finally, the navicular is reconstituted. Because healing occurs spontaneously, only symptomatic treatment is necessary. If pain is a significant problem, immobilize the foot in a short-leg walking cast for 8 weeks to reduce inflammation and provide relief of pain. Long-term follow-up studies show no residual disability.

Freiberg disease Metatarsal head osteochondritis, also known as Frieberg disease or infraction, is an idiopathic segmental avascular necrosis of the head of a metatarsal. It most commonly occurs in adolescent girls and involves the second metatarsal. Pain and localized tenderness (Fig. 5.23) are common. If the patient is seen early, a bone scan will show increased uptake and establish the diagnosis. Later, radiographs will show irregularity of the articular surface, sclerosis, fragmentation, and finally reconstitution. Residual overgrowth and articular irregularity may lead to degenerative changes and persistent pain. Treat with rest and immobilization to reduce inflammation. An orthosis to unweight the involved metatarsal head, sole stiffeners to reduce motion of the joint, and even a short-leg walking cast may be useful. For severe persisting pain, operative correction may be necessary. Options include joint debridement, excisional arthroplasty (proximal phalanx), interposition arthroplasty using the tendon of the extensor digitorum longus, and dorsiflexion osteotomy of the metatarsal (often the best choice).

Sever disease Calcaneal apophyseal osteochondrosis, also known as Sever disease, is commonly diagnosed by heel pain and radiographic features of fragmentation and sclerosis of the calcaneal apophysis. These radiographic changes occur commonly in asymptomatic children (Fig. 5.24). Most heel pain in children is due to inflammation of the attachment of the plantar fascia or heel-cord.

Impingement Pain

Os trigonum syndrome Compression of the ossicle in dancers often causes foot pain.

Anterior tarsal impingement Anterior foot pain is sometimes due to compression of articular margins often secondary to tarsal coalitions or heel-cord contracture (Fig. 5.25).

Syndesmosis Disruption

Disruption of the syndesmosis between the primary ossicle and secondary centers of ossification (accessory ossicles) is a common cause of pain in the feet of children and teenagers. This disruption is the equivalent of a stress injury of the cartilaginous or fibrous attachment. This disruption becomes painful unless healing is complete. The condition commonly recurs.

Accessory navicular is an accessory ossification center on the medial side of the tarsal navicular that occurs in about 10% of the population and remains as a separate ossification center in about 2% (Fig. 5.26). Disruptions are common during late childhood and adolescence and are probably due to repetitive trauma. This disruption causes pain and localized tenderness. This pain may cause inhibition of the function of the posterior tibialis muscle with secondary lowering of the longitudinal arch. Radiographs show an accessory ossicle and reduction of the calcaneal pitch in some cases.

Manage with a short-leg cast or splint. If the problem persists, excision of the accessory navicular may be necessary. Simple excision with or without plication of the posterior tibialis tendon is as effective as the more extensive Kidner procedures, which require rerouting the tendon.

Malleolar ossicles Ossification centers occur below the medial and lateral malleoli. Persisting ossicles under the lateral malleolus are most likely to be painful (Fig. 5.27). Manage first by cast immobilization. Rarely, excision or stabilization by internal fixation is necessary.

Idiopathic Disorders

Osteochondritis dissecans talus Ankle pain, swelling, stiffness, and a trauma history suggest this diagnosis. Confirm with radiographs (Figs. 5.28 and 5.29). Manage with activity modification, immobilization, nonsteroidal antiinflammatory drugs (NSAIDs), and time. Most will resolve. Lesions that are lateral with sclerotic margins and seperated are more likely to require surgery. Remove loose bodies. The value of drilling is uncertain. Replace and fix large lesions.

Tarsal tunnel syndrome Foot pain, Tinel's sign over tarsal tunnel, dysesthesias, and delayed nerve condition suggest this diagnosis. This syndrome differs in children. Typically the child is female, walks with the foot in varus, may use crutches, and often requires operative release.

Reflex sympathetic dystrophy This syndrome usually affects the lower limb in girls (Fig. 5.30). Consider this diagnosis when the foot is swollen, stiff, cool, and generally painful. A history of injury is common. See Chapter 3 for management.

Foot Deformities

Foot deformities may cause pain due to pressure over bony prominences (Fig. 5.31) or to altered mechanics of the foot. Pain from deformity is usually not difficult to recognize.

References
1999 Foot and ankle problems in the young athlete. Omey ML and Micheli LJ. Med Sci Sports Exerc 31:470
1999 Natural course of osteochondritis dissecans in children. Sales de Gauzy J, Mansat C, Darodes PH, Cahuzac JP. JPO-B 8:26
1998 Osteochondritis dissecans of the talus during childhood and adolescence. Higuera J et al. JPO 18:328
1996 The os trigonum syndrome: imaging features. Karasick D, Schweitzer ME. Am J Roentgenol 166:125
1995 Köhler's bone disease of the tarsal navicular. Borges JL, Guille JT, Bowen JR. JPO 15:596
1995 Kidner procedure for symptomatic accessory navicular and its relation to pes planus. Prichasuk S, Sinphurmsukskul O. Foot Ankle Int 16:500
1995 Fracture of the cuboid in children. A source of leg symptoms. Simonian PT, et al. JBJS 77B:104
1992 Bone scintigraphy in preschool children with lower extremity pain of unknown origin. Englaro EE, Gelfand MJ, Paltiel HJ. J Nucl Med 33:351
1992 Os trigonum impingement in dancers. Marotta JJ, Micheli LJ. Am J Sports Med 20:533
1992 Reflex sympathetic dystrophy in children. Clinical characteristics and follow-up of seventy patients. Wilder RT, et al. JBJS 74A:910
1991 Freiberg's disease and dorsiflexion osteotomy. Kinnard P, Lirette R. JBJS 73B:864
1991 Tarsal tunnel syndrome. Causes and results of operative treatment. Takakura Y, et al. JBJS 73B:125
1990 Foot growth in children age one to five years. Gould N;, Moreland M, Trevino S, Alvarez R, Fenwick J, Bach N. Foot Ankle 10:211
1990 Surgical treatment of symptomatic accessory tarsal navicular. Bennett GL, Weiner DS, Leighley B. JPO 10:445
1990 Anatomy of the os trigonum. Grogan DP, Walling AK, Ogden JA. JPO 10:618
1990 Accessory ossification patterns and injuries of the malleoli. Ogden JA, Lee J. JPO 10:306
1987 Symptomatic ossicles of the lateral malleolus in children. Griffiths JD, Menelaus MB. JBJS 69B:317
1982 The tarsal tunnel syndrome in children. Albrektsson B, Rydholm A, Rydholm U. JBJS 64B:215

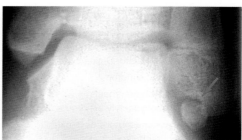

Fig. 5.27 Lateral malleollar ossicle. This ossicle was painful, not improved by casting, and evenutally required fusion with screw fixation.

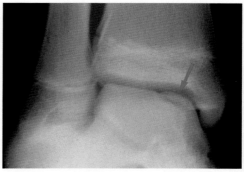

Fig. 5.28 Medial osteochondritis dissecans lesion. Medial lesions are less common and often unassociated with trauma.

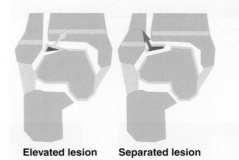

Elevated lesion   **Separated lesion**

Fig. 5.29 Lateral osteochondritis dissecans lesion types. A lesion that is elevated (yellow arrow) or separated (red arrow) may require surgery.

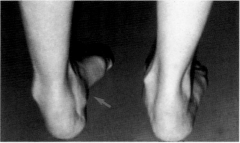

Fig. 5.30. Reflex sympathetic dystrophy. The varus deformity of the left foot is due to reflex sympathetic dystrophy.

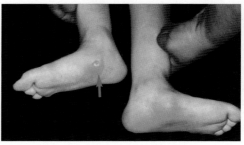

Fig. 5.31 Foot deformities in a child with spina bifida. Prominence of the head of the talus caused skin breakdown in the foot with diminished sensation.

Toe Deformities	Disorders
Polydactyly	Chondoectodermal dysplasia
	Carpenter syndrome
	Oto–Palato–Digital syndrome
Syndactyly	Apert syndrome
Metatarsal hypoplasia	Achondrogenesis
	Brachydactyly syndrome
Broad toe	Acromesomelic dysplasia
	Larsen syndrome
	Rubinstein–Taybi syndrome

Fig. 5.32 Syndromes associated with toe deformities.

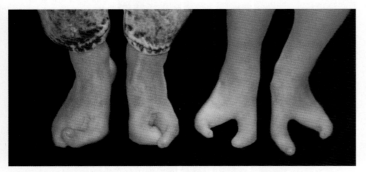

Fig. 5.33 Cleft foot deformity. These deformities are present in both the father and the son. The major problems are difficulties with shoe fitting and the unusual appearance.

Toe Deformities

Generalized Disorders

If a toe deformity is found, carefully examine the hands and feet of the child and of the parents. These deformities are sometimes manifestations of a generalized disorder (Fig. 5.32).

Cleft Foot Deformity

This rare deformity is transmitted as an autosomal dominant trait, is usually bilateral, and often involves the hands and feet (Fig. 5.33). A noninherited form is less common and is often unilateral. If it causes shoe-fitting problems, correct in late infancy or childhood by osteotomy and soft tissue approximation.

Microdactyly

Small toes are often found in Streeter's dysplasia and may be secondary to intrauterine hypotension, causing insufficient circulation to the toes (Fig. 5.34). No treatment is required.

Syndactyly

Fusion of the toes produces no functional disability and treatment is unnecessary. Look for some underlying problem.

Polydactyly

Polydactyly or supernumerary digits are common (Fig. 5.35). They are most common in girls and in blacks and are sometimes inherited as an autosomal dominant trait. Most involve the little toe and duplication of the proximal phalanx with a block metatarsal or wide metatarsal head. Excise the extra digit late in the first year when the foot is large enough to make excision simple and before the infant is aware of the problem. Plan the procedure to minimize the scar, establish a normal foot contour, and avoid disturbing growth. Central duplications often cause permanent widening of the foot. Poor results are more likely for great toe duplications with persistent hallux varus and complex deformities (Figs. 5.36 and 5.37).

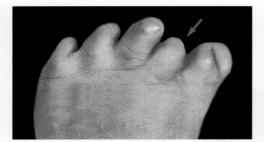

Fig. 5.34 Microdactyly.

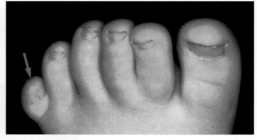

Fig. 5.35 Polydactyly. Polydactyly causes a cosmetic and shoe fitting problem. Excision of the accessory toe is appropriate late in the first year.

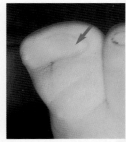
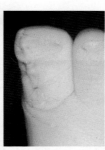
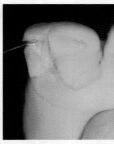

Fig. 5.36 Excision of bifid great toe. Half of the toe is removed. Excision of complex polydactyly is sometimes difficult.

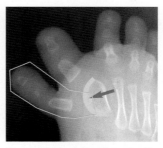

Fig. 5.37 Bracket epiphysis. Toe deformities may be complex. In this case, the metatarsal epiphysis is continuous for both toes. Excise the accessory digit and the adjacent portion of the growth plate.

Curly Toes

Curly toes (Fig. 5.38) are common in infancy and produce flexion and rotational deformities of the lesser toes. These deformities improve with time. Most will resolve spontaneously. Some advise tape splinting (Fig. 5.39), and, rarely, flexor tendinotomy is required for persisting deformity.

Overriding Toes

Overriding toes are common. Overriding of the second, third, and fourth toes usually resolves with time. Overriding of the fifth toe is more likely to be permanent (Fig. 5.40) and cause a problem with shoe fitting. Overriding of the fifth toe is often bilateral and familial. If overriding becomes fixed, persists, and causes shoe-fitting problems, operative correction is appropriate. Correct with the Butler soft tissue alignment procedure.

Hammer Toes

Hammer toes are secondary to a fixed flexion deformity of the proximal interphalangeal (PIP) joint (Fig. 5.41). The distal joint may be fixed or flexible. The condition is often bilateral, familial, and most commonly involves the second toes and less frequently the third and fourth. Operative correction is indicated in adolescence if the deformity produces pain or shoe-fitting problems. Correct by fusing the IP joint.

Claw Toes

Claw toes are usually associated with a cavus foot and are often secondary to a neurologic problem. Correction is usually part of the management of the cavus foot complex.

Hypertrophy

Hypertrophy (Fig. 5.42) is seen in children with Proteus syndrome, neurofibromatosis, or vascular malformation, or it can occur as an isolated deformity. Most show abnormal accumulation of adipose tissue, and some show endoneural and perineural fibrosis and focal neural and vascular proliferation. Management is difficult. Epiphysiodesis, debulking, ray resection, and through-joint amputations are often necessary. Recurrence is frequent, and several procedures are often required during childhood to facilitate shoe fitting.

References

2000 Operative repair of the fixed hammertoe deformity. Coughlin MJ, Dorris J, Polk E. Foot Ankle Int 21:94

1999 Congenital cleft-foot deformity treatment. Abraham E, Waxman B, Shirali S, Durkin M. JPO 19:404

1998 Macrodactyly. Kotwal PP, Farooque M. JBJS 80B:651

1997 Effect of proximal phalangeal epiphysiodesis in the treatment of macrodactyly. Topoleski TA, Ganel A, Grogan DP. Foot Ankle Int 18:500

1993 Butler's operation for congenital overriding of the fifth toe. Retrospective 1-7-year study of 23 cases. De Boeck H. Acta Orthop Scand 64:343

1993 Surgery for curly toe deformity: a double-blind, randomised, prospective trial. Hamer AJ, Stanley D, Smith TW. JBJS 75B:662

1993 Metatarsal epiphyseal bracket: treatment by central physiolysis. Mubarak SJ, O'Brien TJ, Davids JR. JPO 13:5

1992 Polydactyly of the foot: an analysis of 265 cases and a morphological classification. Watanabe H, Fujita S, Oka I. Plast Reconstr Surg 89:856

1991 Anomalies of the fingers and toes associated with Klippel-Trenaunay syndrome. McGrory BJ, et al. JBJS 73A:1537

1990 Pathology of macrodactyly. Desai P, Steiner GC. Bull Hosp Jt Dis Orthop Inst 50:116

1987 Strapping of curly toes in children. Turner PL. Aust N Z J Surg 57:467

1985 Polydactyly of the foot. Phelps DA, Grogan DP. JPO 5:446

1984 Open flexor tenotomy for hammer toes and curly toes in childhood. Ross ER, Menelaus MB. JBJS 66B:770

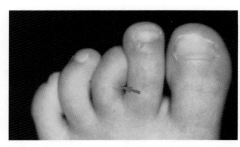

Fig. 5.38 Curly toes. This deformity may involve one or more toes and resolves spontaneously.

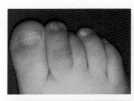 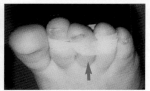

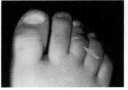

Fig. 5.39 Taping of overlapping curly toes. Paper tape is applied loosely to align toes (red arrow). Regardless of treatment, correction occurs over time (green arrow).

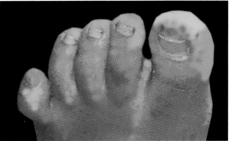

Fig. 5.40 Overlapping toe. This overlapping fifth toe persisted and required operative correction.

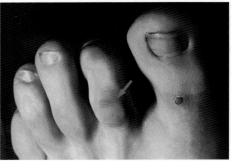

Fig. 5.41 Hammer toe. The fixed flexion deformity of the PIP joint of the second toe causes a callus (arrow) to form over the toe.

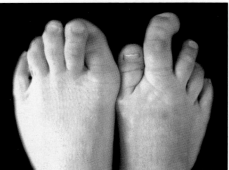

Fig. 5.42 Hypertrophy. Overgrowth may cause severe shoe-fitting problems and require resection, epiphysiodesis, or amputation.

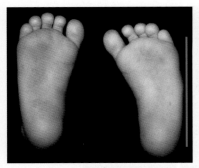
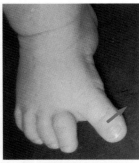

Fig. 5.43 Metatarsus adductus. A convexity of the lateral border of the foot (red line) is the most consistent feature of this deformity.

Fig. 5.44 Great toe abduction. This is a dynamic deformity that resolves with time.

Type	Etiology	Comment
Metatarsus adductus	Late intrauterine, positional deformity	Common form 90% resolve spontaneously
Metatarsus varus	Earlier onset, intrauterine position?	Often rigid Cast correction necessary
Skewfoot	Familial Generalized joint laxity	Hindfoot valgus Abduction midfoot Adduction forefoot Treatment difficult
Abducted great toe	Unknown	Dynamic deformity Resolves spontaneously

Fig. 5.45 Types of forefoot adductus and varus deformities. The differential diagnosis of metatarsus adductus should include the rigid, nonresolving form, and the skewfoot.

Forefoot Adductus

Metatarsus Adductus and Varus

Adductus of the forefoot is the most common foot deformity. It is characterized by a convexity to the lateral aspect of the foot (Fig. 5.43) or a dynamic abduction of the great toe (Fig. 5.44). The deformities fall into four categories (Fig. 5.45).

Metatarsus adductus is a common intrauterine positional deformity. Because it is associated with hip dysplasia in 2% of cases, a careful hip evaluation is essential. Metatarsus adductus is common, flexible, benign, and resolves spontaneously.

Metatarsus varus is an uncommon rigid deformity that often persists and requires cast correction. Metatarsus varus does not produce disability and does not cause bunions, but it does produce cosmetic and occasionally shoe-fitting problems.

Great toe abduction is a dynamic deformity due to overactivity of the great toe abductor. Sometimes called a "searching toe." The condition improves spontaneously. No treatment is required.

Management

Evaluate by performing a screening examination, test for stiffness, and consider the child's age (Fig. 5.46). Manage metatarsus adductus by documentation and observation (Fig. 5.47)

Manage metatarsus varus by serial casting (Figs. 5.48 and 5.49) or bracing (see page 73). Long-leg bracing is useful in the toddler. Serial casting is most effective. The deformity yields much more rapidly when the cast is extended above the flexed knee.

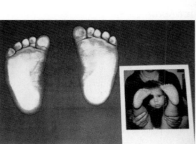
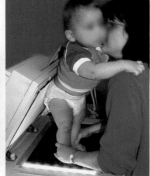

Fig. 5.47 Imaging the adducted foot. The infant's foot shape is recorded on a copy machine. The printout from the copy machine is compared to a photograph.

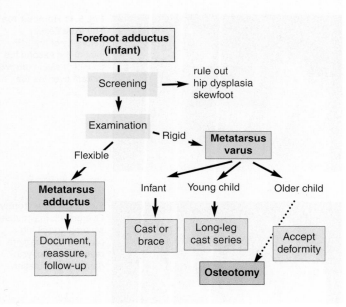

Fig. 5.46 Steps in managing forefoot adductus.

Forefoot adductus (infant) → Screening → rule out hip dysplasia skewfoot

Screening → Examination

Examination — Rigid → **Metatarsus varus**

Examination — Flexible → **Metatarsus adductus** → Document, reassure, follow-up

Metatarsus varus → Infant → Cast or brace

Metatarsus varus → Young child → Long-leg cast series

Metatarsus varus → Older child → Accept deformity

Long-leg cast series → **Osteotomy**

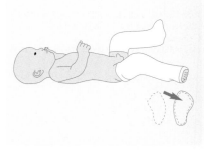
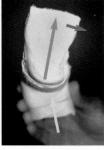

Fig. 5.48 Long-leg cast for metatarsus varus. This treatment of metatarsus varus is most effective, as the flexed knee provides control of tibial rotation. Using the thigh portion of the cast as a point of fixation (yellow arrow), the foot is laterally rotated (green arrow) and abducted (red arrow) to achieve the most effective correction.

The following technique is useful to about age 5 years. Apply a short-leg cast first. As the cast sets, mold the forefoot into abduction. Finally, while holding the short-leg cast in external rotation and with the knee flexed about 30°, extend the cast to include the thigh. This long-leg cast allows both walking and effective correction.

In the older child, it may be best to accept the deformity, as it does not cause disability. If operative correction is selected, correct by osteotomy rather than capsulotomy. Correction is not simple and complications are common.

Skewfoot

Skewfoot, Z-foot, and *serpentine foot* are all terms given to a spectrum of complex deformities. This deformity includes hindfoot plantarflexion, midfoot abduction, and forefoot adduction (Fig. 5.50). A tight heel-cord is usually present in symptomatic cases. Skewfeet are seen in children with myelodysplasia; they are sometimes familial but are usually isolated deformities. There is a spectrum of severity. Some practitioners describe overcorrected clubfeet as skewfeet. Idiopathic skewfeet may persist and cause disability in adolescence and adult life.

Manage idiopathic skewfeet in young children by initial documentation with standing AP and lateral radiographs and observe to determine the effect of growth on the deformity. Most will persist. Plan correction in late childhood with heel-cord lengthening and osteotomies. Lengthen the calcaneus and first cuneiform (Fig. 5.51).

References

1999 Below-knee plaster cast for the treatment of metatarsus adductus. Katz K, David R, Soudry M. JPO 19:49

1996 Magnetic resonance imaging of skewfoot. Hubbard AM, et al. JBJS 78A:389

1995 Abductory midfoot osteotomy procedure for metatarsus adductus. Harley BD, et al. J Foot Ankle Surg 34:153

1995 Calcaneal lengthening for valgus deformity of the hindfoot. Results in children who had severe, symptomatic flatfoot and skewfoot. Mosca VS. JBJS 77A:500

1994 The long-term functional and radiographic outcomes of untreated and non-operatively treated metatarsus adductus. Farsetti P, Weinstein SL, Ponseti IV JBJS 76A:257

1987 The Heyman-Herndon tarsometatarsal capsulotomy for metatarsus adductus: results in 48 feet. Stark JG, Johanson JE, Winter RB. JPO 7:305

1986 A reappraisal of metatarsus adductus and skewfoot. Berg EE. JBJS 68A:1185

1986 Skewfoot (forefoot adduction with heel valgus). Peterson HA. JPO 6:24

1984 Shortening of the first metatarsal as a complication of metatarsal osteotomies. Holden D, et al. JBJS 66A:582

1983 Metatarsus adductus: classification and relationship to outcomes of treatment. Bleck EE. JPO 3:2

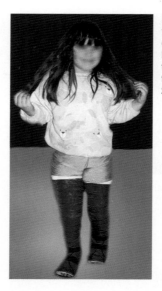

Fig. 5.49 Cast treatment of metatarsus varus. This child with a persisting stiff deformity was corrected using these long-leg casts. The knee is flexed to about 30° to control rotation. The foot is abducted in the casts. The casts are changed every 2–3 weeks until correction is completed.

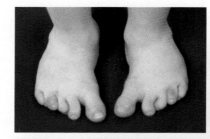
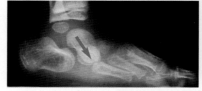
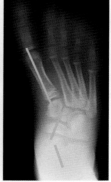

Fig. 5.50 Skewfoot deformity. Note the forefoot adduction in the photograph, the plantar flexed talus (red arrow), and the *Z* alignment (orange lines).

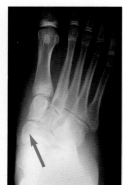
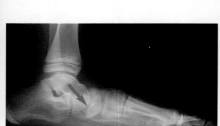
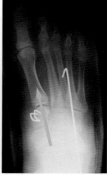
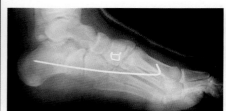

Fig. 5.51 Sequence of correction of skewfoot. Calcaneal and cuneiform osteotomies and a heel-cord lengthening were performed. Note the changes in talar alignment between the preoperative (red arrows) and postoperative (orange arrows) radiographs.

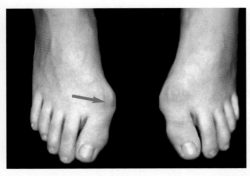

Fig. 5.52 Mild bunion deformities. The bunion is a prominence over the head of the first metatarsal. The right bunion (arrow) is most prominent here, and both are relatively mild. Usually no active treatment is required for bunions of this severity.

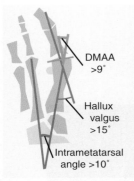

Fig. 5.53 Measurements for bunion assessment.

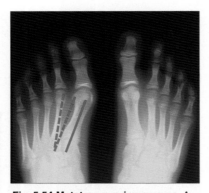

Fig. 5.54 Metatarsus primus varus. An increased intermetatarsal angle (between dotted lines) is present in metatarsus primus varus. The hallux valgus is a secondary deformity.

Forefoot Deformities

Bunion

A bunion is a prominence of the head of the first metatarsal (Fig. 5.52). In children they are usually due to metatarsus primus varus, a developmental deformity characterized by an increased intrametatarsal angle (Fig. 5.53) that exceeds about 9° between the first two rays. Hallux varus is a secondary deformity probably due to the effect of wearing shoes, as the great toe must be positioned in valgus to fit within a shoe. The normal hallux valgus angle is <15°. The combination of primary and secondary deformities cause the typical adolescent bunion (Fig. 5.54).

Bunions are often familial (Fig. 5.55) and may occur in children with neuromuscular disorders (Fig. 5.56). Other factors may include pronation of the forefoot, joint laxity, and pointed shoes. Bunions are rare in barefoot populations.

Evaluation Look for evidence of joint laxity, heel-cord contracture, pes planus, or other skeletal defects. Is the toe rotated? Is there a family history of bunions? Order AP and lateral standing radiographs. Measure the intermetatarsal angle. Measure the distal metatarsal articular angle (DMAA). This is normally less than 8°. Is the metatarsal–phalangeal joint subluxated? Is the cuneiform–metatarsal articulation oblique? Note the relative lengths of the first and second rays.

Management Attempt to delay operative correction until the end of growth to reduce the risk of recurrence.

Shoes Encourage girls to avoid shoes with pointed toes and high heels, as they aggravate the deformity and increase discomfort.

Splints For nighttime use, splints may be effective but are difficult to use because of the required duration of management (Fig. 5.57).

Operative correction Tailor the choice of operation based on the pathology. There are many possible procedures (see Chapter 16).

Complications Ray shortening, elevation or depression of metatarsal heads, subluxation of the metatarsal phalangeal joint, and overcorrection or undercorrection are all possible complications of operative treatment.

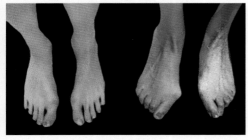

Fig. 5.55 Familial bunions. Both mother and daughter have bunions.

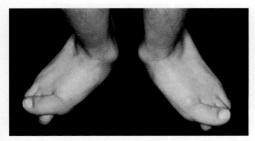

Fig. 5.56 Severe hallux valgus in cerebral palsy. Note the absence of metatarsus primus varus and any prominence of the metatarsal head.

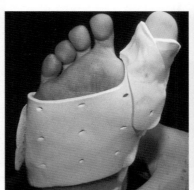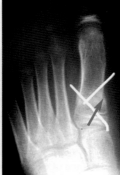

Fig. 5.57 Treatment of juvenile bunions. Night splinting or operations are options. This child had metatarsus primus varus corrected by osteotomy and fixed with crossed pins (arrow).

Dorsal Bunion

The uncommon dorsal bunion (Fig. 5.58) is due to an elevation of the first metatarsal. This elevation is caused by an imbalance between the stronger tibialis anterior and peroneus longus muscles. It is most common in clubfeet. This can be corrected by a plantar flexion osteotomy of the cuneiform or metatarsal and a muscle-balancing procedure.

Bunionette

Bunionette (tailor's bunion) is a painful bony prominence on the lateral side of the fifth metatarsal head, often associated with an inflamed thickened bursa and calluses. These deformities are developmental and involve an increased metatarsalphalangeal angle of the fifth toe, an increased intermetatarsal angle between fourth and fifth toes, and an increased intermetatarsal angle between the great and second toes. Management often requires an osteotomy for correction.

Hallux Rigidus

This is a degenerative arthritis of the first metatarsal phalangeal joint due to repetitive trauma, which causes stiffness, limited dorsiflexion, and pain. Manage by protecting the joint with a shoe stiffener. If severe and persistent, correct by a dorsal dorsiflexion osteotomy (Fig. 5.59) to move the arc of motion into more extension.

Short Metatarsal

Shortening of one or more metatarsals may be due to a developmental abnormality as part of a generalized disorder or from trauma, infection, or tumors. Severe shortening may cause metatarsalgia and a cosmetic disability. Rarely the deformity is severe enough to justify operative correction. This can be done by a single-stage lengthening technique (Fig. 5.60) or by gradual distraction histiogenesis.

References

1998 The treatment of congenital brachymetarsia by one-stage lengthening. Baek GH, Chung MS. JBJS 80B:1040

1998 Dorsal wedge osteotomy in the treatment of hallux rigidus. Blyth MJ, Mackay DC, Kinninmonth AW. J Foot Ankle Surg 37:8

1998 Surgical treatment for bunions in adolescents. Senaris-Rodriguez J, et al. JPO-B 7:210

1997 Metatarsal lengthening: case report and review of literature. Choudhury SN, Kitaoka HB, Peterson HA. Foot Ankle Int 18:739

1997 Mitchell osteotomy for adolescent hallux valgus. Weiner BK, Weiner DS, Mirkopulos N. JPO 17:781

1996 Bunions and deformities of the toes in children and adolescents. Thompson GH. Instr Course Lect 45:355

1995 Applications of the opening wedge cuneiform osteotomy in the surgical repair of juvenile hallux abducto valgus. Lynch FR. J Foot Ankle Surg 34:103

1994 A controlled prospective trial of a foot orthosis for juvenile hallux valgus. Kilmartin TE, Barrington RL, Wallace WA. JBJS 76B:210

1993 Adolescent bunion deformity treated with double osteotomy and longitudinal pin fixation of the first ray. Peterson HA, Newman SR. JPO 13:80

1992 Juvenile hallux valgus. A conservative approach to treatment. Groiso JA. JBJS 74A:1367

1991 Metatarsus primus varus. A statistical study. Kilmartin TE, Barrington RL, Wallace WA. JBJS 73B:937

1990 Radiologic anatomy of the painful bunionette. Nestor BJ, et al. Foot Ankle 11:6

1989 Hohmann-Thomasen metatarsal osteotomy for tailor's bunion (bunionette). Steinke MS, Boll KL. JBJS 71A:423

1989 Osteochondral defects of the first metatarsal head in adolescence: a stage in the development of hallux rigidus. Thomas AP, Dwyer NS. JPO 9:236

1989 Treatment of hallux valgus in adolescents by the chevron osteotomy. Zimmer TJ, Johnson KA, Klassen RA. Foot Ankle 9:190

1988 Relationship between adolescent bunions and flatfeet. Kalen V, Brecher A. Foot Ankle 8:331

1988 Distal metatarsal osteotomy for bunionette deformity. Konradsen L, Nielsen PT. J Foot Surg 27:493

1985 Dorsal bunion following clubfoot surgery. Johnston CE 2d, Roach JW. Orthopedics 8:103

1983 Dorsal bunions in children. McKay DW. JBJS 65A:975

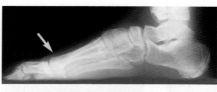

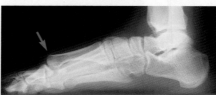

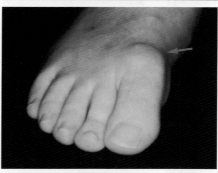

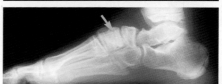

Fig. 5.58 Dorsal bunion. This child's bunion developed between the ages of 14 (yellow arrow) and 18 years (red arrows). The deformity was corrected by a dorsal opening wedge osteotomy (orange arrow) and lateral transfer of the anterior tibialis.

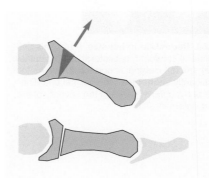

Fig. 5.59 Dorsal osteotomy for hallux rigidus. A dorsal closing wedge osteotomy moved the arc of motion into more plantarflexion at the metatarsal phalangeal joint.

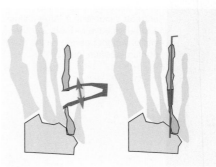

Fig. 5.60 Technique of metatarsal lengthening. This one-stage lengthening is described by Baek and Chung (1998).

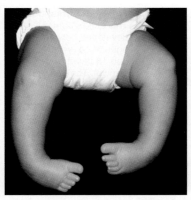

Fig. 5.61 Typical appearance of bilateral clubfeet. The deformity includes equinus, adductus, varus, and medial rotation.

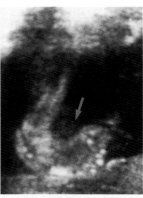

Fig. 5.62 Clubfoot on ultrasound at 16 weeks.

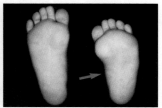

Fig. 5.63. Severe clubfoot. Note the prominent medial crease (arrow).

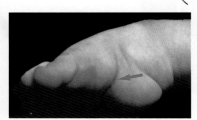
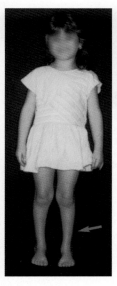

Fig. 5.64 Reduction in leg size. (Left) This girl with bilateral clubfeet has bilateral calf hypoplasia. (Above) The left clubfoot is corrected, but the foot is significantly shorter than the normal one. The degree of hypoplasia parallels the severity of the clubfoot deformity.

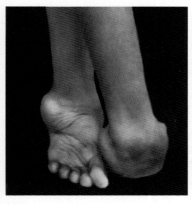

Fig. 5.65 Untreated clubfeet. These are the feet of a 13-year-old Cambodian boy with untreated clubfeet. A large callus and bursa have formed over the site of weight bearing on the dorsum of each foot.

Clubfoot

Clubfoot (CF) is a complex congenital deformity that includes components of equinus, varus, adductus, and medial rotation (Fig. 5.61). Clubfoot is also referred to as *talipes equinovarus* (TEV). Clubfoot occurs in about 1 in 1000 births, is bilateral in half the cases, and affects males more frequently.

Etiology

The cause of clubfeet is multifactorial. In affected families, clubfeet are about 30 times more frequent in offspring. Fetal ultrasound screening shows the deformity in the first trimester (Fig. 5.62). It is frequently associated with other congenital abnormalities such as neural tube defects, anomalies of the urinary or digestive system, and other musculoskeletal abnormalities. Most show polyhydramnios, and amniocentesis often shows abnormal karyotype. The clubfoot deformity can have many etiologies, as evidenced by the variability of expression and response to management.

Mild clubfoot is a late intrauterine deformity (see Chapter 1) and corrects rapidly with cast treatment. At the other end of the severity spectrum, severe clubfoot behaves like a disruption, having an origin earlier in fetal life and requiring operative correction. Severe clubfoot is seen in conditions such as arthrogryposis (Fig. 5.63). Classic or idiopathic clubfoot is a polygenic disorder, is relatively common, and occupies the middle range of the severity spectrum.

Pathology

The pathology of clubfoot is typical of a dysplasia. The tarsals are hypoplastic. The talus is most deformed; the size is reduced and the talar neck is shortened and deviated in a medial and plantar direction. The navicular articulates with the medial aspect of the neck of the talus due to the abnormal shape of the talus. The relationship of the tarsals is abnormal. The talus and calcaneus become more parallel in all three planes. The midfoot becomes more medially displaced and the metatarsals are adducted. In addition to the deformities of cartilage and bone, the ligaments are thickened and the muscles hypoplastic. This results in a generalized hypoplasia of the limb with shortening of the foot and smallness of the calf (Fig. 5.64). Because the hypoplasia primarily involves the foot, limb length discrepancy is usually less than 1 cm. The foot is small, and split size shoes are often required. The amount of foot shortening is proportional to the severity of the clubfoot.

Natural History

Untreated, clubfoot produces considerable disability (Fig. 5.65). The dorsolateral skin becomes the weight-bearing area. Calluses form and walking becomes limited. Treated clubfoot often causes minor disability from excessive loading on the lateral aspect of the foot due to residual varus and stiffness.

Clinical Features

The diagnosis of clubfoot is not difficult and is seldom confused with other foot deformities. Sometimes severe metatarsus varus is confused with clubfoot, but the equinus component of clubfoot makes the differentiation clear. The presence of a clubfoot should prompt a careful search for other musculoskeletal problems.

Examine the back for evidence of dysraphism, the hips for dysplasia, and the knees for deformity. Perform a screening neurologic examination. Note the size, shape, and flexibility of the feet. Take radiographs of the spine or pelvis if abnormalities are found on physical examination. If the infant is 6 months of age or older, initial AP and lateral radiographs are useful to supplement the physical examination. Measure the AP and lateral talocalcaneal angles. Compare these with the normal values (see Chapter 17). MRI studies will show the cartilaginous elements but are not practical for routine use.

Note the degree of stiffness of the foot (Fig. 5.66) and compare the size of the foot with the uninvolved foot. Marked differences in foot length suggest that the deformity is severe and foretell the need for operative correction. Document the components of the clubfoot deformity, the equinus, heel varus, forefoot adductus, and medial rotation. In the child, cavus is common.

Equinus is due to a combination of a plantar flexed talus, posterior ankle capsular contracture, and shortening of the triceps.

Varus results from frontal plane parallelism of the talus and calcaneus, contracture of the medial subtalar joint capsules, and contracture of the posterior tibialis muscle.

Adductus and medial rotation are due to medial deviation of the neck of the talus, medial displacement of the talonavicular joint, and metatarsus adductus. Tibial rotation is normal. Tibial or femoral torsion are not primary features of clubfeet.

Classification

A number of classifications have been proposed.

Etiologic classification This is based on the possible causes of clubfoot and include several types.

Positional clubfeet are flexible and thought to result from intrauterine position late in gestation. These resolve quickly with serial casting.

Idiopathic clubfeet include the classic forms with an intermediate degree of stiffness. They are polygenic in etiology.

Teratologic clubfeet are associated with arthrogryposis, myelodysplasia, and other generalized disorders. These feet are very stiff and difficult to manage.

Dimeglio classification This classification is based on stiffness. Range of motion in equinus, adduction, varus, and medial rotation are the given points. The sum of these points establishes the severity (Fig. 5.67).

Imaging Studies

Radiographs, ultrasound, and MRI imaging are used for assessment. Because active treatment usually occurs during early infancy when ossification is incomplete, the value of radiographic studies is limited. Because MRI studies are expensive and require deep sedation, they are not practical. Ultrasound studies are promising and likely to become more widely used with time. Currently, radiographs are still the most practical. Radiographs become increasingly valuable with increasing age (Fig. 5.68). The common measures are as follows:

Tibial calcaneal angle in maximal dorsiflexion is a measure of equinus. To fall into the normal range, the angle should be >10° beyond a right angle.

Lateral talocalcaneal angle is a measure of varus. Parallelism is a sign of residual heel varus.

AP calcaneocuboid alignment provides an assessment of the severity of the midfoot adduction and varus.

Navicular position Dorsal displacement of the navicular is a sign of malalignment of the midtarsal joints.

The value of radiographs is uncertain because long-term studies suggest that triceps strength, foot mobility, and plantar loading as measured clinically may be more significant than static radiographic measures in assessing results.

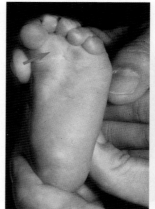
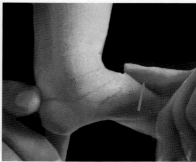

Fig. 5.66 Testing flexibility. Assessing flexibility is a good way to determine the severity of the clubfoot.

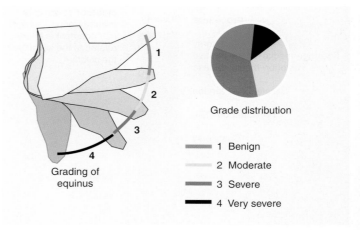

Fig. 5.67 Dimeglio classification. Clubfoot stiffness in equinus (shown here), varus, rotation, and adduction are assessed. The sum of these scores is used to establish severity. The distribution of clubfeet into the four grades of severity are shown in the pie chart. Based on Dimeglio et al. (1995).

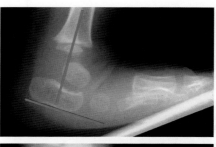
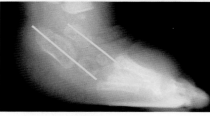

Fig. 5.68 Radiographic evaluation of clubfoot. On a maximum dorsiflexion radiograph, measure the tibial calcaneal angle (red lines). On resting or standing radiographs, note the parallelism between the axes of the talus and calcaneus (yellow lines).

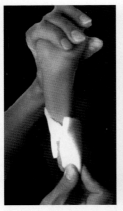
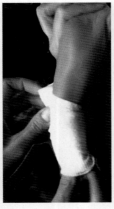
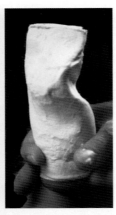

Fig. 5.69 Initial management with corrective casts. Cast treatment is helpful in correcting or reducing clubfoot deformity. Padding is first applied. A well-molded long-leg cast is most effective in correction.

Procedure	Severity
Talectomy	
Posterior–medial–lateral release	
Posterior–medial release	
Transfer of AT tendon	
Percutaneous TAL	
Casts only	

Fig. 5.70 Relating clubfoot severity to management. Clubfoot management is often related to the severity of the clubfoot.

Management

The objective of management of clubfoot is to correct the deformity and retain mobility and strength. The foot should be plantigrade and have a normal load-bearing area. Secondary objectives include the ability to wear normal shoes, satisfactory appearance, and avoidance of unnecessarily complicated or prolonged treatment. The clubfoot is never fully corrected. When compared with a normal foot, all clubfeet show some residual stiffness, shortening, or deformity.

Management trends are influenced by data that suggest that maintaining mobility and triceps strength are more important than judging outcomes on radiographic criteria. Current trends favor casting (Fig. 5.69), passive motion, percutaneous heel-cord tenotomies integrated into the cast management sequence, customized operative procedures (Fig. 5.70), and procedures of less magnitude.

Idiopathic clubfeet Start treatment as soon as possible after birth. Several approaches are used (Fig. 5.71).

The Ponseti approach is becoming increasingly more widely used. Manipulate the foot and then apply a long-leg cast to correct the deformities in a definite sequence. Correct the cavus, rotate the foot from under the talus, and finally correct the equinus (see page 384). Usually a percutaneous tenotomy is performed to facilitate equinus correction (Fig. 5.72), and sometimes a transfer of the anterior tibialis (AT) is performed in early childhood. Rotational splinting is an essential part of management. Flexibility and strength are maintained.

The French approach emphasizes prolonged intense manipulations and splinting.

The traditional approach includes initial casting and then one of several techniques for operative correction. Delay major procedures until the end of the first year of growth. Tailor the extent of the procedure to the severity of deformity (Figs. 5.70, 5.73, and 5.74). Prevent recurrent deformity with night splinting.

Severe clubfeet as seen in conditions such as arthrogryposis are best managed by initial casting, multiple tendon–ligament releases, and a resumption of casting. Often an open postero–medial–plantar release is required at about 1 year of age. Night splinting in the position of maximum correction is essential to reduce the risk of recurrence (Fig. 5.75). Correct recurrent deformities with casts. Avoid repeated major operative procedures. Plan a final bony correction at the end of growth.

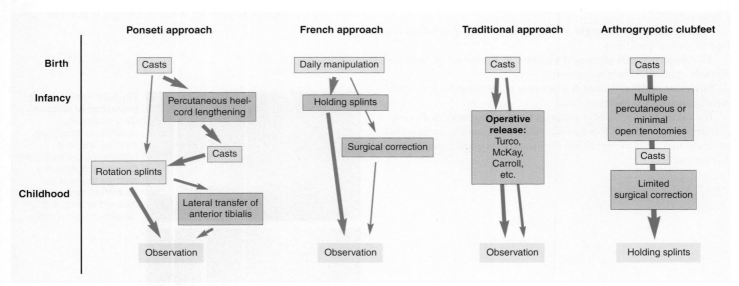

Fig. 5.71 Approaches to management of clubfeet.

Complications of treatment are common.

Recurrence is the most frequent problem. About one-third of clubfeet require more than one procedure.

Stiffness may result from excessive articular pressure during treatment, compartment syndromes complicating surgery, internal fixation, avascular necrosis of the talus, and operative scarring.

Weakness of the triceps jeopardizes function. Overlengthening and repeated lengthening procedures increase this risk.

Varus deformity commonly causes excessive plantar pressure over the base of the fifth metatarsal.

Severe deformity in older children are sometimes best managed with the Ilizarov frame (Fig. 5.76). To release the deformity, use the frame to stretch soft tissues to achieve gradual correction.

Consultants for Clubfoot Section

Alain Dimeglio, e-mail: a-dimeglio@chu-montpellier.fr
John Herzenberg, e-mail: frcsc@aol.com
Vince Mosca, e-mail: vmosca@chmc.org
Ignacio Ponseti, e-mail: ignacio-ponseti@uiowa.edu

References

2000 Predictive value of intraoperative clubfoot radiographs on revision rates. Moses W, Allen BL, Jr., Pugh LI, Stasikelis PJ. JPO 20:529

1999 Clubfoot surgical treatment: preliminary results of a prospective comparative study of two techniques. Manzone P. JPO-B 8:246

1998 Non-surgical treatment of congenital clubfoot with manipulation, cast, and modified Denis Browne splint. Yamamoto H, Muneta T, Morita S. JPO 18:538

1997 2nd Gait analysis and muscle strength in children with surgically treated clubfeet. Karol LA, Concha MC, Johnston CE. JPO 17:790

1997 Management of clubfoot deformity in amyoplasia. Niki H, Staheli LT, Mosca VS. JPO 17:803

1997 Common errors in the treatment of congenital clubfoot. Ponseti IV. Int Orthop 21:137

1996 Antenatal sonographic diagnosis of clubfoot: a six-year experience. Pagnotta G, et al. J Foot Ankle Surg 35:67

1996 Correction of persistent clubfoot deformities with the Ilizarov external fixator. Experience in 10 previously operated feet followed for 2-5 years. Wallander H, Hansson G, Tjernstrom B. Acta Orthop Scand 67:283

1995 Classification of clubfoot. Dimeglio A, et al. JPO-b 4:129

1995 Update on pathologic anatomy of clubfoot. Ippolito E. JPO-b 4:17

1994 Correction of the neglected clubfoot by the Ilizarov method. de la Huerta. CO 301:89

1994 Cause of toe-in gait after posteromedial release for congenital clubfoot. Yamamoto H, Muneta T, Furuya K. JPO 14:369

1993 A single-gene explanation for the probability of having idiopathic talipes equinovarus. Rebbeck TR, et al. Am J Hum Genet 53:1051

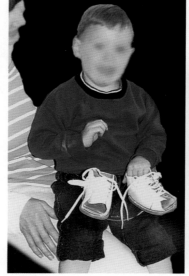
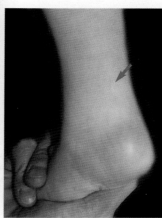

Fig. 5.72 Ponseti management. This child had serial casting, a percutaneous tenotomy (arrow), and an excellent outcome with a flexible, strong, plantigrade foot.

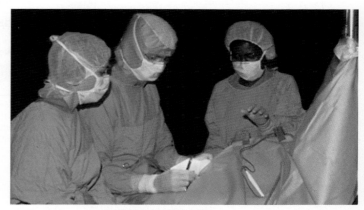

Fig. 5.73 Operative setup for traditional approach. Prone positioning of the patient allows excellent visualization and assistance for clubfoot surgery.

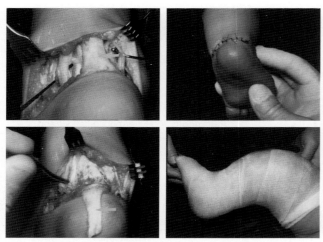

Fig. 5.74 Operative correction. This posterior release includes lengthening of the heel-cord (arrows) and opening of the joint capsule. Immobilization is provided by a long-leg cast.

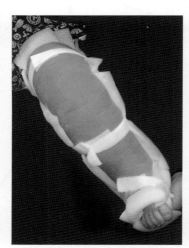

Fig. 5.75 Night splints. These can be made from a bivalved fiberglass cast and can be secured with Velcro closures.

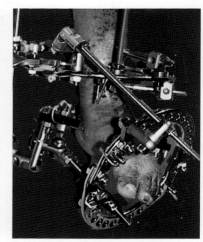

Fig. 5.76 Ilizarov frame. This is an effective method of correcting severe deformity in the older child.

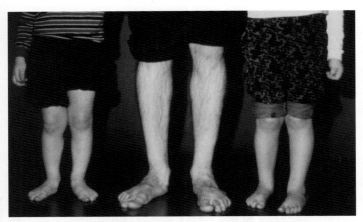

Fig. 5.77 Familial flatfeet. Each member of this family had flexible flatfeet. None were symptomatic. Demonstrating the flatfoot in the asymptomatic adult provides reassurance for the parents.

Flatfeet

The flatfoot (FF), or *pes planus,* is a foot with a large plantar contact area. The flatfoot is often associated with a valgus heel and a reduction in height of the longitudinal arch. Flatfeet are classified as physiologic or pathologic. Physiologic flatfeet are flexible, common, benign, and a variation of normal. Pathologic flatfeet show some degree of stiffness, often cause disability, and usually require treatment. Ankle valgus, as seen in myelodysplasia and poliomyelitis, may be confused with a flatfoot deformity. Valgus is in the subtalar joint. Make the differentiation radiographically.

Flexible Flatfoot

The flexible flatfoot or physiologic flatfoot is present in nearly all infants, many children, and about 15% of adults. Flatfeet often run in families (Fig. 5.77). Flatfeet are most common in those who wear shoes, are obese, or have generalized joint laxity (Fig. 5.78). There are two basic forms. Developmental flatfeet occur in infants and children as a normal stage of development (Fig. 5.79). The hypermobile flatfoot persists as a normal variant. Two studies of military populations have shown that the flexible flatfoot does not cause disability and, in fact, is associated with a reduction in stress fractures.

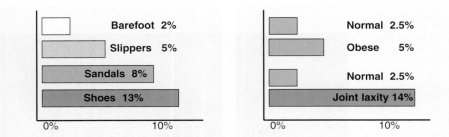

Fig. 5.78 Associations of flexible flatfeet. These studies from India demonstrate that flatfeet are more common in adults who wore shoes as children, the obese, and those with joint laxity. From Roe and Joseph (1993).

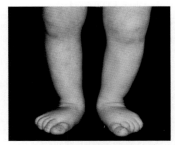

Fig. 5.79 Developmental flatfeet. Most infants and many children have flatfeet. The infant's flatfeet are often due to their thick subcutaneous plantar fatpad and joint laxity.

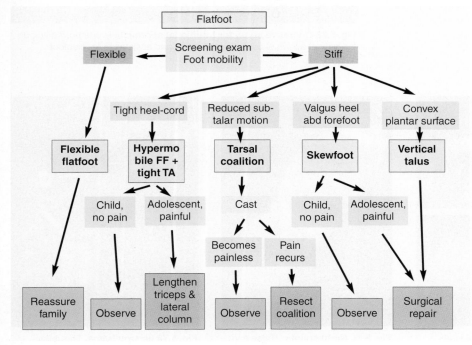

Fig. 5.80 Flatfoot management. This algorithm outlines the evaluation and management of flatfeet.

Category	Disorder
Flexible flatfoot	Developmental flatfoot
	Hypermobile flatfoot
	Calcaneovalgus foot
Pathologic flatfoot	Hypermobile flatfoot and tight tendo-achilles
	Lateral tibial torsion, obesity
	Tarsal coalitions
	Talocalcaneal
	Calcaneonavicular
	Neurogenic flatfoot
	Severed posterior tib tendon
	Vertical talus

Fig. 5.81 Classification of flatfeet. Flatfeet are categorized into physiologic and pathologic types.

Evaluation Evaluate to establish a diagnosis (Fig. 5.80). The screening examination may show generalized joint laxity. On standing, the foot appears flat and the heel may show mild valgus. The arch reappears when the child toe stands or the foot is unweighted. Subtalar and ankle motions are full. Radiographs are unnecessary. Flatfeet can be classified into physiologic (flexible) types and pathologic types (Fig. 5.81).

Management The flexible flatfoot (Fig. 5.82) requires no treatment, as it has been shown that the condition is not a source of disability. Shoe modifications or inserts (Figs. 5.83 and 5.84) are ineffective, expensive, result in a bad experience for the child, and may adversely affect the individual's self-image (see page 40). Operative intervention to create an arch by blocking subtalar motion may establish an arch but may expose the child to risks of an operation (Fig. 5.85), months of postoperative discomfort, and, possibly because of damage to the subtalar joint, cause degenerative arthritis of the subtalar joint in adult life.

Interventions should not be imposed on the child to "satisfy" the parent. Provide reassurance and make copies of the parent education material (see page 416) to show the grandparents and other family members. If the family insists that something be done, encourage the use of flexible shoes, limitation of excess weight, and a healthy lifestyle for the child.

Calcaneovalgus Deformity

This congenital deformity is due to intrauterine crowding, producing both calcaneus and valgus (Fig. 5.86). The condition may be confused with a vertical talus. Differentiation is made by determining the degree of stiffness. The calcaneovalgus foot is very flexible and the calcaneus lies in dorsiflexion. This condition is associated with developmental hip dysplasia, which should be ruled out by a careful examination of the hips. Because the calcaneovalgus flatfoot is a positional deformity, it resolves spontaneously. Treatment is not required.

Hypermobile Flatfoot and Heel-Cord Contracture

Heel-cord contractures cause an obligatory heel valgus, altered tarsal motion, lateral column shortening, and a painful pathologic flatfoot.

Evaluation The patient is usually in the second decade and has vague activity-related foot pain. The foot is flat on standing and the heel-cord contracted. The foot cannot be dorsiflexed beyond neutral with the knee extended (Fig. 5.87). Radiographs often show excessive plantarflexion of the talus. This condition is often confused with simple hypermobile flatfoot and inappropriately called a *symptomatic flexible flatfoot*.

Management Lengthen the contracture of the triceps. If the soleus is contracted, lengthen the heel-cord. If only the gastrocnemius is contracted, perform a recession. Most cases have secondary shortening of the lateral column and require a calcaneal lengthening (see page 392).

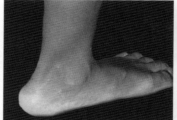
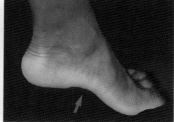

Fig. 5.82 Arch develops on toe standing. This is a characteristic finding in flexible flatfeet.

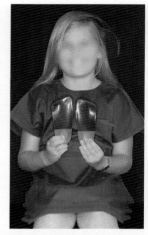

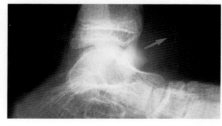

Fig. 5.83 Effect of shoe modifications in flatfeet. This prospective, controlled study compared arch development with various treatments. No difference was found. Talarmetatarsal angles before (light shade) and after (dark shade) treatment. From Wenger et al. (1989).

Fig. 5.84 Orthotics can be discarded. This girl was pleased when she was told she could discard the orthotics. Plastic inserts are uncomfortable and make the child feel abnormal.

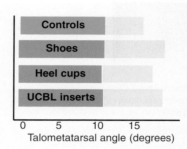

Fig. 5.85 Extrusion of silastic implant. This implant was placed in a child with flexible flatfeet.

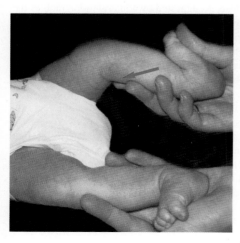

Fig. 5.86 Calcaneovalgus deformity. This is a positional deformity that requires no treatment.

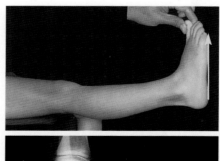
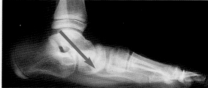

Fig. 5.87 Heel-cord contracture with flexible flatfoot. This child with a flexible flatfoot also has a heel-cord contracture. Note that the foot cannot be dorsiflexed above a neutral position with the knee extended (yellow arrow) and that the foot shows plantarflexion of the talus (red arrow).

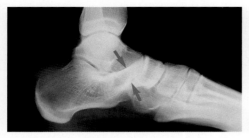

Fig. 5.88 "Anteater sign." The calcaneonavicular coalition is seen in lateral radiographs with this characteristic feature (arrows).

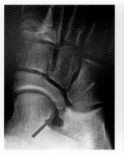
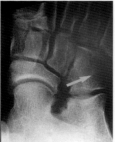

Fig. 5.89 Calcaneonavicular coalition. This T-C coalition is readily seen on oblique radiographs of the foot before resection (red arrows). Surgical resection (orange arrow) reduced discomfort and restored motion.

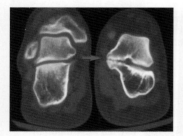
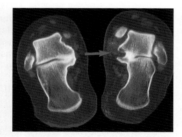

Fig. 5.90 Subtalar coalition. The middle facet subtalar coalition (arrow) is readily identified by CT imaging.

Fig. 5.91 Failed resection. This resection failed because the coalition was not fully resected.

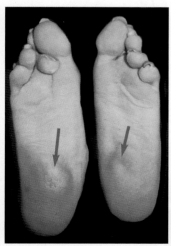
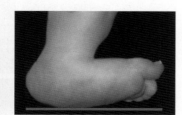

Fig. 5.92 Vertical talus in an adult. Note the prominences on the sole of the foot causing calluses and pain with walking.

Fig. 5.93 Vertical talus in arthrogryposis. Note the convexity to the sole of the foot.

Tarsal Coalitions

Coalitions are fusions between tarsal bones that cause a loss of inversion and eversion motion. They are often familial, may be unilateral or bilateral, and occur in both sexes equally. The fusion imposes increased stress on adjacent joints and sometimes causes degenerative arthritis, pain, and peroneal spasm. These symptoms usually develop during early adolescence. Sometimes coalitions remain silent. Two common forms are present: Be aware that coalitions may involve more than one joint.

Calcaneonavicular coalitions are most common and sometimes identified on a lateral radiograph (Fig. 5.88) but are readily shown by an oblique radiograph of the foot (Fig. 5.89). The coalition may be composed of bone, cartilage, or fibrous tissue. Incomplete coalitions may show only narrowing or irregularity of the calcaneonavicular articulation.

Manage symptomatic coalitions with a trial of immobilization. Apply a short-leg walking cast for 4 weeks. The pain should disappear. If pain recurs soon after removal, operative correction is usually necessary. Resect the coalition (see Chapter 16) and interpose extensor hallicus brevis muscle to prevent recurrence.

Talocalcaneal coalitions (T-C) usually involve the middle facet of the subtalar joint. Conventional radiographs are often normal, but a special calcaneal or "Harris" view may show the fusion. However, the coalition is best demonstrated by CT scans of the foot (Fig. 5.90).

Manage symptomatic coalitions with a trial using a short-leg cast. If pain recurs, consider operative resection. Assess the size of the coalition by CT imaging. Resection is likely to fail if coalitions exceed 50% of the joint. Technical problems are common (Fig. 5.91). Heel valgus may be increased by resection. Sometimes a calcaneal lengthening will be needed to correct this component. Outcomes for resection of subtalar coalitions are much less predictable than for the more common calcaneonavicular fusions. Advise the family of the potential for an unsatisfactory result and the possibility that additional procedures may be necessary.

Other coalitions may occur at the talonavicular and naviculocuneiform joint. More extensive coalitions may be present in children with clubfeet, fibular hemimelia, and proximal focal femoral deficiencies. Be aware that pain and stiffness of the subtalar joint may occur with arthritis, tumors, and articular fractures. Consider these uncommon causes of pain if calcaneonavicular and talocalcaneal fusions are ruled out by radiography.

Vertical Talus

The vertical talus is the most severe and serious pathologic flatfoot (Fig. 5.92). It is a congenital deformity that produces not only flattening but an actual convexity of the sole of the foot (Fig. 5.93).

Evaluation Vertical talus is usually associated with other conditions such as myelodysplasia and arthrogryposis. The foot is stiff, with contractures of both the dorsiflexors and plantarflexors. The head of the talus projects into the plantar aspect of the foot, producing the convexity of the sole. The diagnosis is suggested by a lateral radiograph of the foot showing the vertical orientation of the talus (Fig. 5.94). Vertical talus may be confused with flexible oblique talus, a different condition. Make the differentiation by studying lateral flexion and extension radiographs of the foot. The vertical talus will show stiffness and fixation in contrast to the flexible oblique talus, which shows a freely mobile mid- and hindfoot (Fig. 5.95). Note especially the mobility of the calcaneus. If the calcaneus is fixed in plantarflexion in both views of the foot, the diagnosis is vertical talus.

Management Correct by a single-stage procedure late in the first year of growth. Lengthen the heel-cord and anterior structures and perform a posterolateral release. Elevate the plantarflexed talar head to reestablish the talonavicular joint. Fix with a single smooth longitudinal transcutaneous K wire. Consider transfer of the tibialis anterior to the talus. In the older child, a naviculoectomy or subtalar fusion may be required.

Neuromuscular Flatfeet

Flatfeet are common in cerebral palsy (Fig. 5.96) because of spastic contractures of the heel-cord and muscle imbalance. These flatfeet may require operative stabilization because of skin breakdown on the medial aspect of the foot and to provide more stability in walking (Chapter 16).

Other Causes

Laceration of the posterior tibialis tendon causes flatfeet in children as it does in adults.

Overcorrected clubfeet is a common cause. This complication may occur in children who have clubfeet and ligamentous laxity.

External tibial torsion and obesity are associated with painful flatfeet in adolescence.

Skewfoot produces heel valgus and a flat-appearing foot, as discussed earlier in this chapter.

Ankle valgus occurs in children with myelodysplasia and clubfeet. Correct by tethering distal tibial growth with a screw (Fig. 5.97). Remove it when deformity is slightly overcorrected.

References

1999 Flexible flat feet in children: a real problem? Garcia-Rodriguez A, et al. Pediatrics 103:e84

1999 Planovalgus foot deformity. Current status. Staheli LT. J Am Podiatr Med Assoc 89:94

1999 Pediatric flatfoot: evaluation and management. Sullivan JA. J Am Acad Orthop Surg 7:44

1998 Resection for symptomatic talocalcaneal coalition. Comfort TK, Johnson LO. JPO 18:283

1997 Multiple tarsal coalitions in the same foot. Clarke DM. JPO 17:777

1997 Gait abnormalities following resection of talocalcaneal coalition. Kitaoka HB, Wikenheiser MA, Shaughnessy WJ, An KN. JBJS 79A:369

1997 Talocalcaneal coalition resection: a 10-year follow-up. McCormack TJ, Olney B, Asher M. JPO 17:13

1997 Early one-stage reconstruction of congenital vertical talus. Stricker SJ, Rosen E. Foot Ankle Int 18:535

1997 The sinus tarsi spacer in the operative treatment of flexible flat feet. Verheyden F, et al. Acta Orthop Belg 63:305

1996 Tarsal coalition. Kulik SA Jr, Clanton TO. Foot Ankle Int 17:286

1995 Calcaneal lengthening for valgus deformity of the hindfoot. Results in children who had severe, symptomatic flatfoot and skewfoot. Mosca VS. JBJS 77A:500

1995 Congenital vertical talus: a retrospective and critical review of 32 feet operated on by peritalar reduction. Napiontek M. JPO-b 4:179

1995 Foot deformity and the length of the triceps surae in Danish children between 3 and 17 years old. Reimers J, Pedersen B, Brodersen A. JPO-b 4:71

1994 Talocalcaneal coalition in patients who have fibular hemimelia or proximal femoral focal deficiency. A comparison of the radiographic and pathological findings. Grogan DP, Holt GR, Ogden JA. JBJS 76A:1363

1994 Subtalar coalition: diagnosis with the C sign on lateral radiographs of the ankle. Lateur LM, et al. Radiology 193:847

1994 Pes planus in childhood due to tibialis posterior tendon injuries. Treatment by flexor hallucis longus tendon transfer. Masterson E, et al. JBJS 76B:444

1994 Clubfeet and tarsal coalition. Spero CR, Simon GS, Tornetta P 3rd. JPO 14:372

1994 Tarsal coalition: depiction and characterization with CT and MR imaging. Wechsler RJ, et al. Radiology 193:447

1994 Resection for symptomatic talocalcaneal coalition. Wilde PH, et al. JBJS 76B:797

1992 Osseous and non-osseous coalition of the middle facet of the talocalcaneal joint. Kumar SJ, et al. JBJS 74A:529

1992 The influence of footwear on the prevalence of flat foot. A survey of 2300 children [see comments]. Rao UB, Joseph B. JBJS 74B:525

1990 Calcaneonavicular coalition treated by resection and interposition of the extensor digitorum brevis muscle. Gonzalez P, Kumar SJ. JBJS 72A:71

1990 Computed tomography in suspected tarsal coalition. Examination of 26 cases. Warren MJ, et al. Acta Orthop Scand 61:554

1989 Corrective shoes and inserts as treatment for flexible flatfoot in infants and children [see comments]. Wenger DR, et al. JBJS 71A:800

1988 Foot deformities in the newborn--incidence and prognosis. Widhe T, Aaro S, Elmstedt E. Acta Orthop Scand 59:176

1948 Hypermobile flatfoot with short tendo achillis. Harris RI, Beath T. JBJS 30A:116

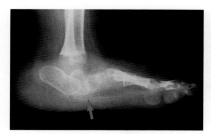

Fig. 5.94 Vertical talus. The talus is positioned in a vertical position (red arrow) as part of the complex deformity of hindfoot equinus and forefoot dorsiflexion.

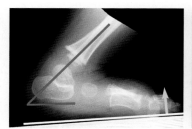
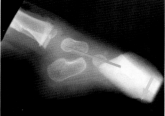

Fig. 5.95 Dorsiflexion–plantarflexion study. This study in an infant shows a dorsiflexion of the calcaneus (red lines) and alignment of the talus and metatarsals (orange line) consistent with a hypermobile foot and inconsistent with a vertical talus.

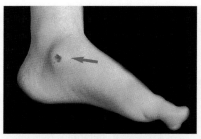

Fig. 5.96 Foot in cerebral palsy. Note the skin breakdown on the medial side of the foot (red arrow). Note the eversion of the foot on the footrests of the wheelchair (yellow arrows).

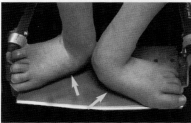

Fig. 5.97 Heel valgus secondary to ankle deformity. Note the valgus ankle (red line) in this 10-year-old child with myelodysplasia. This was managed by placing a tethering medial malleolar screw. Note the improvement early (yellow line) and at 2 years postoperative (orange line). The screw was then removed.

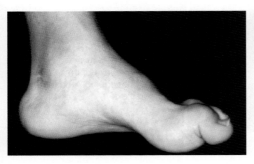

Fig. 5.98 Typical cavus foot. Note the high arch and clawing of the great toe.

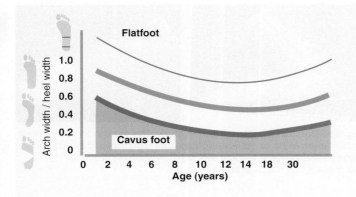

Fig. 5.99 Normal values for foot contact area. Contact area is described by the ratio of the arch width to the heel width. The mean value (green line), and two standard deviation levels for a low arch (blue line) and a high arch (red line) are shown. A foot is considered to have a cavus deformity if the arch contact area falls outside the ±2 SD level (red area).

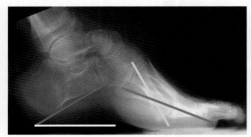

Fig. 5.100 Radiographic features of cavovarus deformity. Note the calcaneal pitch (red–white angle) and the first (yellow) and fifth (blue) metatarsal alignment.

Cavus Feet

A cavus foot is characterized by increased height of the longitudinal arch and is often associated with clawing of the toes and heel varus (Fig. 5.98). Cavus is most often physiological. It is simply the extreme end of the spectrum of normal variability of the shape of the longitudinal arch. This physiologic form is often familial. Pathologic forms of cavus deformity are usually neurogenic.

Physiologic Cavus

This deformity falls outside the normal range (beyond ±2 SD from the mean) of variability in arch height (Fig. 5.99). Often a parent's feet have a high arch. The parent often volunteers that they have a "good" (high) arch. In fact, these parents are more likely to have pain than those with normal or low arches. The cavus is usually bilateral, with an onset in infancy. They may also have calluses under the metatarsal heads. The child's musculoskeletal and neurologic screening examinations are normal, and clawing of the toes is absent. This is a diagnosis of exclusion. Occasionally the teenager will complain of metatarsal pain. This is best managed by shock-absorbing shoeware and, if necessary, a soft shoe insert to unload the metatarsal heads.

Pathologic Cavus

Pathologic cavus is usually secondary to a neuromuscular disorder causing muscle imbalance. A major objective of management is to determine the underlying cause of the deformity.

Evaluation The neuromuscular disorders causing cavus deformities are often familial, so the family history is important. Look at the parent's feet. Sometimes they may claim their feet are normal when they are clearly deformed. Perform a careful screening examination of the child. Examine the musculoskeletal system for other problems. Look for midline skin lesions over the spine. A careful neurologic examination is essential. Check muscle strength. Examine the foot, noting the severity of the cavus, degree of rigidity, and presence of clawing of the toes and skin changes over the metatarsal heads. Standing radiographs of the feet are useful in documenting the type and severity of the deformity (Fig. 5.100). Special studies such as spine radiographs for spinal dysraphism, electromyography (EMG), DNA blood tests for Charcot–Marie–Tooth (CMT) disease, nerve conduction velocity measurements, and CPK determination for muscular dystrophy assessment may be necessary. Consultations with a neurologist may be appropriate. Establish the etiology of the cavus deformity (Fig. 5.101).

Natural history Because of the reduced area of plantar contact, deformity, and rigidity, cavus feet often cause considerable disability (Fig. 5.102).

Category	Type	Etiology
Physiologic	Cavovarus	Familial
Pathologic	Cavovarus deformity	Clubfoot residual cavus
		Idiopathic
		Neuromuscular disease
		Friedreich's ataxia
		Charcot–Marie–Tooth
		Spinal dysraphism
		Spina bifida
		Poliomyelitis
	Calcaneocavus	Spina bifida
		Poliomyelitis
		Overlengthened heel-cord

Fig. 5.101 Classification of cavus deformity. This classification includes the majority of causes of cavus feet. Pathologic cavus is often associated with neurologic disorders.

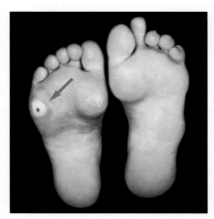

Fig. 5.102 Skin irrigation with cavus deformity. The cavus deformity increases the load on the metatarsal heads. If sensation is poor, as in the child with spina bifida, skin breakdown is common (arrow).

Types of Cavus Deformities

Congenital cavus is a rare deformity that may be due to intrauterine constraint or fixed deformity (Fig. 5.103). Assess the effect of growth.

Calcaneocavus results from weakness of the triceps, an increase in the calcaneal pitch, and a cavus deformity. Correct muscle imbalance if possible. This deformity is seen in poliomyelitis (Fig. 5.104), in spina bifida, and following overlengthening of the triceps.

Cavovarus is the most common form. Muscle imbalance results in a mild increased calcaneal pitch and plantarflexion of the forefoot. This deformity is seen in CMT disease. Clawing of the toes is often seen.

Management

Follow a flowchart to manage (Fig. 5.106). The teenager will often complain of difficulty in fitting shoes, calluses over the claw toes and under the metatarsal heads, and pain.

Mild deformity Order shock-absorbing footwear and soft molded shoe inserts to broaden the load-bearing area of the foot.

Moderate or severe deformity This requires operative correction. Operations improve muscle balance, flatten the arch to broaden the weight-bearing surface, and correct toe deformity.

Flexible deformities or those in young children are best managed by a plantar medial release and appropriate tendon transfers. Plan serial postoperative casting starting at 2 weeks following surgery. Continue until the deformity is resolved. If performed during childhood, be prepared for recurrence.

Fixed deformities require correction in two stages. First, perform a soft tissue release as described above. Follow this by osteotomies to correct bony deformity and tendon transfers to balance the foot. In most cases, perform a calcaneal osteotomy (Fig. 5.105) for calcaneocavus deformity and a plantar flexion medial cuneiform osteotomy for cavovarus correction. Avoid arthrodesis whenever possible to maintain mobility and reduce the risk of degenerative arthritis of adjacent joints.

References

2000 Personal communication. Mosca V.

2000 Function after correction of a clawed great toe by a modified Robert Jones transfer. Breusch SJ, Wenz W, Doderlein L. JBJS 82B:250

1996 The foot in hereditary motor and sensory neuropathies in children. Ghanem I, Zeller R, Seringe R. Rev Chir Orthop Reparatrice Appar Mot 82:152

1994 The modified Robert Jones tendon transfer in cases of pes cavus and clawed hallux. Tynan MC, Klenerman L. Foot Ankle Int 15:68

1993 Evaluation and treatment of diastematomyelia. Miller A, Guille JT, Bowen JR. JBJS 75A:1308

1993 Computed tomographic analysis of pes cavus. Price AE, Maisel R, Drennan JC. JPO 13:646

1993 Tarsal coalition presenting as a pes cavo-varus deformity: report of three cases and review of the literature. Stuecker RD, Bennett JT. Foot Ankle 14:540

1989 The cavovarus foot deformity. Etiology and management. McCluskey WP, Lovell WW, Cummings RJ. CO 247:27

1988 Congenital "high-arched (cavus) forefoot"--a newly described deformity and surgical correction. Rosman M. JPO 8:418

1985 The Akron midtarsal dome osteotomy in the treatment of rigid pes cavus: a preliminary review. Wilcox PG, Weiner DS. JPO 5:333

1981 Plantar release in the correction of deformities of the foot in childhood. Sherman FC, Westin GW. JBJS 63A:1382

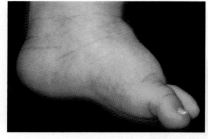
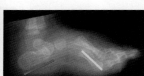

Fig. 5.103 Congenital cavus. This deformity gradually resolved during the first 2 years of growth. Note the calcaneal pitch (red line) and first metatarsal (yellow line) alignments.

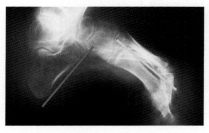

Fig. 5.104 Hindfoot cavus deformity. This severe deformity was secondary to weakness of the triceps from poliomyelitis. Note the calcaneal pitch (red line) and first metatarsal (yellow) alignments.

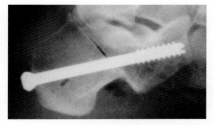

Fig. 5.105 Calcaneo-varus deformity. This patient underwent a calcaneal lengthening to reduce deformity of the calcaneus.

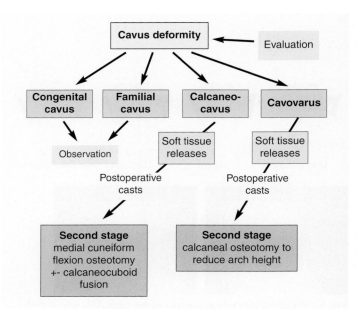

Fig. 5.106 Cavus management flowchart. From Mosca (2000).

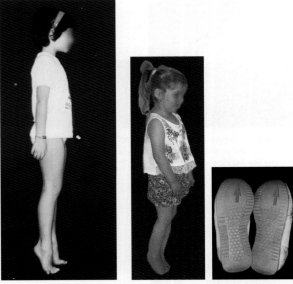

Fig. 5.107 Idiopathic toe walking. (Left) This girl has a contracture of the gastrocnemius causing an equinus gait. (Middle and right) This girl's shoes show excessive wear on the toes (arrows).

Category	Diagnosis
Congenital	Clubfoot
Idiopathic	Gastroncnemius contracture
	Accessory soleus muscle
	Generalized triceps
	contracture
Neurologic	Cerebral palsy
	Poliomyelitis
Myogenic	Muscular dystrophy
Functional	Hysterical toe walking

Fig. 5.108 Toe walking classification. This classification includes the common causes of an equinus gait.

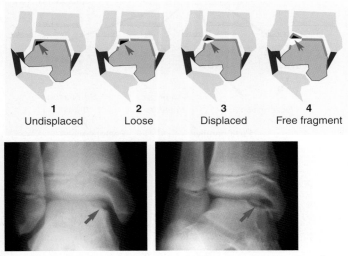

1	2	3	4
Undisplaced	Loose	Displaced	Free fragment

Fig. 5.109 Osteochondritis dissecans of the talus. This Berndt and Hartly classification is based on Giguera et al. (1998). Most can be diagnosed with conventional radiographs (red arrows). The degree of displacement can be demonstrated by CT studies.

Other Foot Conditions

Toe Walking

Toe walking, or *equinus gait,* may occur in otherwise normal children (Fig. 5.107) or in children with neuromuscular disorders (Fig. 5.108).

Neurogenic equinus This deformity is common in children with cerebral palsy, muscular dystrophy, and incompletely treated clubfeet. Correction usually requires lengthening of the heel-cord and sometimes opening of the ankle joint capsule.

Idiopathic toe walking Persistent toe walking in infants and young children is uncommon and usually due to shortening of the triceps muscle. Toe walking can be classified into three distinct clinical categories.

Gastrocnemius contracture is the most common form. This isolated deformity is often familial and varies in severity. Ankle dorsiflexion is limited with the knee extended. The sole shows wear under the toes. Physical therapy and stretching exercises are ineffective, and although casting will correct the contracture, recurrence is common. Operative lengthening of the gastrocnemius aponeurosis is effective.

Accessory soleus is a rare congenital deformity in which the body of the soleus muscle extends to the ankle. This produces equinus and a fullness on the medial side of the ankle. Operative lengthening may be necessary.

General triceps contracture is a rare condition that may result in fibrosis and shortening of the triceps muscle group. Ankle dorsiflexion is limited regardless of knee position. Operative correction by heel-cord lengthening may be necessary.

Osteochondritis Dissecans of the Talus

These lesions are regions of avascular bone that occur most commonly on the anterolateral and posteromedial aspects of the talar dome. The lateral lesions are more likely to be associated with an ankle sprain and to be traumatic in origin.

The causes of these lesions may vary. Some follow trauma, while most occur spontaneously and may represent variations in ossification or idiopathic avascular necrosis. They are most common during adolescence in both genders. Most lesions are medial in location.

Evaluation Order AP, lateral, and mortise radiographs. CT and MRI may be helpful to assess the extent of the lesions and cartilage status if operative management is being considered.

Classification As with other osteochondritis lesions, these are classified into four categories (Fig. 5.109).

Management This is based on the type of lesion.

Type 1 and 2 lesions Manage in a short-leg cast for 4–6 weeks.

Type 3 lesions Manage by reduction and immobilization of the fragment with bioabsorbable pegs. Approach by arthroscopy or with the aid of a transmalleolar osteotomy.

Type 4 lesions Excise if small or old. Replace and fix if feasible.

Prognosis Good to excellent in the 90% range.

Ball-and-Socket Ankle

Ball-and-socket ankle is a rare deformity associated with conditions such as extensive tarsal coalitions (Fig. 5.110), congenital shortening of the lower limb, absent digital rays, and aplasia or hypoplasia of the fibula. The deformity causes little or no disability, and no treatment is required.

Calcaneal Prominence

This deformity is seen in adolescence, is often bilateral, and is thought to be related to irritation from shoewear (Fig. 5.111). Manage most cases with thoughtful shoe selection. Rarely, exostectomy is required. Operative results are often poor.

Tumors of the Foot

Accessory soleus is a rare variation in the soleus causing a swelling just medial to the achilles tendon. The mass is smooth, round, and non-tender and grows proportionately with the foot. No treatment is required.

Plantar fibromatosis is a rare tumor with a characteristic location on the anteromedial portion of the heel pad (Fig. 5.112). As recurrence following resection is common and many resolve spontaneously, observational management is usually indicated.

Subungal exostosis is a benign bone tumor of the distal phalanx occurring beneath or adjacent to the nail (Fig. 5.113). This rare tumor occurs in late childhood or adolescence and most commonly affects the great toe. Its characteristic location and radiographic appearance establish the diagnosis. Manage by careful and complete excision to avoid recurrence.

Other tumors Many other benign and malignant tumors occur in the foot and usually have no unusual features that are unique to the foot (Fig. 5.114).

Chapter Consultant Vince Mosca, e-mail: vmosca@chmc.org

References

2000 Serial casting in idiopathic toe-walkers and children with spastic cerebral palsy. Brouwer B, Davidson LK, Olney SJ. JPO 20:221

2000 Idiopathic toe-walking: does treatment alter the natural history? Eastwood DM, et al. JPO-B 9:47

1999 Idiopathic toe-walking: a review. Sala DA, Shulman LH, Kennedy RF, Grant AD, Chu ML. Dev Med Child Neurol 41:846-8

1998 Osteochondritis dissecans of the talus during childhood and adolescence. Higuera J et al. JPO 18:328

1998 Idiopathic toe walking: a comparison of treatment methods. Stricker SJ, Angulo JC. JPO 18:289

1997 Accessory soleus muscle. A report of 4 cases and review of literature. Brodie JT, et al. CO 337:180

1997 Muscle abnormalities in idiopathic toe-walkers. Eastwood DM, et al. JPO-b 6:215

1997 Plantar fibromatosis of the heel in children: a report of 14 cases. Godette GA, O'Sullivan M, Menelaus MB. JPO 17:16

1997 The kinematic patterns of toe-walkers. Kelly IP, et al. JPO 17:478

1997 Effect of persistent toe walking on ankle equinus. Analysis of 60 idiopathic toe walkers. Sobel E, Caselli MA, Velez Z. J Am Podiatr Med Assoc 87:17

1995 Osteochondritis dissecans of the talus in identical twins. Woods K, Harris I. JBJS 77B:331

1993 Results of excision of calcaneal prominence. Biyani A, Jones DA. Acta Orthop Belg 59:45

1992 Prominence of the calcaneus: late results of bone resection. Huber HM. JBJS 74B:315

1986 Electromyography of idiopathic toe walking. Kalen V, Adler N, Bleck EE. JPO 6:31

1986 Genesis of the ball-and-socket ankle. Takakura Y, Tamai S, Masuhara K. JBJS 68B:834

1984 Ball-and-socket ankle joint: anatomical and kinematic analysis of the hindfoot. Hiroshima K, et al. JPO 4:564

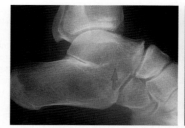
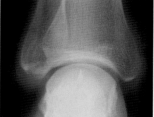

Fig. 5.110 Ball and socket ankle. Note the subtalar fusion (red arrow) and the spherical shape of the ankle (yellow arrow).

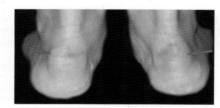

Fig. 5.111 Calcaneal prominences. This teenage girl has bilateral prominences with some discomfort.

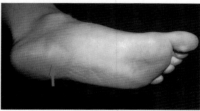

Fig. 5.112 Plantar fibromatosis.

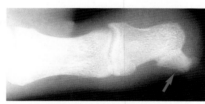

Fig. 5.113 Subungal exostosis

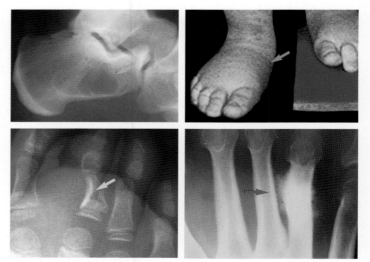

Fig. 5.114 Tumors of the foot. Numerous tumors occur about the foot. Some are benign, such as cysts of the calcaneus (orange arrow) and vascular tumors (green arrow). Less common are malignant tumors, such as desmoid tumors (yellow arrow) and osteogenic sarcoma (red arrow).

Berman A, Gartland JJ. Metatarsal osteotomy for the correction of adduction of the fore part of the foot in children. J Bone Joint Surg 1971;53A:498-506.

Bigos SJ, Coleman SS. Foot deformities secondary to gluteal injection in infancy. J Pediatr Orthop 1984;4:560-563.

Canale ST, Belding RH. Osteochondral lesions of the talus. J Bone Joint Surg 1980;62A:97-102.

Chambers RB, Cook TM, Cowell HR. Surgical reconstruction for calcaneonavicular coalition: Evaluation of function and gait. J Bone Joint Surg 1982;64A:829-836.

Coleman SS, Chestnut WJ. A simple test for hindfoot flexibility in the cavovarus foot. Clin Orthop 1977;123:60-62.

Cowell HR, Wein BK. Genetic aspects of club foot. J Bone Joint Surg 1980;62A:1381-1384.

Crawford AH, Marxen JL, Osterfeld DL. The Cincinnati incision: A comprehensive approach for surgical procedures of the foot and ankle in childhood. J Bone Joint Surg 1982;64A:1355-1358.

Cummings RJ, Lovell WW. Operative treatment of congenital idiopathic club foot. J Bone Joint Surg 1988;70A:1108-1112.

DeRosa GP, Ahlfeld SK. Congenital vertical talus: The Riley experience. Foot Ankle 1984;5:118-124.

Evans D. Calcaneo-valgus deformity. J Bone Joint Surg 1975;57B:270-278.

Fulford GE, Cairns TP. The problems associated with flail feet in children and their treatment with orthoses. J Bone Joint Surg 1978;60B:93-95.

Gould N; Moreland M; Trevino S; Alvarez R, Fenwick J, Bach N. Foot growth in children age one to five years. Foot Ankle 1990, 10:211-3

Griffin PP, Wheelhouse WW, Shiavi R et al. Habitual toe-walkers: A clinical and electromyographic gait analysis. J Bone Joint Surg 1977;59A:97-101.

Harris RI, Beath T. Etiology of peroneal spastic flat foot. J Bone Joint Surg 1948;30B:624-634.

Harris RI, Beath T. Hypermobile flat-foot with short tendo achillis. J Bone Joint Surg 1948;30A:116-140.

Herzenberg JE, Goldner JL, Martinez S et al. Computerized tomography of talocalcaneal tarsal coalition: A clinical and anatomic study. Foot Ankle 1986;273-288.

Hsu LC, O'Brien JP, Yau AC, et al. Batchelor's extra-articular subtalar arthrodesis: A report on sixty-four procedures in patients with poliomyelitic deformities. J Bone Joint Surg 1976;58A:243-247.

Hutchins PM, Foster BK, Paterson DC, et al. Long-term results of early surgical release in club feet. J Bone Joint Surg 1985;67B:791-799.

Inglis G, Buxton RA, Macnicol MF. Symptomatic calcaneonavicular bars: The results 20 years after surgical excision. J Bone Joint Surg 1986;68B:128-131.

Ippolito E, Ponseti IV. Congenital club foot in the human fetus: A histological study. J Bone Joint Surg 1980;62A:8-22.

Ippolito E, Ricciardi Pollini PT, Falez F. Köhler's disease of the tarsal navicular: Long-term follow-up of 12 cases. J Pediatr Orthop 1984;4:416-417.

Irani RN, Sherman MS. The pathological anatomy of clubfoot. J Bone Joint Surg 1963;45A:45-52.

Jahss MH. Tarsometatarsal truncated-wedge arthrodesis for pes cavus and equinovarus deformity of the fore part of the foot. J Bone Joint Surg 1980;62A:713-722.

Karlholm S, Nilsonne U. Operative treatment of the foot deformity in Charcot-Marie-Tooth disease. Acta Orthop Scand 1968;39:101-106.

Karp MG. Köhler's disease of the tarsal scaphoid: An end-result study. J Bone Joint Surg 1937;19:84-96.

Katz MM, Mubarak SJ. Hereditary tendo Achillis contractures. J Pediatr Orthop 1984;4:711-714.

Keck SW, Kelly PJ. Bursitis of the posterior part of the heel: Evaluation of the surgical treatment of eighteen patients. J Bone Joint Surg 1965;47A:267-273.

Laaveg SJ, Ponseti IV. Long-term results of treatment of congenital club foot. J Bone Joint Surg 1980;62A:23-31.

Luba R, Rosman M. Bunions in children: Treatment with a modified Mitchell osteotomy. J Pediatr Orthop 1984;4:44-47.

Mann RA. Decision-making in bunion surgery. In Greene, WB (ed): AAOS Instruct Course Lect, 1990;39:3-13.

McKay DW. New concept and approach to clubfoot treatment: Section I: Principles and morbid anatomy. J Pediatr Orthop 1982;2:347-356; Section II: Correction of the clubfoot. J Pediatr Orthop 1983;3:10-21; Section III: Evaluation and results. J Pediatr Orthop 1983;3:141-148.

McMaster MJ. The pathogenesis of hallux rigidus. J Bone Joint Surg 1978;60B:82-87.

Mosier KM, Asher M. Tarsal coalitions and peroneal spastic flat foot: A review. J Bone Joint Surg 1984;66A:976-984.

Olney BW, Asher MA. Excision of symptomatic coalition of the middle facet of the talocalcaneal joint. J Bone Joint Surg 1987;69A:539-544.

Paulos L, Coleman SS, Samuelson KM. Pes cavovarus: Review of a surgical approach using selective soft-tissue procedures. J Bone Joint Surg 1980;62A:942-953.

Peterson HA. Skewfoot (forefoot adduction with heel valgus). J Pediatr Orthop 1986;6:24-30.

Rushforth GF. The natural history of hooked forefoot. J Bone Joint Surg 1978;60B:530-532.

Scranton PE Jr. Treatment of symptomatic talocalcaneal coalition. J Bone Joint Surg 1987;69A:533-539.

Seimon LP. Surgical correction of congenital vertical talus under the age of 2 years. J Pediatr Orthop 1987;7:405-411.

Simons GW. Complete subtalar release in club feet: Part I: A preliminary report. J Bone Joint Surg 1985;67A:1044-1055; Part II: Comparison with less extensive procedures. J Bone Joint Surg 1985;67A:1056-1065.

Staheli LT, Chew DE, Corbett M. The longitudinal arch: A survey of eight hundred and eighty-two feet in normal children and adults. J Bone Joint Surg 1987;69A:426-428.

Stark JG, Johanson JE, Winter RB. The Heyman-Herndon tarsometatarsal capsulotomy for metatarsus adductus: Results in 48 feet. J Pediatr Orthop 1987;7:305-310.

Turco VJ. Resistant congenital club foot: One-stage posteromedial release with internal fixation. A follow-up report of a fifteen-year experience. J Bone Joint Surg 1979;61A:805-814.

Vander Wilde R, Staheli LT, Chew DE, et al. Measurements on radiographs of the foot in normal infants and children. J Bone Joint Surg 1988;70A:407-415.

Wenger DR, Mauldin D, Speck G, et al. Corrective shoes and inserts as treatment for flexible flatfoot in infants and children. J Bone Joint Surg 1989;71A:800-810.

Wetmore RS, Drennan JC. Long-term results of triple arthrodesis in Charcot-Marie-Tooth disease. J Bone Joint Surg 1989;71A:417-422.

Williams GA, Cowell HR. Köhler's disease of the tarsal navicular. Clin Orthop 1981;158:53-58.

Zinman C, Reis ND. Osteochondritis dissecans of the talus: Use of the high resolution computed tomography scanner. Acta Orthop Scand 1982;53:697-700.

Chapter 6—Knee and Tibia

In this chapter, disorders of the knee and tibia are addressed. In all age groups, knee problems account for over one-fourth of musculoskeletal complaints. In children, knee complaints are substantially less common but increase in frequency during the teen years. Osteomyelitis and osteogenic sarcoma develop more often about the knee than at any other site due to the rapid growth rate of the distal femoral and upper tibial physes.

Introduction

Nomenclature

The fully extended knee is the neutral or zero position. The normal range of motion extends from neutral to about 140°, with most activities performed in the 0°–65° segment of the flexion arc. In the child, hyperextension of up to 10°–15° is normal (Fig. 6.1). The difference between active and passive motion is termed *lag*.

Hyperextension, if associated with stiffness, is called a *recurvatum deformity*. Restricted motion is described by specifying the arc of motion. For example, a stiff knee may be described as having an "arc of motion from 20°–55°." The arc of motion in hyperextension is preceded by a minus sign. A child with a hyperextension deformity may have a range from –20° to 30°, giving a 50° arc of motion.

The knee angle is the thigh–leg angle or femoral–tibial angle (see Chapter 4). Changes in the knee angle that represent normal variations are physiological and cause bowlegs or knock-knees. Deformities, those falling outside the normal range (±2 SD) and those due to pathological processes, are termed *genu varum* or *genu valgum*.

Normal Development

The knee develops as a typical synovial joint during the third to fourth fetal months. The secondary centers of ossification for the distal femur form between the sixth and ninth fetal months and for the upper tibia between the eighth fetal and first postnatal months. The patella ossification center appears between the second and fourth years in girls and the third and fifth years in boys.

Developmental Variations

Variations of ossification or development may cause confusion in assessing radiographs.

Bipartite patella is due to an accessory ossification center of the patella that usually occurs in the superior–lateral corner (Fig. 6.2).

Fibrocortical defects are usually insignificant developmental variations that are most common about the knee. They are eccentric and show sclerotic margins and radiolucent centers. They resolve spontaneously (Fig. 6.3).

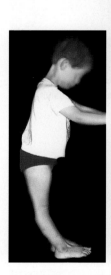
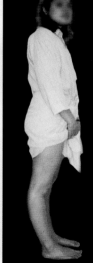

Fig. 6.1 Hyperextension deformities of the knee. The boy's knees hyperextend due to generalized joint laxity. The girl's have a hyperextension deformity due to a knee injury with loss of knee flexion.

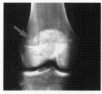
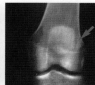

Fig. 6.2 Bilateral bipartite patellae. Secondary centers may appear on both knees. They are usually asymptomatic.

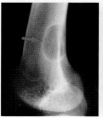
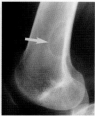

Fig. 6.3 Fibrocortical defect. Typical large lesion in distal femur (red arrow). Two years later, spontaneous healing has occurred (yellow arrow).

Clinical Feature	Disorder
Patellar hypoplasia	Nail-patella syndrome Beals syndrome Diastrophic dysplasia Neurofibromatosis
Genu varum	Rickets Achondroplasia TAR syndrome Metaphyseal dysplasia
Genu valgum	Rickets Morquio syndrome Poliomyelitis Ellis-Van Creveld syn.
Genu recurvatum	Myelodysplasia Arthrogryposis Larsen syndrome
Flexion contracture	Arthrogryposis Pterygium syndrome Myelodysplasia
Patellofemoral disorders	Nail-patella syndrome Rubinstein-Taybi syn.

Fig. 6.4 Syndromes associated with knee deformity. These are examples that illustrate the relationship of knee deformities in various generalized disorders.

Evaluation

Evaluating the child's knee is different from that of the adult because disorders are more likely to be due to some underlying generalized dysplasia or to focal congenital or developmental deformity.

Screening Examination

Screen for some underlying abnormality (Fig. 6.4), such as nail–patella syndrome (Fig. 6.5). Dislocation of the patella is common in Down syndrome. Dimpling over the knee is common in arthrogryposis. Recurvatum occurs in spina bifida and in arthrogryposis. Genu varum and valgum are common in ricketic disorders, and genu valgum is common in Morquio's and Ellis–Van Creveld syndromes.

Physical Examination

The physical examination usually provides the diagnosis or at least the basis for ordering further studies.

General inspection Look for obvious deformity, check the knee angle, and perform a rotational profile (Fig. 6.6).

Knee Observe the child standing and note symmetry, knee angle, position of patella, masses, joint effusion, muscle definition and atrophy (Fig. 6.7), and signs of inflammation. Is there full extension or hyper-extension?

Patellar tracking Ask the child to sit and slowly flex and extend the knee. Observe the tracking of the patella. Does it move in a linear fashion or displace laterally as the knee extends (Fig. 6.8)? Does the knee fully flex and extend?

Q angle is the angle formed by a line connecting the anterior superior iliac spine with the midportion of the patella and a second line from the patellar mid-point to the tibial tubercle. Normally the enclosed angle is less than about 15°. A larger angle may or may not be associated with patellofemoral instability.

Point of maximum tenderness Locate the PMT by systematically examining the entire knee and tibia. The PMT often establishes a working diagnosis (Fig. 6.9).

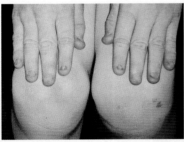
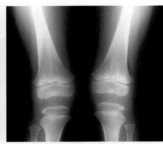

Fig. 6.5 Nail–patella syndrome. Note the nail dysplasia and absence of the patella.

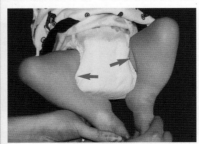

Fig. 6.6 Inspection. The screening examination of this standing child shows the shortening and bowing of the left tibia (yellow arrow) and the café-au-lait spots of neurofibromatosis. Severe flexion contractures are present in the popliteal pterygium syndrome (red arrows).

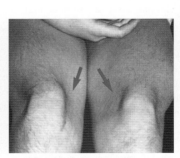

Fig. 6.7 Hypoplasia of the quadriceps. Hypoplasia is a common dysplastic feature in patellofemoral disorders in children and adolescents. Note the lack of definition of the VMO (arrows).

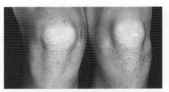
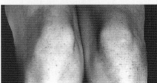
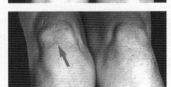

Fig. 6.8 Patellar tracking. As the child slowly extends the knee, the patella normally tracks vertically. Lateral patellar displacement as the knee becomes fully extended (arrow) is described as "J" tracking.

Palpate   to assess temperature, swelling, and tenderness. Is the affected knee warmer than the other knee? Is a joint effusion present (Fig. 6.10)? Parapatellar fullness suggests a joint effusion. Evaluate any fullness by extending the knee, compressing the suprapatellar region, and checking for a fluid wave in the knee. A posttraumatic effusion is a sign of a significant intraarticular injury such as a torn peripheral meniscus, anterior cruciate ligament (ACL) injury, or osteochondral fracture.

Manipulate   to determine if the patella is displaceable. In loose-jointed children, the patella is very mobile and more likely to dislocate.

Patellar apprehension is elicited by extending the knee and attempting to displace the patella laterally. Patients with recurrent dislocations who sense that this may cause the patella to dislocate may become apprehensive and may reach out to stop the examination.

Knee motion   Is the arch of motion free and unguarded? Is crepitation or snapping present?

Knee tests   Anteroposterior laxity can be assessed with the Lachman test. Flex the knee about 15°–20° and attempt to displace the tibia anterior in its relationship to the femur. Normally a firm endpoint will be felt. Check for instability with varus and valgus stress (Fig. 6.11). With the knee flexed to a right angle, evaluate for anterior or posterior drawer signs.

Imaging Studies

Special radiographic projects such as sunrise and notch views (Fig. 6.12) may be useful. If conventional radiographs are not adequate, order special imaging studies (Fig. 6.13). Bone scans may be helpful in determining the location or activity of lesions, and MRI studies are most useful for tumors or meniscal abnormalities. Be aware that because of the sensitivity of these tests, overreading is common.

Arthroscopy

Arthroscopy is essential for assessing meniscal injuries and for other ligamentous and osteochondral problems in children. It is less valuable for assessing pain.

References

2000 Objective evaluation of knee laxity in children. Flynn JM, et al. JPO 20:259

1998 Instability of the patellofemoral joint in Rubinstein-Taybi syndrome. Mehlman CT, Rubinstein JH, Roy DR. JPO 18:508

1997 Knee arthroscopy in Chinese children and adolescents: an eight-year prospective study. Maffulli N, et al. Arthroscopy 13:18

1996 Magnetic resonance imaging of knee injuries in children. King SJ, Carty HM, Brady O. Pediatr Radiol 26:287

1994 Larsen's syndrome: review of the literature and analysis of thirty-eight cases. Laville JM, Lakermance P, Limouzy F. JPO 14:63

1993 Arthroscopy of the acute traumatic knee in children. Prospective study of 138 cases. Vahasarja V, Kinnuen P, Serlo W. Acta Orthop Scand 64:580

1991 Arthroscopy in children. Hope PG. J R Soc Med 84:29

1990 Knock-knee deformity in children. Congenital and acquired. Cozen L. CO 258:191

1990 Popliteal pterygium syndrome: an orthopaedic perspective. Oppenheim WL, et al. JPO 10:58

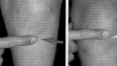
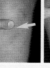
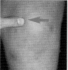

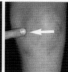

Arrow	PMT	Condition
Red	Tibial tubercle	Osgood–Schlatter disease
Yellow	Distal pole patella	Sinding–Larsen–Johansson syn.
Green	Medial patellar margin	Patellar instability
Blue	Medial joint line	Meniscal lesion
White	Medial collateral ligament	Ligament injury

Fig. 6.9 Point of maximum tenderness. Evaluate the PMT for common painful conditions about the knee.

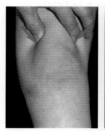
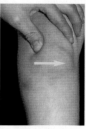

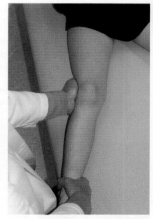

Fig. 6.10 Knee tests. Compressing the suprapatellar bursa (red arrows) displaces any joint fluid into the joint to demonstrate an effusion. Displacing the patella laterally (yellow arrows) may elicit the patellar apprehension sign.

Fig. 6.11 Knee stability. Test for medial lateral instability with the knee flexed to 30°. Test the opposite or normal knee to determine what is normal for the child.

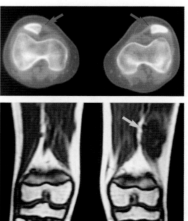
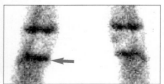

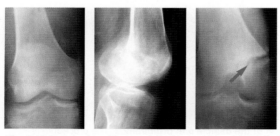

Fig. 6.12 Notch view. The condylar fracture is seen only in the notch view (red arrow).

Fig. 6.13 Special imaging studies. These special studies demonstrate lateral patellar positioning (red arrows), a hemangioma by MRI (yellow arrow), and increased uptake of the proximal medial tibial physis in tibia vara (blue arrow).

Category	Disorder
Referred	SCFE, other hip problems
	Tumor
Stress	Osgood–Schlatter disease
	Sinding–Larsen–Johansson
	Stress fractures
	Proximal tibia
	Patella
	Distal femur
	Medial collateral ligament
Bursitis	Prepatellar
	Pes anserina
Intraarticular	Meniscus
	Ligaments
	Osteochondritis dissecans
Tumors	Popliteal cyst
	Miscellaneous
Arthritis	Septic
	Pauciarticular
	Juvenile rheumatoid arthritis
	Rheumatoid spondylitis

Fig. 6.14 Classification of knee pain. Knee pain has many causes. Some examples are listed.

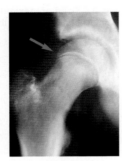

Fig. 6.15 Pitfalls in evaluating knee pain. Referred pain can occur from this slipped capital femoral epiphysis (arrow).

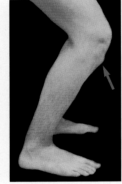
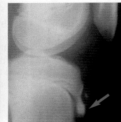
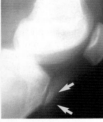

Fig. 6.16 Osgood-Schlatter disease. Note the prominence and the ossification over the tibial tubercle (red arrows). Persisting tenderness over an ossicle in the mature knee (yellow arrows) is an indication for excision.

Knee Pain

Knee pain is a common presenting complaint (Fig. 6.14).

Referred Pain

First consider the possibility of referred pain from slipped capital femoral epiphysis (Fig. 6.15) or pain from a tumor. These conditions require urgent treatment.

Osgood–Schlatter Disease

Osgood–Schlatter disease (OSD) is a traction apophysitis of the tibial tubercle due to repetitive tensile microtrauma. It occurs between ages 10 and 15 years, with the onset in girls about 2 years before that in boys. OSD is usually unilateral and occurs in 10–20% of children participating in sports. OSD is associated with patella alta. Whether this association is a cause or an effect of OSD is not known. The tibial tubercle maybe enlarged on the asymptomatic side.

Physical examination will demonstrate swelling and localized tenderness over the tibial tubercle (Fig. 6.16) and no other abnormalities. Order a radiograph if the condition is unilateral or atypical. Radiographs usually show soft tissue swelling and sometimes a separate ossicle over the tubercle.

Natural history OSD resolves with time in most children (Fig. 6.17). In about 10% of knees, some residual prominence of the tibial tubercle or persisting pain from an ossicle may cause problems.

Manage by ordering modifications of activities, use of NSAIDs, and a knee pad to control discomfort. If OSD is severe or persists, apply a knee immobilizer for a week or two to relieve inflammation. Injection of steroids is not recommended. Often quadriceps and hamstring flexibility exercises are prescribed. To reduce apprehension, consider referring to ODS as a *disorder* or *condition* rather than a *disease* when discussing the problems with the patient and family. Make certain that they are aware that resolution is usually slow, often requiring 12–18 months. Persisting disability from tenderness and tubercle prominence may be sufficient to require excision of the ossicle and prominence (Fig. 6.18).

Complications are rare and include growth arrest with recurvatum deformity and rupture of patellar tendon or avulsion of the tibial tubercle.

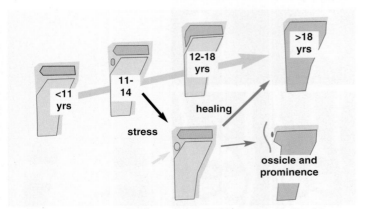

Fig. 6.17 Natural history of OSD. The normal development of the apophysis is shown by the green arrow. Excessive traction (yellow) of the patellar tendon causes inflammation. Usually this process heals. In some cases, inflammation and a separate ossicle persist (red). Based on Flowers and Bhadreshwar (1995).

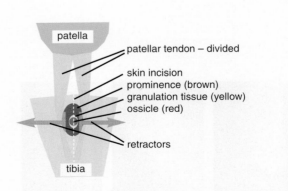

Fig. 6.18 Excision of the ossicle and prominence. The procedure is performed through a midline incision to the ossicle and prominence. Sometimes inflammatory granulation tissue is present in active lesions.

Sinding–Larsen–Johansson Syndrome

Sinding–Larsen–Johansson syndrome is a traction apophysitis of the distal pole of the patella (Fig. 6.19). The condition is most common in males at or before puberty. Resolution occurs in 6–12 months. Rest the knee to resolve the pain and tenderness. Quadriceps flexibility exercises are commonly prescribed. No residual disability has been reported.

Pes Anserina Bursitis

Inflammation of the pes anserina bursa causes pain and tenderness over the hamstring tendon insertions on the posterior medial aspect of the upper tibial metaphysis. This uncommon condition occurs during the teen years. Manage the bursitis with rest and nonsteroidal antiinflammatory medications.

Medial Collateral Ligament Pain

Medial collateral ligament pain is an overuse condition causing pain and tenderness over the medial collateral ligament. This ligament lies on the posteromedial aspect of the knee at or above the joint line.

Bipartite Patella

Accessory centers of ossification of the patella (Fig. 6.20) may produce a bipartite patella. The separate ossicle is attached to the body of the patella by fibrous or cartilaginous tissue. Trauma may disrupt this attachment, and the ossicle then becomes painful. The disruption may heal with rest. In others, healing fails to occur and the ossicle remains chronically painful. Small painful ossicles may be removed. Larger ossicles should be fixed with a screw to the patella and grafted to promote union.

Osteochondritis Dissecans

Osteochondritis dissecans may involve the medial or lateral condyle or patella (Fig. 6.21). The lateral side of the medial condyle is involved in 75% of cases. Symptoms include pain, a mild effusion, or later mechanical symptoms. Image by a notch view. Classify based on degree of displacement (Fig. 6.22). A good prognosis is related to a younger age and to a small lesion in a nonweight-bearing location without displacement.

Manage type 1 and 2 lesions with activity modification, isometric exercises, and a knee immobilizer. Manage based on symptoms rather than on radiographic appearance. Radiographic healing takes many months. Manage type 3 lesions by drilling and stabilizing with K wires (Fig. 6.23) or absorbable pins. Manage type 4 lesions if small by excision. Replace large lesions or those involving the weight-bearing areas and fix internally if adequate subchondral bone exists on the fragment.

Prognosis For large lesions involving the weight-bearing surfaces, osteoarthritis is common in adult life.

References

1999 Osteochondritis dissecans: a Multicenter Study of the European Pediatric Orthopedic Society. Hefti F, et al. JPO-b 8:231

1997 Radiologic study of patellar height in Osgood-Schlatter disease. Aparicio G, et al. JPO 17:63

1996 Pes anserinus syndrome due to solitary tibial spurs and osteochondromas. Fraser RK, et al. JPO 16:247

1995 Tibial tuberosity excision for symptomatic Osgood-Schlatter disease. Flowers MJ, Bhadreshwar DR. JPO 15:292

1994 Painful bipartite patella. A new approach to operative treatment. Ogata K. JBJS 76A:573

1991 Tibia recurvatum as a complication of Osgood-Schlatter's disease: a report of two cases. Lynch MC, Walsh HP. JPO 11:543

1991 Osteochondritis dissecans of the knee. A long-term study. Twyman RS, Desai K, Aichroth PM. JBJS 73B:461

1990 Natural history of Osgood-Schlatter disease. Krause BL, Williams JP, Catterall A. JPO 10:65

1989 Results of drilling osteochondritis dissecans before skeletal maturity. Bradley J, Dandy DJ. JBJS 71B:642

1987 Arthroscopy of the knee in children. Eiskjaer S, Larsen ST. Acta Orthop Scand 58:273

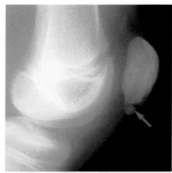
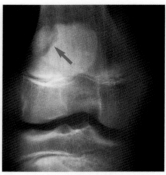

Fig. 6.19 Sinding–Larsen–Johansson syndrome. Note the separate lesion of the distal pole of the patella. This should be differentiated from the uncommon type of bipartite patella involving the inferior pole of the patella.

Fig. 6.20 Bipartite patella. Note the separate ossicle on the superolateral aspect of the patella. The lesion was painful.

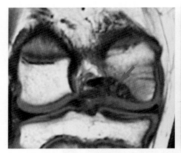
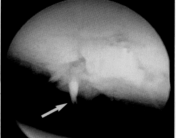

Fig. 6.21 Osteochondritis dissecans. MRI demonstrates a large defect (red arrow) with intact cartilage. Arthroscopy shows a lesion with overlying irregular cartilage (yellow arrow).

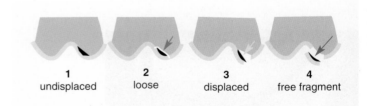

1	2	3	4
undisplaced	loose	displaced	free fragment

Fig. 6.22 Classification of osteochondritis dissecans. The lesion (black) may be undisplaced or loosely in place (blue arrow). Displacement may may be partial (yellow arrow) or complete (red arrow), allowing the fragment to be free.

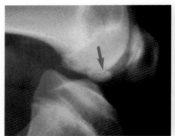
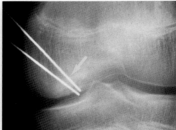

Fig. 6.23 Treatment of osteochondritis dissecans. The lesion (red arrow) was treated with drilling and fixation by diverging pins (yellow arrow). Cannulated screw fixation can also be used.

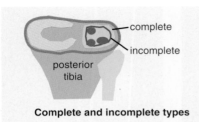

Complete and incomplete types

Fig. 6.24 Complete and incomplete types of discoid meniscus. These menisci are fixed to the tibia both in front and back of the knee (brown spots). The most vulnerable site for injury is posterior (red spot). Based on Dickhaut and DeLee (1982).

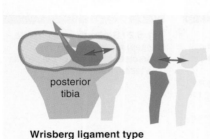

Wrisberg ligament type

Fig. 6.25 Wrisberg ligament type of discoid meniscus. The ligament is attached to the Wrisberg ligament (green arrow). This ligament (meniscofemoral ligament) attaches to the femur. With knee flexion and extension, the meniscus moves (red arrow) because it has no fixation to the tibia.

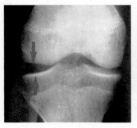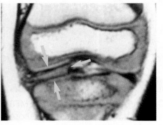

Fig. 6.26 Discoid lateral meniscus. Note the widening of the lateral joint space (red arrows) and the bow-tie-shaped discoid meniscus on MRI (yellow arrows).

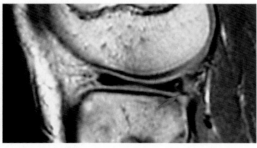

Fig. 6.27 Meniscal tear. Note the meniscal tear on this MRI (arrow).

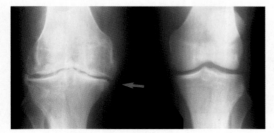

Fig. 6.28 Long-term effect of meniscectomy. At age 13 years, this 29-year-old man had a total meniscectomy of the right knee. Note the degenerative changes compared to the unoperated knee.

Intraarticular Disorders

Meniscal and ligamentous lesions are relatively rare in children but become more common during adolescence.

Discoid Meniscus

Three types of discoid meniscus occur.

Complete and incomplete types are thicker than normal and cover all or part of the tibial surface (Fig. 6.24).

Wrisberg ligament type is attached to the meniscofemoral ligament posteriorly (Fig. 6.25). This meniscus has no other fixation and is mobile. It is most likely to cause snapping and symptoms in the younger child. Because of its mobility, it may be caught between the femoral condyles and become torn or eroded.

Diagnosis Symptoms include pain, snapping or locking, loss of knee extension, and giving way. Tenderness and fullness may be present over the lateral joint line, and crepitation may be present with motion. In the young child, snapping may be the only complaint. Radiographs may show widening of the joint space (Fig. 6.26). MRI studies are usually diagnostic and usually allow differentiation of the type of lesion. Arthroscopic confirmation should be delayed until operative treatment is considered necessary.

Management depends on the type, symptoms, and activity level of the child. Be conservative. Meniscoplasty is indicated for the meniscus with posterior attachments. Attempt to preserve the meniscus whenever possible. Total meniscectomy is the last resort. Long-term outcomes are poor due to premature osteoarthritis.

Tears of Medial Meniscus

These lesions become more common during the teen years. The findings are similar to tears seen in adults (Fig. 6.27). Tears are usually longitudinal in type. Preserve the meniscus by repairing reduceable outer third lesions. Perform a partial meniscectomy for inner third or comminuted lesions. Avoid total meniscectomy to preserve the stress shielding function of the meniscus. Meniscectomy in childhood leads to premature osteoarthritis (Fig. 6.28).

Cruciate Ligament Deficiencies

Cruciate ligament insufficiency is seen in a variety of conditions in children.

Congenital deficiencies are common in fibular hemimelia and proximal focal femoral deficiencies. These deficiencies complicate limb lengthening procedures in these children. Isolated absence of both anterior and posterior cruciate ligaments have been reported.

Acquired deficiencies occur from traumatic rupture of the ligament (Fig. 6.29), attenuation associated with tibial spine fractures, and sometimes in association with diaphyseal femoral shaft fractures without known knee injury.

Management ACL tears are repaired in traumatic ruptures that cause disability, especially when associated with meniscal injuries (see Chapter 11).

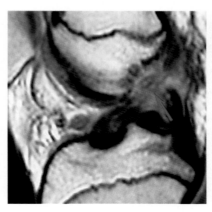

Fig. 6.29 Traumatic ACL tear in adolescent. This 15-year-old boy has a tear in his ACL as shown on the MRI.

Tumors of the Knee

Meniscal Cysts

Meniscal cysts are uncommon lesions that usually occur over the lateral aspect of the knee and may be associated with a meniscal tear. Image with ultrasound or by MRI (Fig. 6.30). Manage by arthroscopic excision or repair.

Popliteal Cysts

These cysts are different in children than in adults. The cysts seldom communicate with the joint and are not related to intraarticular defects. The natural history is of spontaneous resolution.

Diagnosis is usually not difficult (Fig. 6.31). Most cysts are found by the parents through observation. The cysts are usually nontender, smooth, cystic to the touch, and located between the medial head of the gastrocnemius and the semitendinosis. Translumination demonstrates that the mass is a cyst. Ultrasound shows the lesion well, so that MRI is seldom necessary.

Management Reassure the family that the condition is benign and will resolve with time. If the family is still nervous, consider confirming the diagnosis by aspirating the cyst. Advise the family that the aspiration is only to confirm the diagnosis and not for treatment because the cyst will recur. Aspiration reassures the family that it is not cancer. Cysts resolve spontaneously over a period of several years. Resection is indicated only with large painful cysts. Recurrence following resection is common.

Synovial Disorders

Intraarticular hemangiomata These lesions infiltrate and thicken the synovium, making it subject to injury and bleeding (Fig. 6.32). The diagnosis can be made by aspirating blood from the joint and confirmed by biopsy done concurrently with a synovectomy. Warn the family that recurrence during growth is likely.

Juvenile rheumatoid arthritis causes chronic synovitis with stiffness, overgrowth of the tibia and femur, contractures, and eventually joint destruction. Steroid injections, arthroscopic synovectomies, and contracture releases supplement medical management.

References

2000 Long-term follow-up of conservatively treated popliteal cysts in children. Van Rhijn LW, Jansen EJ, Pruijs HE. JPOB 9:62

1998 Popliteal cysts in children: a retrospective study of 62 cases. De Greef I, Molenaers G, Fabry G. Acta Orthop Belg 64:180

1997 Meniscal injury in children: long-term results after meniscectomy. Dai L, Zhang W, Xu Y. Knee Surg Sports Traumatol Arthrosc 5:77

1997 Anterior cruciate ligament tears in children: an analysis of operative versus nonoperative treatment. Pressman AE, Letts RM, Jarvis JG. JPO 17:505

1996 Ligamentous instability of the knee in children sustaining fractures of the femur: a prospective study with knee examination under anesthesia. Buckley SL, et al. JPO 16

1996 Discoid meniscus in children: magnetic resonance imaging characteristics. Connolly B, et al. Can Assoc Radiol J 47:347

1995 Discoid lateral meniscus in children. Long-term follow-up after excision. Washington ER 3rd, Root L, Liener UC. JBJS 77A:1357

1994 Juvenile rheumatoid arthritis of the knee: evaluation with US. Sureda D, et al. Radiology 190:403

1992 Management of congenital fibular deficiency by Ilizarov technique. Miller LS, Bell DF. JPO 12:651

1992 Meniscal cyst and magnetic resonance imaging in childhood and adolescence. Van der Wilde RS, Peterson HA. JPO 12:761

1991 Congenital discoid lateral meniscus in children. A follow-up study and evolution of management. Aichroth PM, Patel DV, Marx CL. JBJS 73B:932

1990 Tumors about the knee in children. Gebhardt MC, Ready JE, Mankin HJ. CO 255:86

1989 Isolated posterior cruciate ligament injury in a child: literature review and a case report. Frank C, Strother R. Can J Surg 32:373

1986 Congenital aplasia of the cruciate ligaments. A report of six cases. Kaelin A, Hulin PH, Carlioz H. JBJS 68B:827

1986 Soft tissue release for knee flexion contracture in juvenile chronic arthritis. Rydholm U, Brattstrom H, Lidgren L. JPO 6:448

1983 Missing cruciate ligament in congenital short femur. Johansson E, Aparisi T. JBJS 65A:1109

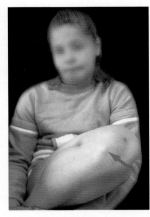
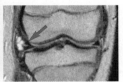

Fig. 6.30 Lateral meniscal cyst. Note the cyst upon physical examination of the knee and on the MRI.

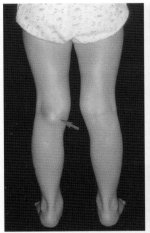
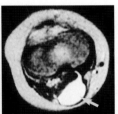
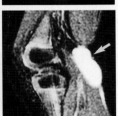
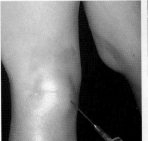
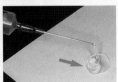

Fig. 6.31 Popliteal cyst. Note the classic location (red arrow) and MRI appearance (yellow arrows) of the cyst. Aspiration treatment (green arrow) removes viscous fluid (blue arrow) from within the cyst.

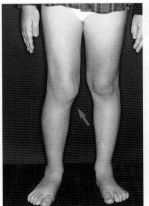

Fig. 6.32 Intraarticular hemangioma. Note the swelling of the knee. This boy had repeated synovectomies for recurrent hemangiomata of the knee.

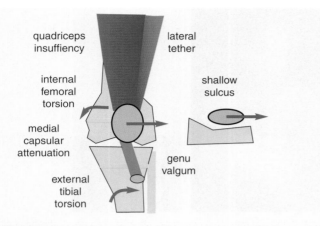

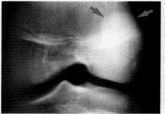

Condition	Effect
Femoral and tibial torsion	Increases Q angle
	Overall limb malalignment
Genu valgum	Increases Q angle
Condylar hypoplasia	Promotes lateral subluxation or dislocation
Patella alta	Results in less lateral stability
Quad insufficiency	Produces imbalance in quadriceps
Med. cap. attenuation	Inadequate medial check-rein
VL contracture	Tethers patella laterally

Fig. 6.33 Factors contributing to patellofemoral instability. These factors combine to increase the risk of patellar subluxation or dislocation.

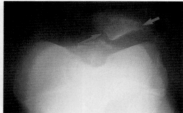

Fig. 6.34 Patellar hypoplasia. This deformity was part of the nail–patella syndrome.

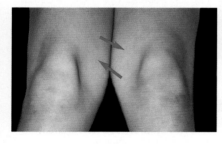

Fig. 6.35 Quadriceps hypoplasia. Note the loss of delineation of the VMO. The hypoplasia and weakness contribute to patellar instability.

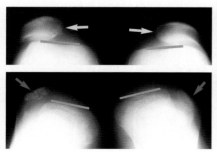

Fig. 6.36 Sunrise views. These projections show subluxation (yellow arrows) and dislocations (red arrows) of the patella. Note the position of the anterior femoral articular surface (green lines).

Patellofemoral Disorders

Many factors may contribute to patellofemoral instability (Fig. 6.33).

Systemic Disorders

Patellofemoral instability is more common in children with (1) knee dysplasias, such as occurs in nail–patella syndrome (Fig. 6.34), Rubinstein–Taybi syndrome, and Turner syndrome; and (2) conditions with increased joint laxity such as Down syndrome. These underlying conditions complicate management.

Congenital Dislocation

Congenital patellar dislocation is a rare condition that causes a progressive flexion, valgus, and tibial external rotational deformities of the knee. Reduce the dislocation and realign the quadriceps mechanism late in the first year. An extensive lateral release is often required.

Patellar Subluxation or Dislocation in Childhood

So-called *habitual* subluxation or dislocation is usually due to a dysplastic knee with contracture of the lateral portion of the quadriceps mechanism. This causes the patella to displace laterally whenever the knee is flexed. Early operative realignment is appropriate, but because the dysplastic features are severe, recurrence is common.

Traumatic Patellar Subluxation or Dislocation

Traumatic patellar dislocations cause an articular fracture. If the injury is severe, producing a tense hemarthrosis, arthroscopic evaluation may be appropriate (see Chapter 10, Trauma).

Adolescent Recurrent Dislocation

Most recurrent dislocations occur in individuals with dysplastic knees. They may show generalized joint laxity, lateral tibial torsion, genu valgum, hypoplasia of the quadriceps (Fig. 6.35), attenuation of the medial joint capsule, limited medial mobility of the patella, and abnormal patellar tracking. Observe the tracking of the patella as the patient slowly extends the knee. Lateral displacement of the patella as the knee nears full extension is described as *J tracking*. J tracking is a common finding. Sometimes the patella becomes subluxated with a sudden lateral shift. The patellar apprehension sign may also be positive. The patient becomes fearful that the patella will dislocate when the examiner applies lateral pressure to the patella. Radiographs may show lateral displacement of the patella (Fig. 6.36).

Management Manage first by ordering isometric quadriceps exercises. If the instability persists, operative correction is often necessary. Identify and correct each dysplastic component. In the growing child, often a lateral release, a medial plication, and a transfer of the semitendinosis to the patella are required. After growth is completed, reposition the tibial tubercle more medial and anterior to align and to optimize quadriceps alignment (see page 396).

Anterior Knee Pain

Anterior knee pain is common during the teen years. It may be associated with some underlying patellofemoral malalignment or may be idiopathic, occurring in individuals without evidence of any underlying abnormality.

Idiopathic anterior knee pain is common in adolescent girls. The pain is often activity related, is poorly localized, and may cause disability. It has been described as the *headache of the knee*. About one-third of these patients have features of the MMPI found in individuals with nonorganic back pain. Its natural history is one of spontaneous improvement over a period of years.

Manage by NSAIDS, isometric exercises, activity modification, and reassurance. Avoid arthroscopy and lateral release procedures.

Structural anterior knee pain is more serious and often requires operative correction.

Identify the underlying dysplastic features such as lateral tibial torsion, genu valgum, patella alta, vastus medialis hypoplasia, lateral tether, shallow sulcus, or excessive joint laxity. Consider imaging the patellofemoral joint with a CT scan to rule out maltracking (Fig. 6.37).

Manage first with NSAIDS and isometric exercises. During the first visit, introduce the possible need for a realignment procedure (Fig. 6.38). Identify and, if possible, quantitate the severity of each dysplastic feature. Thoughtfully place the operative incision (Fig. 6.39). See page 396).

Correct obvious manageable deformities early. In other cases, the decision is difficult. For example, bilateral double-level osteotomies are necessary to correct severe rotational malalignment.

Chapter Consultant Carl Stanitski, e-mail: stanitsc@musc.edu

References

1999 Dysplasia of the patellofemoral joint in children. Eilert RE. Am J Knee Surg 12:114

1998 Sonography of patellar abnormalities in children. Miller TT, et al. AJR Am J Roentgenol 171:739

1998 Patellar tendon-to-patella ratio in children. Walker P, Harris I, Leicester A. JPO 18:129

1997 Treatment of patellofemoral instability in childhood with creation of a femoral sulcus. Beals RK, Buehler K. JPO 17:516

1996 External tibial torsion: an underrecognized cause of recurrent patellar dislocation. Cameron JC, Saha S. CO 328:177

1996 Treatment of severe torsional malalignment syndrome. Delgado ED, et al. JPO 16:484

1996 Axial radiography or CT in the measurement of patellofemoral malalignment indices in children and adolescents? Vahasarja V, et al. Clin Radiol 51:639

1995 Articular hypermobility and chondral injury in patients with acute patellar dislocations. Stanitski CL. Am J Sports Med 23:146

1994 The value of computed tomography for the diagnosis of recurrent patellar subluxation in adolescents. Stanciu C, et al. Can J Surg 37:319

1992 Congenital dislocation of the patella and its operative treatment. Langenskiold A, Ritsila V. JPO 12:315

1992 Patellofemoral stress. A prospective analysis of exercise treatment in adolescents and adults. O'Neill DB, Micheli LJ, Warner JP. Am J Sports Med 20:151

1992 Patellofemoral pain in the pediatric patient. Thabit G 3d, Micheli LJ. Orthop Clin North Am 23:567

1990 Patellofemoral pain in children. Yates CK, Grana WA. CO 255:36

1988 Treatment of patellofemoral instability in Down's syndrome. Mendez AA, Keret D, MacEwen GD. CO 234:148

1986 Acute patellar dislocations. The natural history. Hawkins RJ, Bell RH, Anisette G. Am J Sports Med 14:117

1985 Recurrent dislocation of the patella treated by the modified Roux-Goldthwait procedure. A prospective study of forty-seven knees. Fondren FB, Goldner JL, Bassett FH 3d. JBJS 67A:993

1985 The natural history of anterior knee pain in adolescents. Sandow MJ, Goodfellow JW. JBJS 67B:36

1981 Functional versus organic knee pain in adolescents. A pilot study. Fritz GK, Bleck EE, Dahl IS. Am J Sports Med 9:247

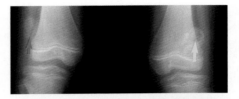
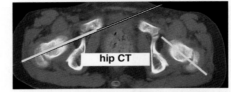
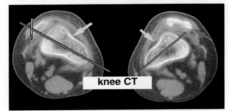
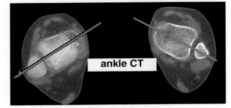

Fig. 6.37 Rotational malalignment syndrome. This child had habitual dislocations at age 5 years. Realignment was performed on the worse left side. She was not seen again until age 10 years. At this time, she is asymptomatic. Her left patella is subluxated and right patella dislocated. The child has severe rotational malalignment as demonstrated by CT scans. Note that the bicondylar axis is medially rotated 30° (yellow lines). This results in 60° of anteversion (red lines) and about 75° of lateral tibial torsion (blue lines). Note the displaced patella (red arrows) and the shallow condylar grooves (yellow arrows). It was elected not to attempt operative repair because rotational osteotomies of both femora and tibiae and realignment would be necessary. The chance of success was considered too poor to justify the magnitude of the procedures. This case demonstrates the complex pathology of some types of congenital development patellofemoral disorders.

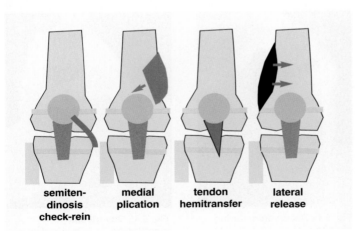

semiten-
dinosis
check-rein

medial
plication

tendon
hemitransfer

lateral
release

Fig. 6.38 Components of operative repair. These components are usually combined to correct all dysplasic features. The lateral release alone is usually inadequate.

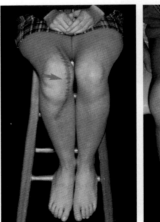
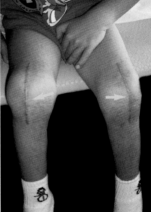

Fig. 6.39 Operative knee scars. Knee scars cause considerable disability (red arrow). A mid-line vertical incision is optimal for extensive realignment procedures (yellow arrows).

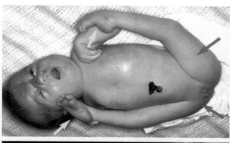

Fig. 6.40 Typical hyperextension deformity in the newborn. This deformity is common in breech presentations and is often associated with other deformities such as dislocated hips (red arrows) and clubfeet (yellow arrows).

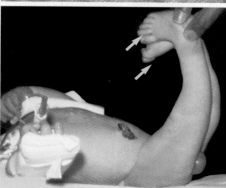

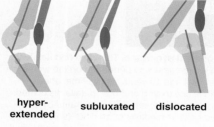

Fig. 6.41 Classification of extension deformities. These deformities can be classified by severity. Based on Curtis and Fisher (1969).

hyper-extended   subluxated   dislocated

Knee Flexion and Extension Deformities

Knee flexion and extension deformities are common and disabling. They have many causes, including congenital contractures, deformities from neuromuscular disorders, trauma, and infection.

Congenital Hyperextension

This deformity is often associated with other conditions (Fig. 6.40) such as arthrogryposis, spina bifida, developmental hip dysplasia, and clubfeet. In many cases, the child was born breech.

Pathology depends upon severity. In dislocated knees, fibrosis of the quadriceps muscle, absence of the suprapatellar pouch, and valgus deformity of the knee are often present.

Evaluation Look for other abnormalities. Make a radiograph of the pelvis to make certain the hips are not dysplastic or dislocated. Ultrasound or MRI imaging may be necessary to assess the knee. Grade the severity of the deformity (Fig. 6.41).

Management Manage by gentle stretching and casting (Fig. 6.42) or by using the Pavlik harness if the knee can be flexed to 60°. For knee dislocations, perform a quadriceps lengthening at about 1–3 months of age (Fig. 6.43). Immobilize in 90° of flexion for about one month. Consider correction of other deformities such as hip dislocations and clubfeet concurrently.

If treatment is delayed (Fig. 6.44), management is more difficult. Limited quadriceps lengthening may move the arc of motion into a more functional plane. In older children or adolescents, bony deformity may require flexion osteotomy to improve alignment.

Prognosis is determined by severity (Fig. 6.45). It is generally better for unilateral cases with early operative correction.

Acquired Recurvatum Deformity

Bony deformity of the upper tibia usually results from trauma to the anterior proximal tibial physis (Fig. 6.46). This portion of the physis is vulnerable to arrest. Recurvatum has been reported following traction, spica cast immobilization, proximal tibial traction pin placement, femoral shaft fractures, and meningococcal infections.

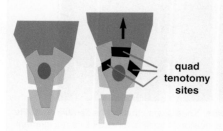

Fig. 6.42 Nonoperative management. Serial cast correction is usually effective in hyperextended or subluxated hips.

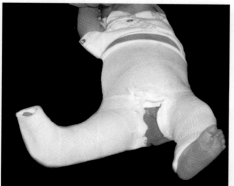

quad tenotomy sites

Fig. 6.43 Percutaneous quadriceps recession. This procedure is performed in early infancy through three percutaneous incisions. The infant is immobilized in a spica cast for 4–6 weeks. From Roy and Crawford (1989).

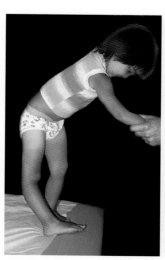

Fig. 6.44 Recurvatum during childhood. This deformity has been present since birth. It causes the child considerable disability.

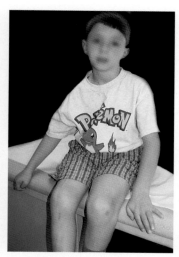

Fig. 6.45 Quadriceps lengthening. This child had an open quadriceps lengthening of the right knee through a vertical midline approach.

Evaluation Make radiographs of the upper tibia. Note that the tibia is usually inclined posteriorly by about 9°. Assess the status of the growth plate with MRI or CT scans.

Management Consider resection of physeal bars of the anterior tibia if 2 years of growth remain. At the end of growth, correct the deformity with a opening wedge osteotomy just proximal to the insertion of the patellar tendon (Fig. 6.47).

Flexion Deformity in Neuromuscular Disorders
Congenital and acquired flexion contracture deformities are common in children with neuromuscular problems. Acquired deformities result from imbalance between the quadriceps and hamstrings. Flexion deformity is common in arthrogryposis (Fig. 6.48), cerebral palsy (Fig. 6.49), and myelodysplasia.

Manage by restoring muscle balance and correcting secondary bone deformity (see Chapter 14).

Consultant Bill Oppenheim, e-mail: woppenhe@ucla.edu

References

1999 Congenital dislocation of the knee: overview of management options. Muhammad KS, LA Koman, JF Mooney, 3rd, BP Smith. J South Orthop Assoc 8:93

1994 Larsen's syndrome: review of the literature and analysis of thirty-eight cases. Laville JM, Lakermance P, Limouzy F. JPO 14:63

1993 Congenital dislocation of the knee. Its pathologic features and treatment. Ooishi T, et al. CO 287:187

1991 Natural history of knee contractures in myelomeningocele. Wright JG, et al. JPO 11:725

1990 The knee in arthrogryposis multiplex congenita. Sodergard J, Ryoppy S. JPO 10:177

1989 Congenital dislocation of the knee. Bensahel H, et al. JPO 9:174

1989 Percutaneous quadriceps recession: a technique for management of congenital hyperextension deformities of the knee in the neonate. Roy DR, Crawford AH. JPO 9:717

1987 Congenital dislocation of the knee. Johnson E, Audell R, Oppenheim WL. JPO 7:194

1969 Congenital hyperextension with anterior subluxation of the knee. Curtis BH, Fisher RL. JBJS 51A:255

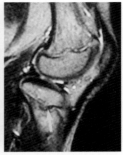
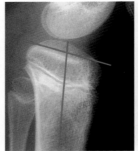
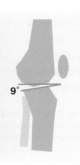

Fig. 6.46 Recurvatum from physeal injury. Note the anterior inclination of the proximal tibia (red line) and irregular physis on the MRI (yellow arrow). Normally the tibial articular surface inclines posteriorly by about 9° (green lines).

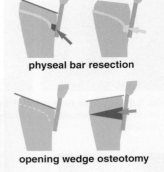

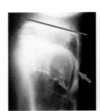
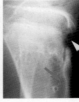

physeal bar resection

opening wedge osteotomy

Fig. 6.47 Correction of physeal bar. This child was treated with a proximal tibial pin (blue arrows) causing a physeal bar (red arrow) and a secondary recurvatum deformity (red lines). This bar was resected and the defect filled with fat (yellow arrows). The established deformity at the end of growth can be corrected by an opening wedge osteotomy (green arrow) just proximal to the tibial tubercle.

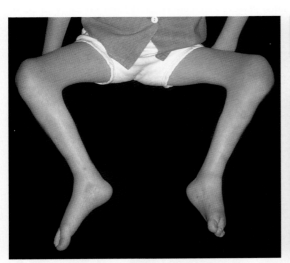
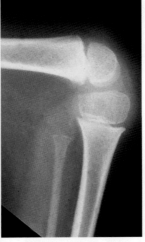

Fig. 6.48 Knee flexion in arthrogryposis. This child was unable to walk because of the knee flexion contracture. Following correction by soft tissue releases and femoral shortening, the child became ambulatory.

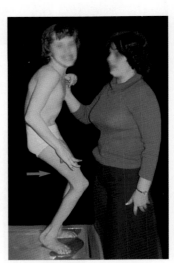

Fig. 6.49 Flexion deformity in cerebral palsy. This is part of the crouch gait (red arrow). See page 332.

Direction	Comment	Natural history
Lateral	Physiological in infancy	Resolves
Anterior	With other deformities	Persists
Posteromedial	Classic pattern	Resolves incompletely
Anterolateral	Pre-pseudoarthrosis	Progressive deformity

Fig. 6.50 Patterns of tibial bowing. The direction of the apex of the tibial bow determines the prognosis and management. Simple lateral bowing is benign in contrast with anterolateral bowing, which often leads to pseudoarthrosis of the tibia.

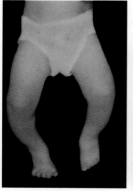
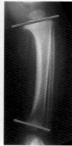

Fig. 6.51 Physiologic bowing. This physiologic lateral tibial bowing resolves spontaneously in late infancy. Radiographs are usually not necessary.

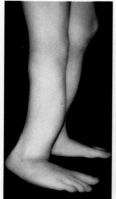
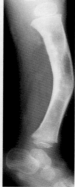
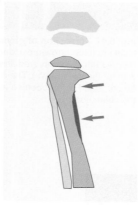

Fig. 6.52 Anterior bow in fibular deficiency.

Fig. 6.53 Focal fibrocartilagenous dysplasia. Note the lucency (red arrow) and the sclerosis (blue arrow).

Tibial Bowing

Tibial bowing is common and varied. The prognosis varies depending upon the direction of the apex or convexity of the bowing (Fig. 6.50).

Lateral Tibial Bowing

Lateral tibial bowing is common in infants and is simply a variation of normal (Fig. 6.51). The condition is usually mild, symmetrical, and unassociated with other problems. Reassure the family and provide a follow-up if necessary. Radiographs are usually unnecessary.

Anterior Tibial Bowing

Anterior bowing is often associated with fibular hemimelia (Fig. 6.52). Sometimes a dimple is present over the apex. Limb shortening is the major problem.

Focal Fibrocartilagenous Dysplasia

This rare deformity has a characteristic radiographic appearance (Fig. 6.53). The lesions tend to heal with growth.

Posteromedial Tibial Bowing

Posteromedial bowing (Fig. 6.54) is a rare condition associated with a calcaneal deformity of the foot and mild limb shortening. The condition may be due to abnormal intrauterine position. The calcaneal foot deformity resolves with time. The bowing improves with growth. Shortening tends to increase with time and correction by epiphysiodesis or lengthening is often necessary.

Anterolateral Tibial Bowing

Anterolateral bowing is a serious form of tibial bowing (Fig. 6.55). The bowing may increase spontaneously and fracture at its apex. This leads to a pseudoarthrosis of the tibia that is difficult to manage. Anterolateral bowing is managed by protection with a cast or brace to prevent fracture or by operatively augmenting the bone strength to reduce the risk of fracture.

Pseudoarthrosis of the Tibia

Pseudoarthrosis of the tibia results from a pathological fracture (Fig. 6.56) that may occur before or after birth. It may be preceded by an anterolateral bowing of the tibia and is sometimes associated with neurofibromatosis. The pseudoarthrosis occurs in the distal tibial diaphysis and can be graded by severity (Fig. 6.57).

Management is extremely difficult, and some patients eventually require amputation because of a failure to achieve union. Operative correction is necessary, with several options available (Fig. 6.58). First, stabilize with an intramedullary (IM) rod and a graft to promote union (Fig. 6.59). If this fails, place a vascularized graft from the other fibula or

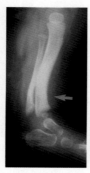
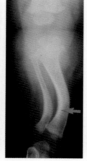
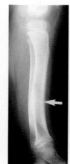
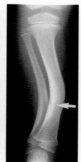
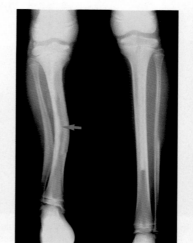
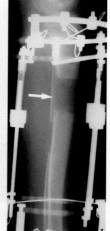

Fig. 6.54 Posteromedial tibial bowing. This bow was present at birth (red arrows). The bowing improved gradually throughout childhood, as shown at age 3 years (yellow arrows) and 10 years (blue arrow). This is an unusually severe form with persistent bowing and shortening of 4.5 cm. The deformity was corrected by an osteotomy and lengthening (white arrow) with a circular frame at age 12 years.

immobilize with an Ilizarov device. The Ilizarov fixator allows a segment of diaphysis to be transported. The pseudoarthrosis is compressed while the proximal metaphysis is lengthened. If successful, union without sacrificing length is achieved. Place an IM rod to prevent recurrent deformity. Trials using electrical stimulation to promote union have had limited success.

Union may not be achieved even after several procedures. In other cases, only a tenuous union is obtained. The tibia is dysplastic and may refracture, and the leg is short and weak. The outcome is unsatisfactory and amputation is required.

Isolated Fibular Pseudoarthrosis

Rarely, only the fibula is affected by the pseudoarthrosis (Fig. 6.56). Manage by plate fixation, autogenous grafting, and correcting ankle valgus. If the pseudoarthrosis persists, create a synostosis between the distal fragment and the tibia to prevent further shortening.

Consultant Perry Schoenecker, e-mail: pschoenecker@shrinenet.org

References

2000 The fibula in congenital pseudoarthrosis of the tibia: the EPOS multicenter study. European Paediatric Orthopaedic Society. Keret D, et al. JPOb 9:69

2000 Functional results at the end of skeletal growth in 30 patients affected by congenital pseudoarthrosis of the tibia. Tudisco C, et al. JPOb 9:94

1997 Ilizarov technique in the treatment of congenital pseudoarthrosis of the tibia. Ghanem I, Damsin JP, Carlioz H. JPO 17:685

1995 Congenital pseudoarthrosis of the tibia. Long-term followup of 29 cases treated by microvascular bone transfer. Gilbert A, Brockman R. CO 314:37

1995 MRI of focal fibrocartilaginous dysplasia. Meyer JS, et al. JPO 15:304

1993 Late-onset pseudoarthrosis of the dysplastic tibia. Roach JW, Shindell R, Green NE. JBJS 75A:1593

1992 Use of an intramedullary rod for the treatment of congenital pseudoarthrosis of the tibia. Anderson DJ, et al. JBJS 74A:161

1992 Treatment of congenital pseudoarthrosis of the tibia using the Ilizarov technique. Paley D, et al. CO 280:81

1991 Prophylactic bypass grafting of the prepseudoarthrotic tibia in neurofibromatosis. Strong ML, Wong-Chung J. JPO 11:757

1988 Tibia vara due to focal fibrocartilaginous dysplasia. The natural history. Bradish CF, Davies SJ, Malone M. JBJS 70B:106

1984 Congenital posteromedial bowing of the tibia and fibula. Pappas AM. JPO 4:525

1982 Pathology and natural history of congenital pseudoarthrosis of the tibia. Boyd HB. CO 166:5

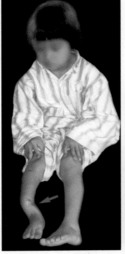
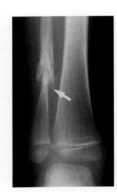

Fig. 6.55 Anterolateral bowing and pseudoarthrosis of the tibia. This girl has a pseudoarthrosis of the right tibia (arrows).

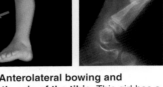

Fig. 6.56 Fibular pseudoarthrosis.

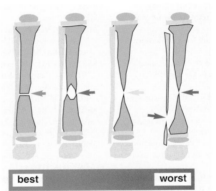

Fig. 6.57 Prognosis of tibial pseudoarthrosis. outlook is best for simple pseudoarthrosis (green arrow), cystic (blue arrow), scerlotic (yellow arrow) and worst for sclerotic type with pseudoarthrosis of the fibula (red arrows)

best   worst

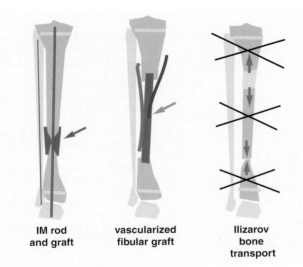

IM rod and graft   vascularized fibular graft   Ilizarov bone transport

Fig. 6.58 Pseudoarthrosis tibia treatment methods. The most successful methods for treating this defect are the intermedullary rod and autogenous bone graft (red arrow), the vascularized fibular graft (green arrow), and the Ilizarov method with compression of the lesion and lengthening of the proximal tibia.

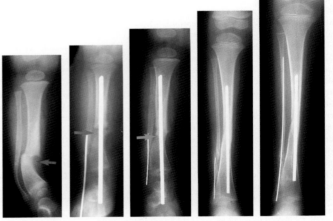

Fig. 6.59 Management by intramedullary fixation and grafting. This infant was born with an anterolateral bow. He was managed in a clam-shell brace. While bathing without the brace, the infant fell and fractured the dysplastic tibia (red arrows). This was treated with IM rod fixation and grafting (blue arrow). Tenuous union was achieved (green arrow). The fibula remained unhealed at age 4 years, and ankle valgus developed. A distal tibial–fibular fusion was created to avoid further valgus from developing.

Andrish J. Meniscal injuries in children and adolescents: Diagnosis and management. J Am Acad Ortho Surg 1996;4:231-237.

Batten J, Menelaus MB. Fragmentation of the proximal pole of the patella: Another manifestation of juvenile traction osteochondritis? J Bone Joint Surg 1985;67B:249-251.

Baxter MP. Assessment of normal pediatric knee ligament laxity using the genucom. J Pediatr Orthop 1988;8:546-550.

Bellier G, Dupont JY, Larrain M, et al. Lateral discoid menisci in children. Arthroscopy 1989;5:52-56.

Bergman NR, Williams PF. Habitual dislocation of the patella in flexion. J Bone Joint Surg 1988;70B:415-419.

Bergström R, Gillquist J, Lysholm J, et al. Arthroscopy of the knee in children. J Pediatr Orthop 1984;4:542-545.

Boyd HB, Pathology and natural history of congenital pseudarthrosis of the tibia. Clin Orthop 1982;166:5-13.

Bradley J, Dandy DJ. Osteochondritis dissecans and other lesions of the femoral condyles. J Bone Joint Surg 1989;71B:518-522.

Cahill BR, Berg BC. 99m-Technetium phosphate compound joint scinitigraphy in the management of juvenile osteochondritis dissecans of the femoral condyles. Am J Sports Med 1983;11:329

Cash JD, Hughston JC. Treatment of acute patellar dislocation. Am J Sports Med 1988;16:244-249.

Clark CR, Ogden JA. Development of the menisci of the human knee joint: Morphological changes and their potential role in childhood meniscal injury. J Bone Joint Surg 1983;65A:538-547.

Crossett LS, Beaty JH, Betz RR, et al. Congenital pseudarthrosis of the tibia: Long-term follow-up study. Clin Orthop 1989;245:16-18.

Curl WW. Popliteal Cysts. 1996;J Am Acad Ortho Surg 4 #3:129-132.

Dal Monte A, Donzelli O, Sudanese A, et al. Congenital pseudarthrosis of the fibula. J Pediatr Orthop 1987;7:14-18.

Dickhaut SC, DeLee JC. The discoid lateral-meniscus syndrome. J Bone Joint Surg 1982;64A:1068-1073.

Dinham JM. Popliteal cysts in children: The case against surgery. J Bone Joint Surg 1975;57B:69-71.

Dugdale TW, Renshaw TS. Instability of the patellofemoral joint in Down syndrome. J Bone Joint Surg 1986;68A:405-413.

Fabry G, Lammens J, Van Melkebeek J, et al. Treatment of congenital pseudarthrosis with the Ilizarov technique. J Pediatr Orthop 1988;8:67-70.

Fairbank JC, Pynsent PB, van-Poortvliet JA, et al. Mechanical factors in the incidence of knee pain in adolescents and young adults. J Bone Joint Surg 1984;66B:685-693.

Flowers MJ, Bhadreshwar DR. Tibial tuberosity excision for wymptomatic Osgood-Schlatter disease. J Ped Orthop 1995;15:292-297.

Glynn MK, Regan BF. Surgical treatment of Osgood-Schlatter disease. J Pediatr Orthop 1983;3:216-219.

Gordon JE, Schoenecker PL. Surgical treatment of congenital dislocation of the patella. J Ped Orthop 1999;19:260-264.

Green JP, Waugh W, Wood H. Congenital lateral dislocation of the patella. J Bone Joint Surg 1968;50B:285-289.

Guidera KJ, Satterthwaite Y, Ogden JA, et al. Nail Patella Syndrome: A review of 44 Orthopedic patients. J Ped Orthop 1991;11:737-742.

Hall JE, Micheli LJ, McManama GB Jr. Semitendinosus tenodesis for recurrent subluxation or dislocation of the patella. Clin Orthop 1979;144:31-35.

Hayashi LK, Yamaga H, Ida K, et al. Arthroscopic meniscectomy for discoid lateral meniscus in children. J Bone Joint Surg 1988;70A:1495-1500.

Hofmann A, Wenger DR. Posteromedial bowing of the tibia: Progression of discrepancy in leg lengths. J Bone Joint Surg 1981;63A:384-388.

Inoue M, Shino K, Hirose H, et al. Subluxation of the patella: Computed tomography analysis of patellofemoral congruence. J Bone Joint Surg 1988;70A:1331-1337.

Insall J. Current concepts review: Patellar pain. J Bone Joint Surg 1982;64A:147-152.

Jakob RP, von Gumppenberg S, Engelhardt P. Does Osgood-Schlatter disease influence the position of the patella? J Bone Joint Surg 1981;63B:579-582.

Johnson RP. Lateral facet syndrome of the patella: Lateral restraint analysis and use of lateral resection. Clin Orthop 1989;238:148-158.

King AG. Meniscal lesions in children and adolescents: A review of the pathology and clinical presentation. Injury 1983;15:105-108.

Kort JS, Schink MM, Mitchell SN, et al. Congenital pseudarthrosis of the tibia: Treatment with pulsing electromagnetic fields. The international experience. Clin Orthop 1982;165:124-137.

Kujala UM, Kvist M, Heinonen O. Osgood-Schlatter disease in adolescent athletes: Retrospective study of incidence and duration. Am J Sports Med 1985;13:236-241.

Laville, JM. Knee Deformities in Larsen's syndrome. 1994;J Ped Orthop B 3:180-184

Lo, IKY, Fowler P, Miniaci A. The outcome of operative treated anterior cruciate disruptions in the skeletally immature child. Arthroscopy 1997;13:627-634.

Lonner LH, Parisien JS. Arthroscopic treatment of meniscal cysts. Operative Techniques in Ortho. 1995;5(1):72-77.

Manzione M, Pizzutillo PD, Peoples AB, et al. Meniscectomy in children: A long-term follow-up study. Am J Sports Med 1983;11:111-115.

McDermott MJ, Bathgate B, Gillingham BL, Hennrikus WL. Correlation of MRI and arthroscopic diagnosis of knee pathology in children and adolescents. J Ped Orthop 1998;18:675-678.

McManus F, Rang M, Heslin DJ. Acute dislocation of the patella in children: The natural history. Clin Orthop 1979;139:88-91.

Medlar RC, Lyne ED. Sinding-Larsen-Johansson disease: Its etiology and natural history. J Bone Joint Surg 1978;60A:1113-1116.

Minami A, Ogino T, Sakuma T, et al. Free vascularized fibular grafts in the treatment of congenital pseudarthrosis of the tibia. Microsurgery 1987;8:111-116.

Mintzer C, Richmond J, Taylor J. Meniscal repair in the young athlete. Am J Sports Med 1998;26:630-633.

Mital MA, Matza RA, Cohen J. The so-called unresolved Osgood-Schlatter lesion: A concept based on fifteen surgically treated lesions. J Bone Joint Surg 1980;62A:732-739.

Morrissey RT, Riseborough EJ, Hall JE. Congenital pseudarthrosis of the tibia. J Bone Joint Surg 1981;63B:367-375.

Morrisy RT, Eubanks RG, Park JP, et al. Arthroscopy of the knee in children. Clin Orthop 1982;162:103-107.

Mori Y, Okumo H, Iketani H, et al. Efficacy of Lateral Retinacular Release for painful bipartite patella. Am J Sports Med 1995;23 #1 13-16.

Murray HH, Lovell WW. Congenital pseudarthrosis of the tibia: A long-term follow-up study. Clin Orthop 1982;166:14-20.

Nimon G, Muray D, Sandow M, Goodfellow J. Natural history of anterior knee pain: A 14-20 year follow-up of nonoperative management. J Ped Orthop 1998;18:118-122.

Ogden JA, Southwick WO. Osgood-Schlatter disease and tibial tuberosity development. Clin Orthop 1976;116:180-189.

Ohno O, Naito J, Iguchi T, et al. An electron microscopic study of early pathology in chondromalacia of the patella. J Bone Joint Surg 1989;70A:883-899.

Paletta GA, Bednarz P, Stanitski CL, et al. The Prognostic value of quantitative bone scan in knee osteochondritis dissecans. 1998;Am J Sports Med 26 #1, 7-11.

Pappas AM. Congenital posteromedial bowing of the tibia and fibula. J Pediatr Orthop 1984;4:525-531.

Paterson D. Congenital pseudarthrosis of the tibia. Clin Orthop 1989;247:44-54.

Pho RW, Levack B, Satku K, et al. Free vascularised fibular graft in the treatment of congenital pseudarthrosis of the tibia. J Bone Joint Surg 1985;67B:64-70.

Sally P, Poggi J, Speer K, et al. Acute dislocation of the patella. Am J Sports Med 1996;24:52-60.

Sandow MJ, Goodfellow JW. The natural history of anterior knee pain in adolescents. J Bone Joint Surg 1985;67B:36-38.

Sanpera I, Fixen J, Sparks LT, et al. Knee in Congenital Short Femur. J Ped Orthop 1995;4:159-163.

Schenck RC, Goodnight JM. Osteochondritis dissecans. Current concepts review. J Bone Joint Surg 1996;78A:439-456.

Schoenecker PL et al. Dysplasia of the knee associated with the syndrome of thrombocytopenia and absent radius. J Bone Joint Surg 1984;66A 421-427.

Schutzer SF, Ramsby GR, Fulkerson JP. The evaluation of patellofemoral pain using computerized tomography: A preliminary study. Clin Orthop 1986;204:286-293.

Scuderi G, Cuomo F, Scott WN. Lateral release and proximal realignment for patellar subluxation and dislocation: A long-term follow-up. J Bone Joint Surg 1988;70A:856-861.

Shim SS, Leung G. Blood supply of the knee joint: A microangiographic study in children and adults. Clin Orthop 1986;208:119-205.

Søballe K, Hansen AJ. Late results after meniscectomy in children. Injury 1987;18:182-184.

Stanisavljevic S, Zemenick G, Miller D. Congenital, irreducible, permanent lateral dislocation of the patella. Clin Orthop 1976;116:190-199.

Stanitski CL. Anterior cruciate ligament injury in the skeletally immature athlete. Operative Techniques in Sports Medicine 1998;6(4):228-233.

Stanitski CL, Paletta GA. Articular injury with acute patellar dislocation in adolescents. Am J Sports Med 1998;26:52-55.

Stanitski CL. Correlation of arthroscopic and clinical examinations with magnetic resonance imaging findings of injured knees in children and adolescents. Am J Sports Med 1998;26:2-6.

Stanitski CL. Patellar Instability in the School Age Athlete Instructional Course Lectures Vol 47 p345-350 1998 D. Cannon, ed Amer Acad Orthop Surg Pub, Rosemont, Il 60018.

Suman RK, Stother IG, Illingworth G. Diagnostic arthroscopy of the knee in children. J Bone Joint Surg 1984;66B:535-537.

Takeda Y, Ikata T, Yoshida S, et al. MRI high signal intensity in the menisci of asymptomatic children. J Bone Joint Surg 1998;80B:463-467.

Yadav SS, Thomas S. Congenital posteromedial bowing of the tibia. Acta Orthop Scand 1980;51:311-313.

Ziv I, Carroll NC. The role of arthroscopy in children. J Pediatr Orthop 1984;4:243-247.

Chapter 7—Hip

General

Problems of the hip account for about 15% of the practice of orthopedists. Many hip problems in adults have their origin during growth.

Development

Ossification of the ischium, ilium, pubis, femoral shaft, and distal femoral epiphysis occur before birth. The femoral head ossifies between the second and eighth postnatal months. (Fig. 7.1) and fuses with the neck between 15 and 21 years in boys and one year earlier in girls.

Growth of the upper femur occurs not only in the capital epiphysis and trochanteric epiphysis but also along the neck of the femur (Fig. 7.2). Trauma to specific sites causes specific types of deformities (Fig. 7.3).

Most growth of the acetabulum occurs from the triradiate cartilage. Closure will cause severe progressive dysplasia. Additional growth of the acetabulum occurs from the acetabular epiphysis. This growth is especially important late in childhood and during adolescence.

Damage to these growth centers, either from trauma or as a complication of treatment, is a common source of deformity and disability. The upper femur is very susceptible to vascular or epiphyseal injury.

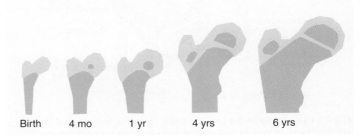

Birth   4 mo   1 yr   4 yrs   6 yrs

Fig. 7.1 Ossification of proximal femur. This sequence shows ossification in the normal child. Redrawn from Tönnis (1984).

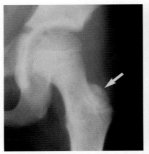
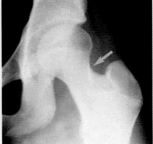

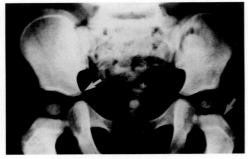

Fig. 7.2 Pelvic growth. This child had a phosphorolized oil dietary supplement as a child. Growth patterns are shown. Note the growth that occurs in the triradiate cartilage (orange arrow) and upper femur (red arrow). Courtesy I. Ponseti.

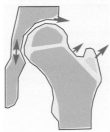

Fig. 7.3 Proximal femoral growth. Note that growth (red arrows) occurs at many sites about the upper femur, including appositional growth of the femoral neck. Damage to the greater trochanteric apophysis from curettage for a bone cyst (yellow arrow) or from reaming to place an IM nail (orange arrow) causes deformity.

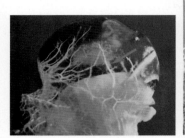

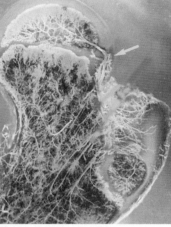

Fig. 7.4 Vascularity of the femoral head. In infancy, transepiphyseal vessels are often present (red arrow). In childhood, the femoral head is supplied by the lateral retinacular vessels that must traverse the joint (yellow arrow). From Chung (1976).

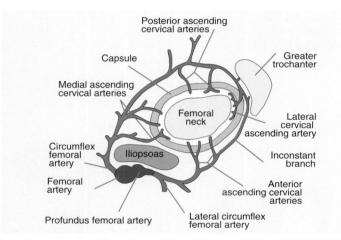

Fig. 7.5 Vascularity of the femoral head. Note that the proximal femur is supplied by an arcade of vessels that arise from the profundus femoral artery.

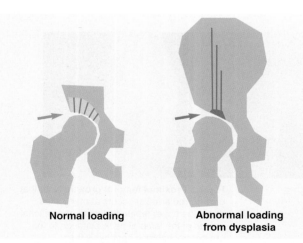

Fig. 7.6 Biomechanics of the hip. In the normal hip, loading (green arrow) is low and well distributed. In dysplasia, loading is concentrated (red arrow), resulting in eventual cartilage degeneration.

Vascularity

Disturbances in blood supply to the upper femur are a common cause of many serious deformities and subsequent disability.

The femoral head may receive blood through the ligamentum teres, epiphyseal vessels, or metaphysis. The femoral head in the infant is supplied by epiphyseal vessels and vessels that traverse the epiphyseal plate (Fig. 7.4). These transepiphyseal vessels disappear as ossification develops in the femoral head. Circulation in the child is primarily through the metaphyseal vessels. Only in late childhood and adolescence do the ligamentum teres vessels make a significant contribution. After closure of the capital epiphyseal plate, the metaphyseal vessels contribute to the circulation.

During most of childhood, two anastomotic rings formed by the medial and lateral circumflex vessels provide blood (Fig. 7.5). These signs are variable and deficiencies may contribute to the development of avascular necrosis.

Biomechanics

Loading within the joint is affected by the load-bearing area (Fig. 7.6). Increased loading is prominent when the hip is subluxated or shallow. Increased loading leads to osteoarthritis in adult life.

Operative procedures, especially osteotomies of the pelvis and femur, dramatically affect the biomechanics of the hip. The hip joint normally carries about four times its body weight. Hip joint loading is reduced by varus femoral osteotomy or by medializing the joint, as done in the Chiari osteotomy. When reconstructing a hip, try to achieve as normal anatomy as possible.

Term	Definition
Coxa	**Refers to Joint**
Vara	Reduction neck–shaft angle
Valga	Increased neck–shaft angle
Plana	Flattening femoral head
Magna	Enlarged femoral head
Breva	Shortened femoral neck
Hip dysplasia	**Abnormal features of hip joint**
Acetabular	Dysplastic acetabulum
Femoral	Dysplastic femur
Joint status	**Acetabulofemoral relationship**
Congruous	Concentric reduction
Subluxated	Loss of concentricity
Dislocated	No joint elements in contact
Joint fit	**Joint surface relationship**
Spherical	Round femoral head
Congruous	Congruous fit
Incongruous	Incongruous
Aspherical	Femoral head nonspherical
Congruous	Congruous fit
Incongrous	Incongruous

Fig. 7.7 Nomenclature for deformity. These terms are commonly used to describe various patterns of hip deformity.

Nomenclature

Hip terminology is reasonably straightforward (Fig. 7.7). The most significant recent change was the replacement of the term *congenital* with *developmental* in hip dysplasia. Congenital hip disease (CDH) thus becomes developmental hip dysplasia (DDH). Hip disorders caused by muscle disorders secondary to neurologic disorders such as cerebral palsy are called *neurogenic* dysplasia of the hip (NDH). The term *dysplasia* is a broad term covering disorders that may involve the acetabulum, upper femur, or both elements.

Evaluation

A thorough evaluation of the hip is important due to the vulnerability of the hip joint to damage, especially from impaired blood supply. Delays in diagnosis of DDH, septic arthritis, and slipped epiphysis are relatively common and sometimes result in joint destruction. The deep position of the hip joint makes evaluation more difficult than most extremity joints such as the knee or ankle. This, together with its tenuous vascularity, places the hip at special risk.

History

Is there a family history of hip problems? DDH occurs in families. Has the child complained of pain? Night pain suggests a neoplastic origin. Remember that hip pain may be referred to the knee (Fig. 7.8). Has the child limped? Were there systemic signs? Has the problem been getting worse or plateaued? Be certain to rule out septic arthritis and slipped epiphysis as acute disorders and DDH as a long-term problem.

Physical Examination

Observation Does the child appear ill? Is there spontaneous movement of the limb? Pseudoparalysis is common in trauma and infections. Does the child limp? Limping from hip problems is usually antalgic or due to an abductor lurch.

Palpation Palpate for tenderness over the bony prominences. Tenderness is often found in the adolescent with bursitis, tendonitis, or overuse syndromes. By determining the point of maximum tenderness exactly, a presumptive diagnosis can often be made.

Range of Motion Hip disorders often result in loss of motion. Inflammatory disorders usually cause a reduction in internal hip rotation early on and eventually flexion and adduction contracture of the hip.

Hip rotation Assess with the child prone. Assessing the range of medial rotation is a valuable screening test (Fig. 7.9). The finding of asymmetric hip rotation is abnormal and indicates the need for a radiograph of the pelvis.

Flexion Detect the presence of a contracture using the Thomas or prone extension test (Fig. 7.10). The prone extension test is most accurate, especially in children with neuromuscular disorders.

Abduction–Adduction Assess while stabilizing the pelvis with one hand.

Trendelenburg Test

Assess an abductor lurch using the Trendelenburg test (Fig. 7.11). Ask the child to lift one leg at a time. The pelvis should rise on the elevated side. A drop of that side is a positive sign and suggests that the abductor mechanism is weak on the opposite side. This lurch may be due to weakness of the muscles, a change in shape of the upper femur, or inflammation of the joint.

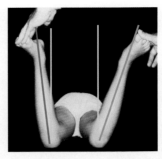

Fig. 7.9 Hip rotation test. Position the child prone with the knees flexed to 90°. Rotate the hips internally and note any guarding and the extent of rotation. Asymmetry of rotation is usually abnormal. In this child with Legg–Calvé–Perthes disease on the left hip, rotation was limited as compared to the right hip.

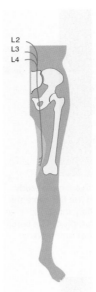

Fig. 7.8 Hip pain referred to knee. The obturator nerve supplies articular branches to the hip and cutaneous coverage about the knee. Hip disorders may present with knee pain.

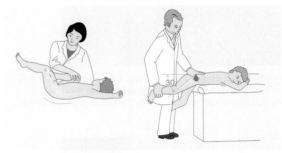

Fig. 7.10 Hip flexion contracture assessment. The Thomas test (left) is performed with the contralateral hip flexed. Extend to measure the degree of contracture. The prone extension test (right) is performed with the child prone. Gradually extend the hip until the hand on the pelvis begins to rise. The horizontal–thigh angle indicates the degree of contracture.

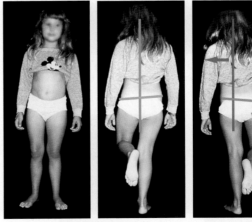

Fig 7.11 Trendelenburg test This girl has DDH with weakness of the left hip abductors. When standing on her right leg, right hip abductors contract to elevate the left pelvis to maintain the head centered over the body (green lines). When standing on the weaker left leg, abductor weakness allows the right pelvis to fall (blue arrow). She must then shift her weight over the left leg (red lines).

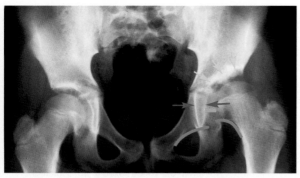

Fig. 7.12 AP X-ray of pelvis. Much can be learned from this simple study. The right hip is normal. Acetabular dysplasia is present on the left. Note the triangular shape of the tear drop (red arrows). Note that the joint space (orange line) is widened. Shenton's line (green lines) is disrupted. The sercil (yellow arrows) is sclerotic. The left hip joint is slightly higher and more laterally positioned than the normal side.

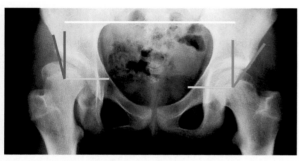

Fig 7.13 Center–edge (CE) angle. This child has a normal left hip with a CE angle of 30˚. The right hip is aspherical and subluxated and the CE angle is 10˚. Note that measures are made with the pelvis level (white line).

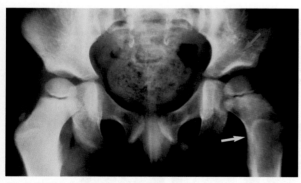

Fig 7.14 Hemideossification. Note the bone loss of the left hemipelvis (red arrow) due to an osteoid osteoma (yellow arrow) of the proximal femur.

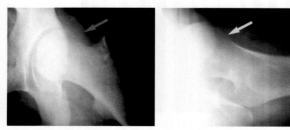

Fig. 7.15 Lateral X-rays of the proximal femur. Frog-leg lateral (red arrow) is only an oblique view. A true lateral (yellow arrow) requires special positioning but provides more information as it is made at right angles to the AP view.

Laboratory Studies

A CBC and ESR are often helpful in evaluating hip disorders. The ESR and CRP are useful in differentiating septic arthritis from toxic synovitis. Infections usually elevate the ESR above 25–30 mm/hr. Toxic synovitis causes only a slight elevation in the ESR and CRP. Hematologic disorders such as leukemia and sickle cell disease may cause pelvic pain.

Hip Joint Aspiration

The aspiration of the hip is the most certain method of establishing the diagnosis of septic arthritis. Aspirate the joint promptly if the diagnosis of septic arthritis is seriously included in the differential. Although a negative aspirate (even when documented by an arthrogram) is not absolutely definitive, it is highly suggestive that the problem is not within the joint.

Delays in diagnosing septic arthritis may be catastrophic because it jeopardizes the vascularity to the femoral head and articular cartilage. Joint aspiration does not affect bone scans and should not be delayed by plans to perform imaging procedures.

Imaging

Imaging is required to evaluate hip disorders in children. Imaging is the only way to establish a prognosis. The vast majority of hip problems in children can still be managed adequately by careful examination and conventional radiographs.

Conventional radiography Evaluate most hip problems with conventional radiography. Except for the initial study, use a gonad shield. Obtain a single AP study (Fig. 7.12). Several useful measures may be made from this simple study (Fig. 7.13). Note any asymmetry in ossification of the pelvis. A painful condition such as an osteoid osteotomy results in hemideossification (Fig. 7.14). Be aware of the situations in which false negative studies are commonly misleading. A negative study does not rule out DDH in the neonate or an early septic arthritis. An AP radiograph may not show a mild slipped capital femoral epiphysis (SCFE).

Add other views as necessary. The frog-leg lateral allows comparison of both upper femora. The true lateral is useful in assessing the degree of slip in SCFE or the degree of involvement in Legg–Calvé–Perthes disease (Fig. 7.15).

Useful special views include the abduction–internal rotation study for hip dysplasia (Fig. 7.16), maximum abduction and adduction views for assessing hinge abduction problems, and anteversion studies. Femoral anteversion measurement is seldom necessary.

The load-bearing area of the hip significantly affects its longevity. A reduction in this area may be due to one or more of the following factors:

1. Simple hip dysplasia. The hip joint is either maldirected or shallow. Both reduce contact area. The depth of the acetabulum is often assessed by the CE angle. This angle increases during childhood as the joint ossifies. At the end of growth, values are like those of adults with a normal range of 25°– 45˚. Features of the normal hip are used as a basis for assessing deformity (Fig. 7.17) and planning reconstruction.

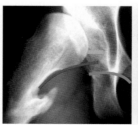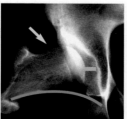

Fib 7.16 Abduction internal rotation (AIR) view. The resting position (red arrow) shows the hip in a 14-year-old child with cerebral palsy. The hip is subluxated (orange lines), and Shenton's line (green arc) is disrupted (red arc). The AIR view (yellow arrow) shows improved congruity and less subluxation and restoration of Shenton's line.

2. Incongruity reduces contact area. The femoral head is normally round and matches the shape of the acetabulum (Fig. 7.18). An aspherical femoral head is usually due to vascular problems. In the young child, the acetabulum usually remodels to become congruous and the hip become aspherical and congruous (Fig. 7.19). If acetabular remodeling fails to occur, the hip may be aspherical and incongruous—a bad combination.

3. Displacement of the femoral head. The relationship between the femoral head and acetabulum is normally congruous. If the head is displaced, it becomes subluxated. If all cartilage contact is lost, the joint is dislocated.

Ultrasonography (US) Ultrasound studies are of greatest value when readily available and performed by an orthopedist in conjunction with the overall evaluation. Cost, restricted assess, and operator inexperience may limit value. Ultrasound's greatest potential usefulness is in assessing DDH in early infancy. Assessing joint effusion, localizing abscesses, and assessing the severity of SCFE, head size in LCP disease, and neck continuity in coxa vara are other applications. This imaging technique is underutilized in North America.

Scintography Bone scans (BS) are useful in localizing inflammatory processes about the pelvis (Fig. 7.20) and in assessing the circulation of the femoral head. Order high-resolution or pinhole-collimated AP and lateral scans of both proximal femora when assessing avascular necrosis (AVN). The bone scan is useful in confirming a preslip and assessing bone tumors.

Arthrography The usefulness of this procedure is limited, as it is invasive and requires sedation or anesthesia. Arthrography is appropriate to confirm joint penetration in negative taps for suspected joint sepsis and for special situations in managing DDH. The role in LCP disease is more controversial.

Magnetic resonance imaging (MRI) These studies are the most expensive and require sedation for infants and young children. MRI studies are most useful in assessing intrarticular disorders of the hip. Cartilagenous loose bodies or fracture fragments, deformity of the cartilagenous femoral head, status of the growth plate, and avascular necrosis are usually definable.

Computerized tomography (CT) Order CT studies to evaluate inflammatory conditions such as an iliopsoas abscess or the configuration of the upper femur and acetabulum. CT scans have replaced tomography in assessing AVN and physeal bridges.

Three-dimensional CT reconstructions are often helpful in visualizing complex deformities of the hip necessary when planning reconstructive surgery (Fig. 7.21).

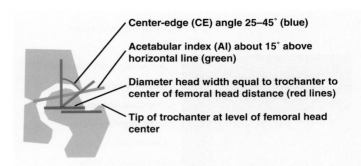

Center-edge (CE) angle 25–45° (blue)

Acetabular index (AI) about 15° above horizontal line (green)

Diameter head width equal to trochanter to center of femoral head distance (red lines)

Tip of trochanter at level of femoral head center

Fig. 7.17 Normal measurements. These are measurements of the normal adolescent hip.

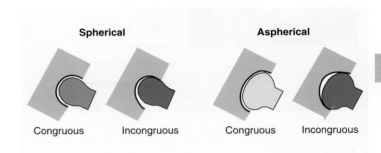

Spherical   Aspherical

Congruous   Incongruous   Congruous   Incongruous

Fig. 7.18 Congruity. Congruity of the hip may be either sypherical or aspherical and congruous or incongruous. Incongruity (red) results in areas of excessive load, causing excessive cartilage wear and eventually osteoarthritis.

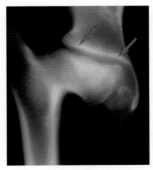

Fig. 7.19 Aspherical congruity. This deformity resulted from Legg–Calvé–Perthes disease during middle childhood. The head became flattened and the acetabulum remodeled to become congruous.

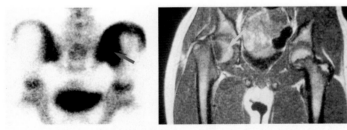

Fig. 7.20 Imaging options. This bone scan shows inflammation of the sacroiliac joint (red arrow), and the MRI shows a slipped epiphysis (yellow arrow).

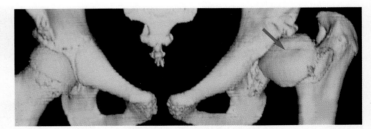

7.21 Three-dimensional CT reconstruction. Reconstructions are useful in assessing complex hip deformity prior to reconstruction. This deformity is secondary to avascular necrosis associated with DDH management in infancy.

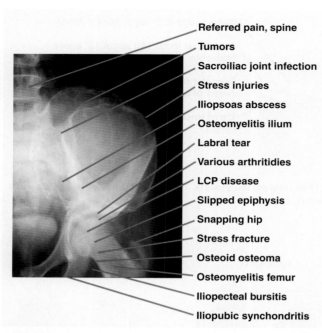

Referred pain, spine
Tumors
Sacroiliac joint infection
Stress injuries
Iliopsoas abscess
Osteomyelitis ilium
Labral tear
Various arthritidies
LCP disease
Slipped epiphysis
Snapping hip
Stress fracture
Osteoid osteoma
Osteomyelitis femur
Iliopecteal bursitis
Iliopubic synchondritis

Fig. 7.22 Causes of hip pain in children. The differential diagnosis is extensive.

Hip and Pelvic Pain

The causes of hip and pelvic pain are numerous (Fig. 7.22), sometimes making the diagnosis difficult.

Diagnosis

Detailing these features may help establish the diagnosis.

Age LCP disease is most common in boys in middle childhood (Fig. 7.23). SCFE must be considered in the older child or adolescent. Overuse syndromes are most common in the adolescent.

Onset Acute onset is suggestive of injury or a rapid onset of infection. SCFE may be chronic or sudden. Acute slips are characterized by a mild injury and inability to walk. LCP disease onset is usually insidious. Overuse syndromes are most painful when active.

Spontaneous movement The most consistent physical finding for septic arthritis of the hip is a loss of spontaneous movement of the affected limb.

Systemic illness The child is ill with septic arthritis, and less sick with toxic synovitis, rheumatoid spondylitis, and tumors.

Resting position of the limb Intraarticular hip disorders usually result in the spontaneous positioning in slight flexion and lateral rotation (Fig. 7.24). This position reduces the intraarticular pressure.

Tenderness Palpate to determine the site of tenderness (Fig. 7.25).

Hip rotation test Guarding and a loss of medial rotation suggest the problem is within the joint (Fig. 7.26).

Night pain Nocturnal pain suggests the possibility of a malignant tumor.

Back stiffness Limitation of forward bending suggests that the disorder may be referred from the spine.

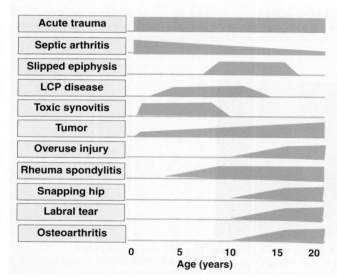

Acute trauma		
Septic arthritis		
Slipped epiphysis		
LCP disease		
Toxic synovitis		
Tumor		
Overuse injury		
Rheuma spondylitis		
Snapping hip		
Labral tear		
Osteoarthritis		

0   5   10   15   20
Age (years)

Fig. 7.23 Hip pain causes by usual age of onset. These are ages when conditions are most common.

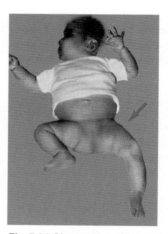

Fig. 7.24 Observation. Observation revealed pseudoparalysis of the left leg, and the left hip is positioned in slight flexion and external rotation. These findings are typical for septic arthritis of the left hip.

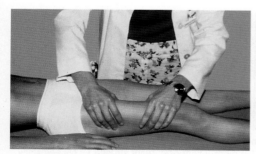

Fig. 7.25 Thigh tenderness. Palpate for localized tenderness.

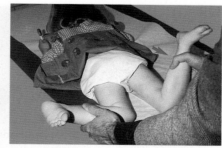

Fig. 7.26 Hip rotation test. This child has reduced medial rotation of the right hip due to toxic synovitis.

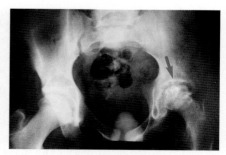

Fig. 7.27 Joint damage from septic arthritis. Note the severe joint damage from septic arthritis treated 2 weeks after onset.

Causes

Establish the diagnosis by considering the features and the common causes of hip pain (Fig. 7.28).

Infection is a common cause of pelvic pain. The early diagnosis of septic arthritis is critical because it may severely damage or destroy the hip joint (Fig. 7.27). Because of the tenuous vascularity of the hip, joint infections must be diagnosed and drained promptly. Soft tissue abscess, such as the psoas abscess, may be suspected by the finding of tenderness on rectal examination and soft tissue swelling on the AP radiograph of the pelvis. Confirm the diagnosis by CT or MRI studies. Sacroiliac infections are identified by bone scans.

Stress injuries or repetitive microtrauma may cause hip pain. Such pain is most common during the second decade and often follows vigorous activity. It may involve the upper femur but more commonly involves the origin of muscles such as the greater trochanter and iliac spines. The diagnosis is usually suggested by the history, physical findings of well-localized tenderness, and negative radiographs but a positive bone scan.

Tumors A variety of tumors occur about the hip and pelvis. Osteoid osteoma is common in the proximal femur and produces pain in a pattern that is nearly diagnostic. The pain is nocturnal and relieved by aspirin. The tumor produces reactive bone with a radiolucent nidus on conventional radiographs (Fig. 7.29).

Toxic synovitis (or transient synovitis) is a idiopathic benign inflammation of the hip joint (Fig. 7.30) that occurs in children. This condition is important, as it may be confused with septic arthritis and less commonly with LCP disease. The condition causes pain and irritability of the hip. It subsides over several days spontaneously.

Idiopathic chrondolysis This uncommon condition is seen in late childhood or adolescence. The hip becomes painful, and stiff and joint space narrowing is present (Fig. 7.31). See page 157.

Rheumatoid spondylitis Unlike juvenile rheumatoid arthritis, hip involvement may be the first sign of rheumatoid spondylitis. Establish the diagnosis with serologic tests.

References

2000 Towards evidence based emergency medicine: best BETs from the Manchester Royal Infirmary. Diagnostic imaging of the hip in the limping child. Wright N, Choudhery V. J Accid Emerg Med 17:48

1999 Idiopathic chondrolysis of the hip: long-term evolution. del Couz Garcia A et al. JPO 19:449

1999 Differentiating between septic arthritis and transient synovitis of the hip in children: an evidence-based clinical prediction algorithm. Kocher MS, Zurakowski D, Kasser JR. JBJS 81A:1662

1995 Differential diagnosis and management of hip pain in childhood. Hollingworth P. Br J Rheumatol 34:78

1990 Ultrasound examination of the irritable hip. Bickerstaff DR, et al. JBJS 72B:549

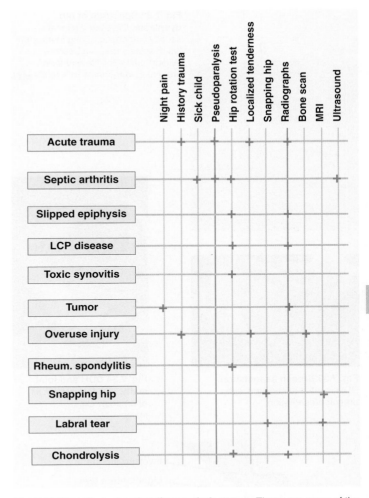

	Night pain	History trauma	Sick child	Pseudoparalysis	Hip rotation test	Localized tenderness	Snapping hip	Radiographs	Bone scan	MRI	Ultrasound
Acute trauma		+									
Septic arthritis			+	+	+						+
Slipped epiphysis					+			+			
LCP disease					+			+			
Toxic synovitis					+						
Tumor	+							+			
Overuse injury						+					
Rheum. spondylitis					+						
Snapping hip							+			+	
Labral tear										+	
Chondrolysis					+			+			

Fig. 7.28 Hip pain and major diagnostic features. These are some of the major clinical features that differentiate each cause of pain.

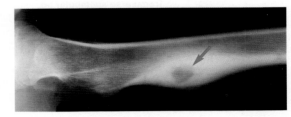

Fig. 7.29 Osteoid osteoma. These lesions are common in the proximal femur and cause night pain.

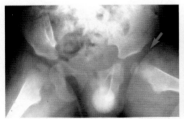
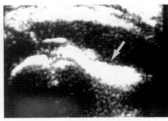

Fig. 7.30 Toxic synovitis. The hip is often positioned in slight flexion and external rotation (red arrow). Ultrasound studies often show an effusion (yellow arrow).

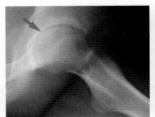
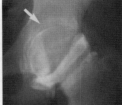

Fig. 7.31 Chondrolysis. This hip shows narrowing of the joint space on conventional radiographs (red arrow), and the arthrogram (yellow arrow) shows thinning of the cartilage on the femoral head.

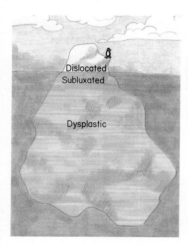

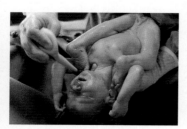

Fig. 7.32 Spectrum of hip dysplasia. Dislocated hips are usually diagnosed during infancy but hip dysplasia may not become evident until adult life and then present as degenerative arthritis.

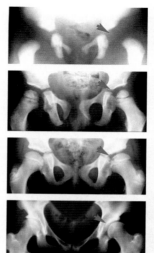

Fig. 7.33 Breech association. DDH is often associated with breech presentation.

Fig. 7.34 DDH and joint laxity. Children with DDH often show excessive joint laxity.

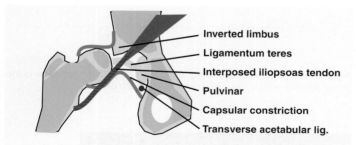

- Inverted limbus
- Ligamentum teres
- Interposed iliopsoas tendon
- Pulvinar
- Capsular constriction
- Transverse acetabular lig.

Fig. 7.35 Structures blocking reduction in DDH. These interpositions may block reduction of the hip.

Developmental Hip Dysplasia

Developmental hip dysplasia (DDH) is a generic term describing a spectrum of anatomic abnormalities of the hip that may be congenital or develop during infancy or childhood. The spectrum covers mild defects such as a shallow acetabulum to severe defects such as *teratologic* dislocations. Teratologic dislocations occur before birth and include severe deformity of both the acetabulum and proximal femur.

Incidence

DDH incidence depends on how much of the spectrum is included (Fig. 7.32). At birth, hip instability is noted in 0.5–1% of joints, but classic DDH occurs in about 0.1% of infants. The incidence of mild dysplasia contributing to adult degenerative arthritis is substantial. It is thought that half of the women who develop degenerative arthritis have pre-existing acetabular dysplasia.

Etiology

DDH is considered to be inherited by a polygenic mode. DDH is more common in breech deliveries (Fig. 7.33), in children with joint laxity (Fig. 7.34), and in girls.

Pathology

The acetabulum is often shallow and maldirected. The proximal femur shows antetorsion and coxa valga. Structural interpositions between the displaced femoral head and acetabulum are common (Fig. 7.35). The iliopsoas tendon is insinuated between the femoral head and acetabulum, causing a depression in the joint capsule. This gives the capsule an hour-glass configuration. The acetabular labrum is inverted into the joint, the ligamentum teres is enlarged, and the acetabulum may contain fat (pulvinar).

Natural History

Residual acetabular dysplasia is common in DDH. This may occur even following an apparently good early reduction (Fig. 7.37). The disability from dysplasia is related to the degree of displacement (Fig. 7.36). Greater displacement causes more function disability. Pain is most common with severe subluxation or articulation in a false acetabulum (Fig. 7.38).

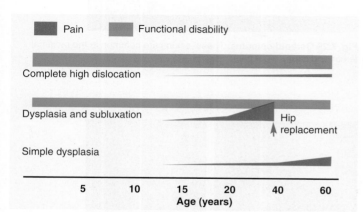

Fig. 7.36 Conceptual chart showing disability from DDH. Pain, altered function, and cosmetic problems often result from persisting hip deformity due to DDH.

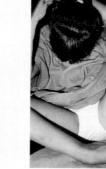

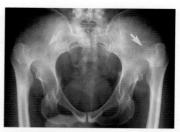

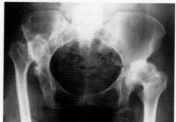

Fig. 7.37 DDH with residual acetabular dysplasia. Radiographs at birth, 3, 10, and 19 years (top to bottom) show persisting dysplasia.

Fig. 7.38 Adult degenerative arthritis. Note that arthritis is most severe in the subluxated (red arrow) hip as compared with the totally dislocated hips (yellow arrows).

Diagnosis

The early diagnosis of DDH is critical to a successful outcome. Acetabular development is abnormal if a hip is subluxated or dislocated. Delays in management result in residual abnormalities and eventual degenerative arthritis.

Neonatal Examination Every newborn should be screened for signs of hip instability. The hip should be examined using both the Barlow and Ortoloni techniques (Figs. 7.39 and 7.40). Examine one hip at a time. The infant should be quiet and comfortable so the muscles about the hip are relaxed. Use no force. Test for instability in several positions.

Changing manifestations of DDH The signs of DDH change with the infant's age (Fig. 7.41). For example, the incidence of hip instability declines rapidly, 50% within the first week. The classic findings of stiffness and shortening increase over the first few weeks of life. These signs become well established in the older infant (Fig. 7.42).

Repeated examinations The hip should be examined during each "well baby" examination. In the neonatal period, DDH is detected by different signs based on the infant's age. In early infancy, instability is the most reliable sign. Later, limitation of abduction and shortening are common. Beware of the bilateral dislocations, as they are more difficult to identify (Fig. 7.43). If hip abduction is less than about 60° on both sides, order an imaging study.

Mother's intuition Although not proven, a common clinical experience is the accuracy of the mother's sense that *something is wrong*. Take the mother's intuition seriously (Fig. 7.44).

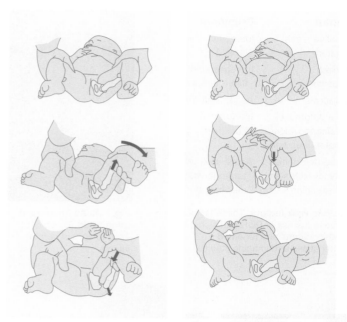

Fig. 7.39 Barlow's sign. Hip instability is demonstrated by attempting to gently displace the hip out of the socket over the posterior acetabulum.

Fig. 7.40 Ortoloni's sign. The thigh is first adducted and depressed to subluxate the hip. The thigh is then abducted. The hip reduces with a palpable "clunk."

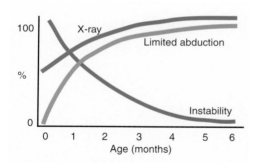

Fig. 7.41 Changing signs of DDH. With increasing age, signs change.

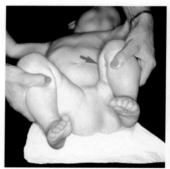
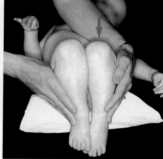

Fig. 7.42 DDH in older infant. Note the limited abduction (red arrow) and shortening (blue arrow) on the affected left side.

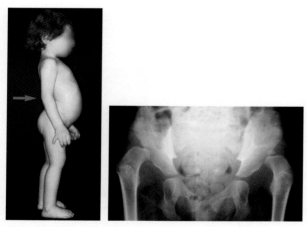

Fig. 7.43 Bilateral DDH. This girl has symmetrical bilateral dislocations. The hip symmetry makes early diagnosis more difficult. Note the typical lumbar lordosis (arrow) that occurs with high dislocations.

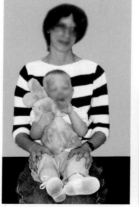
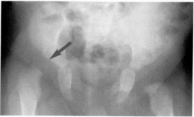

Fig. 7.44 Mother's intuition. This mother had DDH as a child. She suspected that her son's hip was abnormal, but the primary care physician found nothing on examination. She insisted on a radiograph. This study demonstrated a dislocation (red arrow). This scenario is not uncommon.

Factor	Comment
Positive family history	Increases risk tenfold
Breech position	Increases risk five – tenfold
Torticollis	Assoc. deformity
Foot deformities Calcaneovalgus Metatarsus add.	Intrauterine constraint
Knee deformities Hyperextension Dislocation	Associated with teratogenic type dislocation

Fig. 7.45 Risk factors. These factors increase the risk of DDH and signal the need for careful and repeated examinations and imaging studies.

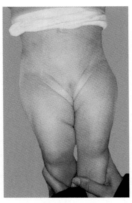

Fig. 7.46 Asymmetrical thigh folds. These occur in up to 20% of normal infants.

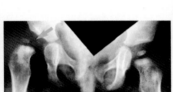

Fig. 7.47 DDH and torticollis. This infant showed the typical features of muscular torticollis with a sternocleidomastoid tumor (red arrow). The physical examination of the hip was normal. The screening radiograph showed DDH (orange arrow).

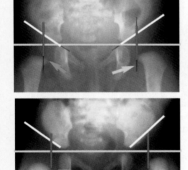

Fig. 7.48 Assessing radiographs in early infancy. Before the ossific nuclei are developed, assessing hip dysplasia is more difficult. These two radiographs show how such hips can be assessed. Draw the horizontal reference line (yellow) through the triradiate cartilage space. Construct the acetabular line (white). The inclination of this line measures the acetabular index. Draw vertical lines at the lateral acetabular edge (red). If the proximal femoral metaphysis lies medial to the vertical line, the hip is reduced (green arrow). If on the vertical line, the hip is subluxated (yellow arrows), and lateral to the line, the hip is dislocated (red arrow).

Hip-at-risk factors. The presence of several factors increase the risk of DDH (Figs. 7.45 and 7.47). When risk factors are present, the infant should be examined repeatedly and the hip imaged by ultrasound or radiography.

Hip "clicks" and asymmetrical thigh folds. Hip clicks are fine, short-duration, high-pitched sounds that are common and benign. These are to be differentiated from "clunks," the sensation of the hip being displaced over the acetabular margin. Clicks and asymmetrical thigh folds are common in normal infants (Fig. 7.46).

Radiography Radiographs become progressively more diagnostic with increasing age. By 2–3 months of age, radiography is reliable and is the optimum age for screening by this method. A single AP radiograph is adequate. Draw the reference lines and measure the acetabular index (AI). Normally, the AI in early infancy falls below 30°, is questionable in the 30°–40° range, and abnormal if above 40°. Hip subluxation or dislocation may often be demonstrated by the metaphysis of the femur positioned lateral to the lateral acetabular marginal line (Fig. 7.48).

Ultrasound imaging The effectiveness of ultrasound imaging depends upon the skill and experience of the examiner. The skillful ultrasound evaluation is an effective screening technique for DDH (Fig. 7.49). The major problem with this screening is the interpretation of the findings. If the hip is unstable, imaging is unnecessary. Imaging is appropriate to evaluate a suspicious finding, when hip-at-risk factors are present, and to monitor the effectiveness of treatment.

Documentation Document your hip evaluation. The failure to diagnose DDH is a common cause of suits against physicians. If the diagnosis is delayed, a record showing that appropriate examinations were made of the hip provides the best defense. DDH may be missed by even the most skilled examiners. Failure to screen for DDH is not acceptable by current standards.

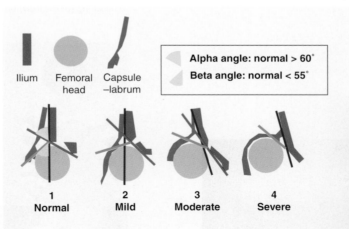

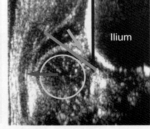

Fig. 7.49 Graf grading of DDH by ultrasound. (Left) Drawing shows how the hips can be graded by measurements based on the ultrasound evaluation. The grades shown are divided by Graf into four types. Each is subdivided into subtypes (not shown). Reference lines are drawn to show the iliac margin (blue), the joint inclination (red), and the line head-joint relationship (green). The alpha and beta angles can be constructed to show severity. (Right) The ultrasound image shows a severe displacement (red arrow) of the femoral head (tan circle) in an infant with DDH. The displaced femoral head compresses the labrum and preossified cartilage (orange arrow) against the ilium (blue line).

Management

The management of DDH is challenging. Delays in diagnosis or problems in management often lead to residual anatomic defects and subsequent degenerative arthritis. The objectives of management include early diagnosis, reduction of the dislocation, avoidance of avascular necrosis, and correction of residual dysplasia.

Birth to 6 months

This is the ideal age for management (Fig. 7.50). Treat DDH in this age group first with an abduction orthosis such as the Pavlik harness.

Pavlik harness This orthosis is most widely used and allows motion in flexion and abduction. Be certain that it is fitted properly (Fig. 7.51) both initially and as applied by the parents. Advise the family on ways of transporting the infant (Figs. 7.52 and 7.54).

See the infant weekly in the brace. Make certain the brace is being fitted properly (Fig. 7.53) and progress is being made. The hip should become progressively more stable.

If harness treatment is successful, continue full-time bracing for 6–8 weeks to allow the hip to become stable. Monitor with ultrasound imaging or by AP radiographs of the pelvis about every 2–4 weeks. Continue the brace at night until the radiographs are normal.

Failure of Pavlik harness treatment If a dislocated hip has not reduced by 3–4 weeks, abandon orthotic treatment. Persisting in orthotic management may cause head deformity and posterior fixation, and make closed reduction impossible. Proceed with closed or open reduction. Manage as is described for infants over 6 months of age.

Night splinting After the hip is reduced and stable, continue with night splinting to facilitate acetabular development. Continue until the radiographs are normal. A simple abduction splint is inexpensive and well accepted by the infant.

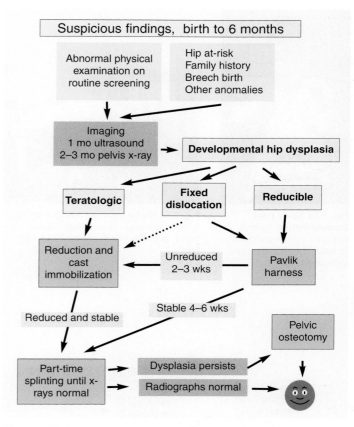

Fig. 7.50 DDH management flowchart, birth to 6 months.

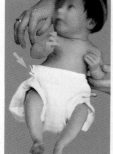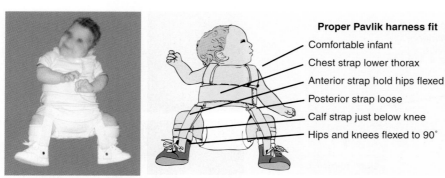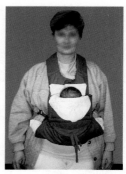

Proper Pavlik harness fit
Comfortable infant
Chest strap lower thorax
Anterior strap hold hips flexed
Posterior strap loose
Calf strap just below knee
Hips and knees flexed to 90°

Fig. 7.51 Proper fit of Pavlik harness. The harness should be carefully fitted. Make certain it is the proper size for the infant. The harness must be comfortable. See the fit after the parent applies the harness to assess problems before the parent leaves the clinic.

Fig. 7.52 DDH mobility. These carriers are ideal, as they provide abduction, mobility, and comfort for the infant and parent.

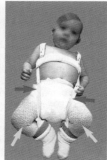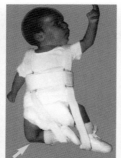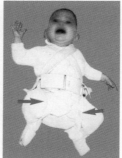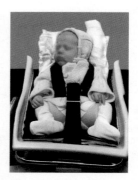

Fig. 7.53 Pitfalls in management. Triple diaper management (orange arrow) is ineffective and gives a false sense that treatment has been initiated. Pavlic harness errors are common. Make certain that the straps are not too tight (red arrows), the calf strap is not too low, the knees are flexed, not the hips (yellow arrows), and the infant is comfortable.

Fig. 7.54 DDH splints and car transportation. These splints should fit into standard infant car seats.

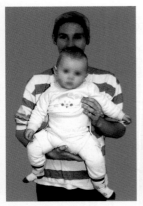

Fig. 7.55 Spica cast immobilization. Infants require cast immobilization to retain the reduction of a dislocated hip.

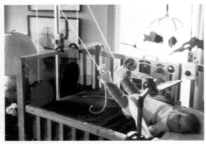

Fig. 7.56 Home traction. Setup at home is less expensive, less stressful for the infant, and often more convenient for the family.

6 to 18 Months

In this age group, most cases of DDH can be managed by closed reduction and spica cast immobilization (Fig. 7.55 and 7.57).

Traction The need for traction is controversial. The current practice is to omit traction in most cases. Traction may be useful if the hip is stiff and closed treatment is planned. Use home traction when possible. Maintain for about 3 weeks with the legs flexed and abducted about 45° with 2–3 pounds of traction applied to each limb (Fig. 7.56).

Scheduling Schedule and obtain consent for a closed, possible open reduction.

Reduction by closed means is first tried. If unsuccessful, open reduction is required. These procedures are outlined on pages 406 and 407.

Arthrography is useful when the quality of reduction is uncertain or the decision regarding management is difficult (Fig. 7.58).

Follow-up Following reduction, the infant should be followed carefully to assess the effect of time on growth, reduction, and acetabular development. Follow with AP radiographs made quarterly through infancy, yearly though early childhood, and then about every third year during middle and late childhood. The frequency of follow-up studies should be individualized based on the severity of any residual dysplasia.

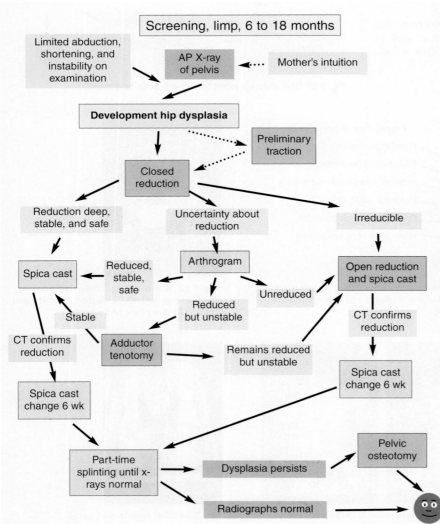

Fig. 7.57 DDH management flowchart, 6 to 18 months.

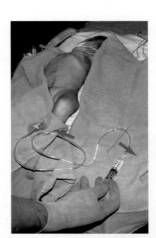

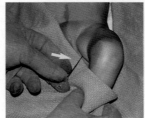

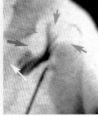

Fig. 7.58 Arthrography. An arthrogram can be very helpful in difficult cases. It outlines the femoral head, defines the obstacles to reduction, and establishes relationships in the joint. It also offers visualization during maneuvers to reduce the hip. Fill a syringe and tubing with 50% diluted dye (red arrows). Fill a second syringe with saline. Guided by the imaging, make a medial approach to the joint with a 3-inch, 20# needle (yellow arrow). Confirm joint entry by injecting a small amount of saline, remove the hub, and observe drainage back from the joint. Once joint entry is confirmed, inject a small amount of dye. Note the large labrum (blue arrow), the femoral head (green arrows), and the pool of dye in the acetabulum (white arrow).

18 to 30 Months

In this age group, operative management is usually required (Fig. 7.59). Occasionally, an infant with a "loose dislocation" can be managed as described in the flowchart for infants 6–18 months of age (Fig. 5.57). If the hip is unusually stiff, be prepared to add femoral shortening as described for management of children over 30 months of age.

Management Manage with an open reduction through an anterolateral approach and perform a concurrent Salter or Pemberton osteotomy. The open reduction is technically challenging. Add the pelvic osteotomy to improve results and save the child a second procedure.

Open reduction is the most difficult part of the procedure. The pelvic osteotomies are relatively simple, but the reduction can sometimes be difficult. The open reduction requires good exposure, careful dissection to minimize the risk of avascular necrosis, and a concentric reduction. The obstacles to reduction must be corrected (Fig. 7.60).

Iliopsoas tendon This tendon is interposed between the femoral head and acetabulum and must be released.

Capsular constriction Open the capsule widely to ensure a complete release.

Transverse acetabular ligament This structure lies across the base of the acetabulum and will block a deep concentric reduction unless released.

Pulvinar is fatty fibrous tissue that often fills the depth of the acetabulum. Remove with a rongeur.

Ligamentum teres is elongated and sometimes hypertrophied. Removal is usually required. The vascular contribution through this ligament is minimal.

Limbus is often inverted and hypertrophied. Do not excise this structure. Once the hip is concentrically reduced, the limbus will remodel and form the labrum, an important structure for hip stability and longevity.

Concurrent osteotomy This choice may be based on the pathology and on the experience and preference of the surgeon.

Femoral osteotomy Proximal femoral varus osteotomy is becoming less commonly used because the acetabular dysplasia is the more significant deformity. Include only minimal rotational correction.

Salter innominate osteotomy is suitable for unilateral mild to moderate dysplasia. The procedure is simple, risks are few, and results good. See page 403.

Pemberton pericapsular osteotomy (Fig. 7.61) is more versatile because it can be performed bilaterally, does not destabilize the pelvis, provides greater correction, and requires no internal fixation. Avoid overcorrection. Stiffness is more common with this procedure, as the operation changes the shape of the acetabulum (see page 402).

Postoperative care is determined by the treatment. If closed or open reduction is performed with an osteotomy, plan at least 12 weeks of spica cast immobilization. Usually the cast is changed once or twice during this period. If a concurrent osteotomy is performed, stability is improved and only 6 weeks of immobilization is necessary.

Follow-up must be continued until the end of growth. Usually a single AP radiograph of the pelvis is made every 6 months for 3 years, then yearly for 3 years, then every 3 years until maturity. At each visit, compare the current study with previous radiographs to determine the effect of time and growth on the development of the hip.

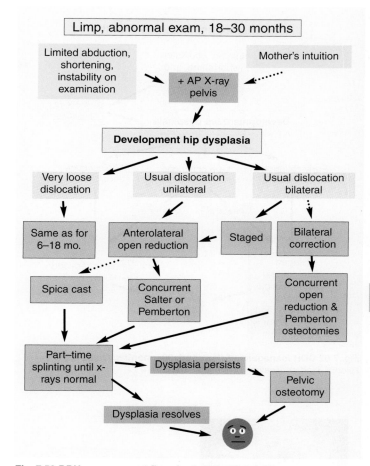

Fig. 7.59 DDH management flowchart, 18 to 30 months.

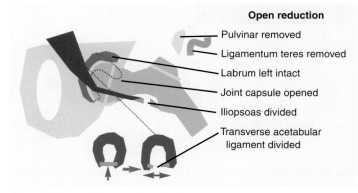

Fig. 7.60 Open reduction. The open reduction is often difficult, and obstruction must be corrected.

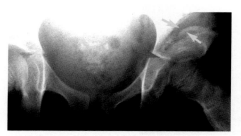

Fig. 7.61 Pemberton pericapsular osteotomy. The osteotomy hinges at the triradiate cartilage (red arrow) and a graft wedges open the osteotomy (yellow arrows).

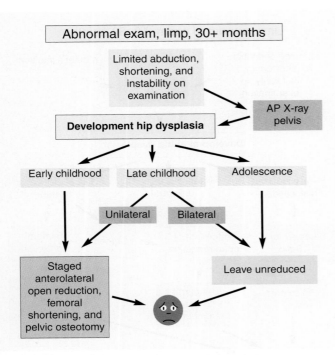

Fig. 7.62 — flowchart boxes:

Abnormal exam, limp, 30+ months

Limited abduction, shortening, and instability on examination

Development hip dysplasia

AP X-ray pelvis

Early childhood | Late childhood | Adolescence

Unilateral | Bilateral

Staged anterolateral open reduction, femoral shortening, and pelvic osteotomy

Leave unreduced

Fig. 7.62 DDH management flowchart, 30+ months. Outcomes are seldom good or excellent in this age range.

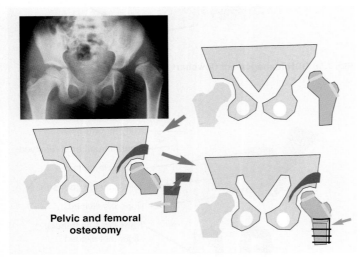

Pelvic and femoral osteotomy

Fig. 7.63 Unilateral open reduction and pelvic and femoral osteotomy. This combination of procedures is necessary in the child. Femoral shortening (red arrow) must be added to allow tension-free reduction. The distal fragment is aligned (yellow arrow) and fixed (green arrow).

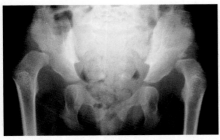

Fig. 7.64 Bilateral DDH in the child. Staged corrections can be done in early childhood. In late childhood or adolescence, leaving the hips unreduced may be prudent.

30+ Months

Manage DDH in this age range by open reduction, femoral shortening, and pelvic osteotomy (Figs. 7.62 and 7.63). If the dislocations are bilateral, correct one side at a time. Allow 6 months between procedures to allow the child to recover. Manage bilateral dislocations on the basis of the age of the child (Fig. 7.64).

Selection of pelvic osteotomies Select the type of osteotomy based on the severity of deformity and the age at the time of treatment. Salter osteotomies are good choices because they can be performed at any age, they do not change the shape of the acetabulum, and when combined with a femoral osteotomy, they usually provide adequate correction.

Femoral osteotomy Femoral shortening osteotomy is nearly always necessary. If the deformity is severe, the femoral shortening is performed first, then the open reduction, followed by the pelvic osteotomy. The femoral fragments are then aligned, with gentle traction on the limb. The overlap is then determined and the overlapping distal femoral segment is resected. The procedure is primarily shortening. Slight varus and no rotation are usually appropriate.

References

2000 Developmental dysplasia of the hip from birth to six months. Guille JT, Pizzutillo PD, MacEwen GD. JAAOS 8:232

2000 At the crossroads--neonatal detection of developmental dysplasia of the hip. Jones D, et al. JBJS 82B:160

2000 Test of stability as an aid to decide the need for osteotomy in association with open reduction in developmental dysplasia of the hip. Zadeh HG, et al. JBJS 82B:17

1999 Soft-tissue interposition after closed reduction in developmental dysplasia of the hip. The long-term effect on acetabular development and avascular necrosis. Hattori T, et al. JBJS 81B:385

1998 Retrospective review at skeletal maturity of the factors affecting the efficacy of Salter's innominate osteotomy in congenital dislocated, subluxed, and dysplastic hips. Morin C, Rabay G, Morel G. JPO 18:246

1998 Selective treatment program for developmental dysplasia of the hip in an epidemiologic prospective study. Poul J, et al. JPO-b 7:135

1998 Pemberton osteotomy for the treatment of developmental dysplasia of the hip in older children. Vedantam R, Capelli A, Schoenecker P. JPO 18:254

1997 Imaging of developmental dysplasia of the hip. Donaldson J, Feinstein K. Pediatr Clin North Am 44:591

1997 Three-dimensional characteristics of cartilaginous and bony components of dysplastic hips in children: three-dimensional computed tomography quantitative analysis. Lin C, et al. JPO 17:152

1997 Postreduction computed tomography in developmental dislocation of the hip: part II: predictive value for outcome. Smith B, et al. JPO 17:631

1997 The predictive value of the development of the acetabular teardrop figure in developmental dysplasia of the hip. Smith J, et al. JPO 17:165

1997 Natural history and treatment outcomes of childhood hip disorders. Weinstein S. CO 227:42

1996 Congenital dislocation of the hip in the older child. The effectiveness of overhead traction. Daoud A, Saighi-Bououina A. JBJS 78A:30

1996 Avascular necrosis and the Pavlik harness. The incidence of avascular necrosis in three types of congenital dislocation of the hip as classified by ultrasound. Suzuki S, et al. JBJS 78B:631

1995 Long-term results of congenital dislocation of the hip treated with the Pavlik harness. Fujioka F, et al. JPO 15:747

1995 The prognosis in untreated dysplasia of the hip. A study of radiographic factors that predict the outcome. Murphy S, et al. JBJS 77A:985

1994 Prognosticating factors in acetabular development following reduction of developmental dysplasia of the hip. Chen I, Kuo K, Lubicky J. JPO 14:3

1993 Pemberton osteotomy for residual acetabular dysplasia in children who have congenital dislocation of the hip. Faciszewski T, Kiefer G, Coleman S. JBJS 75A:643

1993 Acetabular development after closed reduction of congenital dislocation of the hip. Noritake K, et al. JBJS 75B:737

1990 Acetabular dysplasia in the adolescent and young adult. Murphy S, et al. CO 214:23

Avascular Necrosis

Next to achieving a concentric reduction, preventing avascular necrosis (AVN) is of utmost importance. Unless the necrosis is mild, this complication causes altered proximal femoral growth, creates deformity, and often leads to premature degenerative arthritis.

Types The spectrum of AVN (Fig. 7.65) includes severe necrosis, extensive physeal bridge formation, and shortening of the femoral neck, which leads to degenerative arthritis during adult life. At the other end of the spectrum is the mild resolving form characterized by irregular ossification but without physeal bridge formation and subsequent deformity.

Prevention Attempt to prevent AVN by using preliminary traction and open reduction in stiff hips with an obstructing limbus, percutaneous adductor tenotomy, femoral shortening in the child, and immobilization in the "safe" or human position. Despite all precautions, AVN may still occur.

Early signs The early signs of AVN (Salter) are often followed by evidence of a growth disturbance. Type 1 deformity is most common and often mild. Type 2 deformity is more severe, causing a profound shortening of the neck.

Deformity The type and severity of the deformity is related to the location and extent of the physeal bridge. Often bridges and deformity are not apparent in early childhood but become obvious toward the end of growth. These bridges cause a tethering of growth and, if eccentric, a tilting of the growth plate (Fig. 7.66). Central large bridges cause total arrest with shortening of the femoral neck, relative trochanteric overgrowth, and mild femoral shortening (Fig. 7.67).

Management If prevention fails, manage the deformity based on its severity and the type of deformity (Fig. 7.68).

References

2000 Avascular necrosis of the hip: a complication following treatment of congenital dysplasia of the hip. Barkin SZ, Kondo KL, Barkin RM. Clin Pediatr 39:307

1999 Avascular necrosis after treatment of DDH: the protective influence of the ossific nucleus. Segal LS, et al. JPO 19:177

1999 Intraobserver and interobserver reliability of Kalamchi and Macewen's classification system for evaluation of avascular necrosis of the femoral head in developmental hip dysplasia. Omeroglu H, et al. Bull Hosp Jt Dis 58:194

1996 Avascular necrosis of the proximal femur in developmental dislocation of the hip. Incidence, risk factors, sequelae and MR imaging for diagnosis and prognosis. Kruczynski J. Acta Orthop Scand Suppl 268:1

1986 Factors relating to hip joint arthritis following three childhood diseases--juvenile rheumatoid arthritis, Perthes disease, and postreduction avascular necrosis in congenital hip dislocation. Cooperman DR, Emery H, Keller C. JPO 6:706

1980 Avascular necrosis following treatment of congenital dislocation of the hip. Kalamchi A, MacEwen G. JBJS 62A:876

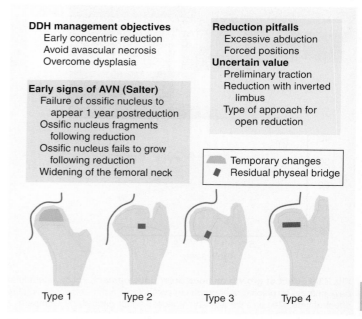

DDH management objectives
  Early concentric reduction
  Avoid avascular necrosis
  Overcome dysplasia

Reduction pitfalls
  Excessive abduction
  Forced positions
Uncertain value
  Preliminary traction
  Reduction with inverted limbus
  Type of approach for open reduction

Early signs of AVN (Salter)
  Failure of ossific nucleus to appear 1 year postreduction
  Ossific nucleus fragments following reduction
  Ossific nucleus fails to grow following reduction
  Widening of the femoral neck

  ▨ Temporary changes
  ▪ Residual physeal bridge

Type 1   Type 2   Type 3   Type 4

Fig. 7.65 Classification of AVN patterns. These patterns depend upon the severity and location of the ischaemic necrosis. Based on Kalamchi and MacEwen (1980) classification.

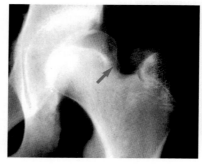

Fig. 7.66 Type 2 deformity. This deformity results from a lateral physeal bridge (red arrow) causing a lateral tilting of the epiphysis (*tilted hat deformity*).

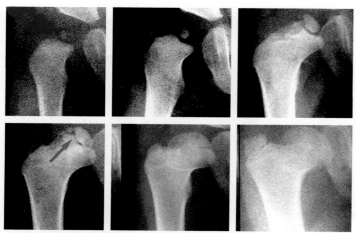

Fig. 7.67 Type 4 deformity. Note the progressive changes throughout infancy and childhood from a central physeal bridge (red arrow) with shortening of the femoral neck and relative trochanteric overgrowth.

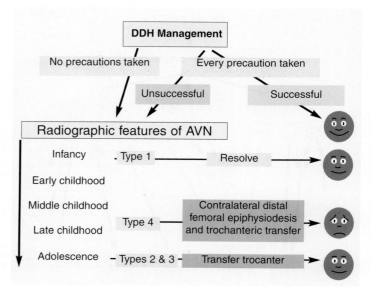

DDH Management

No precautions taken   Every precaution taken

Unsuccessful   Successful

Radiographic features of AVN

Infancy	Type 1 ——— Resolve
Early childhood	
Middle childhood	Contralateral distal femoral epiphysiodesis and trochanteric transfer
Late childhood	Type 4
Adolescence	Types 2 & 3 — Transfer trocanter

Fig. 7.68 Management of AVN occurring as a complication of DDH treatment.

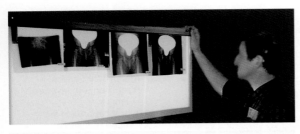

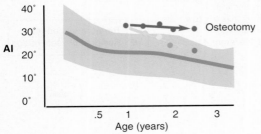

Fig. 7.69 Effect of growth on acetabular development. Follow acetabular development by placing radiographs in chronologic order and assessing the effect of time. Measure the acetabular index (AI) for each study. Compare this sequence of measurements with the chart of normal AI measurements. If improvement occurs (yellow arrow) and the values become normal, treatment is not required. If AI values remain elevated (red dots and arrow), then pelvic osteotomy will be necessary.

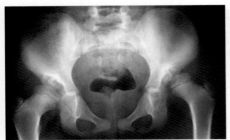

Fig. 7.70 Severe acetabular dysplasia. Attempt to correct acetabular dysplasia before it becomes this severe.

Persisting Dysplasia

The third objective in DDH management is the correction of persisting hip dysplasia. Dysplasia should be corrected during growth to prevent osteoarthritis.

Dysplasia may involve the femur, the acetabulum, or both. The most pronounced deformity is in the acetabulum. The most severe dysplasia includes subluxation. Subluxation and dysplasia cause osteoarthritis, which may begin during the teen years. Disability occurs later with simple dysplasia.

Femoral Dysplasia The proximal femur is anteverted and the head may not be spherical due to the dislocation. The deformity may be due to ischaemic necrosis.

Acetabular dysplasia is the most pronounced deformity and includes shallowness and anterolateral orientation of the socket.

Acetabulofemoral relationship The femoral head is subluxated if not concentric with the acetabulum. The head may also be lateralized following growth with the head subluxated. The acetabulum often becomes saucer shaped, causing instability.

The femoral head may be spherical or aspherical as a result of ischaemic necrosis. The fit with the acetabulum may be congruous or incongruous. Aspherical incongruity is common because over years of growth, the acetabulum assumes a shape to match that of the femoral head.

Timing of correction Correct hip dysplasia as soon as it is evident that the rate of correction is unsatisfactory, preferably before age 5 years. Establish a time line of a series of AP radiographs (Fig. 7.69) of the pelvis taken at 4–6 month intervals during infancy and early childhood. Measure the acetabular index, note the smoothness of the acetabular roof (sercil), and observe the development of the medial acetabulum (tear drop). Assess by studying the sequence of films. Perform a pelvic osteotomy if the AI remains abnormal and the other features remain dysplasic after 2–3 years of observation. Avoid delaying an obvious need for correction (Fig. 7.70).

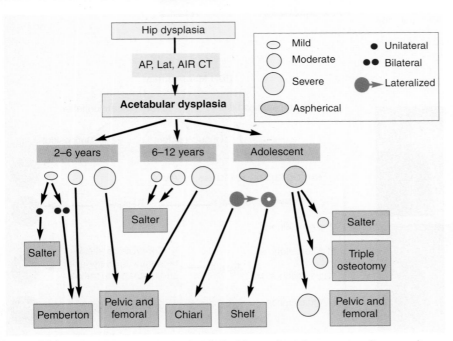

Fig. 7.71 Management of acetabular dysplasia. Manage based on age, severity, congruity, and lateralization.

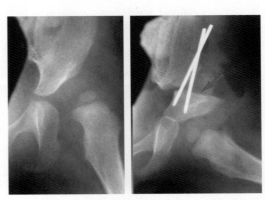

Fig. 7.72 Salter osteotomy. This procedure is useful at any age for mild to moderate dysplasia.

Principles of correction Proper correction of hip dyplasia in DDH follows these certain basic principles:

1. Correct the primary or most severe deformity. This is usually the acetabular deformity.

2. Correction should be adequate. If the deformity is severe, combine a pelvic and femoral osteotomy or perform a shelf operation.

3. Avoid creating incongruity. Avoid the Pemberton procedure in the older child. Consider the shelf or Chiari procedure if aspherical congruity is present.

4. Medialize the lateralized hip in the older child with a Chiari osteotomy.

5. Articular cartilage is more durable than fibrocartilage as develops in the shelf and Chiari procedures.

Procedures Select the appropriate procedure based on the site of deformity, age, severity, and congruity (Fig. 7.71). The choices are numerous (Fig. 7.73). Several procedures are most commonly performed (see details in Chapter 16).

Femoral osteotomy Femoral shortening is essential in the older child with unreduced DDH. Remove just enough bone to allow reduction. Reduce the neck–shaft angle by about 20°. Limit rotational correction to about 20°.

Salter osteotomy This is the best choice for correcting mild deformities at any age (Fig. 7.72). The osteotomy will reduce the AI about 10°–15° and the CE angle by 10°.

Pemberton osteotomy This is the best choice for bilateral or moderate to severe dysplasia (Fig. 7.75) in children under age 6 years.

Triple osteotomies This is the best choice for the adolescent (Fig. 7.74) with moderate dysplasia when spherical congruity is present. Procedures are demanding and risk of complications are significant.

Chiari osteotomy This is appropriate when the hip is lateralized and severely dysplasic. It may be used with aspherical congruity. Avoid over-medialization. It covers with fibrocartilage.

Shelf procedures This enlarges the acetabulum with fibrocartilage. It is versatile and the best choice for severe dysplasia without lateralization when aspherical congruity exists. This is the least risky of the major procedures.

DDH Consultant Michael Benson, e-mail: michael.benson@iname.com

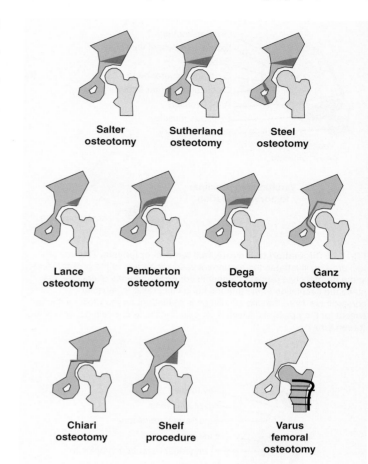

Fig. 7.73 Options for osteotomies of the hip.

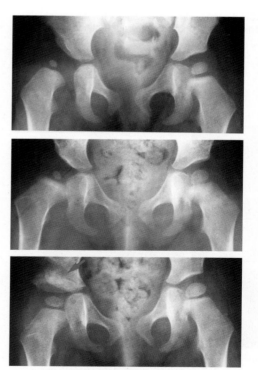

Fig. 7.75 Pemberton osteotomy. This infant showed little improvement with time so correction at age 30 months was preformed. Note that the osteotomy extends into but not through the triradiate cartilage.

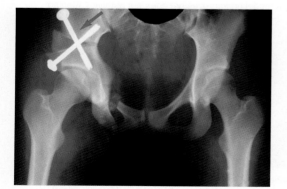

Fig. 7.74 Triple innominate osteotomy. This procedure is useful in correcting dysplasia in the older child or adolescent.

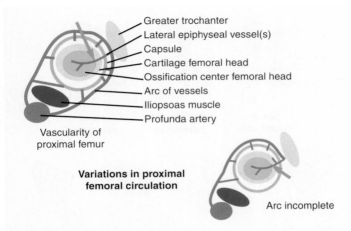

Greater trochanter
Lateral epiphyseal vessel(s)
Capsule
Cartilage femoral head
Ossification center femoral head
Arc of vessels
Iliopsoas muscle
Profunda artery

Vascularity of
proximal femur

**Variations in proximal
femoral circulation**

Arc incomplete

Fig. 7.76 Circulation to the proximal femoral epiphysis. This conceptual drawing illustrates the redundant vascular arcade of the proximal femur in the normal child (upper). Congenital or developmental alterations may make the circulation to the femoral head vulnerable to vascular compromise. Note that the circulation is redundant for the proximal femur except for the epiphysis, which is supplied by the lateral retinacular vessels (green arrow).

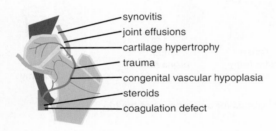

synovitis
joint effusions
cartilage hypertrophy
trauma
congenital vascular hypoplasia
steroids
coagulation defect

Fig. 7.77 Causes of LCP disease. These are some of the causes of LCP disease. They may act alone or in combination to cause ischaemic of the femoral head.

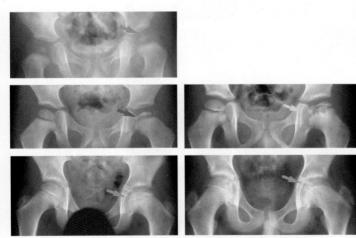

Fig. 7.78 Natural history of early onset LCP disease. These radiographs were taken at ages 2, 3, 5, 8, and 15 years. Note at age 3 years (red arrow) how total head avascular necrosis is evident. Without treatment, healing (yellow arrow) and remodeling (green arrows) occur.

Legg-Calvé-Perthes Disease

Legg–Calvé–Perthes (LCP), or simply Perthes, disease is an idiopathic juvenile avascular necrosis of the femoral head. Synonyms include Waldenström's disease and coxa plana. It affects about 1 in 10,000 children. Males are affected four times more often than girls, and it is bilateral in 10–15% of subjects.

Etiology

The cause of LCP disease is unknown. Affected children are small and delayed in maturation, suggesting a constitutional disorder. Vascularity is tenuous in early childhood, and developmental variations in vascular pattern (Fig. 7.76) are more common in boys, predisposing some individuals. In addition, trauma, alterations in the coagulability of blood, and endocrine and metabolic disorders may be contributing factors (Fig. 7.77). Possibly several factors combine to cause the disease.

Pathology

The pathology is consistent with repeated bouts of infarction and subsequent pathologic fractures. Synovitis and effusion, cartilagenous hypertrophy, bony necrosis, and collapse are present. Widening and flattening of the femoral head follow. Most deformity occurs in the "fragmentation phase." If necrosis is extensive and the support of the lateral pillar is lost, the head collapses, mild subluxation occurs, and pressure from the lateral acetabular margin creates a depression, or "furrow" in the femoral head.

Healing requires replacement of dead bone with living bone. Over time in young children, the deformity remodels and the acetabulum becomes congruous. At maturation, the head is reasonably round and the prognosis fair to good. If growth arrest occurs, or the child is older, remodeling is limited. Thus, the capacity of the acetabulum to remodel to congruity is reduced and osteoarthritis is likely in adult life.

Natural History

The prognosis for LCP disease is fair. The most important prognostic factor is the sphericity of the femoral head at skeletal maturation. This sphericity is related to the age of onset. The younger age, the more likely the head will be spherical (Figs. 7.78, 7.79, and 7.80). The longer the period between the completion of healing and skeletal maturity, the

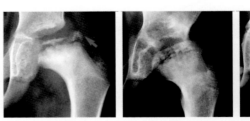

Fig. 7.79 Extrusion with residual coxa plana. Note the extrusion in this 7-year-old child. Remodeling improves but does not resolve flattening.

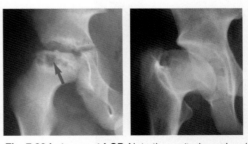

Fig. 7.80 Late onset LCP. Note the metaphyseal–epiphyseal cyst at age 11 years (arrow). The head is aspherical and flat at age 18 years (right).

longer the period of remodeling. This remodeling cannot occur if a physeal bridge develops (Figs. 7.80 and 7.81). Physeal bridging may occur in young patients and accounts for the occasional poor result seen in these young children. Physeal bridging is most likely in the older child.

Factors affecting prognosis are many, complicating assessment of treatment methods. During late childhood and adolescence, children may experience episodes of pain with vigorous activity. These episodes are transient, often lasting a day or two. More persistent disability may develop during middle to late adult life due to osteoarthritis. The need for joint replacement increases with advancing age and is most likely when the onset of LCP disease occurs after the age of 8 or 9 years (Fig. 7.82).

Diagnosis

LCP occurs between 2 and 18 years of age, but most commonly develops in boys between ages 4 and 8 years. Bilateral involvement occurs with usually more than a year interval between onsets. The disease rarely follows toxic synovitis. An antalgic limp is usually the first sign. Pain may be present but is usually mild. Frequently, the child has recurring pain and a limp for several months before being seen by a physician.

Physical examination The child is comfortable, and the screening examination is normal except for the involved leg. The limp is antalgic, a Trendelenburg sign may be present, and mild atrophy is often present. The most prominent find is stiffness (Fig. 7.83). The loss of hip internal rotation is the earliest sign. The hip rotation test is positive. Abduction is nearly always limited. Flexion is least affected.

Imaging studies The stage of the disease determines the findings on imaging. Early in the disease, radiographs may be normal, show slight widening of the cartilage space, or often a pathognomonic radiolucent cleft in the femoral head viewed from a lateral position. Radiographic features are largely determined by the stage of the disease at the first visit (Fig. 7.84). Ultrasound will show a joint effusion. The bone scan often shows reduced uptake on the affected side early in the disease (Fig. 7.85). The MRI shows evidence of marrow necrosis, irregularity of the femoral head, and a loss of the signal on the affected side (Fig. 7.86). In the vast majority of cases, only conventional radiographs are necessary to establish the diagnosis and provide management.

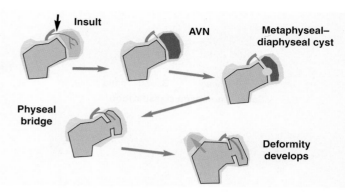

Fig. 7.81 Physeal bridge formation. Cysts may fill in with bone across the growth plate. This creates a bony bridge that tethers growth and causes progressive deformity. The deformity includes shortness of the femoral neck, relative overgrowth of the greater trochanter, and persistence of flattening of the femoral head.

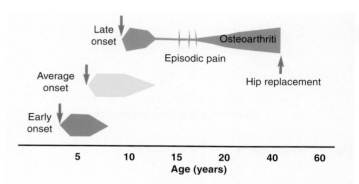

Fig. 7.82 Pain and age of onset of LCP disease. Pain occurs during the acute disease. This lasts for 2–3 years. Pain occurs when deformity persists as episodic incongruity pain during activity and later persistent pain due to osteoarthritis (red).

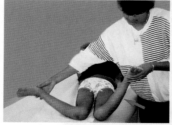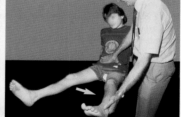

Fig. 7.83 Limited range of motion. Note the reduction of medial rotation on the affected right side (red arrow) consistent with a positive *hip rotation test*. Examine with one hand spanning the iliac spines as a basis to estimate hip abduction that is reduced in LCP disease (yellow arrow).

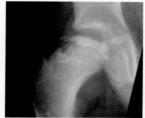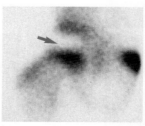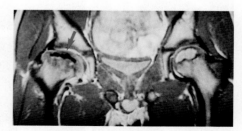

Fig. 7.84 Radiograph. Various features are shown based on the stage of the disease.

Fig. 7.85 Bone scan. Decreased uptake is seen over the region of the femoral head (arrow).

Fig. 7.86 MRI. Marrow necrosis corresponding to the extent of the necrosis (arrow) is evident.

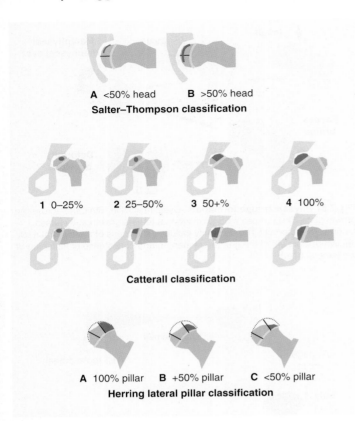

A <50% head   **B** >50% head
Salter–Thompson classification

1 0–25%   **2** 25–50%   **3** 50+%   **4** 100%

Catterall classification

A 100% pillar   **B** +50% pillar   **C** <50% pillar
Herring lateral pillar classification

Fig. 7.87 Classifications of LCP disease severity.

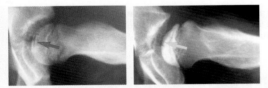

Fig. 7.88 Salter–Thompson classification. Note the extent of the cleft (red arrow), which shows the area of necrosis (yellow arrow), as evident in the radiograph taken 1 year later.

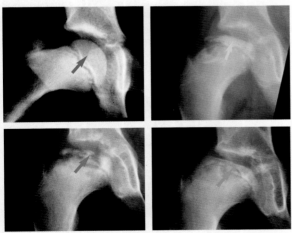

Fig. 7.89 Stages of LCP disease. The disease progresses through the stage of synovitis (red), necrosis (yellow), fragmentation (blue), and reconstitution (green).

Classification

LCP disease is classified by the extent of head involvement and by the stage of the disease.

Extent of involvement Several classification systems are in use for assessing the severity of involvement (Fig. 7.87). Salter–Thompson and Catterall grade the extent of involvement of the epiphysis and Herring grades on the "lateral pillar." The Salter–Thompson classification is based on showing a cleft in the lateral radiograph (Fig. 7.88). This cleft is a fracture line between the living and dead bone and shows the minimum extent of necrosis. This can be observed early in the disease. The other signs may progress into the fragmentation phase of the disease.

Stage of Disease The disease is divided into four stages: synovitis, necrosis or collapse, fragmentation, and reconstitution (Fig. 7.89). The disease progresses through each stage and part of the healing process. In some classifications, the first stage is omitted.

1. Synovitis This stage is of short duration (weeks) and shows the effect of ischemia. Synovitis produces stiffness and pain. Radiographs may show a slight lateralization of the epiphysis (cartilage hyperplasia), bone scans show reduced uptake, and the MRI shows a reduced signal.

2. Necrosis or collapse The necrotic portions of the femoral head undergo collapse, and radiographs show a reduction in size and an increased density of the head. This stage lasts 6–12 months.

3. Fragmentation In this healing stage, avascular bone is resorbed, producing the patchy deossification seen on conventional radiographs. Deformation of the femoral head often occurs during this stage. This stage persists for 1–2 years.

4. Reconstitution New bone is formed. Overgrowth often produces coxa magna and a widening of the neck.

Head-at-risk signs (Fig. 7.90) include extrusion or ossification lateral to the femoral head, metaphyseal changes of rarification or cyst formation, and a radilucency on the lateral aspect of the physis (Gage's sign).

Differential Diagnosis

Disorders that cause clinical and radiographic changes such as LCP disease are numerous (Fig. 7.92). Although these other causes are relatively rare, they should be at least considered before establishing the diagnosis. The most likely diagnoses to miss are hypothyroidism and epiphyseal dysplasia. Dysplasias usually affect both hips with symmetrical degrees of involvement (Fig. 7.91). Bilateral symmetrical involvement is very rare in LCP disease.

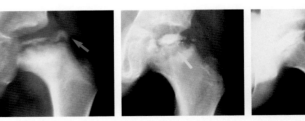

Fig. 7.90 Head-at-risk signs. Extrusion (red arrow), metaphyseal reaction (yellow arrow), and lateral rarification or Gage sign (white arrow).

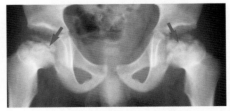

Fig. 7.91 Symmetrical involvement suggests another diagnosis. This child has epiphyseal dysplasia.

Management

The objective of management of LCP is to preserve the sphericity of the femoral head to reduce the risk of stiffness and degenerative arthritis while preserving the emotional well-being of the child.

The management of LCP is very controversial. In the past, treatment regimens have varied from operating on every case to no treatment at all. Children have been subjected to years of hospitalization in recumbency and various types of ineffective bracing (Fig. 7.93) and operative treatments. Remember our humbling history of management in managing the next patient.

Management Principles The following is a list of currently accepted principles of managing LCP:

1. Avoid treatment of patients who will do well without treatment. The young child and children of any age with minimal involvement do not require treatment.

2. Consider the psychosocial situation (Fig. 7.94). The emotionally dysfunctional child should not be subjected to orthotic management. Due to the long duration of the disease, treatment often imposes severe emotional stress for the child. Be sensitive to the child's overall well-being.

3. Provide "containment" to maintain or improve the sphericity of the femoral head (Fig. 7.95). The acetabulum is used as a mold to contain the plastic femoral head. This requires positioning the hip in abduction in a brace or a surgical procedure that increases acetabular coverage of the femoral head.

4. Attempt to maintain or gain a satisfactory range of motion (Fig. 7.96). Motion is nearly always reduced. The degree of stiffness is related to the severity of the disease and the activity level of the child. Gaining motion by curtailing activity has its limits. What constitutes a satisfactory range of motion is seldom defined. A minimum is about 20° of abduction.

5. Control the cost of management. Inpatient traction, MRI studies, arthrography, and operative procedures are most expensive. Conventional radiographs, rest at home, and the selective use of imaging and procedures provides optimum care at least cost.

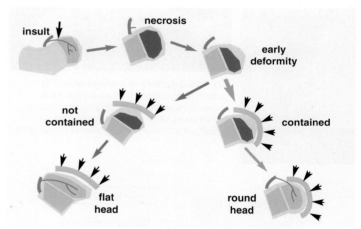

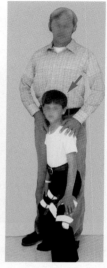

Fig. 7.93 Adaptive boy. The boy circumvented treatment by dropping the brace (arrow).

Fig. 7.94 *Head* at risk. This is a difficult disease for children.

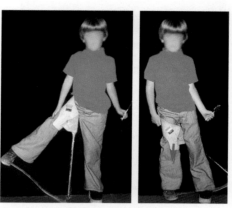

Fig. 7.95 Concept of containment treatment. Containment is provided by positioning the leg or the acetabulum to encompass the femoral head. Without containment (red arrows), the head becomes flattened. The contained head (green arrows) becomes round. Both heads become revascularized.

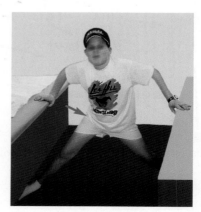

Fig. 7.96 Tight abductors. Note the stiffness of the right hip. Attempt to maintain as much abduction as possible.

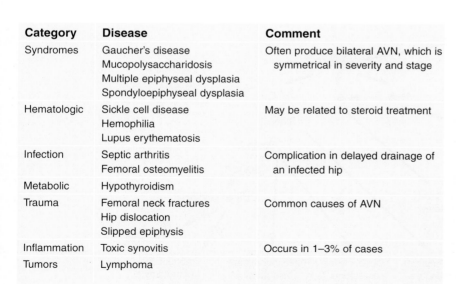

Category	Disease	Comment
Syndromes	Gaucher's disease Mucopolysaccharidosis Multiple epiphyseal dysplasia Spondyloepiphyseal dysplasia	Often produce bilateral AVN, which is symmetrical in severity and stage
Hematologic	Sickle cell disease Hemophilia Lupus erythematosis	May be related to steroid treatment
Infection	Septic arthritis Femoral osteomyelitis	Complication in delayed drainage of an infected hip
Metabolic	Hypothyroidism	
Trauma	Femoral neck fractures Hip dislocation Slipped epiphysis	Common causes of AVN
Inflammation	Toxic synovitis	Occurs in 1–3% of cases
Tumors	Lymphoma	

Fig. 7.92 Differential diagnosis of LCP. Several disorders may be confused with LCP. Often the primary disease makes the cause of the avascular necrosis clear.

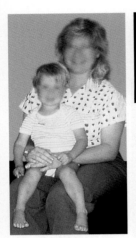

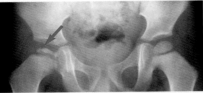

Fig. 7.97 LCP disease in a young child. This 3-year-old girl was managed without treatment. The outcome was good.

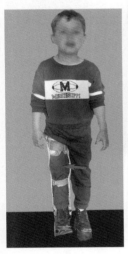

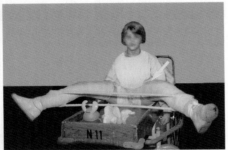

Fig. 7.98 Extremes in management. The pattern bottom brace (red arrow) has been shown to increase hip loading and provides no containment. Wide abduction casts (yellow arrow) are effective but very difficult for the child.

Management Algorithm

The flowchart below (Fig. 7.99) is an approach to management. The management of LCP disease is one of the most controversial in orthopedics. This is one of many approaches. Consider each of the following variables in planning management.

Severity The flowchart (Fig. 7.99) is based on the Herring A, B, and C categories. Be aware that the Salter–Thompson cleft sign when visible will predict severity earlier than either the Herring or Catterall methods. The Herring method does not become fully clear until the stage of late necrosis or early fragmentation.

Operative choices These choices (Fig. 7.99) demonstrate the many options in management. The choices do not include brace management. This option is still viable but poorly accepted by most children and families due to the long duration required.

Age is the most important variable and the first consideration. Prognosis is most dependent on the age of onset. Divide ages into the young child (0–5 years), the middle age group (5–8 years), and the older age group (8+ years). This older group has a much poorer prognosis.

Early childhood The prognosis is usually excellent (Fig. 7.97) unless a physeal bridge develops. The development of bridging is not preventable. In this age group, treatment is not necessary or helpful. Asking the parents to limit the child's activity is asking the parent to do the near impossible. It is not fair or helpful. Simply ask the parents to redirect the child's activity when feasible into some activity that is less physical. If metaphyseal cysts develop, follow the child with an AP radiography every 2 years to assess growth, as physeal bridging may occur. If this complication develops, it may be necessary to transfer the trochanter in late childhood or adolescence.

Middle childhood Avoid treatments that are either ineffective or present special hardships for the child (Fig. 7.98). Manage those with H–A and H–B (H = Herring) without containment. Encourage abduction exercises. Provide follow-up. Consider treating H–C by containment (Fig. 7.100). Such treatment is controversial.

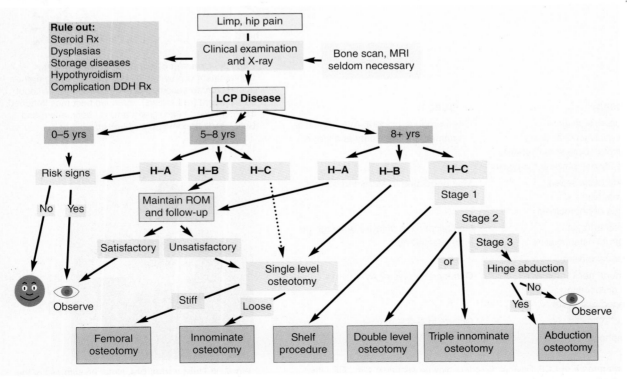

Fig. 7.99 Management of LCP disease. This flowchart considers age, severity, ROM, and stage of disease in determining appropriate management.

Late childhood Consider operative containment in H–B and H–C hips if seen during stage 1 or 2. An option is abduction casts or braces, but most children find this treatment very difficult (Fig. 7.98 right). In stage 1, the shelf procedure (Fig. 7.101) is effective and least invasive. In stage 2, the double-level osteotomy (Fig. 7.102) is often necessary. The head is still plastic and will remodel when well contained. In stage 3, the deformity is permanent. If hinge abduction is present, an abduction osteotomy may improve motion and reduce discomfort (Fig. 7.103). If motion is satisfactory and not painful, accept the deformity (Fig. 7.104).

LCP Consultant Tony Herring, e-mail: johnher@ix.netcom.com

References

2000 The role of coagulation abnormalities in the development of Perthes' disease. Kealey WD, et al. JBJS 82B:744

1999 Legg-Calvé-Perthes disease: MR imaging evaluation during manual positioning of the hip--comparison with conventional arthrography. Jaramillo D et al. Radiology 212:519

1999 Perthes' disease after the age of twelve years. Role of the remaining growth. Mazda K, et al. JBJS 81B:696

1999 Prognosis in Perthes' disease. Meiss L. JBJS 81B:179

1999 Stulberg classification system for evaluation of Legg-Calve-Perthes disease: intra-rater and inter-rater reliability. Neyt JG. JBJS 81A:1209

1999 Perthes' disease and the relevance of thrombophilia [see comments]. Thomas DP, Morgan G, Tayton K. JBJS 81B:691

1998 Prognosis in Perthes' disease: a comparison of radiological predictors. Ismail AM, Macnicol MF. JBJS 80B:310

1998 Relationship between lateral subluxation and widening of medial joint space in Legg-Calvé-Perthes disease. Song HR, et al. JPO 18:637

1997 Acetabulum augmentation for Legg-Calve-Perthes disease. 12 Children (14 hips) followed for 4 years. Dimitriou JK, Leonidou O, Pettas N. Acta Orthop Scand Suppl 275:103

1997 Natural history and treatment outcomes of childhood hip disorders. Weinstein SL. CO 227

1996 Management of Perthes' disease [editorial]. Herring JA. JPO 16:1

1996 Combination trochanteric arrest and intertrochanteric osteotomy for Perthes' disease. Matan AJ, et al. JPO 16:10

1996 Early diagnosis and treatment of hinge abduction in Legg-Perthes disease. Reinker KA. JPO 16:3

1995 The Herring lateral pillar classification for prognosis in Perthes disease. Late results in 49 patients treated conservatively. Farsetti P, et al. JBJS 77B:739

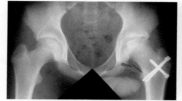
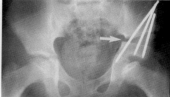

Fig. 7.100 Moderate containment. Containment is provided by a varus osteotomy (red arrow) or a single innominate osteotomy (yellow arrow).

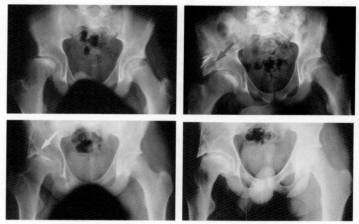

Fig. 7.101 Shelf containment in LCP disease. This 10-year-old girl is H–C and in stage 1. A shelf procedure was performed. Radiographs are shown at age 10 years (red arrow), 11 years (yellow arrow), and 12 years (orange arrow).

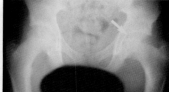
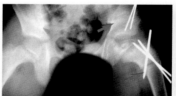

Fig. 7.102 Double-level osteotomy for LCD disease. Containment in this 10-year-old child with H–C was provided by an innominate and femoral osteotomy (red arrow)s. A round head is shown at age 15 years (yellow arrow).

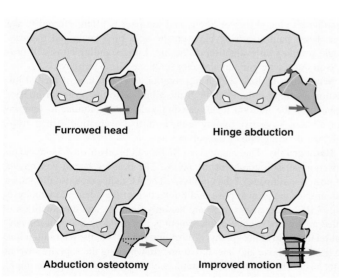

Furrowed head

Hinge abduction

Abduction osteotomy

Improved motion

Fig. 7.103 Hinge abduction. With flattening or furrowing of the femoral head, adduction is full but abduction causes the lateral margin of the femoral head to hinge on the pelvis, in turn causing widening of the medial joint space and pain. Pain and motion may be improved by an abduction osteotomy.

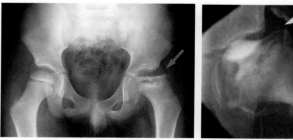

Fig. 7.104 Severe deformity. Severe deformity on AP radiograph (red arrow) and by arthrogram (yellow arrow) in an 11-year-old boy in stage 3. The deformity was established and no treatment was recommended.

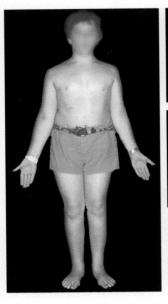

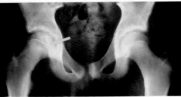

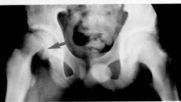

Fig. 7.105 Slipped capital femoral epiphysis. Typical habitus (left). Upper radiograph in orthopedist's office where diagnosis of SCFE was made. Acute slip (red arrow) occurred in the parking lot on the way to the hospital.

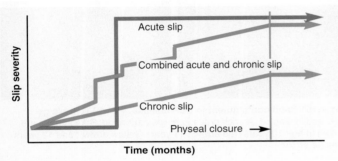

Fig. 7.106 Patterns of slippage. Slipping occurs over a period of months. At physeal closure, progression ceases.

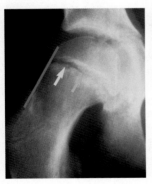

Fig. 7.107 Classic AP radiographic features. Note that the head is displaced inferior to a line (red) drawn along the superior margin of the neck. Metaphyseal rarifaction (yellow arrow) and slight widening of the growth plate (orange arrow) are seen.

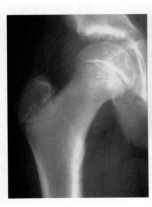

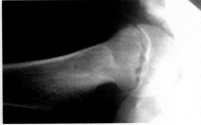

Fig. 7.108 Very early slip. Note that on the AP view, no change is seen in the head–neck relationship. The slight slip is clearly evident on the lateral view.

Slipped Capital Femoral Epiphysis

Slipped capital femoral epiphysis (SCFE) is a displacement of the upper femoral epiphysis on the metaphysis (Fig. 7.105). SCFE is the most common adolescent hip disorder. It occurs in about 1 in 50,000, most commonly in obese boys. The peak age for boys is 13 years and for girls 11 years, with a range from middle childhood to maturity. SCFE is bilateral in about one-fourth of cases, with possibly slight silent slippage in even more.

Etiology

The cause of SCFE is complex. In early adolescence, the growth plate is relatively weaker, as evident from the incidence of physeal injuries at other sites at this age. The hip is vulnerable, as it carries about four times its body weight. Retroversion or a reduced neck shaft angle may increase the verticality of the plate, making it mechanically less stable. The risk is further increased by any constitutional disorder that adds to this physeal weakness. Endocrine disorders such as hypothyoidism, hypopituitarism, or hypogonadism and metabolic disorders such as rickets or treatment with radiation or chemotherapy may contribute. If obesity (Fig. 7.105, left) or trauma are added to this, the plate may fail, either gradually, acutely, or as a combination of gradual and acute components.

Natural History

Failure of physis and slipping may occur from age 6 years until the plate is fused. Most slips are gradual over a period of many months (Fig. 7.106). Often the progress on the slip is variable; acute episodes are superimposed on gradual slipping. Closure of the plate as the result of treatment or as it occurs naturally at the end of growth halts the process. Following slipping, remodeling may reduce the deformity. The risk of osteoarthritis is increased when the slip is more severe, the child is older, and especially if avascular necrosis or chondrolysis complicate management.

Patients with SCFE have a normal acetabulum and the articular cartilage is often preserved. Thus, despite the presence of significant deformity, many do well for many decades. Chondrolysis and avascular necrosis cause early degeneration.

An enigma is the significance of the so-called pistol grip deformity. This deformity is often seen in males who develop osteoarthritis. Speculation suggests that this deformity is secondary to unappreciated SCFE. Why such mild deformity should cause early degeneration is unclear.

Diagnosis

The diagnosis of SCFE is made more difficult because the onset of the common chronic slip is insidious and the pain is often referred to the knee. Knee pain occurring between the ages of 6 years and maturity should promote an evaluation of the hip. Long-standing slips will produce an out-toeing gait, an abductor lurch, and limb atrophy.

Screening is done with a hip rotation test. The loss of medial hip rotation is due to inflammation of the joint and to the posterior inferior slippage of the femoral head, causing a deformity similar to femoral retroversion. A positive finding requires further evaluation with a "frog-leg" lateral radiograph of the pelvis.

Radiography The diagnosis of SCFE can nearly always be made on conventional radiographs of the pelvis. The frog-leg lateral best shows the posterior slippage of the epiphysis. The AP radiograph usually shows widening of the growth plate and rarefaction of the adjacent metaphysis (Fig. 7.107). Sometimes these are the only findings, and the condition is called a "preslip." Subtle displacement is identified by a loss of the normal relationship at the epiphysis–neck interphase. On the AP radiograph, the head lies above and lateral to a line drawn along the superior margin of the neck. On the lateral radiograph, any slipping will disrupt this alignment (Fig. 7.108). On the AP radiograph, assess severity by the percentage of contact between the head and neck. For a more accurate assessment, obtain a true lateral view and measure the slip angle (Fig. 7.109).

Other imaging Pinhole (high-resolution) lateral bone scans of both femoral heads will show increased uptake in preslips (Fig. 7.110). Ultrasound imaging will demonstrate the "step off" at the site of displacement. The MRI shows AVN or altered head position (Fig. 7.111).

Management

The objective of management is to stabilize the growth plate to prevent further slippage and to avoid complications (see flowchart in Fig. 7.114, next page). Achieve this by a screw, pins, epiphysiodesis, or immobilization with a spica cast.

Stable SCFE Fix mild and moderate stable slips *in situ* with a single screw (see page 408). This prevents further slippage and leads to fusion of the growth plate (Fig. 7.112). In the child under age 8 years, fix with smooth pins to allow growth.

For severe slips, the choice is *in situ* fixation or osteotomy. *In situ* fixation is sometimes difficult, and it is necessary to place the entry point of the screw far forward on the neck of the femur. If motion is unsatisfactory, an osteotomy can be performed later. The other choice is an osteotomy to correct deformity and stabilize the slip.

Osteotomy The procedure may be performed at the neck, the base of the neck, intertrochanteric, or subtrochanteric location.

1. Cervical osteotomy Osteotomies of the neck include shortening, are correct at the site of deformity, but carry a significant risk of AVN. Unless the surgeon has considerable experience with the technique it is wisely avoided.

2. Base of the neck osteotomy This provides safety with good correction. Through an anterolateral approach, the capsule is opened. An anterolaterally based wedge of bone is removed at the base of the neck. Any prominences are shaved off. Fixation is simply achieved with screws or Steinmann pins.

3. Intertrochanteric osteotomy This is safe, and involves fixing with a nail plate.

4. Subtrochanteric osteotomy Far from the deformity, this fixation is more difficult.

The base of the neck or the intertrochanteric level osteotomy levels are preferred because correction is good and risks are fewer.

Osteoplasty Residual prominence of the anterior portion of the femoral neck is a common cause of loss of hip flexion. Removal is simple and safe.

Prophylactic pinning Bilateral slips occur in about one-fourth of patients. Always carefully evaluate the apparently uninvolved side. Pin the other side if you are suspicious that an early slip is present or if some underlying metabolic disorder such as renal osteodystrophy is present.

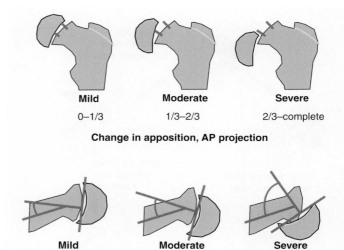

Mild
0–1/3

Moderate
1/3–2/3

Severe
2/3–complete

Change in apposition, AP projection

Mild
0–30°

Moderate
30°–60°

Severe
60°–90°

Slip angle, true lateral projection

Fig. 7.109 Grading severity of SCFE. Severity can be expressed as a grade based on the displacement seen in the AP projection. A more accurate measurement is the slip angle measured from a true lateral radiograph.

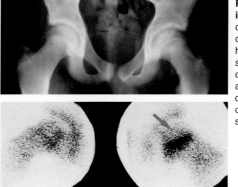

Fig. 7.110 Bone scan in preslip. The diagnosis of a preslip can be confirmed by a high-resolution bone scan. Increased uptake of the physis (red arrow) is noted as compared to the opposite uninvolved side.

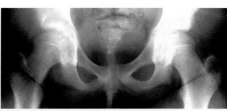
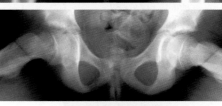
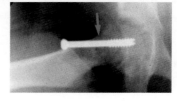

Fig. 7.112 Pinning stable SCFE *in situ*. This mild slip was pinned *in situ* with a single pin (red arrow).

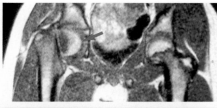

Fig. 7.111 MRI view of SCFE. This study shows a severe slip (red arrows).

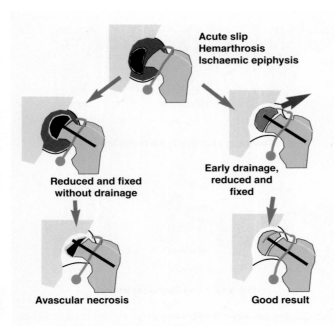

Acute slip
Hemarthrosis
Ischaemic epiphysis

Reduced and fixed
without drainage

Early drainage,
reduced and
fixed

Avascular necrosis

Good result

Fig. 7.113 Prevention of AVN by early drainage. This concept of Parsch and Swintkowski recommends early emergency decompression, reduction, and fixation to prevent AVN in acute SCFE.

Unstable Slips Acute slips (5–10% of all slips) cause instability and increase the risks of avascular necrosis (AVN). They occur suddenly, causing an inability to walk. As the slip is unstable, any movement of the leg causes pain.

Unstable slips are often more severe than gradual slips. Management is difficult and controversial, and the outcome is sometimes poor. Acute management choices include traction, manipulation, cast immobilization, acute decompression, reduction, and fixation. Mounting evidence suggests that early decompression and fixation reduces the risk of AVN (Fig. 7.113).

Admit the patient. Arrange for pin fixation. If the procedure is delayed, consider applying skin traction with the limb supported on a pillow. Reduction may occur from traction or when the limb is in position in the operating room for fixation. Fix as with a stable slip. Supplement the fixation with a second screw if the first pin is not optimal or if the patient is obese or even more unreliable about self-care than most adolescents. Encourage bedrest for 3 weeks and then non-weight-bearing activity until early callus is seen. Follow-up to observe for AVN.

Complications

Complications are common in SCFE. Some can be avoided.

Avascular necrosis AVN is a serious complication that often follows management of unstable slips (Fig. 7.115). Do everything possible to prevent this disastrous outcome. Avoid manipulative reductions. In unstable slips, consider emergency drainage and pin in the position that results from traction or operative positioning. Follow the patient's progress clinically (Fig. 7.118). Be suspicious if hip rotation becomes guarded or progressively more restricted. Necrosis is usually clear radiographically in 6–12 months or earlier on MRI studies (Fig. 7.116).

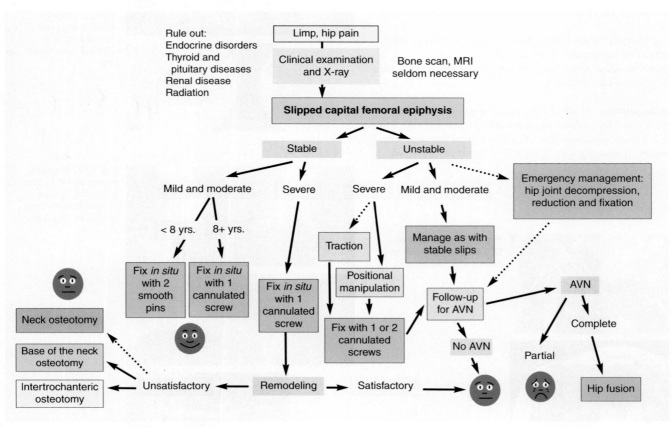

Fig. 7.114 Management flowchart for SCFE.

If AVN occurs, remove or exchange protruding pin(s), prescribe crutch walking, and encourage motion with activities such as swimming. If the AVN is only partial, attempt to salvage function. Procedures such as drilling or coring are not effective. Fuse the hip if pain and disability are unacceptable. Avoid fusion techniques (such as cobra plates) that jeopardize the outcome of conversion to a prosthetic joint later in life.

Chrondolysis may occur with or without treatment (Fig. 7.117). Joint penetration by guide pins or screws is a doubtful cause. The joint space narrows, hip motion decreases, and an abduction contracture often develops (Fig. 7.119). Relieve weight bearing and encourage motion. The value of aspirin, hospital traction, and capsulotomy is uncertain. Most improve with time. Rarely the disease progresses to joint destruction and arthrodesis. The combination of chondrolysis and AVN is devastating and usually ends in hip fusion.

SCFE Consultant Randy Loder, e-mail: rloder@shrinenet.org

References

2000 Follow-up study of severe slipped capital femoral epiphysis treated with Dunn's osteotomy. [In Process Citation]. Fron D, et al. JPO 20:320

2000 Subclinical slipped capital femoral epiphysis. Relationship to osteoarthrosis of the hip [letter]. Hoaglund F,Steinbach L. JBJS 82A:142

1999 Knee pain as the initial symptom of slipped capital femoral epiphysis: an analysis of initial presentation and treatment. Matava M, et al. JPO 19:455

1999 Intertrochanteric corrective osteotomy for moderate and severe chronic slipped capital femoral epiphysis. Parsch K, et al. JPO-b 8:223

1999 Chondrolysis of the hip complicating slipped capital femoral epiphysis: long-term follow-up of nine patients. Tudisco C, et al. JPO-b 8:107

1997 Does a single device prevent further slipping of the epiphysis in children with slipped capital femoral epiphysis? Jerre R, et al. Arch Orthop Trauma Surg 116:348

1997 Slipped capital femoral epiphysis. The prevalence of late contralateral slip [letter; comment]. Pritchett J. JBJS 79A:470

1996 Stable slipped capital femoral epiphysis: Evaluation and Management. [Record Supplied By Publisher]. Aronsson D, Karol L. J Am Acad Orthop Surg 4:173

1996 Natural history of untreated chronic slipped capital femoral epiphysis. Carney B, Weinstein S. CO p.43

1996 Slipped capital femoral epiphysis. The prevalence of late contralateral slip [see comments]. Hurley J, et al. JBJS 78A:226

1996 The demographics of slipped capital femoral epiphysis. An international multicenter study. Loder R. CO p.8

1996 Prevention of secondary coxarthrosis in slipped capital femoral epiphysis: a long-term follow-up study after corrective intertrochanteric osteotomy. Schai P, Exner G, Hansch O. JPO-b 5:135

1995 Slipped capital femoral epiphysis associated with endocrine disorders. Loder R, et al. JPO 15:349

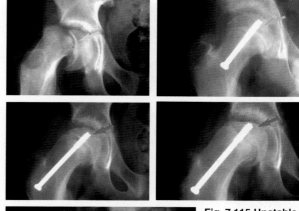

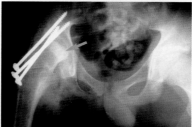

Fig. 7.115 Unstable slip with avascular necrosis. This acute slip (yellow arrow) was reduced and pinned (orange arrow) without drainage. The hip underwent AVN (red arrows) and eventually required a hip fusion (green arrow).

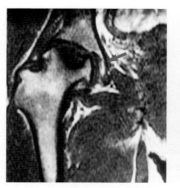

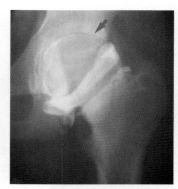

Fig. 7.116 MRI view of AVN. Note the large area of involvement in the femoral head (red arrow).

Fig. 7.117 Chondrolysis. Note the narrowing of the cartilage space as demonstrated by this arthrogram.

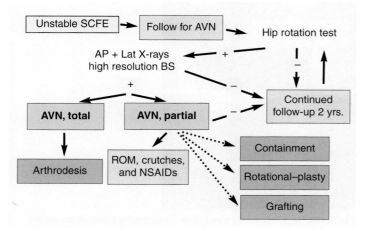

Fig. 7.118 Management of AVN in SCFE.

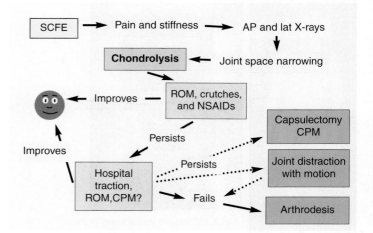

Fig. 7.119 Management of chondrolysis in SCFE.

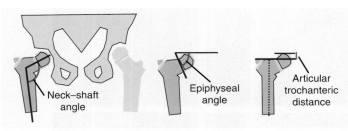

Fig. 7.120 Measurements of the proximal femur. These measurements are often used in discussion of changes in the neck–shaft angle.

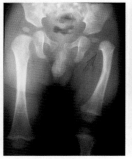

Primary coxa vara
   Congenital:
      Isolated defect
      Bone dysplasias
   Developmental
Secondary coxa vara
   Trauma, malunion
   Avascular necrosis, DDH management
   Tumors
      Fibrous dysplasia
      Bone cysts
   Osteopenic
   Iatrogenic, post-varus osteotomy
Functional coxa vara, coxa breva
   LCP disease
   Total physeal arrest, DDH treatment

Fig. 7.121 Causes of coxa vara.

Uncommon Hip and Femoral Disorders
Coxa Vara

Coxa vara (CV) describes a deformity in which the neck–shaft angle is reduced below 110° (Fig. 7.120). CV has many causes (Fig. 7.121) and can be a primary isolated deformity or associated with other disorders.

Measurements Measurements of the shape of the upper femur in addition to the neck–shaft angle include the epiphyseal angle and the articular trochanteric distance (ATD). The ATD is an important measurement in assessing abductor muscle deficiencies. Normally the center of the femoral head lies at the level of the tip of the trochanter. The ATD is positive. A reduction in the ATD may be due to coxa vara or relative trochanteric overgrowth from loss of growth of the capital femoral epiphysis.

Disability Coxa vara causes limb shortening and abductor muscle weakness. As the deformity increases the epiphyseal angle, the deformity is sometimes progressive.

Congenital coxa vara is often associated with a short femur (Fig. 7.122) or it can be associated with a skeletal dysplasia such as spondyloepiphyseal dysplasia.

Developmental coxa vara may develop over time (Fig. 7.124).

Secondary coxa vara may be associated with other problems, as is common in fibrous dysplasia, or it may be iatrogenic, as may occur after a varus osteotomy treatment of LCP disease.

Management is based on the category of deformity.

Progressive coxa vara may be congenital or developmental. Perform a valgus osteotomy (Fig. 7.123) that reduces the epiphyseal angle to less than about 40°. This more horizontal position provides stability and reduces the risk of recurrence.

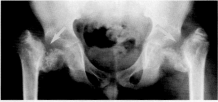

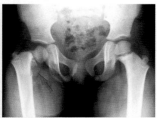

Fig. 7.122 Congenital coxa vara. This deformity is often associated with congenital short femur (red arrow) or may occur as a feature of a bone dysplasia (yellow arrows).

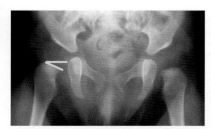

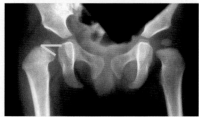

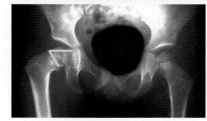

Fig. 7.124 Developmental coxa vara. Radiographs show progressively increasing epiphyseal angle (yellow angles) at 3 months (top), 12 months (middle), and 3 years (bottom).

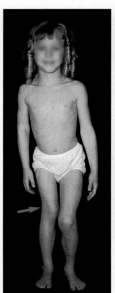

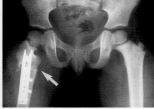

Fig. 7.123 Valgus osteotomy. Note the shortening of the right leg (blue arrow). The varus deformity (red arrow) was corrected with a valgus osteotomy (yellow arrow).

Varus osteotomy Residual deformity is most common when the procedure is performed late in childhood when the time for remodeling is limited (Fig. 7.125). The effect of this osteotomy is sometimes minimized by a concurrent greater trochanteric arrest.

Fibrous dysplasia The deformity is often progressive (Fig. 7.126), producing a shephard's crook deformity. Manage early with a valgus osteotomy, stabilized by permanent intramedullary fixation.

Coxa Valga

An increased neck shaft angle is seldom a problem. Coxa valga is seen in cerebral palsy and other neuromuscular disorders. This deformity may be confused with antetorsion because both can increase the *apparent* neck shaft angle (Fig. 7.127). The *true* neck shaft angle can be assessed by rotating the hip under image intensification until the proximal femur is in profile.

Idiopathic Chondrolysis

This idiopathic disorder is characterized by chondrolysis with a spontaneous onset resulting in pain, stiffness, and narrowing of the joint space (Fig. 7.128). Its natural history is variable. Often restoration of the joint space occurs over several years. In others, the hip becomes ankylosed and fusion is required.

Manage by weight release with crutches while encouraging active motion through activities such as swimming.

Protrusio Acetabula

Protrusio is rare in children. It occurs in Marfan syndrome, seronegative spondyloarthropathy, and conditions that weaken bone. Pain, stiffness, medial displacement of the acetabulum (Fig. 7.129) and an increased CE angle are typical features. Manage the underlying disease. Consider early fusion of the triradiate cartilage in Marfan syndrome or in severe deformity. An osteotomy of the pelvis to shift the loading more laterally (reverse triple innominate osteotomy) may be required.

Snapping Hip

Snapping hip may occur in the adolescent. The iliopsoas tendon subluxates, creating a snap and causing pain. The subluxation can be demonstrated by ultrasound. Manage with rest, injection, or rarely with tendon lengthening.

Labral Tears

Labral tears can occur in adolescents spontaneously following trauma or associated with acetabular dysplasia. The diagnosis can be made by MRI, arthroscopy, or arthrography. Management is difficult. Limited debridement may provide relief.

References

1999 Acetabular labral tear: arthroscopic diagnosis and treatment. Hase T, Ueo T. Arthroscopy 15:138

1998 Coxa vara in childhood: evaluation and management. Beals R. J Am Acad Orthop Surg 6:93

1997 Coxa vara: surgical outcomes of valgus osteotomies. Carroll K, Coleman S, Stevens P. JPO 17:220

1997 Ultrasonographic diagnosis of hip snapping related to iliopsoas tendon. Hashimoto BE, et al. J Ultrasound Med 16:433

1997 Genu valgum in children with coxa vara resulting from hip disease. Shim J, et al. JPO 17:225

1996 Protrusio acetabuli: its occurrence in the completely expressed Marfan syndrome and its musculoskeletal component and a procedure to arrest the course of protrusion in the growing pelvis [see comments]. Steel HH. JPO 16:704

1995 Acetabular labrum tears. Diagnosis and treatment. Fitzgerald RH, Jr. CO p.60

1995 Surgical release of the 'snapping iliopsoas tendon'. Taylor GR, Clarke NM. JBJS 77B:881

1993 Protrusio acetabuli in seronegative spondyloarthropathy. Gusis SE, et al. Semin Arthritis Rheum 23:155

1990 Evaluation of the measurement methods for protrusio acetabuli in normal children. Gusis SE, et al. Skeletal Radiol 19:279

1988 Torn acetabular labrum in young patients. Arthroscopic diagnosis and management. Ikeda T, et al. JBJS 70B:13

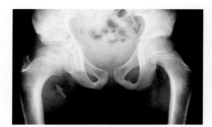

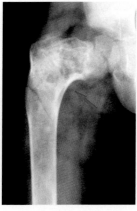

Fig. 7.125 Postoperative coxa vara. This varus deformity followed a varus osteotomy for treatment of LCP disease.

Fig. 7.126 Secondary coxa vara. This varus deformity is secondary to fibrous dysplasia..

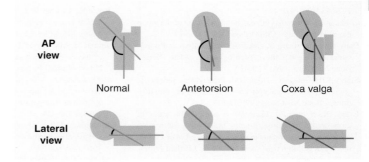

Fig. 7.127 Effect of rotation on neck–shaft angle. Note that the neck–shaft angles (black arcs) on the AP projections are increased both by antetorsion (blue lines) and coxa valga (red lines).

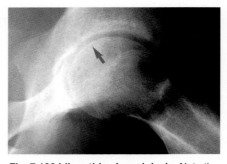

Fig. 7.128 Idiopathic chrondolysis. Note the narrowing of the joint space

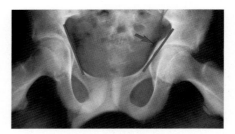

Fig. 7.129 Acetabular protrusion. Note the deepening of the acetabulum.

Ando M, Gotoh E. Significance of inguinal folds for diagnosis of congenital dislocation of the hip in infants aged three to four months. J Pediatr Orthop 1990;10:331-334.

Betz RR, Steel HH, Emper WD, et al. Treatment of slipped capital femoral epiphysis. Spica-cast immobilization. J Bone Joint Surg 1990;72:587.

Bialik V, Fishman J, Katzir J, et al. Clinical assessment of hip instability in the newborn by an orthopedic surgeon and a pediatrician. J Pediatr Orthop 1986;6:703-705.

Bialik V, Reuveni A, Pery M, et al. Ultrasonography in developmental displacement of the hip: A critical analysis of our results. J Pediatr Orthop 1989;9:154-156.

Bos CF, Bloem JL, Obermann WR, et al. Magnetic resonance imaging in congenital dislocation of the hip. J Bone Joint Surg 1988;70B:174-178.

Boyer DW, Mickelson MR, Ponseti IV. Slipped capital femoral epiphysis: Long-term follow-up study of one hundred and twenty-one patients. J Bone Joint Surg 1981;63A:85-95.

Castillo R, Sherman F. Medial adductor open reduction for congenital dislocation of the hip. J Pediatr Orthop 1990;10:335-340.

Cherney DL, Westin GW. Acetabular development in the infant's dislocated hips. Clin Orthop 1989;242:98-103.

Chung SM. The arterial supply of the developing proximal end of the human femur. J Bone Joint Surg 1976;58A:961-970.

Coleman SS. Diagnosis of congenital dysplasia of the hip in the newborn infant. Clin Orthop 1989;247:3-12.

Dahlstrom H, Friberg S, Oberg L. Stabilisation and development of the hip after closed reduction of late DDH. J Bone Joint Surg 1990;72:186.

Emery RJH, Todd RC, Dunn DM. Prophylactic pinning in slipped upper femoral epiphysis. Prevention of complications. J Bone Joint Surg 1990;72:217.

Evans IK, Deluca PA, Gage JR. A comparative study of ambulation abduction bracing and varus derotation osteotomy in the treatment of severe Legg-Calvé-Perthes disease in children over six years of age. J Pediatr Orthop 1988;8:676-682.

Galbraith RT, Gelberman RH, Hajek PC, et al. Obesity and decreased femoral anteversion in adolescence. J Orthop Res 1987;5:523-528.

Galpin RD, Roach JW, Wenger DR, et al. One-stage treatment of congenital dislocation of the hip in older children, including femoral shortening. J Bone Joint Surg 1989;71A:734-741.

Graf R. Fundamentals of sonographic diagnosis of infant hip dysplasia. J Pediatr Orthop 1984;4:735-740.

Hadlow V. Neonatal screening for congenital dislocation of the hip: A prospective 21-year survey. J Bone Joint Surg 1988;70B:740-743.

Haueisen DC, Weiner DS, Weiner SD, et al. The characterization of "transient synovitis of the hip" in children. J Pediatr Orthop 1986;6:11-17.

Henderson RC, Renner JB, Sturdivant MC, Greene WB. Evaluation of magnetic resonance imaging in Legg-Perthes disease: A prospective, blinded study. J Pediatr Orthop 1990;10:289-297.

Ilfeld W, Westin GW, Makin M. Missed or developmental dislocation of the hip. Clin Orthop 1986;203:276-281.

Kalamchi A; MacEwen GD. Avascular necrosis following treatment of congenital dislocation of the hip. J Bone Joint Surg 1980 62A:876-878

Kasser JR, Bowen JR, MacEwen GD. Varus derotation osteotomy in the treatment of persistent dysplasia in congenital dislocation of the hip. J Bone Joint Surg 1985;67A:195-202.

Klisic P, Rakic K, Pajic D. Triple prevention of congenital dislocation of the hip. J Pediatr Orthop 1984;4:759-761.

Kloiber R, Pavlosky W, Portner O, et al. Bone scintigraphy of hip joint effusions in children. AJR 1983;140:995-999.

Koval KJ, Lehman WB, Rose D, et al. Treatment of slipped capital femoral epiphysis with a cannulated-screw technique. J Bone Joint Surg 1989;71:1370.

Kumar SJ, MacEwen GD, Jaykumar AS. Triple osteotomy of the innominate bone for the treatment of congenital hip dysplasia. J Pediatr Orthop 1986;6:393-398.

Lohmander LS, Wingstrand H, Heinegard D. Transient synovitis of the hip in the child: Increased levels of proteoglycan fragments in joint fluid. J Orthop Res 1988;6:420-424.

McAndrew MP, Weinstein SL. A long-term follow-up of Legg-Calvé-Perthes disease. J Bone Joint Surg 1984;66A:860-869.

McHale KA, Corbett D. Noncompliance with Pavlik harness treatment of the infantile hip problems. J Pediatr Orthop 1989;9:649-652.

Mickelson MR, Ponseti IV, Cooper RR, et al. The ultrastructure of the growth plate in slipped capital femoral epiphysis. J Bone Joint Surg 1977;59A:1076-1081.

Mukherjee A, Fabry G. Evaluation of the prognostic indices in Legg-Calvé-Perthes disease: Statistical analysis of 116 hips. J Pediatr Orthop 1990;10:153-158.

Pavlov H, Goldman AB, Freiberger RH. Infantile coxa vara. Radiology 1980;135;631-640.

Pritchett JW, Perdue KD. Mechanical factors in slipped capital femoral epiphysis. J Pediatr Orthop 1988;8:385-388.

Salter RB. The present status of surgical treatment for Legg-Calvé-Perthes disease. J Bone Joint Surg 1984;66A:961-966.

Salter RB, Thompson GH. Legg-Calvé-Perthes disease: the prognostic significance of the subchondral fracture and a two-group classification of the femoral head involvement. J Bone Joint Surg 1984;66A:479-489.

Simons GW. A comparative evaluation of the current methods for open reduction of the congenitally displaced hip. Orthop Clin North Am 1980;11:161-181.

Sponseller PD, Desai SS, Millis MB. Comparison of femoral and innominate osteotomies for the treatment of Legg-Calvé-Perthes disease. J Bone Joint Surg 1988;70A:1131-1139.

Staheli LT, Coleman SS, Hensinger RN, et al. Congenital hip dysplasia. In Murray JA (ed): AAOS Instruct Course Lect 1984;33:350-363.

Thomas CL, Gage JR, Ogden JA. Treatment concepts for proximal femoral ischemic necrosis complicating congenital hip disease. J Bone Joint Surg 1982;64A:817-828.

Thomas IH, Dunin AJ, Cole WG, et al. Avascular necrosis after open reduction for congenital dislocation of the hip: analysis of causative factors and natural history. J Pediatr Orthop 1989;9:525-531.

Tönnis D. Congenital dysplasia and dislocation of the hip. Springer–Verlag. Berlin, 1984.

Tönnis D, Storch K, Ulbrich H. Results of newborn screening for DDH with and without sonography and correlation of risk factors. J Pediatr Orthop 1990;10:145-152.

Tredwell SJ, Davis LA. Prospective study of congenital dislocation of the hip. J Pediatr Orthop 1989;9:386-390.

Trueta J. The normal vascular anatomy of the human femoral head during growth. J Bone Joint Surg 1957;39B:358-394.

Weinstein JN, Kuo KN, Millar EA. Congenital coxa vara: A retrospective review. J Pediatr Orthop 1984;4:70-77.

Yngve D, Gross R. Late diagnosis of hip dislocation in infants. J Pediatr Orthop 1990;10:777-779.

Chapter 8 – Spine and Pelvis

Spine problems in children have the potential to cause considerable disability and must be taken seriously. Whereas the majority of adults have back pain at times, back pain in children is less common and often due to some specific organic disease that requires treatment. Deformity is of greater concern in the child because of the potential for progression with growth. Conversely, minor truncal asymmetry is common in children and may cause undue concern leading to unnecessary apprehension and treatment.

Normal Development

The vertebral bodies form in the usual sequence from mesenchyme to bone (Fig. 8.1). In the frontal projection, the spine is relatively straight throughout growth. In the lateral projection, the spine evolves from a single curve at birth to a triple curve pattern in the child (Fig. 8.2). Although this triple curve pattern is necessary to assume an upright posture, the obliquity imposes an added load on the lumbar spine. This load contributes to development of spondylolysis in the child, intervertebral disc herniation in the adolescent, and degenerative arthritis in the adult.

Terminology and Normal Variability

Sagittal plane The normal range for dorsal kyphosis falls between about 20° and 45°. Kyphosis between 45° and 55° is marginal. Kyphosis below 20° is referred to as *hypokyphosis,* and above 55° as *hyperkyphosis.* Hyperkyphosis is sometimes referred to as a "round back" deformity. Normal levels for lumbar lordosis fall between 20° and 55°. Likewise, reduced lordosis is termed *hypolordosis,* and increased lordosis, *hyperlordosis.* Hypolordosis is called a "flat back" and hyperlordosis either a "lordotic deformity" or a "swayback."

Frontal plane Mild curves that cause truncal asymmetry are usually normal variants (Fig. 8.3). These variations are <10° by Cobb and < 5° by scoliometer measure. These asymmetries have not been shown to cause any disability in childhood or adult life.

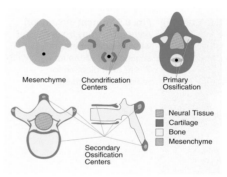

Fig. 8.1 Vertebral development. Vertebrae develop first as mesenchyme, then cartilage, and finally bone. Secondary ossification centers develop during childhood and fuse during adolescence or early adult life. From Moore (1988).

Neural Tissue
Cartilage
Bone
Mesenchyme

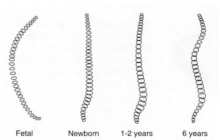

Fig. 8.2 Normal spine development (sagittal plane). The spine changes from a single curve at birth to a triple curve during childhood.

Fetal   Newborn   1-2 years   6 years

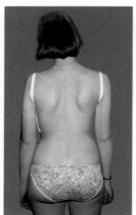

Fig. 8.3 Mild truncal asymmetry. These mild asymmetries are variations of normal, do not require treatment, and cause no disability.

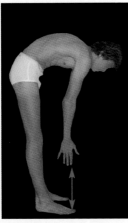
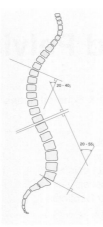

Fig. 8.4 Limited forward bending. Limited forward bending (red arrow) is seen in a variety of diseases. It is an important sign that suggests the need for additional studies.

Fig. 8.5 Method of measuring spinal alignment. Select the endplate of the upper and lower vertebrae with greatest deviation from the horizontal plane. Construct an endplate and right angle line (red). The enclosed angle is the degree of kyphosis or lordosis (red lines).

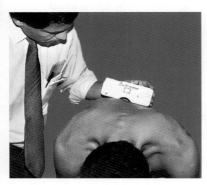

Fig. 8.6 Truncal inclination. Asymmetry may be assessed with an inclinometer or scoliometer. Measures above 5-7° are an indication for radiographic studies.

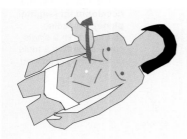

Fig. 8.7 Abdominal reflexes. Stroke each quadrant of the abdomen with the base of a reflex hammer to assess the symmetry of the reflex.

Imaging Method	Condition
Radiography	Initial study
PA	36-inch standing for scoliosis
Lateral	36-inch standing for kyphosis or lordosis
Oblique lumbar	Spot L-S spine for spondlyolysis
CT scans	Fracture, tumors
Bone scans	Back pain, infection, tumors
MRI	Spinal dysraphism, cord lesions, tumors, abscesses

Fig. 8.8 Uses of imaging methods for spinal disorders. Avoid ordering a battery of studies, as this is expensive and often exposes the child to unnecessary radiation.

Evaluation

The spine is evaluated as part of a screening examination or to assess pain or deformity. The screening examination was detailed in Chapter 2.

History and Physical Examination

Screening examination Is there some underlying disorder? Marfan syndrome, neurofibromatosis, ostoeochondrodystrophies, or mucopoly-saccharidoses are readily obvious in the older child but may not be so apparent in the infant.

History Inquire about the onset, progression, disability, and duration. The family history is of great importance, because scoliosis and hyperkyphosis are often familial. Back pain is also familial.

Posture Note asymmetry of shoulder height, scapular prominence, flank crease, or asymmetry of the pelvis. Note any skin lesions, especially those in the midline. The presence of midline skin lesions such as dimples, hemangioma or hair patches, cavus feet, or leg atrophy are often associated with underlying spinal lesions. Café au lait spots are associated with neurofibromatosis, a cause of scoliosis.

Be aware that minor truncal asymmetries occur in about 10% of children. These are benign, cause no disability, and require no treatment. Avoid calling attention to such normal asymmetries because it only worries the patient and family.

Forward bending Perform the forward bending test (Fig. 8.4). This is best done with the examiner seated in front of the child. Control her forward bend by holding her hands together. Slowly guide her forward bending while observing the symmetry of each level of her spine. Any significant scoliosis will be readily apparent. Assess asymmetry with a scoliometer (Fig. 8.6), which measures inclination. Minor degrees of asymmetry are usually only a variation of normal, but require follow-up examination. If any abnormalities are found, a detailed physical and screening neurological examination is essential to avoid diagnostic errors. Hesitation, a list to one side, or restricted motion is abnormal. Lesions such as spinal cord tumors, spondylolisthesis, disc herniations, or discitis limit the mobility or symmetry on forward bending.

Side view As viewed from the side, the back should curve evenly without any sharp angulation. A sharp angular segment of the spine is seen in Scheuermann kyphosis.

Neurological examination should be part of the examination. In addition to the routine assessment, assess abdominal reflexes. Abdominal reflexes are assessed by gently stroking each quadrant of the abdominal wall (Fig. 8.7). Absence or asymmetry suggests a subtle neurological abnormality that may indicate the need for more intensive neurological investigation such as MRI.

Imaging Studies

Radiographs and other imaging studies are indicated to measure the vertebral curves and to further assess specific problems identified by the physical examination (Figs. 8.5 and 8.8).

Radiographs Make PA and lateral spine films in the upright position on 36-inch film using shielding and techniques that avoid excessive radiation exposure. Order oblique lumbosacral views to assess the pars if spondylolysis is suspected and not seen on lateral view.

Bone scans are usual in assessing back pain when radiographs are negative or equivocal. SPECT imaging is useful to assess subtle pars reactions.

CT studies are useful to detail bony deformities or lesions.

MR imaging is used to study patients with neurological findings, those with unexplained progression of deformity, and certain types of deformity as well as preoperatively for children with neurological impairment. These studies are helpful in evaluating tumors, congenital abnormalities such as Chiari malformation, various cysts, tethered cords, and filum terminale anomalies.

Spine and Pelvis Congenital Deformities

Diastematomyelia

This is a congenital defect with a central cartilagenous-bony projection that divides the spinal cord (Fig. 8.9).

Diagnosis Cutaneous lesions occur in most with a hairy patch, dimple, hemangioma, subcutaneous mass, or teratoma at or near the level of the diastematomyelia. Other deformites are common. Nearly all have some associated anomaly like spinal dysraphism, asymmetry of the lower extremities, club foot, or a cavus foot. Two-thirds have congenital scoliosis. Two-thirds are located in the lumbar spine. Half have neurological abnormalities.

Management Resect the spur in patient with progressive neurological findings. Follow the others and consider resection should neurological findings develop or if correction of spinal deformity is planned.

Sacral Agenesis

Caudal regression or sacral agenesis includes a spectrum of abnormalities (Fig. 8.10) with hypoplasia or aplasia of the sacrum, which is most common in offspring of diabetic mothers.

Clinical features include knee-flexion contractures with popliteal webbing, dislocations and flexion contractures of the hips, scoliosis, equinovarus deformities of the foot, and instability at the spinal-pelvic junction. These deformities vary in severity with the level of the agenesis and the resulting loss of motor power. Neurological features may be most predictive of progression and MR imaging is helpful in assessment.

Management is often difficult and depends upon the deformity, motor, and sensory status. Knee flexion deformities are difficult to correct, and recurrence is common. The combination of limited operative procedures, orthotic or mobility aids are tailored to the child. Spine–pelvic instability and hip dislocations are often better tolerated than the stiffness caused by surgical stabilization or reduction.

Exstrophy Bladder

A failure of anterior closure of the pelvis results in pelvic diastasis and an open bladder (Fig. 8.11).

Clinical features include pelvis diastasis, acetabular retroversion, and lateral rotation of limbs with out-toeing gait. This out-toeing tends to improve with age.

Management Orthopedic disabilities are insufficient to require correction. Pelvic osteotomy may be required during bladder reconstruction to facilitate closure. Perform bilateral supra-acetabular osteotomies and stabilize with a spica cast following urological repair.

References

2000 Clinical results with anterior diagonal iliac osteotomy in bladder exstrophy. Ozcan C, et al. J Urol 163:1932

1999 Bilateral posterior pelvic resection osteotomies in patients with exstrophy of the bladder. Gugenheim JJ, et al. CO p. 70

1998 Nuclear medicine in pediatric orthopedics. Mandell GA. Semin Nucl Med 28:95

1997 Natural history of distal spinal agenesis. Van Buskirk CS, Ritterbusch JF. JPO-b 6:146

1996 High-resolution multi-detector SPET imaging of the paediatric spine. Kriss VM, et al. Nucl Med Commun 17:119

1995 Agenesis and dysgenesis of the sacrum: neurosurgical implications. O'Neill OR, et al. Pediatr Neurosurg 22:20

1995 The anatomy of the pelvis in the exstrophy complex. Sponseller PD, et al. JBJS 77A:177

1994 Iliac osteotomy: a model to compare the options in bladder and cloacal exstrophy reconstruction. McKenna PH, et al. J Urol 151:182

1994 Hip function and gait in patients treated for bladder exstrophy. Sutherland D, et al. JPO 14:709

1993 Evaluation and treatment of diastematomyelia. Miller A, Guille JT, Bowen JR. JBJS 75A:1308

1982 Orthopaedic management of lumbosacral agenesis. Long-term follow-up. Phillips WA, et al. JBJS 64A:1282

1978 Sacral agenesis. Renshaw TS. JBJS 60A:373

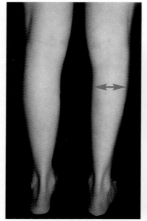
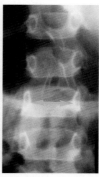
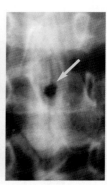

Fig. 8.9 Spinal dysraphism. Diastematomyelia and other congenital spine defects should be considered in children with cavus feet or limb hypoplasia (red arrow). The interpedicular distance is widened (orange arrow) and a midline bony bar bisects the spinal cord as shown on myelography (yellow arrow).

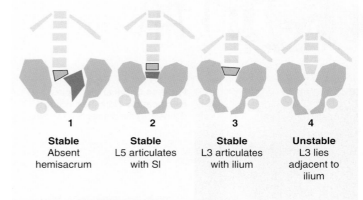

1	2	3	4
Stable	**Stable**	**Stable**	**Unstable**
Absent hemisacrum	L5 articulates with SI	L3 articulates with ilium	L3 lies adjacent to ilium

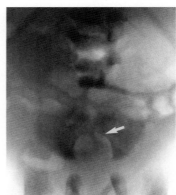

Fig. 8.10 Sacral agenesis classification by Renshaw. The sacrum may be hypoplastic or completely absent (red). The spine–pelvic relationship may be stable or unstable. Radiographs show a type 3 deficiency (yellow arrow). Based on Renshaw (1978).

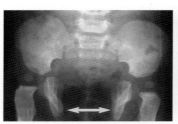
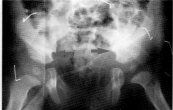

Fig. 8.11 Bladder exstrophy. This is associated with separation of the pubic bones (yellow arrow) and retroversion of the acetabula. Bilateral iliac osteotomies (red arrows) were performed to facilitate bladder reconstruction.

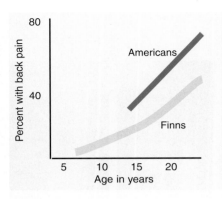

Fig. 8.12 Percentage of children with back pain. Back pain increased from about 1% at 7 yrs. to nearly 20% in adolescents of Finnish children and 56 % in adults. From Taimela (1997). In Americans incidence is about 30% in adolescence, and about 75% in adults. From Olson (1992) and Balague (1995).

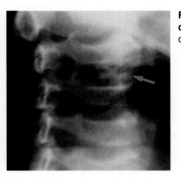

Fig. 8.13 Familial back pain. The child may learn about back pain from siblings and parents.

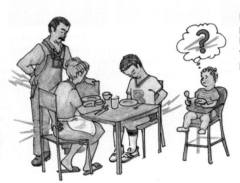

Fig. 8.14 Cervical disc space calcification. Note the calcium deposits in the disc space (arrow).

Vertebral Tumors
Benign
Eosinophilic granuloma
Osteoid osteoma
Aneurysmal bone cyst
Osteoblastoma
Neurofibromatosis
Osteochondroma
Malignant
Ewing sarcoma
Lymphoma bone
Leukemia

Spinal Cord Tumors
Benign
Neurofibroma
Lipoma
Spinal cysts
Malignant
Astrocytoma
Ependymona
Mixed glioma
Ganglioglioma

Fig. 8.15 Vertebral (bone) and spinal cord tumors.

Metastatic tumors
Ewing sarcoma
Rhabdomyosarcoma
Adenocarcinoma
Neuroblastoma
Misc. other tumors

Cord compression
Neuroblastoma
Sarcomas
Astrocytomas
Lymphomas

Fig. 8.16 Metastatic tumors to spine. From Freiberg (1993).

Fig. 8.17 Tumors causing cord compression in children. From Conrad (1992).

Back Pain

Back pain in children is usually caused by some significant organic disease.

Prevalence
Back pain becomes increasingly common during childhood (Fig. 8.12). By mid-teens recurrent or chronic pain occurs in about a quarter of boys and a third of girls.

Evaluation
Be concerned about a history of back pain in children. Sometimes the presenting symptoms of serious conditions may be misleadingly mild, and the spectrum of causes and mode of presentation differ from adults.

Worrisome features include onset before age 4 years, symptoms persisting beyond 4 weeks, interference with function, systemic features, increasing pain, neurological findings, and recent onset of scoliosis.

Examine with a focus on mobility, symmetry, tenderness, neurological status, and hamstring tightness.

Image first with conventional radiographs. Supplement with a bone scan as necessary. High-resolution SPET imaging may be useful in assessing adolescent stress injuries. Add MRI if tumor or infection is suspected.

Idiopathic Back Pain
Adolescent benign back pain Back pain without physical abnormalities accounts for an increasingly large proportion of the category with advancing age. Overall about half of children's and adolescents back pain falls into this category.

Management may be difficult. Some suggest limiting backpacks to less than 20% of body weight (not evidence based). Encourage activity, a healthy lifestyle, and weight control. Provide reassurance. Consider this as a *backache* that is common, requires no treatment, and is best ignored.

Prognosis If back pain is present in adolescence together with a positive family history of back pain, nearly 90% of adolescents will have back pain in adult life. Psychosocial problems are more significant than structural abnormalities in determining the likelihood that back pain will become chronic (Fig. 8.13).

Conversion reaction Reflex sympathetic dystrophy or conversion hysteria may underlie back pain. The typical patient presents with gross, bizarre, and disabling symptoms. Most are adolescent girls. As this type of back pain is very difficult to manage, consider referring to an adolescent medicine specialist or pediatric rheumatologist who has experience in managing this problem. Management often includes physical therapy, psychotherapy, and supportive measures.

Rheumatoid Spondylitis
Rheumatoid disorders may cause back and pelvic pain. The age of onset is usually between 4 and 16 years. More than 90% of patients are HLA-B27 positive with the absence of RF and ANA. About a third will have a family history. Symptoms include peripheral arthritis, usually pauciarticular and asymmetric, involving big joints of the lower limbs. Many complain of heel, back, or sacroiliac pains. An acute iridocyclitis may occur. Most patients develop radiographic sacroilitis. Refer to a rheumatologist.

Cervical Disc Space Calcification
Cervical disc space calcification is a rare, idiopathic, inflammatory condition with clinical manifestations of fever, neck pain and stiffness, and eventual disc space calcification (Fig. 8.14). The pain and fever resolve spontaneously; calcification is seen at the end of the inflammatory phase. Often residual narrowing and irregularity of the disc space is seen if radiographs are made. Manage with rest, a cervical collar, and a nonsteroidal antiinflammatory agent. Resolution of the acute symptoms usually occurs within 7–10 days.

Tumors

Tumors may be metastatic or primary. Primary tumors may arise from the cord or bone (Fig. 8.15).

Metastatic Tumors

These tumors are most common in the thoracic, lumbar, then cervical spine (Fig. 8.16). Manage with chemotherapy and radiation. Mortality is high. Those who survive are likely to have deformity. Early stabilization may prevent progression of the deformity.

Primary Tumors

Primary tumors may occur in the vertebrae or cord. Most vertebral tumors are benign, most cord tumors are malignant. Either type may cause spinal cord compression (Fig. 8.17).

Spinal cord tumors cause diagnostic difficulties. They may present to the orthopedist with torticollis, scoliosis, gait disturbances, foot deformities, or back pain. Often forward bending is limited and asymmetrical. Perform a careful neurological examination. Study with plain radiographs first. Look for changes in intrapedicular distance. MRI studies are usually diagnostic.

Vertebral tumors are more common. Most are benign. Most present with pain. Duration of symptoms from benign tumors is usually longer than those from malignant tumors. Most may be diagnosed by conventional radiographs.

Osteoid osteoma and osteoblastoma cause classic night pain, usually secondary scoliosis, limited spinal mobility (Fig. 8.18), often tenderness, and sometimes classic radiographic features (Fig. 8.19). Bone scans are often diagnostic. Excision is often necessary. Exactly localize with preoperative imaging.

Eosinophilic granuloma causes pain, tenderness, limited mobility, and usually a focal lesion. The classic vertebrae plana (Fig. 8.20) is often absent. For solitary, uncomplicated lesions, observational management is appropriate. If lesions are multiple or if neurological invovement is present, operative resection may be necessary.

Aneurysmal bone cysts cause pain, rarely cord or root compression, sometimes deformity, and limited mobility. Radiographs are often diagnostic with expansion and ballooning of the cortex (Fig. 8.21). Management is often difficult. Manage with preoperative selective arterial embolization, intralesional excision curettage, bone grafting, and fusion of the affected area if instability is present.

References

1999 Back pain in childhood and adolescence. Richards BS, McCarthy RE, Akbarnia BA. Instr Course Lect 48:525

1999 Back pain in children who present to the emergency department. Selbst SM, et al. Clin Pediatr (Phila) 38:401

1999 Nonspecific back pain in children. A search for associated factors in 14-year-old schoolchildren. Viry P, et al. Rev Rhum Engl Ed 66:381

1998 At what age does low back pain become a common problem? A study of 29,424 individuals aged 12-41 years. Leboeuf-Yde C, Kyvik KO. Spine 23:228

1997 Primary tumors of the spine in children. Natural history, management, and long-term follow-up. Beer SJ, Menezes AH. Spine 22:649

1997 Eosinophilic granuloma of the spine. Floman Y, et al. JPO-b 6:260

1997 Are low back pain and radiological changes during puberty risk factors for low back pain in adult age? A 25-year prospective cohort study of 640 school children. Harreby MS, et al. Ugeskr Laeger 159:171

1997 The prevalence of low back pain among children and adolescents. A nationwide, cohort-based questionnaire survey in Finland. Taimela S, et al. Spine 22:1132

1996 The natural history of low back pain in adolescents. Burton AK, et al. Spine 21:2323

1996 Back pain in children. Hollingworth P. Br J Rheumatol 35:1022

1996 Back pain in children and adolescents. Payne WK 3rd, Ogilvie JW. Pediatr Clin North Am 43:899

1995 Juvenile spondyloarthropathies: clinical manifestations and medical imaging. Azouz EM, Duffy CM. Skeletal Radiol 24:399

1993 Metastatic vertebral disease in children. Freiberg AA, et al. JPO 13:148

1992 Pediatric spine tumors with spinal cord compromise. Conrad EU 3d, et al. JPO 12:454

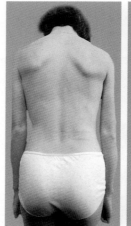
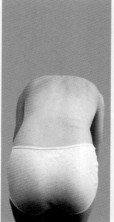
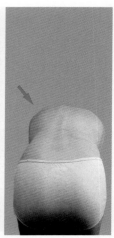

Fig. 8.18 List on forward bending. This boy with an osteoid osteoma shows asymmetrical forward bending. Bending is restricted on the right side (arrow).

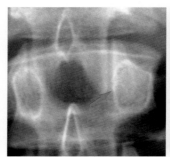
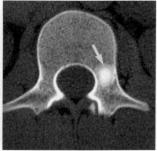
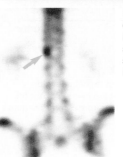

Fig. 8.19 Osteoid osteoma spine. This lesion caused severe night pain. Enlargement of pedicle is seen on radiographs (red arrow). The bone scan showed a focal hot spot (yellow arrow) and the CT scan shows the sclerotic lesion (orange arrow). Excison was curative.

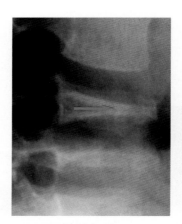
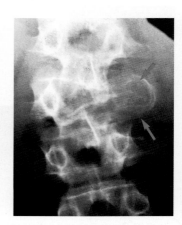

Fig. 8.20 Disc collapse from eosinophic granuloma. Note the vertebral collapse. The appearance is classic.

Fig. 8.21 Aneurysmal bone cyst in 15-year-old boy. Note the expansile cystic lesion (red arrows).

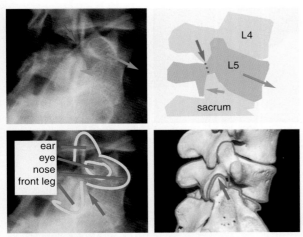

Fig. 8.22 Spondylolysis. The fracture through the pars is shown by red arrows. Note the fracture through the pars as shown on the oblique radiograph (upper left) and diagram (upper right). The *scotty dog* analogy is often used (lower left) to describe the vertebral elements (yellow lines). The neck is the site of fracture. On the model (lower right), the site of fracture is shown.

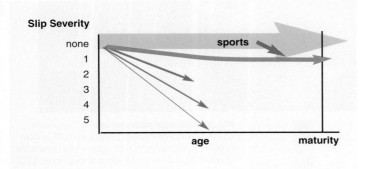

Fig. 8.23 The natural history of pars defects. Most defects develop during early childhood and remain mild. Others develop in late childhood usually due to repetitive trauma from certain sports or less commonly acute trauma.

Spondylolysis and Spondylolisthesis

Bilateral or unilateral defects of the pars interarticularis cause spondylolysis (Fig. 8.22). This defect may allow displacement of the vertebrae which is called spondylolisthesis. These lesions are the most common cause of structural back pain in children and adolescents.

Pathogenesis

In children these conditions are usually due to a stress fracture through a congenitally dysplastic pars interarticularis (Fig. 8.23). This inherent weakness occurs more commonly in certain races (such as Inuit peoples), families, or individuals. Often the defects are associated with spina bifida occulta. Spondylolisthesis occurs in about 4% of 4-year-old children and increases to about 6% by maturity. Spondylolisthesis occurs in about a third of those with pars defects, especially in those with mechanical instability. These lesions occur more commonly in children with abnormal bone or connective tissue, as occurs in conditions such as Marfan syndrome and osteopetrosis. Lesions are common in children who participate in certain sports that cause hyperextension of the lumbar spine with rotation such as gymnastics, wrestling, diving, and weight lifting. Progression after adolescence is unusual.

Clinical Features

History and physical examination The child usually complains of back pain. Tenderness may be present at the L5-S1 level. If the displacement is severe, a prominence is palpable over the defect (Fig. 8.24). Straight leg raising and forward bending may be limited. The neurological examination is usually normal. If the condition is acute, secondary scoliosis may be present.

Imaging First, order a standing lateral radiograph of the lumbosacral spine. A forward displacement of the body of L5 or L4 establishes the diagnosis. If no displacement is present, order oblique radiographs of the lower lumbar spine to assess the status of the pars. Spina bifida occulta is common in children with the defect. A bone scan may show reaction (Fig. 8.25) before radiographs show a defect and may be used to determine the activity and healing potential of the lesion (Fig. 8.26). Even more sensitive is the SPECT scan or MR imaging in demonstrating bone reaction. Rarely the slippage is severe and a noticeable deformity is present.

Classification Wiltse classifies spondylolisthesis into two types:

Dysplastic is a congenital facet deficiency allowing slippage.

Isthmic allows slippage due to a defect in the pars interarticularis. These lesions may be due to a fatigue fracture, a stress fracture, or elongation without fracture.

Grade the degree of slip in severity and activity (duration).

Severity Grade on the basis of slip angle (Fig. 8.27) and displacement (Fig. 8.28). Slip angle changes usually occur with slips greater than 50%.

Activity Grade on the duration or activity (Fig. 8.26). Recent fractures are active and show increased uptake on bone scan. Cold lesions are chronic, inactive, and less likely to heal.

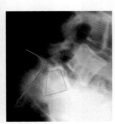

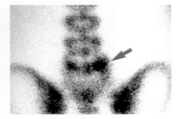

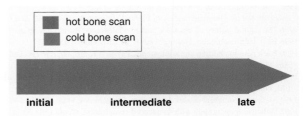

Fig. 8.24 Grade 5 spondylolisthesis. The severe slip produces a flattening of the back (yellow arrow) and complete forward displacement of L5 on the sacrum (red outlines).

Fig. 8.25 Unilateral spondylolysis. This bone scan shows (arrow) an active unilateral defect.

Fig. 8.26. Activity of spondylolysis. Stages of activity. Acute stage following trauma (red), intermediate stage, and late stage (blue).

Progression Pain is most pronounced at the time of onset or fracture. Most isthmic lesions become stable and painless with time. Pain is aggravated by activity, especially competitive sports. Often lesions are symptomatic in adolescence but become painless in adult life when activity levels are reduced. The incidence of back pain is comparable to normal population levels.

Management

Management is based on the patient's age, degree of deformity, type of lesion, activity, and physical activity level.

Spondylolysis management depends upon the activity of the lesion.

Acute lesions from an acute injury or recent overuse experience are managed by reduction of activity and usually an under-arm brace. Often these lesions will heal.

Established lesions Manage symptoms with NSAIDS and activity modification. Operative stabilization is seldom necessary.

Spondylolisthesis is managed based on severity of the slip considering the displacement and slip angle. If fusion is required it is often performed without reduction (Fig. 8.29).

Grade 1–2 slips Manage with NSAIDS, activity modification, and TLSO as necessary to control symptoms. Follow with standing lateral radiographs.

Grade 3 slips Most require operative stabilization in children. Fuse L4–S1 level with posterolateral autogenous grafting. See page 411.

Grade 4 slips These slips may require fusion of L4-S1 as the displacement may be significant making identification of the transverse process of L5 difficult. If slip angle is severe, reduction is sometimes elected (Figs. 8.30 and 8.31)

Grade 5 (spondyloptosis) management is controversial. *In situ* fusion provides pain relief and safety but the deformity remains. Reduction incurs greater risk but improves appearance and posture (Fig. 8.24).

Special situations requiring tailoring of management.

L4 spondylolisthesis is less common, more mechanical in etiology, often causes more symptoms, and is more likely to require operative stabilization.

Spondylolysis with persisting symptoms may be managed by repair of the pars defect with grafting and fixation.

References

1999 Management of spondylolysis and spondylolisthesis in the pediatric and adolescent population. Smith JA, Hu SS. CO 30:487

1996 Bone SPET of symptomatic lumbar spondylolysis. Itoh K, et al. Nucl Med Commun 17:389

1995 Lumbar spondylolysis in children and adolescents. Morita T, et al. JBJS 77B:620

1993 Early diagnosis of lumbar spondylolysis by MRI. Yamane T, Yoshida T, Mimatsu K. JBJS 75B:764

1989 Nonoperative treatment for painful adolescent spondylolysis or spondylolisthesis. Pizzutillo PD, Hummer CD 3d. JPO 9:538

1987 Long-term follow-up of patients with grade-III and IV spondylolisthesis. Treatment with and without posterior fusion. Harris IE, Weinstein SL. J BJS 69A:960

1984 The natural history of spondylolysis and spondylolisthesis. Fredrickson BE, et al. JBJS 66A:699

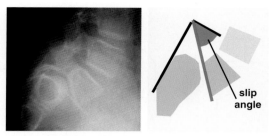

Fig. 8.27 Slip angle. Draw the sacral line (black) as a right angle line to a line along the posterior margin of the sacrum. Draw the L5 body line along the inferior margin of the body of L5 (red line). The slip angle is the angular difference between the sacral and L5 body lines (blue angle).

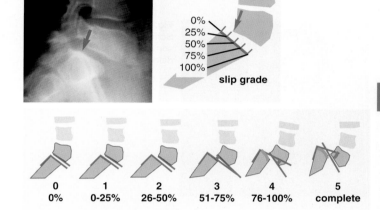

Fig. 8.28 Slip displacement. The severity of the slip is assessed by the degree of displacement of L5 relative to the sacrum (red arrows) and the slip angle (blue arrows). Slips are graded into 5 categories based on degree of displacement. Note that the slip angle increases progressively through grades 3 to 5.

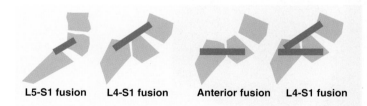

Fig. 8.29 Insitu fusion. The fusion is based on the severity of the slip.

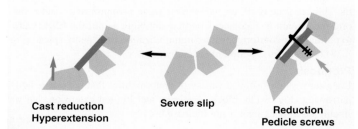

Fig. 8.30. Reduction techniques. Reduction of the severe slip may be done with hyperextension casting (blue arrow) or with pedicle screws (green arrow). Once reduced, a two-level fusion is usually performed.

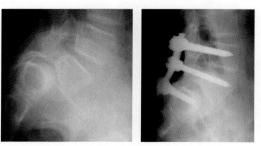

Fig. 8.31 Reduction and fixation. This grade 3 slip was reduced, fixed with pedicle screws, and fused.

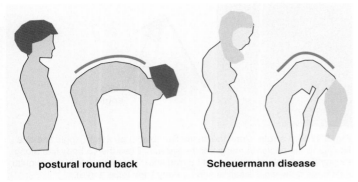

postural round back   **Scheuermann disease**

Fig. 8.32. Differentiating postural round back and Scheuermann disease. Note the smooth contour of the back on forward bending in the child with round back as compared with the angular pattern in the child with Scheuermann disease.

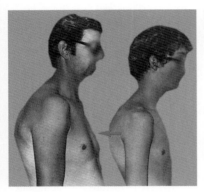

Fig. 8.33. Familial Scheuermann. This father and son have the same fixed deformity.

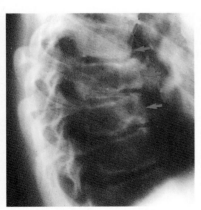

Fig. 8.34. Painful kyphosis. This 16-year-old male has pain and tenderness over the lower thoracic spine. Note the narrow disc spaces, and erosion and deformity of the vertebral bodies (red arrows).

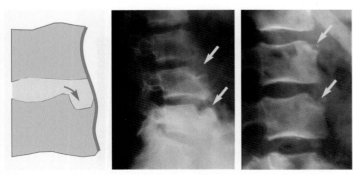

Fig. 8.35 Schmorl nodes. With vertical loading, the nucleus may herniate into the vertebral body (red arrow) producing pain and atypical radiographic defects (yellow arrows).

Scheuermann Disease

Scheuermann disease is a familial disorder of the thoracic spine producing vertebral wedging and kyphosis greater than about 45° (Fig. 8.32).

Clinical Features

A history of heavy physical loading from athletics or work is common. Often the deformity is familial (Fig. 8.33).

Clinical Features

Patients often complain of deformity, fatigue, and sometimes pain. The normal even contour of the spine is lost with an abrupt kyphotic segment at or above the thoracolumbar level. Tenderness over the apex may be present. Radiographs show anterior body wedging. Mild scoliosis is common. The strict definition requires a wedging of at least 5° involving three vertebrae (Fig. 8.34).

Manage

Treat the pain by NSAIDs, rest, and stress reduction. Sometimes a TLSO will be helpful in controlling the pain. Management of the deformity is discussed on page 176.

Schmorl Nodes

These nodes are vertical herniations of the intervertebral disc through the vertebral endplate causing narrowing of the disc space (Fig. 8.35). Sometimes the condition is referred to as *lumbar Scheuermann disease*. This herniation is most common in adolescents, is often associated with trauma, and may be the cause of back pain. The lesions may be seen on plain radiographs, although MR imaging is most sensitive and may be indicated when the diagnosis is uncertain. Manage by rest, NSAIDs, and sometimes a TLSO.

Discitis

Discitis is an inflammation (probably infection) of disc space that involves the lower thoracic or upper lumbar disc spaces in infants and children. Unlike other musculoskeletal infections, discitis usually resolves spontaneously.

Clinical features

The clinical features of discitis are age related. Discitis in the infant is characterized by fever, irritability, and an unwillingness to walk. The child may show constitutional illness with nausea and vomiting. The adolescent may complain of back pain. Because the symptoms are vague and poorly localized, the diagnosis is often delayed. The findings of fever and malaise, a stiff back, unwillingness to walk, and an elevated ESR and CRP are suggestive of discitis.

Imaging Early in the disease, a bone scan may show increased uptake over several vertebral levels (Fig. 8.36). After 2–3 weeks, narrowing of the disc space is seen on a lateral radiograph of the spine. MRI often shows worrisome features and may lead to overtreatment (Fig. 8.37).

Aspiration or biopsy Disc space aspiration is not necessary unless the disease is atypical.

Management

Manage based on the stage and severity of the disease. If the child is systemically ill, antistaphylococcal antibiotic treatment is appropriate. If the child is acutely ill, an intravenous route is appropriate. Otherwise, oral medication is adequate. Continue antibiotics until the ESR returns to normal. For comfort, consider immobilization in a "panty spica" (Fig. 8.38) or brace for a period of several weeks.

Prognosis

Long-term studies show a variety of abnormalities that include residual narrowing (Fig. 8.11), block vertebrae, and limited extension, but the likelihood of back pain is not increased.

Disc Herniation

Disc herniations occur rarely in adolescents. Predisposing features include positive family history, recent trauma, facet asymmetry, spinal stenosis, transitional vertebrae, and spondylolisthesis.

Clinical Features

Herniations usually occur at L4–5 or L5–S1 levels, often producing radicular pain and secondary spinal deformity. The patient may be seen because of scoliosis or a list. Straight leg raising is limited, and neurological changes are variable. Radiographs are usually normal. Occult spina bifida is more common in these patients. MRI studies or myelography show the lesion (Fig. 8.39). Disability is increased if the herniation is associated with spinal stenosis. Be aware that fracture of the lumbar vertebral ring apophysis may be confused with disc herniations.

Management

Manage first with with NSAIDs, rest, limited activities, and a TLSO. Persisting or increasing disability are indications for MR imaging and operative disc excision. Endoscopic or open discectomy are successful in 90% of cases.

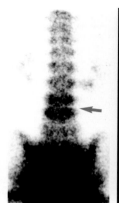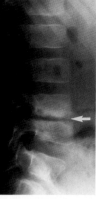

Fig. 8.36 Discitis L4-5. The typical features of discitis are shown on different imaging studies. The bone scan shows increased uptake (red arrow), and later the lateral radiograph shows narrowing (yellow arrow) of the disc space.

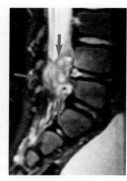

Fig. 8.37. MRI of discitis. The typical intense inflammatory reaction seen on MRI may lead to over-treatment.

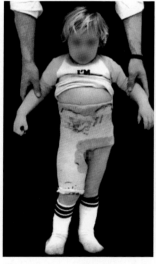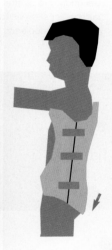

Fig. 8.38. Immobilization of the back reduces discomfort. Most complete immobilization includes the back and one limb to immobilize the lumbosacral spine (left). Adequate immobilization is often achieved with a custom TLSO that extends well down over the pelvis (arrow).

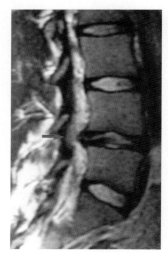

Fig. 8.39. MRI in disc herniation. The posterior bulging disc at L4-5 is clearly demonstrated on MRI.

References

Scheuermann disease
1999 Natural history of congenital kyphosis and kyphoscoliosis. A study of one hundred and twelve patients. McMaster MJ, Singh H. JBJS 81A:1367
1999 Scheuermann kyphosis. Wenger DR, Frick SL. Spine 24:2630
1993 Bone scintigraphy in patients with atypical lumbar Scheuermann disease. Mandell GA et al. JPO 13:622
1992 Familial Scheuermann disease: a genetic and linkage study. McKenzie L, Sillence D. J Med Genet 29:41
1987 Lumbar Scheuermann's. A clinical series and classification. Blumenthal SL, Roach J, Herring JA. Spine 12:929

Schmorl nodes
1994 Schmorl's nodes on magnetic resonance imaging. Their incidence and clinical relevance. Hamanishi C, et al. Spine 19:450
1991 Magnetic resonance imaging of acute symptomatic Schmorl's node formation. Walters G, et al. Pediatr Emerg Care 7:294

Discitis
2000 Discitis and vertebral osteomyelitis in children: an 18-year review. Fernandez M, Carrol CL and Baker CJ. Pediatrics 105:1299
1997 Contiguous discitis and osteomyelitis in children. Song KS, et al. JPO 17:470
1995 Pyogenic infectious spondylitis in children: the convergence of discitis and vertebral osteomyelitis. Ring D, Johnston CE 2nd, Wenger DR. JPO 15:652
1993 Discitis in childhood. 12-35-year follow-up of 35 patients. Jansen BR, Hart W, Schreuder O. Acta Orthop Scand 64:33
1993 Nonspecific diskitis in children. A nonmicrobial disease? Ryoppy S, et al. CO 297:95
1991 Diskitis in children. Crawford AH et al. CO 266:70

Disc herniation
1997 Facet joint asymmetry as a radiologic feature of lumbar intervertebral disc herniation in children and adolescents. Ishihara H, et al. Spine 22:2001
1997 Lumbar intervertebral disc herniation in children less than 16 years of age. Long-term follow-up study of surgically managed cases. Ishihara H, et al. Spine 22:2044
1997 Lumbar disc herniations in children: a long-term clinical and magnetic resonance imaging follow-up study. Luukkonen M, Partanen K, Vapalahti M. Br J Neurosurg 11:280
1996 Endoscopic discectomy in pediatric and juvenile lumbar disc herniations. Mayer HM, Mellerowicz H, Dihlmann SW. JPO-b 5:39
1994 Hamstring tightness and sciatica in young patients with disc herniation. Takata K, Takahashi K. JBJS 76B:220
1992 Familial predisposition and clustering for juvenile lumbar disc herniation. Matsui H, et al. Spine 17:1323
1991 Fracture of the lumbar vertebral ring apophysis imitating disc herniation. Albeck MJ, et al. Acta Neurochir 113:52

Category	Disease

Secondary	Muscle spasm
	  Leg length inequality
	  Functional disorders

Congenital	Failure formation or segmentation Neural tissue disorders

Neuromuscular	Upper neuron, such as
	  cerebral palsy
	Lower neuron (polio)
	Myopathic, such as
	  muscular dystrophy

Constitutional	Syndromes Metabolic disorders Arthritides
Idiopathic	Infantile (0–3 years) Juvenile Adolescent
Miscellaneous	Traumatic Neoplastic Secondary to contractures Iatrogenic, such as radiation and thoracoplasty

Fig. 8.40 Classification of scoliosis. Scoliosis is classified into general categories.

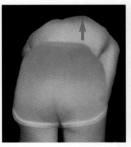
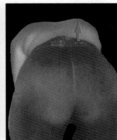

Fig. 8.41 Familial scoliosis. Scoliosis runs in families. Perform a forward bending test on the parents and siblings. This mother (right) was unaware of her scoliosis.

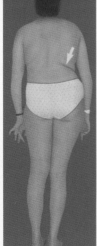
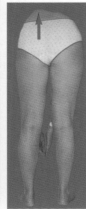

Fig. 8.42 Adolescent idiopathic right thoracic left lumbar scoliosis. The flank crease (yellow arrow) and thoracic prominence (red arrow) are shown.

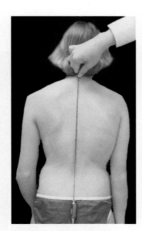

Fig. 8.43 Classification of scoliosis. Scoliosis is classified into general categories.

Scoliosis

Scoliosis is often defined as simply a frontal plane deformity of the spine >10°. The deformity is much more complex and includes significant transverse and sagittal plane components. The causes of scoliosis are numerous (Fig. 8.40). Mild truncal asymmetry occurs in as much as 10% of the population and may be considered as a variation of normal. Curves greater than 10° are abnormal and in the growing child may progress to cause a significant problem. Scoliosis is the most common back deformity.

Evaluation

The evaluation should establish the diagnosis, determine the severity, and allow an estimation of the potential for progression of the scoliosis.

History Inquire about the age of onset, progression, and previous management. A family history of deformity (Fig. 8.41) or pain is important as both run in families. Painful scoliosis in the child suggests an inflammatory or neoplastic basis for the scoliosis.

Screening examination Start with a screening examination. Look for conditions such as Marfan syndrome or the café au lait spots of neurofibromatosis. Assess the child's limb lengths and gait, and perform a neurological examination.

Back examination Note truncal symmetry (Fig. 8.42). Note differences in shoulder height, scapular prominence, flank crease, and pelvic symmetry. Ask the patient to bend forward. Be concerned about stiffness or a list as these suggest an underlying neoplastic or inflammatory process.

Perform the forward bending test. Visually scan each level of the spine to assess symmetry. If a "rib hump" is present, measure it with a scoliometer. This simple device measures the tilt of the rib hump. Assess the balance of the spine using a plumb line (Fig 8.43). The displacement of the weight from the buttock crease is recorded.

Radiographs Radiographs are indicated if the scoliometer reading is greater than 7° or if progression is likely. Progression is more likely if the child is under 12 years, when others in the family have significant curves, or if any findings suggest that the curve may not be simply idiopathic. Radiographs should be made on 36-inch film and taken standing with shielding. A single PA radiograph is satisfactory for screening or a baseline study.

Measure the curve by the Cobb method (Fig. 8.44). Measure the level with the greatest tilt. Note the "apical vertebra" as this defines the level of the curve (Fig. 8.48). Curves greater than 10° are considered significant.

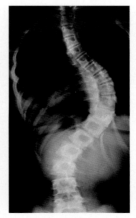
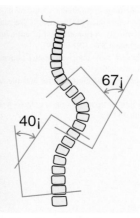

Fig. 8.44 Cobb method for measuring curves. The endplate of the most deviated vertebrae are marked and a right angle line drawn. The angle created by the intersecting lines indicates the degree of curvature.

Secondary or Functional Scoliosis

This type of scoliosis can also be described as "functional" because it is secondary to some other problem. The scoliosis usually resolves when the underlying problem is corrected. The scoliosis is usually flexible and nonstructural. There are no bony changes and the rotational elements are minimal. The common causes of functional scoliosis are leg length inequality and muscle spasm.

Leg length discrepancy Differences in limb length produce a transient functional scoliosis. As discussed in Chapter 4, this type of scoliosis seldom becomes rigid or structural, presumably because the scoliosis is present only when the child is standing on both feet. Thus with lying, sitting, and walking, the spine is straight. The fear of causing a structural scoliosis or other back problems is not a valid reason for ordering a shoe lift or for performing limb length equalization procedures.

Muscle spasm Scoliosis may be the presenting sign for several inflammatory or neoplastic disorders (Fig. 8.45). The spinal curvature often functions to relieve discomfort. Thus, the back is curved to reduce pressure on a nerve root from a herniated disc. Management is directed at the underlying disorder. Scoliosis will disappear once the underlying problem is corrected.

Infantile Scoliosis

Idiopathic scoliosis is the most common spinal deformity. Idiopathic scoliosis is often divided into three subgroups based on time of onset infantile, juvenile, and adolescent categories or simply into either *early* or *late* onset types. Each group has a different natural history and potential for disability (Fig. 8.46). Scoliosis is often classified simply by the site of the most severe curve (Fig. 8.48).

Infantile idiopathic scoliosis occurs in infants and children under 3 years of age. Because the deformity often is associated with plageocephaly and hip dysplasia it is thought to be a positional deformity. Like other position deformities, spontaneous resolution usually occurs. In some cases, the scoliosis is secondary to an underlying spinal abnormality. These cases progress to become severe. Infantile scoliosis is rare in North America.

Evaluation

Truncal asymmetry and scoliosis by radiography establish the diagnosis. Most are boys with left thoracic curves. Measure the apical-rib-vertebral angle difference or RVAD (Fig. 8.47). If the RVAD exceeds 20°, study with an MRI as about a quarter will show a significant neuroanatomical abnormality such as Chiari-1 malformations.

Management

Curves with angles of <20° resolve and require only observation. Follow closely curves >20°. If curves progress and exceed a Cobb angle of about 25° manage with a brace. Curves uncontrolled by bracing that exceed 40° may require operative correction. This correction may include instrumentation without fusion to preserve growth, or anterior and posterior fusion to arrest progression and prevent crankshaft deformity. Be aware that following fusion trunk height will be lost at about 0.03 cm per level fused times the years of remaining growth. Operative

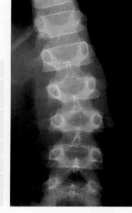

Disease	Comment
Spondylolisthesis	Only with severe displacement
Herniated Disc	Commonly causes scoliosis
Osteoid Osteoma	Focal benign lesion
Intraspinal Tumor	Most serious cause
Discitis	Older child

Fig. 8.45 Underlying causes of scoliosis due to muscle spasm. These conditions should be ruled out if the scoliosis is atypical, associated with pain, list, stiffness, tenderness, or obvious muscle spasm.

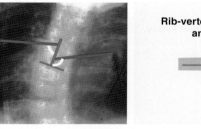

Fig. 8.46 Natural history of idiopathic scoliosis. Progression is related to the age of onset of the scoliosis.

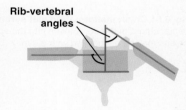

Fig. 8.47 Rib-vertebral angle difference. This is the angle between the axis of the ribs (red lines) and a right angle to the body of the vertebrae (blue lines). The differences is the RVAD.

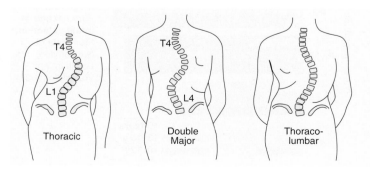

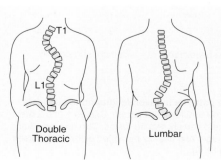

Fig. 8.48 Classification of scoliosis. Scoliosis is classified into general categories.

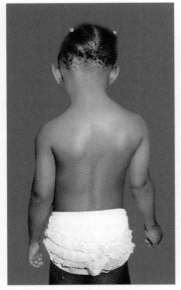

Fig. 8.49 Juvenile scoliosis. This girl shows an elevated right shoulder and thoracic asymmetry.

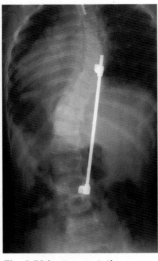

Fig. 8.50 Instrumentation without fusion. This distraction rod was placed to prevent progression while allowing the spine to continue to grow.

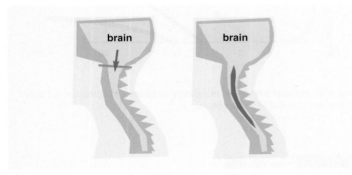

Fig. 8.51 Chiari malformation and syrinx. This malformation is a displacement of the cerebellum into the spinal canal (red arrow). These lesions may be associated with a syrinx (blue).

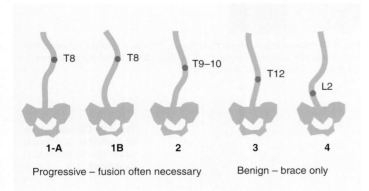

1-A 1B 2 3 4

Progressive – fusion often necessary   Benign – brace only

Fig. 8.52 Progressive curve patterns in juvenile idiopathic scoliosis. Pattern of curves and apex (red dot) level are shown. Curves 1 and 2 are common, often progressive, and usually require fusion. Curves types 3 and 4 are less common, more benign, and usually managed by bracing. Based on Robinson and McMaster (1996).

Juvenile Scoliosis

This form of scoliosis is identified between the 3 and 10 years of age (Fig. 8.49). The course of this early-onset scoliosis is more progressive than the adolescent form and most require bracing.

Etiology

This early-onset scoliosis is more likely to be secondary to some underlying pathology such as a Chiari I malformations (Fig. 8.51) or tumors than curves with onset at puberty.

Evaluation

Hypokyphosis with values <20° suggests a poorer prognosis and complicates orthotic management. In addition to the standard measures, for children with curves >20° study with a full spine MRI as 20–25% will show a significant spinal abnormality that accounts for the early onset and progressive course of this type of scoliosis. Measure the RVAD. Curves with RVAD <10° are usually benign.

Management

Follow for progression. A few curves resolve spontaneously. Institute orthotic management for progressive curves that exceed 20°.

Bracing Manage curves with an apex below T7 with a TLSO. A Milwaukee brace is necessary for more proximal curves. Considering the long duration of bracing necessary, balance brace time with tolerance. Avoid bracing for too many years as the child must endure many years of brace treatment as well as the final surgical correction.

Operative correction is indicated for curves exceeding 40°– 50°. Anterior and posterior fusion are necessary for young children to prevent the crankshaft deformity. Be certain to correct or maintain normal sagittal alignment. Instrumentation without fusion may be considered in very young children (Fig. 8.50) but this is controversial.

Adolescent Scoliosis

Idiopathic scoliosis with an onset after age 10 years is the most common and classic form.

Etiology

The causes of scoliosis are probably multiple. Individuals with progressive curves show vestibular, height, and gender differences from unaffected controls. A genetic component is present but the mode of inheritance is uncertain.

Prevalence

Mild truncal asymmetry occurs in about 10% of the population and is a normal variant. The diagnosis of scoliosis is reserved for curves >10° and this occurs in 2–3% of children, with boys and girls equally affected. Progressive curves are more common in girls by 4–7:1 and prevalence of 0.2% with >30° and 0.1% >40°. About 10% of children identified with scoliosis require treatment.

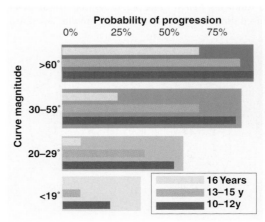

Fig. 8.53 Probability of progression (>5°) based on magnitude of curve at age of initial detection. From data of Nachemson, Lonstein, and Weinstein (1982).

Natural History

The potential for progression depends upon curve type (Fig. 8.52), severity, level of maturation (Fig. 8.53), and Risser sign (Fig. 8.54). In adults, curves <30° progress little, curves 30–50° progress about 10–15° over a lifetime. Curves 50–76° progress about 1° a year. Individuals with scoliosis have normal mortality rates. Curves >100° may reduce pulmonary function. Back pain occurs in about 80%, which is comparable to the general population. Curves at the lumbar and thoracolumbar regions are most likely to be painful.

School Screening

The value of school screening is controversial. The advantage is the earlier detection of deformity. The disadvantage is the large numbers of children with *schooliosis*, those with minimal truncal asymmetry that are referred to physicians, often studied radiographically, and subjected to the anguish of having *scoliosis*. Proposals to be more efficient have included establishing a threshold of 7° scoliometer reading and biannual screening.

Evaluation

Perform an orthopedic evaluation, measure the the Cobb angle (Fig. 8.55), and obtain bending films (Fig. 8.56) if operative correction is planned. Assess the psychosocial situation. Be aware that scoliosis has been shown to increase the risk of suicidal thought, worry, and concern over body image. Try to estimate the tolerance of the child and family to long-term treatment. Exceeding this tolerance results in noncompliance and problems that are sometimes preventable. Support groups, counseling, and special help from family members may be essential.

Management Principles

Manage scoliosis by observation, bracing, or surgery. Exercises, electrical stimulation techniques, and manipulation are ineffective and should be avoided. Ninety percent of curves are mild and require only observation.

Reassurance is an important part of management. Avoid the term *scoliosis* for mild curves and simply refer to the deformity as a "mild truncal asymmetry." This reduces the apprehension that is associated with the diagnosis of *scoliosis*. This diagnosis often causes apprehension as scoliosis is usually equated with treatment either by bracing or surgery.

Indications for treatment should be individualized; however, some generalization can be made.

Brace treatment is indicated for immature patients (Risser 0 or 1) with curves between 25–40°. Boys may be treated with Risser 2–3 if the curve exceeds 30° and is progressive. Observe smaller curves for progression. Progression is defined as a documented increase of 5 or more degrees.

Operative treatment is usually indicated for immature patients with curves of >40° and mature patients with curves >50°.

Brace Treatment

Although the value of bracing is still questioned, evidence suggests that bracing slows or arrests progression of most spinal curvatures in immature patients with progressive curves between 25° and 40°.

Bracing principles apply to most braces. *Immediate effect* should show a reduction of the curve by >50%. *Introduce the brace* over a period of several weeks. *Encourage acceptance* as quickly as possible. *Discomfort* in the brace should be corrected by making necessary modifications early. Continued discomfort reduces compliance, increasing the risk of bracing treatment failure. *Modifications* in the brace will correct this problem. *Encourage normal activities* while being braced (Fig. 8.57). *Schedule follow-up* visits every 4–6 months to assess fit, size, compliance, and curve progression. Obtain a standing PA radiograph out of the brace to assess progress. *Discontinue bracing* about 2 years postmenarcheal or Risser 4 for girls and 5 for boys. Progression while bracing may indicate the need for operative stabilization.

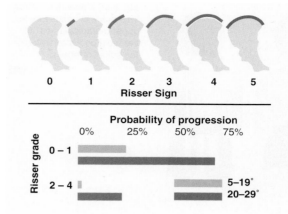
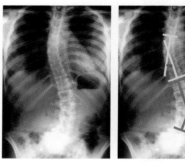

Fig. 8.54 Probability of progression based on curve magnitude and Risser grade. From data of Lonstein and Carlson (1984).

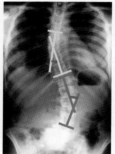

Fig. 8.55 Cobb measure of curve. The degree of scoliosis (red arcs) is the angular difference between right angle lines drawn to the most tilted vertebral bodies. Note the double curve with the thoracic apex at T8 and the lumbar curve at L4.

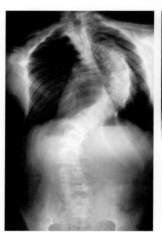
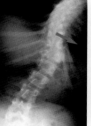
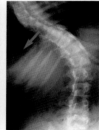

Fig. 8.56 Bending study. To assess the stiffness of the curve, bending films are sometimes used. The degree of correction is a measure of curve flexibility and predictive of correction possible with surgery.

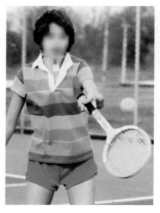

Fig. 8.57 Milwaukee brace. This brace is necessary for higher curves. It is less well tolerated than underarm braces. Encouraging an active lifestyle is especially important in these more restrictive braces.

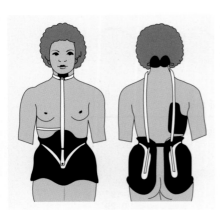

Fig. 8.58 Milwaukee brace. This brace is necessary for upper thoracic curves. It is the most poorly tolerated of the spinal orthoses.

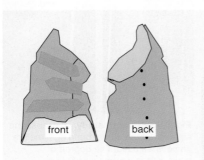

Fig. 8.59 Boston brace. These underarm braces are useful for low thoracic and lumbar curves.

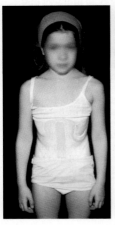
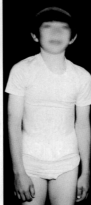

Fig. 8.60 Charleston bending brace. This underarm bending brace is made for nighttime use. Based on Price, et al (1997).

Technique	Comment
Education	Reassurance
Support Groups	Organize or arrange with other patients wearing braces.
Type of Brace	Use underarm braces when possible
Duration: daytime	Part-time bracing per day
	Out of brace for school?
Duration: total	Start weaning early if necessary
Activities	Encourage activities in the brace
	Allow brace-free time for activities
Time out of brace	Be flexible to allow out of brace for special occasions

Fig. 8.61 Adverse effects of bracing. These are techniques that may be used to keep the management within the tolerance limit of the patient.

Bracing options Select the orthosis based on the type and level of curve and the anticipated tolerance of the patient. The most effective bracing types and protocols are most restrictive and cause greatest psychosocial disability. Select a balance that is best for the patient.

Milwaukee brace For upper thoracic curves, the Milwaukee brace is often prescribed. This brace is most restrictive and is compatible with limited activity (Fig. 8.58).

TLSO brace is the most commonly used orthosis. It is appropriate for curves with an apex in the midthorax and below (Fig. 8.59). The Boston brace is prefabricated with custom pads applied by the orthotist. Most include a 15° lordosis correction. The brace may be worn on a 16 or 23 hour per day protocol.

Nighttime braces are best tolerated but effectivenss is contoversial. The Charleston bending brace (Fig. 8.60) is most widely used. The brace is worn only at night allowing the child freedom during the day.

Dealing with compliance Bracing is uncomfortable, often adversely affects self-image, and imposes some difficulties with social and athletic activities. All of these problems further complicate an already difficult time in life. The physician must not exceed the "tolerance limit" of psychological stress on the girl. If this tolerance limit is exceeded, the girl will become noncompliant and may not return for follow-up. She may simply ignore the problem or seek nonconventional methods of treatment that are less demanding.

Improving acceptance Several methods can be used to reduce the adverse effects of brace treatment of scoliosis (Fig. 8.61). The patient should participate in most of her prebracing activities. The bracing schedule may be tailored to the patient. Some patients are already at or beyond their tolerance limit. It may be best to maintain a relationship with the patient and family and to follow the patient without treatment. If the curve is advanced, it may be best to elect an operative option earlier than is normally appropriate.

Operative Treatment Principles

Indications Operative management is the most definitive and effective method of management of scoliosis. It is appropriate for curves that exceed 40–50°.

Risks are early and late.

Early complications include usual operative complications and neural injury. Neural injuries occur in about 0.3% of those with standard posterior fusion.

Late complications include pseudoarthrosis in about 2%, progression in about 1%, late degenerative arthritis at vertebral levels below lumbar fusions, post-fusion back pain, and the *crankshaft phenomenon* if fusions are performed in Risser 0 children.

Fusion levels are important to establish thoughtfully. Fusion too short may result in progression; fusion too long increases the risk of pain and degenerative changes. Inappropriate fusion levels may cause spinal malalignment, changes in posture, and post-fusion back pain.

Classification of curve patterns was established to aid in assessment and determining the appropriate levels for instrumentation and fusion. The curves were classified into five types (Fig. 8.62). Types 1, 2, and 5 are double curves. The level of the apex is established by the degree of angulation of the vertebrae and apex of the curve. The rigidity of the curve may be assessed clinically or by bending radiographs. This classification is becoming less commonly used.

Extent of fusion includes the neutral (or stable) vertebrae above and below the primary curve(s). Attempt to reduce the required number of vertebral levels by considering anterior or selective fusions.

Spinal monitoring is designed to monitor spinal cord function during the operative procedure. The wake-up test has been traditional. Somatosensory evoked potential monitoring is currently being supplemented by monitoring motor function.

Operative Technique

Instrument to reduce the scoliosis and maintain or improve sagittal alignment. Avoid excessive distraction and incorporate solid fixation. Decorticate carefully, excise facet joints when feasible, and add supplemental bone. This supplemental bone may be autogenous, bank bone, or agents that induce osteogenesis.

Harrington instrumentation was the initial standard that incorporated distraction and compression of the ends of the curves (Fig. 8.63). This technique provided little control of sagittal alignment and has been largely replaced.

Luque fixation utilizes sublaminar wires fixed to posterior rods.

Drummond fixation employs spinous processes to posterior rods fixation.

Cotrel and Dubousset (CD) introduced a universal system that provides translation and rotation in addition to distraction that permits a solid 3-dimensional correction. Many modifications of this form such as the Isola and TRSH systems have been developed.

Anterior fixation provides excellent stability when extended to or just beyond the neutral vertebrae (Fig. 8.64). This fixation allows correction with the least number of fused segments.

Video-assisted thoracoscopy These procedures allow anterior releases, rib resection and harvesting, and insertion of correctional implants and fusion with reduced morbidity.

References

Infantile scoliosis

2000 Breast cancer mortality after diagnostic radiography: findings from the U.S. Scoliosis cohort study. Morin Doody M, et al. Spine 25:2052

1999 Infantile and juvenile scoliosis. Dobbs MB, Weinstein SL. OCNA 30:331

1998 Incidence of neural axis abnormalities in infantile and juvenile patients with spinal deformity. Is a magnetic resonance image screening necessary? Gupta P, Lenke LG, Bridwell KH. Spine 23:206

1997 Measurement of rib vertebral angle difference. Intraobserver error and interobserver variation. McAlindon RJ, Kruse RW. Spine 22:198

Juvenile scoliosis

1996 MRI of 'idiopathic' juvenile scoliosis. A prospective study. Evans SC, et al. JBJS 78B:314

1996 Juvenile idiopathic scoliosis. Curve patterns and prognosis in one hundred and nine patients. Robinson CM, McMaster MJ. JBJS 78A:1140

1988 Juvenile idiopathic scoliosis followed to skeletal maturity. Mannherz RE, et al. Spine 13:1087

Adolescent scoliosis

2000 Curve progression and spinal growth in brace treated idiopathic scoliosis. Wever DJ, et al. CO 377:169

2000 Etiology of idiopathic scoliosis: current trends in research. Lowe TG, et al. JBJS 82-A:1157

1999 Adolescent idiopathic scoliosis. Roach JW. OCNA 30:353

1999 Video-assisted thoracoscopy. Crawford AH, Wall EJ, Wolf R. OCNA 30:367

1998 Interobserver reliability and intraobserver reproducibility of the system of King et al. for the classification of adolescent idiopathic scoliosis. Cummings RJ, et al. JBJS 80A:1107

1997 Natural history of adolescent thoracolumbar and lumbar idiopathic scoliosis into adulthood. Cordover AM, et al. J Spinal Disord 10:193

1997 Does scoliosis have a psychological impact and does gender make a difference? Payne WK 3rd, et al. Spine 22:1380

1997 Nighttime bracing for adolescent idiopathic scoliosis with the Charleston Bending Brace: long-term follow-up. Price CT, et al. JPO 17:703

1996 Late-onset idiopathic scoliosis in children six to fourteen years old. A cross-sectional prevalence study. Stirling AJ, et al. JBJS 78A:1330

1995 Boston brace in the treatment of idiopathic scoliosis. Olafsson Y, et al. JPO 15:524

1995 Prediction of progression of the curve in girls who have adolescent idiopathic scoliosis of moderate severity. Logistic regression analysis based on data from The Brace Study of the Scoliosis Research Society. Peterson LE, Nachemson AL. JBJS 77A:823

1990 The epidemiology of "schooliosis." Dvonch VM, et al. JPO 10:206

1986 Idiopathic scoliosis. Natural history. Weinstein SL. Spine 11:780

1984 The prediction of curve progression in untreated scoliosis. Lonstein JE, Carlson JM. JBJS 66A:1061

1983 The selection of fusion levels in thoracic idiopathic scoliosis. King HA, et al. JBJS 65A:1302.

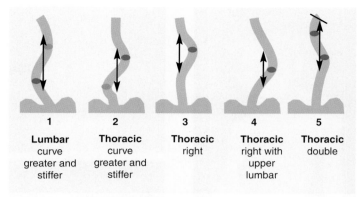

Fig. 8.62 Curve pattern classification. This classification is sometimes still used for classifying curves. Curves may be single or double with the curve apex (shown by red dot or dots) being thoracic, lumbar, or combined. The extent of fusion (arrows) varies with the curve pattern. Based on King, et al (1983).

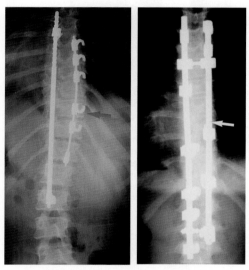

Fig. 8.63 Spinal Instrumentation. Many forms of spinal instrumentation are used. The classic Harrington instrumentation (red arrow) and more modern CD form (yellow arrow) are examples.

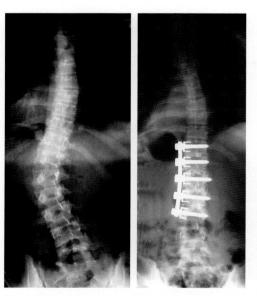

Fig. 8.64 Anterior fixation. This lumbar curve was instrumented and fused involving only 5 vertebrae.

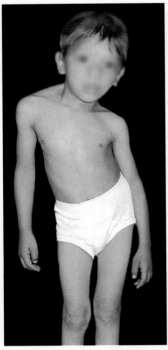

Fig. 8.65 Congenital scoliosis. This child has upper thoracic congenital scoliosis with severe deformity. This type of deformity should be prevented by early surgery.

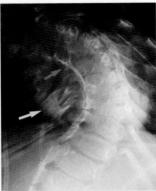

Fig. 8.66 Grades of severity. The hemivertebrae (green arrow) often produces little deformity. On the other extreme, unilateral fusions of the vertebrae (red arrows) and ribs (yellow arrow) causes progressive severe deformity. This curve was fused in infancy to prevent further progression.

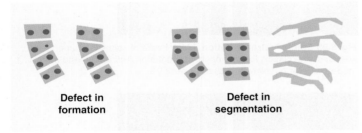

Defect in formation | Defect in segmentation

Fig. 8.67 Types of congenital scoliosis. The common defects are a failure in formation or segmentation. Complex deformities may show mixed patterns.

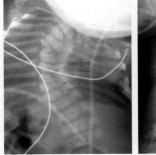 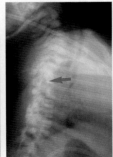 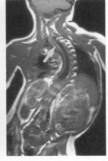

Fig. 8.68 Special imaging in congenital scoliosis. This congenital scoliosis (red arrows) in a newborn was imaged with MRI because of a neurological deficit. Note the hydromyelia (yellow arrow).

Congenital Scoliosis

Congenital structural defects may cause a variety of spinal curves (Fig. 8.65). Such curves are often complex and may require special imaging techniques for assessment. Because these malformations are due to an abnormality of the fetal somite formation, associated lesions in the same somite are common. Thus, the finding of congenital scoliosis, especially one involving the thoracolumbar region, should prompt an ultrasound evaluation of the urinary system and consideration about syndromes such as the VACTERL association (see page 365).

Pathogenesis

Congenital scoliosis is usually caused by a failure of formation or segmentation (Figs. 8.66 and 8.67). The progression of the curve is related to the type of bony defect. Curves that are most likely to progress are those with unilateral unsegmented bars that restrict growth on one side while the opposite side grows normally.

Evaluation

Note the severity, symmetry, and flexibility of the curve. Screen the child for additional disorders of the urinary and cardiovascular systems. Murmurs should be evaluated by a pediatric cardiologist. Order a renal ultrasound as 10–20% will have congenital urinary abnormalities, some of which are life-threatening.

Imaging Study the pattern of the curve on AP and lateral radiographs of the entire spine and additional imaging methods for special situations (Fig. 8.68). Categorize the curve pattern to assess the likelihood of progression. If the curve pattern is ambiguous, CT scans of the apical region are sometimes necessary. MR studies are indicated if neurological abnormalities are found. Plan follow-up and repeat the radiographs in 3–6 months.

Management

The management of congenital scoliosis depends upon the pattern and severity of the curve and rate of progression.

Observation is appropriate when the potential for progression is uncertain. Evaluate every 3 months during the first 3 years and again during puberty when spinal growth is greatest.

Operative treatment is indicated for curves due to unilateral bars. Early in situ fusion prevents progression, or anterior and posterior hemifusion on the convex side may result in some correction of the curve with growth. Problems with growth are less severe than for idiopathic curves as growth is already limited due to the underlying deformity. Operative treatment is required in about half of children with congenital scoliosis.

Orthotic treatment of congenital scoliosis is controversial and less effective than for idiopathic curves. Congenital curves that are long and flexible are most likely to respond to brace treatment.

References

2000 Congenital scoliosis. Jaskwhich D, et al. Curr Opin Pediatr 12:61

1998 Congenital scoliosis caused by a unilateral failure of vertebral segmentation with contralateral hemivertebrae. McMaster MJ. Spine 23:998

1997 Hemivertebral excision for congenital scoliosis. Callahan BC, Georgopoulos G, Eilert RE. JPO 17:96

1995 Variability in Cobb angle measurements in children with congenital scoliosis. Loder RT, et al. JBJS 77B:768

1994 Pulmonary functions in congenital scoliosis. Day GA, et al. Spine 19:1027

1994 Progressive congenital scoliosis treatment using a transpedicular anterior and posterior convex hemiepiphysiodesis and hemiarthrodesis. A preliminary report. Keller PM, Lindseth RE, De Rosa GP. Spine 19:1933

1991 Natural history of scoliosis in congenital heart disease. Farley FA, et al. JPO 11:42

1991 Crankshaft phenomenon in congenital scoliosis: a preliminary report. Terek RM, Wehner J, Lubicky JP. JPO 11:527

Neuromuscular Scoliosis

Most neuromuscular disorders are associated with scoliosis (Fig. 8.69).

Natural History

This scoliosis often occurs early, is rapidly progressive throughout growth, and continues to progress in adult life. Scoliosis often parallels the severity of the neuromuscular disease. Primary curves may interfere with sitting and nursing care. Severe curves may cause cardiopulmonary compromise.

Evaluation

These children have a systemic illness, and a total evaluation is essential.

Physical examination

General evaluation should be thorough. Be certain the diagnosis is accurate to better understand the natural history and potential for disability. Assess the child's motor and mental status, family situation, nutritional status, pulmonary status and general health.

Back examination Observe the child sitting, standing, and walking. Note balance, sagittal alignment, and severity. Examine prone to assess pelvic obliquity (Fig. 8.70). If the scoliosis is secondary to infrapelvic obliquity, focus attention on the hips rather than the spine. Assess sagittal alignment.

Image with PA and lateral 36-inch radiographs. If the hip examination is abnormal, add an AP film that includes the pelvis on the same film to assess the relationship of the hip and spine deformity. Making the spine radiographs with the child sitting is often most helpful.

Laboratory evaluation is essential prior to any surgical procedure. Assess albumen levels (should be > 3.5 g%) for nutritional status, pulmonary function (vital capacity), and lymphocyte levels (above 1500).

Management Principles

Manage with an understanding of the natural history (Fig. 8.71), the potential for disability, and the effectiveness of the various treatment options. As management is often complex, controversial, and long-term, consider what the family values.

Observation is the initial and often primary mode of management for most curves. At each clinic visit, screen for scoliosis with forward bending tests as part of the general physical examination.

Orthotic treatment is controversial (Fig. 8.72). Orthotics are not useful in myelodysplasia or muscular dystrophy and of questionable value in cerebral palsy. Orthotics are often uncomfortable, may cause skin breakdown, decrease pulmonary function, and are expensive for the family. Orthotics may slow progression of the curve in some children and allow a delay in operative correction.

Surgery may be required for progressive curves to provide stability, improve sitting balance, maintain hand function, maintain pulmonary function, facilitate care, and reduce discomfort.

References

2000 The safety and efficacy of Isola-Galveston instrumentation and arthrodesis in the treatment of neuromuscular spinal deformities. Yazici M, Asher MA, Hardacker JW. JBJS 82A:524

1999 Management of neuromuscular scoliosis. McCarthy RE. OCNA 30:435

1997 The outcome of scoliosis surgery in the severely physically handicapped child. An objective and subjective assessment. Askin GN, et al. Spine 22:44

1996 Same-day versus staged anterior-posterior spinal surgery in a neuromuscular scoliosis population: the evaluation of medical complications. Ferguson RL, et al. JPO 16:293

1996 Impact of orthoses on the rate of scoliosis progression in children with cerebral palsy. Miller A, Temple T, Miller F. JPO 16:332

1996 Posterior instrumentation and fusion of the thoracolumbar spine for treatment of neuromuscular scoliosis. Sussman MD, et al. JPO 16:304

1992 Soft Boston orthosis in management of neuromuscular scoliosis: a preliminary report. Letts M, et al. JPO 12:470

1990 Postoperative pulmonary complications in children with neuromuscular scoliosis who underwent posterior spinal fusion. Padman R, McNamara R. Del Med J 62:999

Neuropathic		
Upper motor neuron	cerebral palsy	
	spinocerebellar degen.	
	syringomyelia	
	spinal cord tumors	
	spinal cord trauma	
Lower motor neuron	poliomyelitis	
	trauma	
	spinal muscular atrophy	
	dysautonomia	
Myopathic		
	arthrogryposis	
	muscular dystrophy	
	congenital hypotonia	
	myotonia dystrophica	

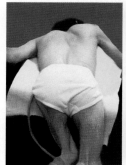
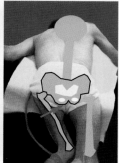

Fig. 8.69 Classification of neuromuscular scoliosis.

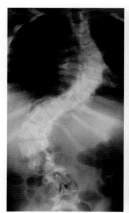
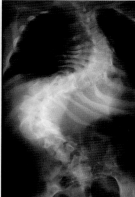

Fig. 8.70 Assess type of pelvic obliquity. Position the child prone over the edge of the exam table. Note that in this patient the spine-to-pelvis relationship becomes neutral or normal. The obliquity is infrapelvic from a dislocated hip.

Fig. 8.71 Progression of neuromuscular scoliosis. This curve progressed significantly between ages 14 and 18 years.

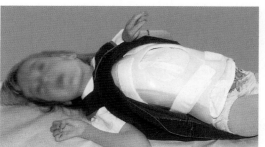

Fig. 8.72 Bracing in cerebral palsy. Bracing in cerebral palsy is controversial.

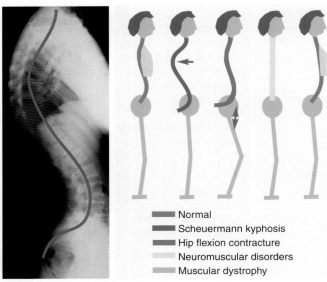

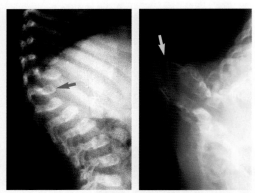

Fig. 8.73 Patterns of sagittal deformity. Normal (green), Scheuermann kyphosis (red); hyperlordosis secondary to hip flexion contracture (blue); flat back (yellow), and thoracic lordosis (brown) with pulmonary compromise.

Fig. 8.74 Congenital kyphosis. Vertebral hypoplasia may lead to paraplegia (red arrow). Kyphosis in spina bifida (yellow arrow) can be very severe, causing skin breakdown over the apex and difficulty in positioning.

Sagittal Alignment

Sagittal alignment (Fig. 8.73) is affected by our upright posture and significantly affects appearance, cardiopulmonary function, and potential for degenerative arthritis of the spine. As the spine has greater mobility in flexion and extension than side bending, sagittal deformities are not complicated by a rotational component as occurs with scoliosis. The spine has three curves, cervical lordosis, thoracic kyphosis, and lumbar lordosis. Upright posture requires that these curves be balanced; they are interrelated. Furthermore, lower extremity alignment affects the spine. For example, excessive lumbar lordosis is usually compensated by hip flexion.

Kyphosis

Kyphosis is a posterior convex angulation of the spine. Kyphosis is normal for the thoracic spine with normal range from about 20°–50°.

Postural Round-back

This is a normal variation. The major problem is cosmetic. It is flexible as the posture can be improved by asking the child to *straighten-up* and does not cause a permanent deformity.

Congenital Kyphosis

Congenital kyphosis may be due to a failure of formation, segmentation, or mixed types (Figs. 8.74 and 8.75). The apex of the curve is most common between T10 and L1. Deformities secondary to a failure of formation are usually progressive and may lead to paraplegia. Assess the apex with high-quality radiographs and a CT study if necessary. Classify the type of deformity. For progressive deformities under about 55°–60° fuse posteriorly. More severe deformities may require anterior and posterior fusions.

Scheuermann Kyphosis

This disease often causes both pain and deformity (Fig. 8.76). The diagnosis is discussed on page 166.

Manage the pain with NSAID and immobilization. Management of the deformity is controversial as long-term disability is mild and effective treatment difficult.

Manage mild deformity curves <60° with observation and encouragement to be physically active.

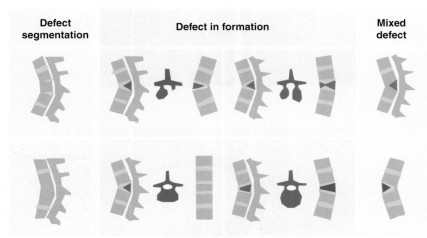

Fig. 8.75 Classification of congenital kyphosis and kyphoscoliosis. Based on McMaster and Singh (1999).

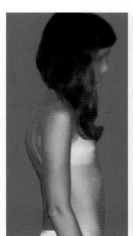
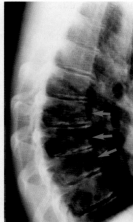

Fig. 8.76 Scheuermann kyphosis. Note the round back deformity and anterior wedging of vertebrae (red arrows).

Curves >60° in skeletally immature children (Risser sign <3) may be improved by brace treatment. Consider applying a preliminary hyperextension plaster cast to improve flexibility. For curves above T7 use a Milwaukee brace (Fig. 8.87). For lower curves use an underarm brace. Brace initially for 20 hrs daily. Once the curve is controlled taper the brace to nighttime use.

Curves >80° uncontrolled by bracing may require operative correction with posterior instrumentation and fusion.

Natural history of this condition is usually benign except in individuals with kyphosis that was upper thoracic and >100° who were likely to have restrictive lung disease.

Postoperative Hyperkyphosis

This serious deformity is common following laminectomy in children for conditions such as tumors or trauma. This deformity is best prevented by decompression or exposures that save posterior elements or early posterior fusion in wide excisions in growing children.

Lordosis

Lordosis is anterior convex angulation of the lumbar spine. The normal range of lordosis is from about 30°–50°.

Developmental Lordosis

This developmental variation is common in the prepubescent child (Fig. 8.88). Parents are concerned. The deformity is flexible, the screening examination normal. Radiographs are not necessary. Resolution occurs with growth.

Functional Hyperlordosis

This deformity is functional, a compensation for fixed deformity above or below the lumbosacral level.

Hyperkyphosis is the primary deformity and the hyperlordosis is compensatory. This compensatory deformity remains flexible and this flexibility is demonstrated by correction of the lordosis on forward bending.

Hip flexion contracture cause a functional increase in lordosis, usually >60°. This deformity is very common in cerebral palsy. Assess with the prone extension test (Fig. 8.89). Lordosis is also common in children with bilateral developmental hip dislocations or coxa vara.

Structural Hyperlordosis or Hypolordosis

Operative procedures that arrest growth of the posterior lumbar vertebrae such as shunting or rhizotomy may result in increasing lordosis with growth.

Spondyloptosis causes a secondary hypolordosis with flattening of the buttocks.

Neuromuscular disorders such as muscular dystrophy may cause hypolordosis.

Fractures with malunion may cause an increase or decrease in lordosis.

References

1999 Congenital spinal deformities. Lonstein JE. OCNA 30:387

1999 Scheuermann's disease. Lowe TG. OCNA 30:475

1999 Natural history of congenital hyphosis and kyphoscoliosis. McMaster MJ, Singh H. · JBJS 81A:1367

1998 Comparison of standing sagittal spinal alignment in asymptomatic adolescents and adults. Vedantam R, et al. Spine 23:211

1996 Severe lumbar lordosis after dorsal rhizotomy. Crawford K, Karol LA, Herring JA. JPO 16:336

1993 The natural history and long-term follow-up of Scheuermann kyphosis. Murray PM, Weinstein SL, Spratt KF. JBJS 75A:236

1987 Scheuermann kyphosis. Follow-up of Milwaukee-brace treatment. Sachs B, et al. JBJS 69A:50

1986 Sagittal profiles of the spine. Voutsinas SA, MacEwen GD. CO 210:235

1983 Radiographic determination of lordosis and kyphosis in normal and scoliotic children. Propst-Proctor SL, Bleck EE. JPO 3:344

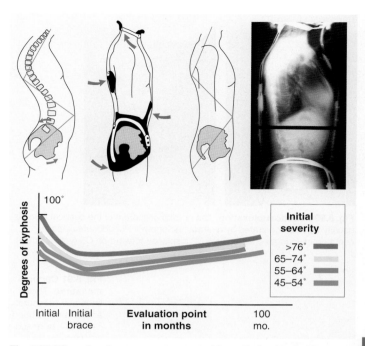

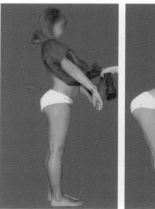

Fig. 8.87 Milwaukee brace management of juvenile kyphosis. The Milwaukee brace is effective in managing kyphosis. The outcome is related to the severity of the curve at the beginning of treatment. Based on Sachs et al. (1987).

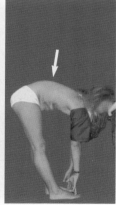

Fig. 8.88 Physiologic lordosis of puberty. This form of lordosis (red arrow) is seen during late childhood just prior to puberty. The spine is flexible and the lordosis disappears on forward bending (white arrow).

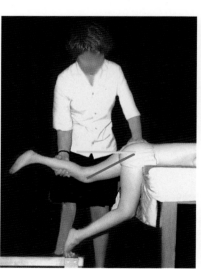

Fig. 8.89 Prone extension test for assessing hip flexion contracture. The thigh is gradually lifted until the pelvis starts to extend. This indicates the limit of hip extension. The contracture is the angle between the thigh (red line) and the horizontal (yellow line).

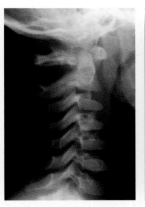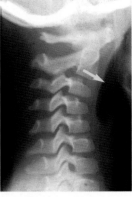

Fig. 8.90 Pseudosubluxation. The normal alignment of the cervical spine is usually well demonstrated by a lateral radiograph. Pseudosubluxation is common in younger children with C2 displaced forward on C3 (yellow arrow).

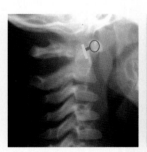

Fig. 8.91 Cervical measures. These lines and measures are commonly used. The SAC, or space available for the cord (yellow), and ADI, or atlanto-dens interval (red line), are expressed in mm.

— McRae line
— McGregor line
— SAC
— ADI

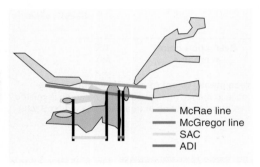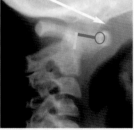

Fig. 8.92 Neutral and flexion views of cervical spine. These studies show the relationship between arch of atlas (red ring) and the front of the odontoid (yellow line). The distance between is the ADI (red line). This relationship changes with neck flexion (right) demonstrating C1-C2 instability with the ADI increasing from 2 to 10 mm due to rupture of the transverse atlantal ligament.

Cervical Spine

Cervical spine problems that often present with neck complaints will be covered in the next chapter.

Radiographs

Conventional radiographs remain the most valuable method of imaging the neck and shoulder.

Pseudosubluxation at C2–3 and less commonly at C3–4 is common in children under the age of 9 years (Fig.8.90).

ADI (atlanto-dens interval) is the distance between the odontoid and anterior arch of axis (Fig. 8.91). This measure is most important in children. This distance is <4–5mm in children. When the ADI >10–12 mm all ligaments have failed. Flexion-extension lateral radiographs (Fig. 8.93) demonstrate instability most graphically.

SAC (space available for the cord) is between the odontoid and the posterior arch of the axis.

Occiput–C1 relationship is often assessed by McRae and McGregor lines (Fig. 8.91).

Special Studies

Additional imaging studies may be appropriate depending upon the evaluation. Look for associated defects. For example, order a renal ultrasound evaluation if the diagnosis of Klippel-Feil syndrome is made. In children with disproportionate dwarfism, prior to any surgical procedure requiring anesthesia, order a screening flexion–extension lateral radiograph of the cervical spine. If instability is demonstrated, special intubation techniques will prevent injury to the cervical spinal cord.

Basilar Impression

Basilar impression is a congenital or acquired deformity in which the cervical spine extends into the foramen magnum. The deformity may be congenital or secondary to osteopenia due to conditions such as rickets or osteogenesis imperfecta. This deformity may cause symptoms during adolescence.

Occipital-Atlantal Instability

Instability at the occiput-C1 level is rare and usually due to a congenital bony defect or marked ligamentous laxity as seen in Down syndrome. Seldom is operative stabilization by fusion necessary.

Atlantoaxial Instability

Instability at the C1–C2 level is relatively common (Fig. 8.92). Instability is due to abnormalities of the odontoid (Figs 8.93 and 8.94) or to ligamentous laxity. Instability results from rupture or attenuation of the transverse atlantal or alar ligaments (Fig. 8.95). Such ligamentous deficiencies are common in Down syndrome and in rheumatoid arthritis. Instability is also common in disproportionate dwarfism. Children with these problems should avoid activities that cause cervical spine stress and have evaluation prior to being administered a general anesthetic.

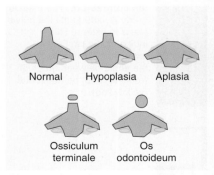

Normal   Hypoplasia   Aplasia

Ossiculum   Os
terminale   odontoideum

Fig. 8.93 Odontoid types. These varied types contribute to varying degrees of instability. Based on Copley and Dormans (1998).

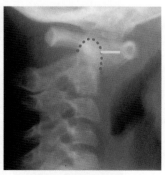

Fig. 8.94 Odontoid hypoplasia. Note the hypoplastic odontoid and the instability as demonstrated by ADI of 8 mm.

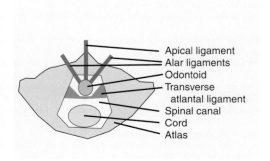

Apical ligament
Alar ligaments
Odontoid
Transverse atlantal ligament
Spinal canal
Cord
Atlas

Fig. 8.95 Constraining ligaments. These multiple ligaments usually prevent the odontoid from compressing the cord.

Polyarticular Juvenile Rheumatoid Arthritis

Clinical stiffness and radiographic changes in the cervical spine occur commonly in polyarticular-onset and systemic-onset disease. Neck problems are rare in pauciarticular-onset disease. Although stiffness and radiographic changes are common, children seldom complain of neck pain.

Klippel–Feil Syndrome

Classically the syndrome includes cervical fusion, low hairline, and stiffness of the neck (Fig. 8.96). The syndrome is now known to be much more generalized.

Clinical features About half have the classic findings of fusions, low hairline, and stiffness. Classify the condition by the levels of fusions. Other clinical associations include congenital scoliosis, renal anomalies, Sprengel deformity, synkinesia, congenital heart disease, and impaired hearing (Fig. 8.97). Other deformities include odontoid abnormalities, occipito-cervical fusion, and basilar impression.

Evaluate carefully with full spine examination, neurological, cardiac, renal, and hearing screening. Make radiographs of the entire spine. Order a renal ultrasound. If neurological findings are present, study with MR imaging.

Management includes advising family of the risks and avoiding activities such as diving, football, and gymnastics, which place excessive loads on cervical spine. Arthrodesis of unstable segments may be required if excessive instability and neurological abnormalities are present.

Natural history Affected individuals have instability problems above and degenerative problems below the levels of fusion. Adults have disability from this syndrome.

Spinal Cord Tumors

Tumors of the cervical spine are similar to those of the rest of the spine. Neurofibromatosis may cause grotesque deformity. Tumors may present with torticollis or cause clumsiness and upper extremity weakness. Some lesions are so slow growing that they remain relatively silent for many years (Fig. 8.98).

Cervical Spine Consultant

Robert Hensinger

References

2000 Radiography of cervical spine injury in children: are flexion-extension radiographs useful for acute trauma? Dwek JR, Chung CB. AJR Am J Roentgenol 174:1617
2000 Reference values for radiological evaluation of cervical vertebral body shape and spinal canal. Remes VM, et al. Pediatr Radiol 30:190
1999 Cervical spine disorders in children. Herman MJ, Pizzutillo PD. OCNA 30:457
1998 Cervical spine disorders in infants and children. Copley LA, Dormans JP. J Am Acad Orthop Surg 6:204
1997 The cervical spine in the skeletal dysplasias and associated disorders. Lachman RS. Pediatr Radiol 27:402
1997 The long-term follow-up of patients with Klippel-Feil syndrome and congenital scoliosis. Theiss SM, Smith MD, Winter RB. Spine 22:1219
1996 The prevalence of nonmuscular causes of torticollis in children. Ballock RT, Song KM. JPO 16:500
1995 The natural history of Klippel-Feil syndrome: clinical, radiographic, and magnetic resonance imaging findings at adulthood. Guille JT, et al. JPO 15:617
1993 Surgically related upper cervical spine canal anatomy in children. Jauregui N, et al. Spine 18:1939
1990 Instability of the upper cervical spine in Down syndrome. Tredwell SJ, Newman DE, Lockitch G. JPO 10:602
1988 Cervical spine disorders in infants and children. Copley LA, Dormans, JP. AAOS 6:204
1986 Changes in the cervical spine in juvenile rheumatoid arthritis. Hensinger RN, De Vito PD, Ragsdale CG. JBJS 68A:189

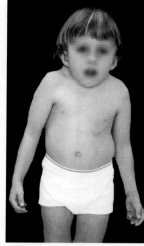
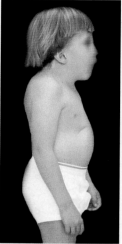
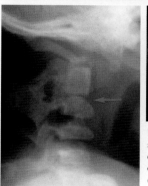
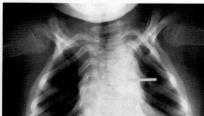

Fig. 8.96 Klippel-Feil syndrome. This syndrome includes shortening of the neck, cervical fusions (red arrow), and various other abnormalities such as scoliosis (yellow arrow).

Disease	Associated Disorders
Klippel-Feil Syndrome	Scoliosis Renal abnormalities Sprengel deformity Deafness Synkinesis Congenital heart disease
Disproportionate Dwarfism	C1-C2 disorders causing instability

Fig. 8.97 Associations. Disorders about the neck are often associated with other congenital defects. Renal and cervical instability problems may not be diagnosed unless special studies are ordered.

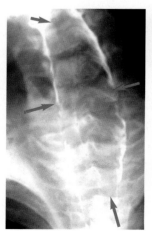

Fig. 8.98 Cervical spinal cord tumor. This myelogram demonstrates an extensive cervical spinal cord tumor (arrows). The boy became progressively weaker over many years before the diagnosis was made.

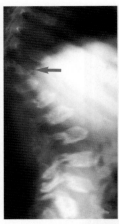
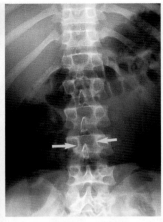

Fig. 8.99 Achondroplasia. Note the kyphosis in the infant (red arrow) and the narrow lumbar canals in the adolescent (yellow arrows).

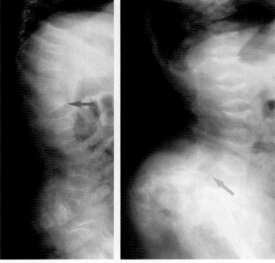

Fig. 8.100 Osteogenesis imperfecta. Note the vertebral deformity (red arrows) and accentuated lumbar lordosis (orange arrow).

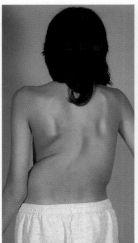
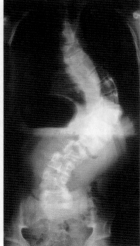

Fig. 8.101 Marfan syndrome. Note the severe right thoracolumbar curve. This curve is not improved by bracing, making instrumention and fusion necessary.

Spine in Generalized Disorders

Many constitutional disorders such as the osteochondrodystrophies and metabolic and chromosomal abnormalities are associated with scoliosis. In these children, during each clinic visit, screen for spinal deformilty.

Achondroplasia

This is a rhizomelic short-limb dwarfism, which is usually readily recognized at birth. Major and disabling spine deformities occur often in these children (Fig. 8.99).

Stenosis of the foramen magnum causes increased hypotonia, sleep apnea, and sudden infant death syndrome. Foramen magnum decompression, duroplasty, and cervical laminectomy may be necessary if symptoms are severe.

Thoracolumbar kyphosis is common in most infants. The deformity is usually flexible. Treat rigid curves >30° with an orthosis. If deformity exceeds 40° after age 5, anterior and posterior fusion may be required.

Spinal stenosis is common and often becomes symptomatic in early adult life. The stenosis may be aggravated by thoracolumbar kyphosis. This deformity is usually treated in adulthood.

Pseudoachondroplasia

This autosomal dominant short-limb dwarfism causes several spinal problems.

Atlantoaxial instability from odontoid deficiencies and generalized laxity is demonstrated by flexion–extension radiographs and MRI if unstable. Decompression and fusion may be required.

Thoracolumbar deformities include kyphosis and scoliosis.

Hyperlordosis may result from hip flexion contracture.

Osteogenesis Imperfecta

Deformity is due to osteopenia (Fig. 8.100), and scoliosis and basiler invagination are serious problems. Bracing is inappropriate as it may cause chest and rib deformity and is unlikely to arrest progression of the curve. Operative stabilization and fusion is indicated for curves exceeding 35°–45°. Instrument with posterior sublaminar segmental fixation and fusion. Add anterior fusion if the deformity is severe and/or associated with kyphosis.

Spondyloepiphyseal Dysplasia

This is a group of short-trunk dwarfism with dysplasia of the spine and long bones.

Atlantoaxial instability occurs in about 40% from odontoid deficiencies, and generalized laxity is demonstrated by flexion–extension radiographs and MRI if unstable. Decompression and fusion may be required.

Thoracolumbar scoliosis and kyphosis are common and may cause back pain in adults. Manage as with idiopathic scoliosis.

Diastrophic Dysplasia

This is an autosomal recessive disorder with short-limb dwarfism. Spine deformities include generalized cervical spina bifida, cervical spine kyphosis, and thoracolumbar kyphoscoliosis. These deformities may be severe and require instrumentation and fusion.

Marfan Syndrome

This is an autosomal dominant disorder of connective tissue.

Scoliosis develops in most patients (Fig. 8.101). Curve patterns are often double major structural right thoracic, left lumbar. Some curves are triple. Curves usually start earlier, and are more progressive, refractory, and rigid.

Brace management is less effective than for idiopathic scoliosis but is used with similar indications and protocols.

Operative management is indicated for curves >50° with segmental fixation using sublaminar wires. Be certain to balance the spine and restore normal sagittal alignment.

Other spinal deformities have included atlantoaxial instability, spondyloptosis, etc.

Morquio Syndrome

This mucopolysaccharidosis type IV is one of a spectrum of lysosomal storage diseases. The spine is normal at birth but deformities develop with growth (Fig. 8.102). Odontoid dysplasia is common and life-threatening. Odontoid aplasia, hypoplasia, or os odontoideum may cause instability. This instability combined with accumulation of mucopolysaccharides within the spinal canal may compromise the cord, causing sudden death or quadriplegia. Manage instability with neurological compromise first with evaluation by dynamic MRI studies. Fuse occiput to C3 or more proximal if posterior elements are adequate. Consider prophylactic stabilization if instability is severe.

Neurofibromatosis

Spine involvement in neurofibromatosis is common (Fig. 8.103). Look for bony dysplasia associated with the scoliosis. If dysplastic features are present, consider MRI or CT studies. Follow carefully as rapid progression may occur with growth.

Nondystrophic scoliosis Manage like idiopathic scoliosis.

Dystrophic scoliosis is often characterized by short angular progressive curves. Brace treatment is ineffective. Correct by combined anterior and posterior spinal fusion. Include the entire structural levels in both the fusion masses.

Rett Syndrome

Rett syndrome is a progressive encephalopathy observed only in girls, who are apparently normal until 6 to 12 months of age. It is characterized by autism, dementia, ataxia, stereotypic hand movements, hyperreflexia, spasticity, seizures, and scoliosis (Fig. 8.104). Scoliosis is usually progressive and seldom responds to brace management. Most require posterior fusion with segmental instrumentation.

Down Syndrome

Trisomy 21 syndrome includes characteristic faces, congenital heart disease, mental retardation, and excessive joint laxity. Upper cervical instability involving the occipito-cervical and the atlantoaxial levels develop in many children. This instability results from joint and ligamentous laxity.

Clinical manifestations of cord compromise from instability include disturbances in gait, exercise intolerance, and neck pain. Mild weakness and hyperreflexia may be found. Screen with flexion-extension radiographs by ages 5–6 years.

Management Be concerned if ADI >5 mm. Follow yearly with examination and every several years with radiographs. Some recommend fusion with ADI >10 mm.

Chapter Consultants

Al Crawford, e-mail: crawa@chmcc.org
Kit Song, e-mail: ksong.chrmc.org
Stuart Weinstein, e-mail: stuart-weinstein@uiowa.edu

References

1999 Cervical spine disorders in children. Herman MJ, Pizzutillo PD. OCNA 30:457
1999 Spinal manifestations of skeletal dysplasias. Kornblum M, Stanitski DF. OCNA 30:501
1997 Spine update. The management of scoliosis in neurofibromatosis. Kim HW, Weinstein SL. Spine 22:2770
1997 Infantile scoliosis in Marfan syndrome. Sponseller PD, et al. Spine 22:509
1996 Occipito-atlanto-axial fusion in Morquio-Brailsford syndrome. A ten-year experience. Ransford AO, et al. JBJS 78B:307
1994 Scoliosis in Rett syndrome. Clinical and biological aspects. Lidstrom J, et al. Spine 19:1632
1991 The spine in diastrophic dysplasia. Poussa M, et al. Spine 16:881
1987 Spinal deformity in Marfan syndrome. Birch JG, Herring JA. JPO 7:546

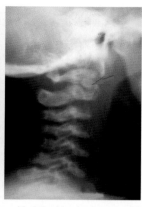

Fig 8.102 Morquio syndrome. Vertebral body changes (yellow arrows) are useful in evaluation. Odontoid hypoplasia (red arrow) is a serious defect.

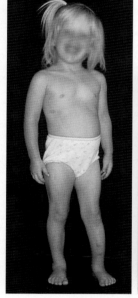
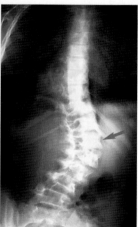

Fig. 8.103 Neurofibromatosis. Curves tend to be sharp and progressive (red arrow).

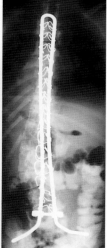
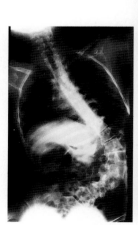

Fig. 8.104 Rett syndrome. Deformity is severe and progressive, often requiring long fusion.

Ascani E, Bartolozzi P, Logroscino CA, et al. Natural history of untreated idiopathic scoliosis after skeletal maturity. Spine 1986;11:784-789.

Ashworth MA (ed). Symposium on school screening for scoliosis: Scoliosis Research Society and British Scoliosis Society. Spine 1988;13:1177-1200.

Blumenthal SL, Roach J, Herring JA. Lumbar Scheuermann's: A clinical series and classification. Spine 1987;12:929-932.

Boachie-Adjei O, Lonstein JE, Winter RB, et al. Management of neuromuscular spinal deformities with Luque segmental instrumentation. J Bone Joint Surg 1989;71A:548-562.

Broom MJ, Banta JV, Renshaw TS. Spinal fusion augmented by luque-rod segmental instrumentation for neuromuscular scoliosis. J Bone Joint Surg 1989;71A:32-44.

Bunnell WP. The natural history of idiopathic scoliosis before skeletal maturity. Spine 1986;11:773-776.

Calvert PT, Edgar MA, Webb PJ. Scoliosis in neurofibromatosis: The natural history with and without operation. J Bone Joint Surg 1989;71B:246-251.

Carr WA, Moe JH, Winter RB, et al. Treatment of idopathic scoliosis in the Milwaukee brace. J Bone Joint Surg 1980;62A:599-612.

DeOrio JK, Bianco AJ Jr. Lumbar disc excision in children and adolescents. J Bone Joint Surg 1982;64A:991-996.

Figueiredo UM, James JI. Juvenile idiopathic scoliosis. J Bone Joint Surg 1981;63B:61-66.

Fredrickson BE, Baker D, McHolick WJ, et al. The natural history of spondylolysis and spondylolisthesis. J Bone Joint Surg 1984;66A:699-707.

Freeman BL III, Donati NL. Spinal arthrodesis for severe spondylolisthesis in children and adolescents: A long-term follow-up study. J Bone Joint Surg 1989;71A:594-598.

Granata C, Merlini L, Magni E, et al. Spinal muscular atrophy: Natural history and orthopaedic treatment of scoliosis. Spine 1989;14:760-770.

Green NE. Part-time bracing of adolescent idiopathic scoliosis. J Bone Joint Surg 1986;68A:738-742.

Hensinger RN. Current concepts review: Spondylolisthesis in children and adolescents. J Bone Joint Surg 1989;1098-1107.

Herman R, Mixon J, Fisher A, et al. Idiopathic scoliosis and the central nervous system: A motor control problem. The Harrington lecture, 1983. Scoliosis Research Society. Spine 1985;10:1-14.

Hoffer FA, Strand RD, Gebhardt MC. Percutaneous biopsy of pyogenic infection of the spine in children. J Pediatr Orthop 1988;8:442-444.

Ippolito E, Ponseti IV. Juvenile kyphosis: Histological and histochemnical studies. J Bone Joint Surg 1981;63A:175-182.

Labelle H, Tohmé S, Duhaime M, et al. Natural history of scoliosis in Friedreich's ataxia. J Bone Joint Surg 1986;68A:564-572.

Lonstein JE, Carlson JM. The prediction of curve progression in untreated idiopathic scoliosis during growth. J Bone Joint Surg 1984;66A:1061-1071.

McMaster MJ. Anterior and posterior instrumentation and fusion of thoracolumbar scoliosis due to myelomeningocele. J Bone Joint Surg 1987;69B:20-25.

McMaster MJ. Occult intraspinal anomalies and congenital scoliosis. J Bone Joint Surg 1984;66A:588-601.

McMaster MJ, David CV. Hemivertebra as a cause of scoliosis: A study of 104 patients. J Bone Joint Surg 1986;68B:588-595.

Mehta MH, Morel G. The non-operative treatment of infantile idiopathic scoliosis. In Zorab PA, Siegler D (eds): Scoliosis. Academic Press, London, 1980, pp 71-84.

Menelaus MB. Diskitis: an inflammation affecting the intervertebral disks in children. J Bone Joint Surg 1964;46B:16.

Mielke CH, Lonstein JE, Denis F, et al. Surgical treatment of adolescent idiopathic scoliosis: A comparative analysis. J Bone Joint Surg 1989;71A:1170-1177.

Miller JA, Nachemson AL, Schultz AB. Effectiveness of braces in mild idiopathic scoliosis. Spine 1984;9:632-635.

Morin B, Poitras B, Duhaime M, et al. Congenital kyphosis by segmentation defect: Etiologic and pathogenic studies. J Pediatr Orthop 1985;5:309-314.

Nash CL Jr, Brown RH. Current concepts review: Spinal cord monitoring. J Bone Joint Surg 1989;71A:627-630.

O'Donnell CS, Bunnell WP, Betz RR, et al. Electrical stimulation in the treatment of idiopathic scoliosis. Clin Orthop 1988;229:107-113.

Peterson HA. Musculoskeletal infections in children: Part VII. Disk-space infection in children. In Evarts CM (ed): AAOS Instruct Course Lect 1983;32:50-60.

Pizzutillo PD, Hummer CD. Non-operative treatment for painful adolescent spondylolysis or spondylolisthesis. J Pediatr Orthop 1989;9:538-540.

Richards BS, Birch JG, Herring JA, et al. Frontal plane and

sagittal plane balance following Cotrel-Dubousset instrumentation for idiopathic scoliosis. Spine 1989;14:733-737.

Rogala EJ, Drummond DS, Gurr J. Scoliosis: Incidence and natural history: A prospective epidemiological study. J Bone Joint Surg 1978;60A:173-176.

Sachs B, Bradford D, Winter R, et al. Scheurmann kyphosis: Follow-up of Milwaukee-brace treatment. J Bone Joint Surg 1987;69A:50-57.

Samuelsson L, Eklof O. Scoliosis in myelomeningocele. Acta Orthop Scand 1988;59:122-127.

Saraste H. Long-term clinical and radiological follow-up of spondylolysis and spondylolisthesis. J Pediatr Orthop 1987;7:631-638.

Smith AD, Koreska J, Moseley CF. Progression of scoliosis in Duchenne muscular dystrophy. J Bone Joint Surg 1989;71A:1066-1074.

Sponseller PD, Cohen MS, Nachemson AL, et al. Results of surgical treatment of adults with idiopathic scoliosis. J Bone Joint Surg 1987;69A:667-675.

Stagnara P, De Mauroy JC, Dran G, et al. Reciprocal angulation of vertebral bodies in a sagittal plane: Approach to references for the evaluation of kyphosis and lordosis. Spine 1982;7:335-342.

Stone B, Beekman C, Hall V, et al. The effect of an exercise program on change in curve in adolescents with minimal idiopathic scoliosis: A preliminary study. Phys Ther 1979;59:759-763.

Sullivan JA, Davidson R, Renshaw TS, et al. Further evaluation of the Scolitron treatment of ideopathic adolescent scoliosis. Spine 1986;11:903-906.

Szalay EA, Green NE, Heller RM, et al. Magnetic resonance imaging in the diagnosis of childhood discitis. J Pediatr Orthop 1987;7:164-167.

Torell G, Nordwall A, Nachemson A. The changing pattern of scoliosis treatment due to effective screening. J Bone Joint Surg 1981;63A:337-341.

Weinstein SL. Idiopathic scoliosis: Natural History. Spine 1986;11:780-783.

Weinstein SL, Ponseti IV. Curve progression in idiopathic scoliosis. J Bone Joint Surg 1983;65A:447-455.

Weinstein SL, Zavala DC, Ponseti IV. Idiopathic scoliosis: Long-term follow-up and prognosis in untreated patients. J Bone Joint Surg 1981;63A:702-712.

Wenger DR, Bobechko WP, Gilday DL. The spectrum of intervertebral disk-space infection in children. J Bone Joint Surg 1978;60A:100.

Chapter 9 – Upper Limb

Because upper limb disorders are less common than those of the lower limbs the topic is covered in one chapter.

Development

The upper limb bud develops between the fourth and eighth fetal week. Most congenital upper limb defects have their origin during this period (Fig. 9.1). During the seventh week, the upper limb flexes at the shoulder and elbow and rotates around a longitudinal axis to account for the dermatomal pattern of the upper extremity. The scapula migrates caudad during development. A failure of the descent of the scapula is a feature of Sprengel deformity. Ossification of the clavicle develops from two centers. A failure of coalescence of these two centers may be the cause of the congenital pseudarthrosis of the clavicle. Upper limb growth occurs most rapidly in the proximal femoral and distal forearm epiphyses (Fig.9.2).

During infancy, hand function progresses in an orderly fashion (Fig. 9.3). Bimanual function becomes refined during the second year. Both fine and gross motor skills improve with age.

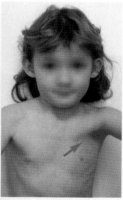

Fig. 9.1 Congenital anomalies. Limb deficiencies (yellow arrow) cause considerable disability. Others, such as Poland syndrome or absence of the pectoralis (red arrow), cause only a cosmetic disability.

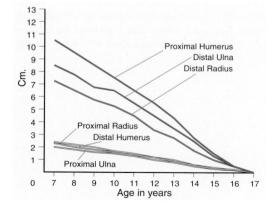

Fig. 9.2 Growth rates for upper limb. The majority of growth of the upper limbs occurs from physes about the wrist and shoulder compared to the elbow. From Pritchett (1988).

Age	Hand Function
1 Month	Hand clenched
2 Months	Opens hands
3 Months	Holds objects
5 Months	Primitive finger grasp
9 Months	Early finger pinch
12 Months	Picks up large objects
18 Months	Piles blocks
3 Years	Buttons clothing
4 Years	Can throw a ball
5 Years	Can catch a ball

Fig. 9.3 Hand function by age. Hand function becomes progressively more skilled with advancing age.

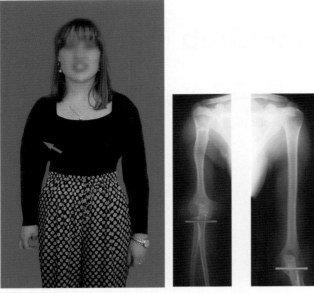

Fig. 9.4 Upper limb length inequality. This girls right arm is shortened due to a cyst of the proximal humerus. Her disability is minimal.

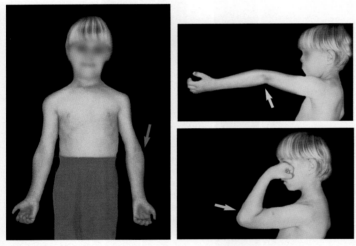

Fig. 9.5 Cubitus varus. This child has a malunion following a supracondylar fracture. In the anatomic position, the child has a cubitus varus deformity (red arrow). Hyperextension deformity (yellow arrow) and limited elbow flexion (orange arrow) are also present.

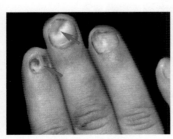

Fig. 9.6 Nail-patella syndrome. Nail dysplasia is seen in the nail-patella syndrome.

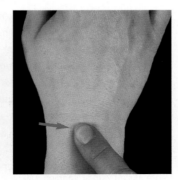

Fig. 9.7 Localize tenderness. Correlate tenderness with anatomic structures.

Upper limb orthopedic problems are less common than those of the lower extremity for several reasons. The upper limb is not subjected to the stresses of load bearing. Upper limb vascularity is less vulnerable than that of the lower limb. For example, the upper humeral circulation is less easily interrupted as that of the proximal femur. The function of each upper limb is more independent than that of the lower limbs. Thus, a short arm causes less functional disability than a short leg (Fig. 9.4).

Evaluation

The physical examination should follow the standard sequence of inspection, palpation, range of motion evaluation, and a careful neurological examination. Imaging should start with conventional radiographs.

Observation

Head and neck Observe the head and neck for abnormalities and asymmetry. The head is normally held in a vertical position by the vestibular and ocular righting mechanisms. Head tilt is common in "wryneck" or torticollis. Describe the deformity in terms of the three planes, flexion-extension, lateral head tilt, and rotation. Observe the shape of the head. Plagiocephaly is common in torticollis and includes a flattening of the malar prominence and a lowering of the position of the eye and ear on the involved side. The ipsilateral occiput is flattened.

Limbs Start with observation of the relationship of the neck and limbs. Note any asymmetry. Observe differences in spontaneous movement. Loss of movement may be due to true paralysis from a nerve injury or more likely from pseudoparalysis due to trauma or infection. The infant with a clavicular fracture or septic arthritis of the shoulder or elbow will spontaneously limit arm movement.

Observe the *carrying angle*, the alignment of the arm and forearm as viewed with the child in the anatomic position. The carrying angle is normally in 0–10° of valgus. A varus carrying angle causes the so-called *gunstock deformity*, which is usually due to malunited supracondylar fracture (Fig. 9.5). An increase in carrying angle is seen in Turner syndrome.

Look for asymmetry or masses and note any finger or nail abnormalities (Fig. 9.6). Nail dysplasia is seen in the nail-patella syndrome. Other syndromes have characteristic finger deformities such as the "hitchhiker's" thumb in diastrophic dysplasia.

Palpation

Palpation is most important if the child complains of pain. Exact localization of the point of maximum tenderness is very important in establishing the cause of pain. This is most feasible about the elbow, wrist (Fig.9.7), and hand, where the bone and joints are subcutaneous.

Range of Motion

Describe the motion of the neck in three planes. The normal child is able to flex the chin to the chest. Lateral head tilt should allow the ear to touch the shoulder. Normal head rotation allows about 90° of motion to the right and left. Assess forearm rotation with the elbow flexed to a right angle. Supination and pronation are each about 90° in the normal child.

Joint Laxity

The upper limb is readily examined to assess joint laxity. Assess the elbow, wrist, and fingers for the ability to hyperextend (Fig. 9.8).

Pain

Pain is usually due to trauma (Fig. 9.9), infection, or neoplasms (Fig. 9.10). Pain is often manifest by pseudoparalysis in the infant and young child. Localization of the site of tenderness is very helpful in narrowing the diagnostic possibilities and in deciding what should be studied radiographically. Sometimes, a bone scan is necessary, localize the problem.

Associations

Certain deformities of the upper extremity are often associated with specific syndromes (Figs. 9.12–9.14). Examples include nail dysplasia in nail-patella syndrome and the various conditions associated with radial and ulnar deficiencies and syndactyly. Carefully examine the whole child. Look for dysmorphic features, and shortness of stature, and assess the child's general health. Inquire about medical problems in the family. Certain findings indicate the need for additional studies. For example, the finding of torticollis is an indication for a radiograph of the pelvis to rule out hip dysplasia. The finding of radial dysplasia is an indication for a hematologic and cardiac evaluation.

Unique Upper Limb Conditions

Chronic clavicular osteomyelitis The response of the clavicle to infection is unique (Fig. 9.11). The clavicle becomes enlarged, sclerotic, and tender suggesting a neoplastic origin. Evaluate with CT scans or MRI to establish the primary focus of the infection. Drain, culture, and biopsy all suspicious portions of the lesion.

Reflex sympathetic dystrophy may occur in the upper extremities of children and adolescents. The condition occurs most commonly in adolescent girls who complain of pain, stiffness, and limited function. Radiographs often show osteopenia and bone scans may show normal, increased, or decreased uptake. See page 58 for a more detailed discription.

References

1997 Osteochondral lesions in the radiocapitellar joint in the skeletally immature: radiographic, MRI, and arthroscopic findings in 13 consecutive cases. Janarv PM, Hesser U, Hirsch G. JPO 17:311

1997 Acute staphylococcal osteomyelitis of the clavicle. Lowden CM, Walsh SJ. JPO 17:467

1995 Septic arthritis of the shoulder during the first 18 months of life. Lejman T, et al. JPO 15:172

1993 Reflex sympathetic dystrophy in children: an orthopedic perspective. Stanton RP, et al. Orthopedics 16:773

1992 Reflex sympathetic dystrophy in children. Clinical characteristics and follow-up of seventy patients. Wilder RT, et al. JBJS 74A:910

1990 Condensing osteitis of the clavicle: does it exist? Jones MW, et al. JBJS 72B:464

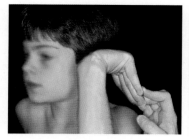

Fig. 9.8 Joint laxity. Joint laxity is commonly assessed in the upper limb.

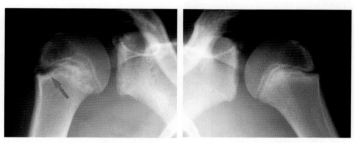

Fig. 9.9 Overuse syndrome shoulder. Note the widening and scolerosis adjacent to the proximal humeral epiphysis in this baseball pitcher.

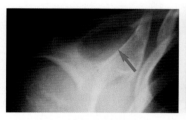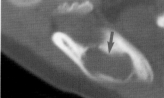

Fig. 9.10 Eosinophilic granuloma. These lesions present in unusual locations such as the scapula (red arrows). They typically cause pain.

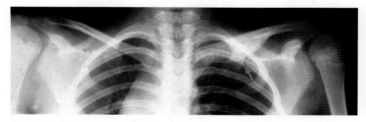

Fig. 9.11 chronic osteomyelitis of the clavicle. Note the swelling and sclerosis of the clavicle (arrow). A low-grade staphylococcal infection was found.

Syndrome	Comment
Craniosynostosis	Form associated with radial aplasia
Fanconi anemia	Bone, skin, hematologic defects
Holt-Oram	Bone and cardiovascular defects
Ladd	Bone and craniofacial
Nagar	Bone and craniofacial
Thrombocytopenia (Tar syndrome)	Associated with radial aplasia

Fig. 9.12 Syndromes associated with radial defects. These syndromes should be considered if radial defects are present.

Syndrome	Comment
Goltz	Bone, skin, eye, anus, retardation
Mammary aplasia	Associated with ulnar hypoplasia

Fig. 9.13 Syndromes associated with ulnar defects. These syndromes should be considered if an ulnar defect is present.

Syndromes with syndactyly

Apert
Carpenter
Noack
Pfeifer
Poland
Summit
Waardenburg
Oculodentodigital
Orofaciodigitial

Fig. 9.14 Syndromes associated with syndactyly.

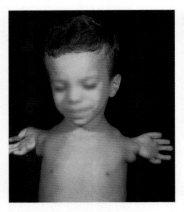

Fig. 9.15 Complete phocomelia. This child has bilateral deficiencies.

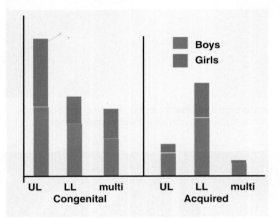

Fig. 9.16 Distribution of pediatric amputees. Distribution for girls (red) and boys (blue) for UL (upper limb), LL (lower limb), or multi (multiple levels) are shown in 1400 cases. From data of Krebs and Fishman (1984).

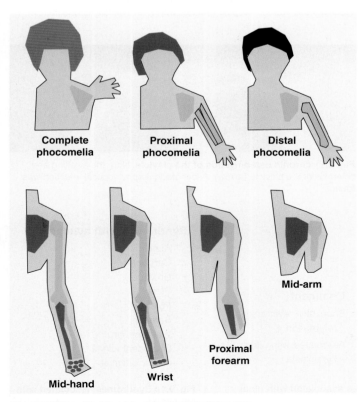

Fig. 9.17 Classification of upper limb deficiencies.

Upper Limb Deficiencies

Upper limb deficiencies may be due to malformations (Fig. 9.15) or disruptions, such as amnionic bands from trauma or result from resections of malignant tumors.

Frequency

Limb deficiencies are most common in the lower limb and in boys (Fig. 9.16). Proximal transverse forearm amputations are the most common congenital upper limb deficiency.

Classification

Classify the congenital limb deficiencies as either intercalary or transverse (Fig. 9.17) and the segmental defect as either longitudinal or transverse. This differentiation has additional diagnostic implications. For example, nearly 90% of children with longitudinal defects of the radius have additional malformations, whereas less than a third of those with transverse defects of the radius have other similiar defects.

Evaluation

Although the diagnosis can usually be made by the physical examination, make radiographs to document and classify the deficiency.

Screening examination is necessary to identify other abnormalities such as radial head dislocations or radioulnar synostoses.

Family situation should be evaluated carefully. Make certain that counseling is available for parents who are having difficulty dealing with the grief and guilt common in parents of limb deficient children. Make a special effort to develop a warm and supportive relationship with the family as management is often difficult. Good rapport improves the child's compliance with treatment and the parent's acceptance of recommendations for management.

Management Principles

The following principles may be helpful in planning management.

Early prosthesthetic fitting is contoversial Some physicians believe that covering the limb with a prosthesis prevents sensory feedback and slows development of bimanual function. Others recommend the fitting of a passive prosthesis between 3 and 6 months of age to promote the development of a more normal self-image by the infant.

First prosthesis is usually passive Convert to an active prosthesis based on the infant's developmental age.

Acceptance is usually less for upper than for lower limb prostheses. The lack of sensibility and fine movement control makes upper limb prostheses less useful than those for the lower limb. Children are most likely to accept an upper limb prosthesis when a specific functional need is recognized. This awareness usually occurs at about 8 years of age.

Myoelectric power is inherently attractive to parents. Because these electrically powered limbs are expensive and difficult to maintain, longterm acceptance is poorer than for the simpler, body powered prostheses.

Congenital and acquired amputations are different. Congenital amputees are more accepting of their disability, develop techniques of compensation, and have fewer painful stumps than those with acquired deficiencies.

Modify prosthesis to facilitate activities of daily living. Make available an experienced occupational therapist to access the child's needs, and make recommendations for modifications that inhance selfcare.

Family support groups are extremely valuable for both the parents and the child. Most childhood amputee clinics have ready access to these support groups and can help families make the necessary contacts.

Allow child natural adaptations Such adaptations are usually practical, effective, and energy efficient (Fig. 9.18).

Replace prosthesis when destroyed, causes discomfort, or becomes suboptimally functional.

Discarding of prosthetics is most common when deficiencies are extensive, prosthetic devices are complex in design, and natural adaptations without a prosthesis are effective.

Operative Procedures

Procedures have limited indications.

Krukenberg procedure separates the radius and ulna to allow grasp with sensibility (Fig. 9.19). The outcome is usually functionally good but cosmetically poor. The procedure is appropriate for blind children who cannot visually position items in their prosthetic hands or hooks or for other children with special needs.

Revisions for overgrowth may be necessary in both congenital and acquired transdiaphyseal amputations (Fig. 9.20).

Prosthetic Options

Terminal devices options include several alternatives.

CAPP (child amputee prosthetic project) includes a closing spring and a frictional resilient covering that enhances control.

Hooks with elastic closures and plastic covering are durable and can be fitted with body-powered opening mechanisms.

Cosmetic hands may be passive, body powered, or myoelectrically controlled.

Powering devices include several options:

Body power is commonly used for both opening of a terminal device and elbow flexion (Fig. 9.21).

Myoelectric power may be provided by single or double electrodes placed over flexor or extensor muscles. Single controls are usually applied during the second year with sensors placed over extensor muscles to activate the opening device. The terminal device stays open as long as the muscle is contracted. A second sensor over the flexors may be applied about age 3 for active flexion.

Upper Limb Deficiencies Consultants

Marybeth Ezaki

Hugh Watts, e-mail: hwatts@ucla.edu

References

2000 Classification of congenital anomalies of the upper limb. Luijsterburg AJ, et al. J Hand Surg [Br] 25:3

2000 The principles of management of congenital anomalies of the upper limb. Watson S. Arch Dis Child 83:10

1997 Scoliosis and trunk asymmetry in upper limb transverse dysmelia. Samuelsson L, Hermansson LL, Noren L. JPO 17:769

1996 Rehabilitation in limb deficiency. 2. The pediatric amputee. Jain S. Arch Phys Med Rehabil 77:S9-13

1995 The prevalence of phantom sensation and pain in pediatric amputees. Krane EJ, Heller LB. J Pain Symptom Manage 10:21

1995 Is body powered operation of upper limb prostheses feasible for young limb deficient children? Shaperman J, et al. Prosthet Orthot Int 19:165

1995 Congenital limb anomalies and amputees in Tayside, Scotland 1965-1994. Stewart CP, Jain AS. Prosthet Orthot Int 19:148

1992 Upper limb deficiencies and associated malformations: a population-based study. Froster UG, Baird PA. Am J Med Genet 44:767

1992 The social and economic outcome after upper limb amputation. Kejlaa GH. Prosthet Orthot Int 16:25

1991 The prosthetic treatment of upper limb deficiency. Curran B, Hambrey R. Prosthet Orthot Int 15:82

1991 3-S prosthesis: a preliminary report. Madigan RR, Fillauer KD. JPO 11:112

1986 Management of the upper-limb-deficient child with a powered prosthetic device. Glynn MK, et al. CO 209:202

1984 Characteristics of the child amputee population. Krebs DE, Fishman S. JPO 4:89

1983 A long-term review of children with congenital and acquired upper limb deficiency. Scotland TR, Galway HR. JBJS 65B:346

1982 Congenital anomalies of the upper limb among the Chinese population in Hong Kong. Leung PC, Chan KM, Cheng JC. J Hand Surg 7A:563

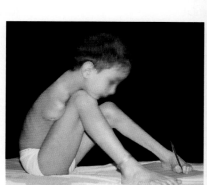
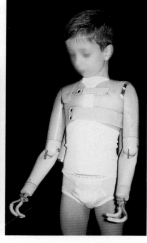

Fig. 9.18 Upper limb amelia. These children become surprisingly proficient in using the feet to duplicate hand function. The prosthetic fitting was marginally successful.

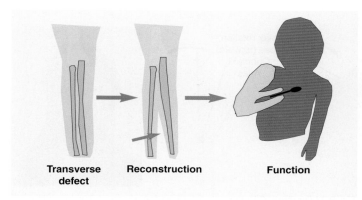

Transverse defect Reconstruction Function

Fig. 9.19 Krukenberg reconstruction. This separation of the distal radius and ulna (red arrow) and repositioning of forearm muscles provides the child with a functional grasp with sensibility.

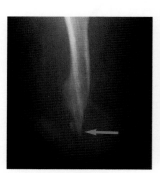
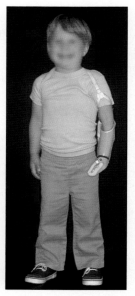

Fig. 9.20 Diaphyseal overgrowth. This is a complication of through-bone amputations.

Fig. 9.21 Upper limb prosthesis. The artificial limb aids function, especially for tasks that are bimanual.

Category	Comments
Muscular torticollis	Most common
Acute torticollis	Acute, resolves
Occipital cervical bony defects	Hemivertebrae
Miscellaneous	Neurogenic–tumors inflammatory Traumatic Ocular: strabismus Hysterical Idiopathic: rotatory displacement

Fig. 9.22 Causes of torticollis. The causes are many, but the vast majority of torticollis are due to disorders listed in the top three categories.

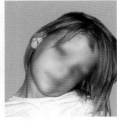

Fig. 9.23 Acute torticollis. This form of torticollis develops suddenly in a previously normal child. Usually the deformity resolves spontaneously in a day or two.

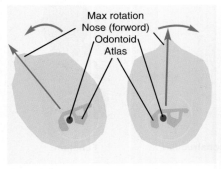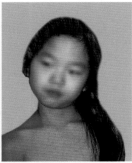

Fig. 9.24 Dynamic CT scans in rotatory displacement. Maximum lateral rotation (blue arrows) CT scans show 45° rotation to the left but no rotation to the right. Note that the asymmetric relationship of the CI and C2 (yellow circle) remains unchanged. Based on Phillips and Hensinger (1989).

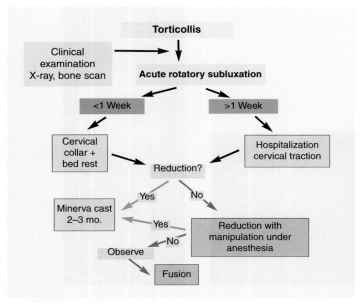

Fig. 9.25 Management of rotatory subluxation. Based on Phillips and Hensinger (1989).

Torticollis

Torticollis, or *wryneck* includes a variety of conditions, that require different management (Fig. 9.22).

Acute Torticollis

Acute torticollis, or wryneck, is relatively common, may occur spontaneously, follow minimal trauma, or occur after an upper respiratory infection. Why the head tilts is uncertain. The tilt may be due to muscle spasm secondary to cervical lymphadenitis or possibly due to a minor subluxation of the cervical vertebrae.

Clinical features Acute torticollis causes the head to tilt, rotate to one side (Fig. 9.23) and become fixed. Radiographs of the cervical spine are difficult to assess because of the lateral flexion and rotation. Laboratory studies are normal.

Manage by immobilizing the neck with a folded towel and encourage rest. Early management is usually provided by the primary care physician. In most children, acute torticollis resolves within 24 hours. If the deformity persists longer than 24–48 hours, be more concerned and manage as rotatory displacement.

Rotatory Displacement

Persistence of acute torticollis is called *rotatory displacement* or *rotatory subluxation*. Treat rotatory displacement early to avoid permanent fixation and residual deformity.

Evaluate Image with conventional and dynamic CT scans. Look for a loss of the ability to rotate the head fully in both directions. In addition, note the relationship between C1 and C2. Fixation of this relationship throughout the arc of rotation is consistent with the diagnosis of rotatory displacement (Fig. 9.24).

Manage First apply traction. If early, head-halter traction is appropriate. Later, halo traction may be required. For displacements that persist beyond a month, repositioning and fusion of C1–2 may be necessary (Fig. 9.25).

Chronic Nonmuscular Torticollis

About 20% of children with chronic torticollis are due to nonmuscular causes. Radiographs may show conditions such as Klippel-Feil anomaly or hemivertebrae. If radiographs are negative and the sternocleidomastoid muscle not contracted, consider an ocular etiology. Refer to an opthalmologist for evaluation. Consider the other conditions that may cause torticollis, such as neonatal brachial plexus palsies and spinal cord tumors.

Consultant Robert Hensinger

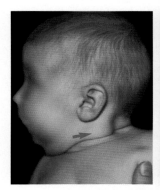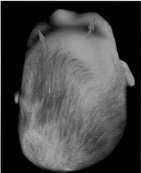

Fig. 9.26 Muscular torticollis and plagiocephaly. The mass (red arrow) develops in early infancy and disappears spontaneously over a period of several months. The plagiocephaly (blue arrows) may persist longer.

Muscular Torticollis

Muscular torticollis is relatively common and presents in two age groups.

Infantile muscular torticollis The infant (Fig. 9.27) is first seen because of a head tilt. Sometimes a history of a breech delivery is given and a firm tumor of the sternocleidomastoid muscle is palpated. Usually only a head tilt and limited neck motion due to a contracture of the muscle are found. Plagiocephaly (asymmetrical head) may be present (Figs. 9.26 and 9.28).

Be certain to rule out developmental hip dysplasia. Even if the hip examination is negative, evaluate the hip by either ultrasound if the infant is seen in the neonatal period or by a single AP radiograph of the pelvis if the infant is older than about 10 weeks of age.

Infantile torticollis resolves spontaneously in about 90% of cases. The value of physical therapy by stretching is uncertain (Fig. 9.27). Of those that persist, operative correction may be necessary. Delay correction until about 3 years of age. Rarely plagiocephaly persists and is a cosmetic problem (Fig. 9.28).

Juvenile muscular torticollis Sometimes muscular torticollis appears to develop during childhood (Fig. 9.29). In this juvenile type, usually both heads of the muscles are contracted causing the head tilt and limiting neck motion. Usually this type of torticollis is permanent and often requires operative correction.

Operative correction Bipolar release (Fig. 9.30) is the most effective procedure for correction of both infantile and juvenile forms of muscular torticollis. See page 410 for details the procedure.

References

2000 Surgical treatment of muscular torticollis for patients above 6 years of age. Chen CE and JY Ko. Arch Orthop Trauma Surg 120:1491

2000 The clinical presentation and outcome of treatment of congenital muscular torticollis in infants--a study of 1,086 cases. Cheng JC, et al. J Pediatr Surg 35:1091

2000 Long-term developmental outcomes in patients with deformational plagiocephaly. Miller RI, Clarren SK. Pediatrics 105:E26

1998 Torticollis and hip dislocation. Walsh JJ, Morrissy RT. JPO 18:219

1996 The prevalence of nonmuscular causes of torticollis in children. Ballock RT, Song KM. JPO 16:500

1996 Difficulties in diagnosing intrinsic spinal cord tumours. Parker AP, Robinson RO, Bullock P. Arch Dis Child 75:204

1996 Torticollis secondary to ocular pathology. Williams CR, et al. JBJS 78B:620

1993 Congenital muscular torticollis: sequela of intrauterine or perinatal compartment syndrome. Davids JR, Wenger DR, Mubarak SJ. JPO 13:141

1989 Torticollis due to a combination of sternomastoid contracture and congenital vertebral anomalies. Brougham DI, et al. JBJS 71B:404

1989 The management of rotatory atlanto-axial subluxation in children. Phillips WA, Hensinger RN. JBJS 71A:664

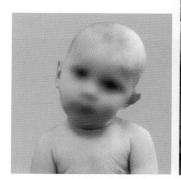
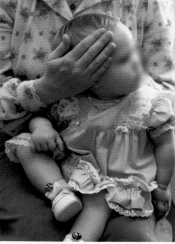

Fig. 9.27 Muscular Torticollis. This is the most common neck problem in childhood. Torticollis is usually seen first in the infant (left). Some advocate treatment by stretching (right), but its value is uncertain.

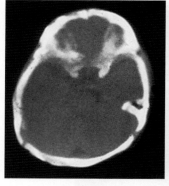
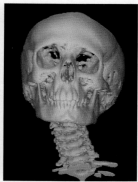

Fig. 9.28 Plagiocephaly torticollis. Cranial deformity is readily shown by CT scans. 3D reconstructions provide graphic documentation of the extent of the deformity.

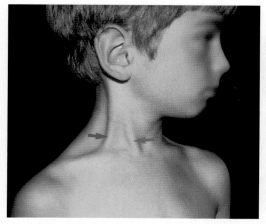

Fig. 9.29 Sternocleidomastoid contracture. Both the clavicular origin (red arrow) and sternal origin (blue arrow) are contracted.

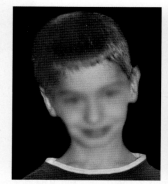
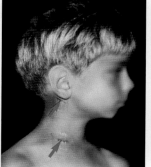
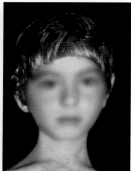

Fig. 9.30 Torticollis release. This 9-year-old with torticollis (left) had a bipolar release (arrows). Note the improvement in head tilt and neck motion followed surgery (right).

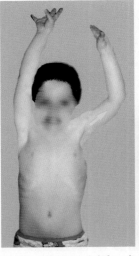
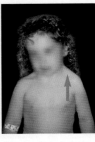
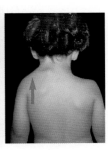

Fig. 9.31 Sprengel deformity. Congenital elevation of the scapula causes a shoulder deformity (red arrows) that cannot be hidden by clothing. Some loss of abduction is a common mild disability (yellow arrow).

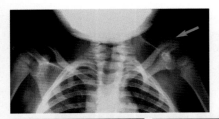
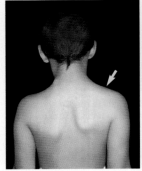
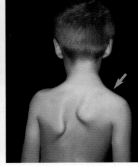

Fig. 9.32 Spectrum of severity. Disability is proportional to the deformity. Shoulder elevation may be severe (red arrow), moderate (yellow arrow), or mild (green arrow).

Sprengel Deformity

Sprengel deformity is a congenital elevation of the scapula (Fig. 9.31). The deformity results from a failure of migration of mesenchyme during the second fetal month.

Clinical Features

The deformity varies in severity (Fig. 9.32), is usually unilateral, and is associated with other abnormalities in 70% of cases. These associated abnormalities include absent or hypoplastic parascapular musculature, abnormalities in the cervicothoracic vertebrae or thoracic rib cage, presence of an omovertebral bone, limited shoulder abduction and multidirectional shoulder instability. Because of restricted scapulothoracic motion, most shoulder motion occurs through the glenohumeral joint.

Management

When the deformity is mild, correction is not appropriate because the operative scar is often more unsightly than the deformity. For moderate deformity, excise the superior pole of the scapula. For severe deformity repositioning of the scapula is necessary. This repositioning requires an extensive soft tissue release, caudad repositioning of the scapula and sometimes excision of the superior portion of the scapula. Perform the correction in early childhood when the scapula is most mobile. This mobility allows maximum correction with the least risk of complications. For correction, several procedures have been described. The Woodward procedure is most widely used.

Green procedure All muscular attachments to the scapula are freed, the omovertebral band is divided, and the scapula is rotated, moved caudad to a more normal position and sutured into a pocket of the latissimus dorsi. In the original description, traction was applied by a wire attached to the scapula to hold it in the corrected position.

Klisic procedure includes performing an osteotomy of the clavicle, extensive muscle releases, excision of the superior scapular margin, and securing the repositioned scapula with sutures to a vertebral spinous process and rib with absorbable sutures (Fig. 9.33).

Woodward procedure exposure is made through a midline incision, the origins of the trapezius and rhomboid muscles are released, the omovertebral bone is excised, and the scapula repositioned (Fig. 9.34). Modifications include excising the superior and medial margins of the scapula.

References

1996 Modified Woodward procedure for Sprengel deformity of the shoulder: long-term results. Borges JL, et al. JPO 16:508
1995 Sprengel's deformity associated with multidirectional shoulder instability. Hamner DL, Hall JE. JPO 15:641
1990 Sprengel deformity. Leibovic SJ, Ehrlich MG, Zaleske DJ. JBJS 72A:192
1981 Relocation of congenitally elevated scapula. Klisic P, et al. JPO 1:43

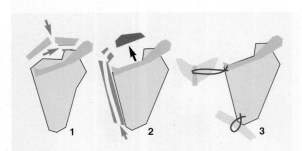

Fig. 9.33 Klisic procedure. 1. The clavicle is divided (blue arrow). 2. The superior pole of the scapula is removed (black arrow) and the muscles are released (red arrows). 3. The repositioned scapula is sutured to the rib and transverse processes (blue sutures). Based on Klisic (1981).

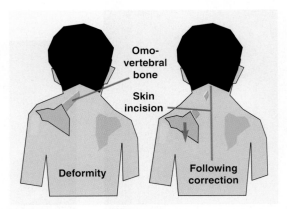

Fig. 9.34 Woodward procedure. Through a midline incision, excise the omovertebral bone, release the soft tissue attachments, and reposition the scapula at a more distal location.

Neonatal Brachial Plexus Palsy

Neonatal palsy (Fig. 9.35) is a traction injury to the brachial plexus that usually occurs during delivery. Risk factors include shoulder or fetal dystocia, obesity, and prolonged labor. The incidence of these injuries has declined due to improved obstetrical practices.

Classification

Severity is determined by the nature and extent of the lesion (Fig. 9.36). Mild lesions are stretch injuries of C5–C6. Severe injuries involve avulsion of nerve roots over multiple levels down to T1. Classically three types of injuries have been described (Fig. 9.37).

Natural History

Recovery depends upon severity. Overall, up to 90% spontaneously completely resolve during the first year. Most improvement occuring in the first 3 months. Failure of recovery of elbow flexion by 3 months or more accurately, a failure of recovery of elbow flexion, wrist, and digital extension by 4 months correlates with a poorer prognosis. Common residual disabilities include loss of external rotation and abduction (Fig. 9.38).

Management

Management may be divided into 4 types.

Range of motion may be helpful to maintain joint mobility. Instruct parents how to gently range joints with each diaper change.

Brachial plexus repair is controversial. Consider repair for infants with early evidence of severe injuries and those without recovery of elbow flexion by 3 months. Evaluate by EMG, nerve conduction, myelography, and CT scans. Root avulsions cannot be repaired. More distal lesions may be repaired or grafted using microsurgical techniques. Results of repairs are unpredictable and should not compromise later orthopedic reconstructive procedures.

Muscle procedures are indicated for children with disabling adduction and internal rotation contractures. The most common procedure is the Sever-L'Episcopo transfer. This procedure includes release of the pectoralis major, subscapularis, and joint capsule if contracted. The teres major and latissimus dorsi tendons are transferred from the anteromedial to the posterolateral aspect of the humerus. Axillary nerve palsy is a potential complication. This procedure is usually performed in early childhood.

Rotational humeral osteotomy is indicated for an internal rotation deformity that limits function. Delay the procedure until mid or late childhood. Rotate the humerus to provide about equal internal and external rotation. Results are predictable, correction is usually permanent, and complications are infrequent.

Should Dislocation

Dislocation of the glenohumeral joint may develop in children with brachial plexus birth palsy as early as 3 months of age. Manage by release of the insertions of the pectoralis major, latissimus dorsi, and teres major followed by a closed reduction of the glenohumeral joint. Transfer the latissimus dorsi and the teres major to the rotator cuff.

Consultant Mark Hoffer, e-mail: sribas@laoh.ucla.edu

References

2000 Emerging concepts in the pathophysiology of recovery from neonatal brachial plexus injury. Noetzel MJ, Wolpaw JR. Neurology 55:5

1999 Tendon transfers about the shoulder and elbow in obstetrical brachial plexus palsy. Bennett JB, Allan CH. JBJS 81A:1612

1998 Closed reduction and tendon transfer for treatment of dislocation of the glenohumeral joint secondary to brachial plexus birth palsy. Hoffer MM, Phipps GJ. JBJS 80A:997

1996 Obstetric brachial plexus palsy. Lindell-Iwan HL, Partanen VS, Makkonen ML. JPO-b 5:210

1995 Functional improvement with the Sever L'Episcopo procedure. Nualart L, Cassis N, Ochoa R. JPO 15:637

1994 The natural history of obstetrical brachial plexus palsy. Michelow BJ, et al. Plast Reconstr Surg 93:675

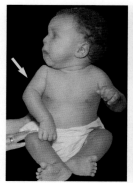
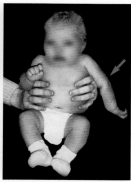

Fig. 9.35 Neonatal palsies. These infants show moderate (yellow arrow) and severe (red arrow) palsies.

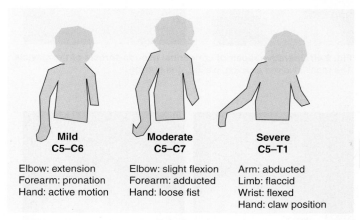

Mild C5–C6	Moderate C5–C7	Severe C5–T1
Elbow: extension	Elbow: slight flexion	Arm: abducted
Forearm: pronation	Forearm: adducted	Limb: flaccid
Hand: active motion	Hand: loose fist	Wrist: flexed
		Hand: claw position

Fig. 9.36 Neonatal palsy classification of severity. Early classification is based on physical position and function. Based on Lidell-Iwan, et al. (1996).

Level	Type	Name
C4, C5, C6	Type I	Erb's palsy
Entire plexus	Type II	Erb-Duchenne-Klumpke
C7, T1	Type III	Klumpke palsy

Fig. 9.37 Classical typing. These palsies are classified by level.

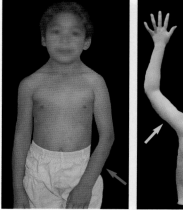
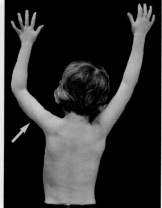

Fig. 9.38 Residual deformites in neonatal palsy. Medial rotation (red arrow) and limited abduction (yellow arrow) are typical deformities that limit function.

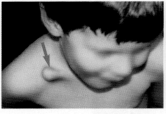

Fig. 9.39 Congenital pseudarthrosis of the clavicle. This pseudarthrosis produced an unsightly lump on the shoulder (red arrow). Note the gap between the ends of the pseudarthrosis (yellow arrows). The defect was operatively corrected.

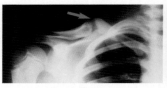

Fig. 9.40 Operative repair of congenital pseudarthrosis of the clavicle. The repair involved excision, plating, and grafting.

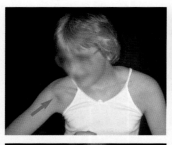

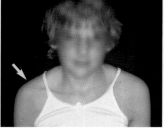

Fig. 9.41 Habitual posterior dislocation of the shoulder. This girl is able to voluntarily dislocate her right shoulder (red arrows). Voluntary reduction occurs easily (yellow arrow).

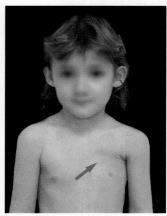

Fig. 9.42 Poland syndrome. Note the deficiency in the pectoralis major muscle (arrow).

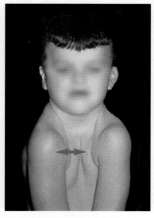

Fig. 9.43 Cleidocranial dysostosis. Absent clavicles allow this boy's shoulders to narrow.

Shoulder

Congenital Pseudarthrosis of the Clavicle

Congenital pseudarthrosis of the clavicle is a rare defect of uncertain cause. The defect may be secondary to a failure of coalescence of the two ossification centers of the clavicle or to erosion of the clavicle from pulsation of the subclavian artery. The lesion practically always occurs on the right side.

Clinical features The pseudarthrosis produces a prominence over the clavicle (Fig. 9.39), and narrowing and slight weakness of the shoulder. Radiographs show a midclavicular defect. Rarely thoracic outlet syndrome is an associated problem. Long-term studies show little functional but some cosmetic disability.

Management Reasonable management options include either accepting or repairing the deformity (Fig. 9.40). Operative repair eliminates the prominence and improves shoulder symmetry but does leave a surgical scar. This scar may be mimized by positioning the incision below the clavicle, limiting its length, and utilizing a subcuticular closure technique.

Early operative correction may be performed in infancy or early childhood by resecting the sclerotic bone ends, careful dissection and preservation of the periosteal sleeve to maintain continuity, and approximating the bone ends using heavy absorbable sutures. No internal fixation or grafting is necessary. Remodeling corrects bony irregularity.

Late operative correction in mid or late childhood usually requires plate fixation and autogenous bone grafting to promote union.

Shoulder Dislocation or Subluxation

Congenital dislocations are very rare. Developmental dislocations may occur with neonatal brachial plexus palsies, or develop spontaneously during childhood. Most dislocations are traumatic.

Traumatic anterior dislocation in children usually recurs regardless of the initial treatment. Prepare the patient and parent for the probability that operative repair will be required.

Recurrent posterior dislocation may occur with minimal trauma or develop spontaneously. If the deformity causes a significant disability, operative stabilization with a bone block or glenoplasty and capsulorraphy may be necessary.

Habitual dislocation occurs in loose-jointed older children or adolescents. One or both shoulders can be voluntarily subluxate or dislocate (Fig. 9.41). Management is difficult. Shoulder exercise, avoidance of voluntary displacement, and counseling maybe helpful. The child should be helped to find a more appropriate method of getting attention. Resolution usually occurs with time. Operative procedures may be necessary for persisting deformity but recurrence poses a significant problem. The condition causes little long-term disability.

Poland Syndrome

This syndrome includes absence of the pectoralis major (Fig. 9.42) and usually finger or forearm abnormalities. The disability is cosmetic, and chest-wall and breast reconstructions is often appropriate.

Cleidocranial Dysostosis

This rare congenital defect is transmitted as a dominant trait. The clavicles are so mobile that they may be approximated (Fig. 9.43). In others the clavicles are simply dysplastic. Associated findings include a large head with a small face, drooping shoulders, coxa vara, narrow chest, and sometimes recurrent shoulder or elbow dislocations. Disability is minimal.

References

2000 Shoulder dislocations in the young patient. Cleeman E, Flatow EL. Orthop Clin North Am 31:217

1997 Recurrent posterior shoulder dislocation in children: the results of surgical management. Kawam M, Sinclair J, Letts M. JPO 17:533

1994 Voluntary subluxation of the shoulder in children. A long-term follow-up study of 36 shoulders. Huber H, Gerber C. JBJS 76B:118

1994 The natural history of congenital pseudarthrosis of the clavicle. Shalom A, Khermosh O, Wientroub S. JBJS 76B:846

1992 The fate of traumatic anterior dislocation of the shoulder in children. Marans HJ, et al. JBJS 74A:1242

Elbow

Panner Disease

This is an osteochondritis of the capitellum that develops spontaneously during late childhood (Fig. 9.44). Clinical features include elbow pain, limitation of motion, and tenderness over the capitellum. Over a period of months, the capitellum fragments and then spontaneously reossifies. The process is usually benign and complete recovery occurs with time. Treatment is seldom necessary.

Adolescent Capitellar Osteochondritis Dissecans

This avascular necrosis of the capitellum is often secondary to repetitive trauma and causes articular damage and often residual long-term disability (Fig. 9.45).

Clinical findings include a history of stiffness, pain, and catching or locking. Examination usually demonstrates a decreased elbow motion and lateral tenderness. Radiography often shows loose articular fragments, flattening of the humeral capitellum, and subchondral cysts. MRI and arthroscopic examination may be helpful. Additional lesions of the radial head may be present.

Management depends upon the clinical findings. Remove loose fragments. The value of debridement and drilling is uncertain. Limit activities until healing is complete.

Prognosis Disability is common in adult life with about half showing join stiffness and degenerative changes, and enlargement of the radial head.

Recurrent Elbow Dislocation

Recurrent dislocations may be secondary to congenital hyperlaxity as occurs in Ehlers Danlos syndrome, a sequela from nonunion of a medial epicondylar fracture or due to residual instability from a previous dislocation. Evaluate with radiography, MRI, and possibly arthroscopy. Tailor operative repair based on the pathology.

Elbow Flexion Contracture

Contractures may be congenital as occurs with some forms of arthrogryposis, or acquired from burn contractures or elbow trauma with articular damage. Individualize management. Posttraumatic contractures may be improved by operative release. Release the anterior and posterior capsules and remove obstacles to motion, and provide a postoperative range of motion and splinting program.

Cubitus Varus Deformity

This deformity is usually due to a malunited supracondylar fracture. When severe, correct with a valgus osteotomy of the distal humerus (Fig. 9.46).

References

2000 Avascular necrosis of the radial head in children. Young S, Letts M, Jarvis J. JPO 20:15

1997 Osteochondral lesions in the radiocapitellar joint in the skeletally immature: radiographic, MRI, and arthroscopic findings in 13 consecutive cases. Janarv PM, Hesser U, Hirsch G. JPO 17:311

1997 Osteochondritis dissecans as a cause of developmental dislocation of the radial head. Klekamp J, Green NE, Mencio GA. CO 338:36

1995 Panner's disease: X-ray, MR imaging findings and review of the literature. Stoane JM, et al. Comput Med Imaging Graph 19:473

1994 Surgical release of elbow-capsular contracture in pediatric patients. Mih AD, Wolf FG. JPO 14:458

1993 Osteochondritis dissecans of the humeral capitellum in children. Jawish R, et al. Eur J Pediatr Surg 3:397

1992 Osteochondritis dissecans of the elbow. A long-term follow-up study. Bauer M, et al. CO 284:156

1992 Excision of the radial head for congenital dislocation. Campbell CC, Waters PM, Emans JB. JBJS 74A:726

1991 Recurrent dislocation of the elbow in a child: case report and review of the literature. Beaty JH, Donati NL. JPO 11:392

1990 Recurrent dislocation of the elbow. Doria A, et al. Int Orthop 14:41

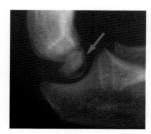

Fig. 9.44 Panner disease. This 8-year-old has pain and tenderness over the capitellum.

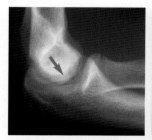
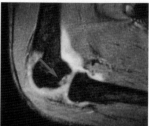

Fig. 9.45 Osteochondritis of the capitellum. When this occurs in the adolescent, the problem is more serious and may cause limitation of motion. Removal of loose bodies is commonly necessary.

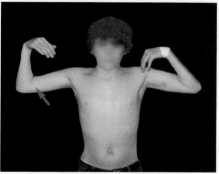

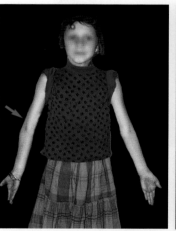
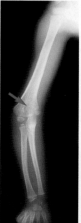

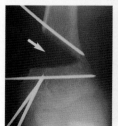
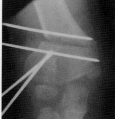
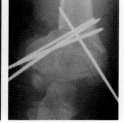

Fig. 9.46 Cubitus varus with operative correction. This girl has cubitus varus (red arrows) secondary to malunion from a supracondylar fracture. This was corrected with a valgus osteotomy (yellow arrow).

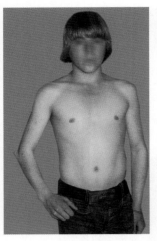

Fig. 9.47. Congenital dislocation of the radial head. This 15-year-old boy has disability from this prominent radial head. The radial head was excised.

Feature	Traumatic	Congenital
Trauma history	Yes	No
Associated defects	No	Often
Direction	Anterior	Posterior
Radial head	Concave end	Round end
Capitellum	Normal	Hypoplastic
Ulna	Normal	Convex

Fig. 9.48 Differentiating congenital and traumatic radial head dislocation. The differentiation can usually be made by the radiographic appearance of the elbow.

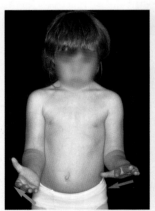

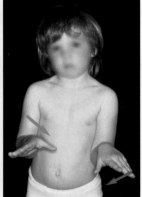

Fig. 9.49 Radioulnar synostosis limiting forearm rotation. The left forearm is fixed in pronation (red arrows). The right forearm rotates freely (green arrows). The synostosis is proximal in location (yellow arrow).

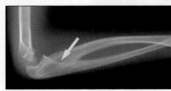

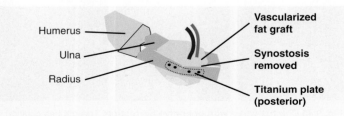

Humerus
Ulna
Radius

Vascularized fat graft

Synostosis removed

Titanium plate (posterior)

Fig. 9.50 Mobilization of radioulnar synostosis. This technique utilizes a free vascularized fascio-fat graft. Based on Kanaya and Ibaraki (1998).

Forearm

Nontraumatic Radial Head Dislocation or Subluxation

The radial head dislocations may be congenital or develop gradually during infancy and childhood. Congenital dislocations are often associated with other defects.

Subluxation or dislocation limits forearm roation and produces a palpable prominence over the displaced radial head (Fig. 9.47). Once dislocated the radial head becomes progressively more prominent with growth. The radial head dislocation causes shortening of the radial side of the forearm, making the ulna more prominent at the wrist. Differentiate congenital and traumatic dislocations (Fig. 9.48) as the management is different. Posterior dislocations are nearly always congenital. Congenital anterior dislocations are usually associated with other congenital defects.

Reduction of the nontraumatic radial head displacement has not been successful. If the radial head becomes unacceptably prominent or painful, excision may be necessary. When possible delay excision until the end of growth. Excision may improve motion and reduce discomfort.

Radioulnar Synostosis

Radioulnar synostosis is usually congenital and occurs in the proximal forearm (Fig. 9.49). Synostoses may be unilateral or bilateral, complete or incomplete, and are usually an isolated defect. Rarely synosteses are familial. Sometimes synostoses develop after fractures of the proximal forearm.

Evaluation The defect may be found during infancy if a screening examination is performed. More often, the defect becomes apparent during early childhood when the loss of forearm rotation is recognized. The position of forearm rotation is variable and determines the degree of disability.

Management is determined by the position of fixation. If rotation is fixed in a relatively neutral position, no treatment is required.

Rotational osteotomy is indicated if the forearm is fixed in more than about 45° of pronation or supination. Correct by a distal osteoclasis or subperiosteal osteotomy and immobilize in a cast with the forearm positioned in neutral or slight pronation.

Vascularized fat graft has been reported to be successful as an interposition tissue following resection of the synostoses in preventing recurrence (Fig. 9.50). Most other techniques of repair have been unsuccessful.

Osteochondromata

Multiple osteochondromata often involve the forearm and often occur at the wrist (Fig. 9.51).

Clinical features Distal lesions of the ulna cause progressive shortening, bowing of the radius and/or ulna, increased ulnar tilt of the distal radial epiphysis, ulnar deviation of the hand, progressive ulnarward translocation of the carpus, and subluxation/dislocation of the proximal radial head.

Management is controversial. Surveys of adults suggest that the deformity causes little disability and is well accepted. Others recommend early excision of the lesions and ulnar lengthening. Be aware that operative gain in motion is usually minimal, recurrence is common, and repeated procedures are often necessary.

References

1998 Mobilization of a congenital proximal radioulnar synostosis with use of a free vascularized fascio-fat graft. Kanaya F, Ibaraki K. JBJS 80A:1186

1997 Management of forearm deformity in multiple hereditary osteochondromatosis. Arms DM, et al. JPO 17:450

1995 A surgical technique of radioulnar osteoclasis to correct severe forearm rotation deformities. Lin HH, et al. JPO 15:53

1994 Deformities and problems of the forearm in children with multiple hereditary osteochondromata. Peterson HA. JPO 14:92

1992 Excision of the radial head for congenital dislocation. Campbell CC, Waters PM, Emans JB. JBJS 74A:726

1987 Ulnar nerve palsy following rotational osteotomy of congenital radioulnar synostosis. Hankin FM, et al. JPO 7:103

1986 Radioulnar synostosis following proximal radial fracture in child. Roy DR. Orthop Rev 15:89

Wrist

Wrist pain

Wrist pain may be due to a number of conditions that are unique to the wrist. These include nonunion of the radial styloid, unrecognized fractures or idiopathic avascular necrosis of the navicular, and overuse syndromes. Most gymnasts experience wrist pain due to overuse. Gymnasts most at risk are older children who are new and participate many hours per week.

Madelung Deformity

Madelung deformity is a defect in the volar, ulnar portion of the distal radial physis, producing a progressive deformity.

Clinical features The deformity when associated with short stature is often inherited as an autosomal dominant defect. Most cases are idiopathic and is most common in girls, usually first noticed during mid to late childhood (Fig. 9.52). The physeal defect causes radial shortening and a tilt of the epiphysis. The deformity is often bilateral but asymmetrical in severity.

Management If the deformity is mild, no treatment is necessary. For more severe deformities, operative correction is necessary to prevent progressive deformity characterized by a decreased radioulnar angle, lunate subluxation, and various degrees of dorsal subluxation of the distal ulnar.

During growth consider closure of the distal ulnar growth plate and resection and fat interposition of the radial physeal bridge.

End of growth consider a corrective osteotomy of the radius and shortening of the ulna. This often improves grip strength. increase range of motion, and reduces pain.

Kienböck Disease

Osteochondritis of the lunate is rare in children. It is thought to be due to repeated minor trauma together with negative ulnar variance (short ulna). The condition sometimes occurs in children with tension athetosis type of cerebral palsy, which combines increased tone and excessive motion. Clinical findings include localized pain and tenderness over the lunate, and typical radiographic features (Fig. 9.53). Manage with rest, NSAIDs, and time. Rarely, symptoms persist making necessary radial shortening to reduce stress on the lunate.

Wrist Ganglia

These cystic lesions occur in adjacently to the joints or tendon sheaths. They are most common on the dorsum of the wrist (Fig. 9.54). Ganglia may cause discomfort and an annoying prominence.

Manage First confirm the diagnosis by translumination or ultrasonography. One alternative is to aspirate the cyst. This confirms the diagnosis but temporarily resolves the symptoms as the cyst usually recurs. If the family and child are patient, allow the cyst to resolve with time. Most cysts will resolve spontaneously. Excise persistent or symptomatic cysts. Excision, especially of the volar ganglia, may be complex, and involve much deeper structures than one might expect. Recurrence is common after all methods of treatment.

References

2000 Long-term follow-up of surgical correction of Madelung's deformity with conservation of the distal radioulnar joint in teenagers. Salon A, Serra M, Pouliquen JC. J Hand Surg [Br] 25:22

1998 Osteotomy of the radius and ulna for the Madelung deformity. dos Reis FB, et al. JBJS 80B:817

1996 Factors associated with wrist pain in the young gymnast. Di Fiori JP, et al. Am J Sports Med 24:9

1993 Aetiology of Kienbock's disease based on a study of the condition among patients with cerebral palsy. Joji S, et al. J Hand Surg 18B:294

1992 Madelung deformity: surgical prophylaxis (physiolysis) during the late growth period by resection of the dyschondrosteosis lesion. Vickers D, Nielsen G J. Hand Surg Br 17: 401

1989 Kienbock's disease in an 8 year old boy. Hosking OR. Aust N Z J Surg 59:92

1989 The natural history of ganglia in children. Rosson JW, Walker G. JBJS 71B:707

1985 Ganglia in children. Satku K, Ganesh B. JPO 5:13

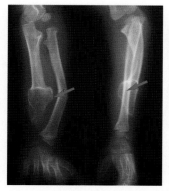

Fig. 9.51 Osteochondromata of the forearm. These are the typical deformities of the typical distal ulnar lesions.

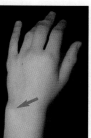

Fig. 9.52 Madelung deformity. This is more common in girls and produces limited wrist motion and prominence of the distal ulna (red arrow) and radial shortening (yellow arrow).

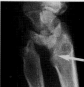

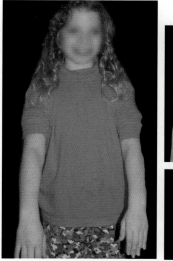

Fig. 9.53 Kienböck disease. This 7-year-old gymnast developed wrist pain. The sclerosis of the lunate is obvious (arrow). Usually this disease occurs in adolescence, producing pain and stiffness.

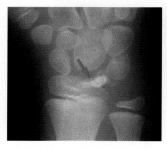

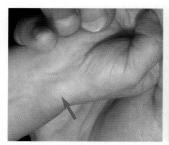

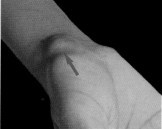

Fig. 9.54 Ganglia. These are the less common volar ganglia (blue arrows).

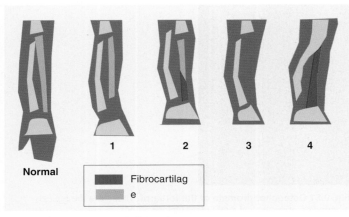

Normal

| Fibrocartilag e |

Fig. 9.55 Types of ulnar deficiencies.

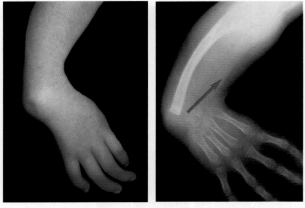

Fig. 9.56 Radial dysplasia. This deformity causes a serious cosmetic as well as functional disability. The hand shifts to the radial side (arrow).

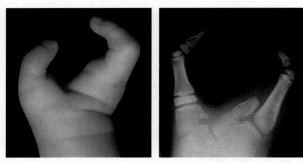

Fig. 9.57 Cleft hand deformities. The child also had deformites of the feet. The condition was familial.

Primary bone tumors	**Soft tissue tumors**
Osteochondromata	Ganglia
Enchondromas	Digital fibromas
Osteoid osteoma	Blood and lymph vessels
Aneurysmal bone cysts	Giant-cell tumors tendon sheath
Ewing sarcoma	Tumeral calcinosis
Epidermoid cysts	Soft tissue chondroma
Bone cysts	Synovial osteochondromatosis
Osteoblastoma	Aggressive fibromatosis
Miscellaneus types	Embryonal rhabdomyosarcoma

Fig. 9.58 Primary bone hand tumors in children. Based on Kozlowski, et al. (1988).

Fig. 9.59 Primary soft tissue hand tumors in children. Based on data from Azouz, et al. (1989).

Hand

Ulnar Dysplasia

The ulnar dysplasia includes an absence or hypoplasia of the ulna (Fig. 9.55). Often the radius is shortened and bowed and the ulna may be fused with the humerus. Finger deformities are common. Look for associated problems. Often function is preserved and reconstruction is not necessary. Tailor management to address the pattern of deformity. Someties resection of the anlage is necessary to prevent progression of radial bowing.

Radial Club Hand

Radial club hand includes an absence or hypoplasia of the radius and associated musculature producing a lateral deviation of the hand (Fig. 9.56). The deficiency may be isolated or part of a generalized skeletal dysplasia. Look for other problems by performing a screening evaluation giving special attention to the hematologic, urinary, and cardiac systems.

Management depends upon the severity of the deformity and the presence of associated defects. Mild hypoplasia may not require any treatment. Treat complete radial aplasia during the first year by first splinting or casting the hand and forearm to stretch the soft tissue contracture followed by operative correction. Operative correction usually include soft tissue release or lengthening and centralization of ulna on the carpals. Plan follow-up throughout infancy and childhood.

Cleft Hand Deformity

The cleft hand or central deficiency is a rare inherited defect that often affects both the hands (Fig. 9.57) and the feet. Operative reconstruction improves both function and appearance.

Hand Tumors

Primary hand tumors in children are extremely varied (Figs 9.58–9.60) and are managed as described in Chapter 13.

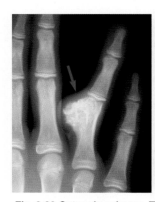
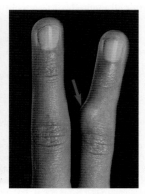

Fig. 9.60 Osteochondroma. This lesion is large and interferes with function.

Dysplasia Epiphysialis Hemimelica

Dysplasia epiphysialis hemimelica (DEH), or Trevor disease, is a rare developmental disorder causing asymmetrical epiphyseal cartilage overgrowth with accessory epiphyseal ossification centers (Fig. 9.61). This overgrowth causes deformity and swelling. DEH of the hand is often confused with other tumors. Manage by excising the lesions and correct secondary deformities by osteotomies. Expect recurrence as long as the child is still growing. These lesions are not premalignant.

Macrodactyly

Overgrowth of the hand (Fig. 9.62) may be secondary to a variety of disorders (Fig. 9.63) or occur as a primary problem. In primary macrodactyly, tissues are normal but growth is accelerated. This overgrowth may be greater, the same, or less than the rest of the limb. In secondary macrodactyly, tissues are abnormal. In some, the tissue type is obvious as with hemangiomata. In others, MRI and biopsies may be required to establish the diagnosis. Management is often difficult. Operative procedures include soft tissue resections, epiphysiodesis, shortening osteotomies, or bone resections and sometimes amputation of digits. Recurrence is distressingly frequent.

Arthritis

Juvenile arthritis (Fig. 9.64), autoimmune disorders, leukemia, sickle cell disease, child abuse, and infections are causes of joint problems in the child's hand. Juvenile arthritis is most common and often includes a loss of wrist extension and radial deviation of the fingers in the metacarpophalangeal joints. Ulnar shortening and involvement of the distal interpahalangeal joints may occur late in the disease. See page 34 for a discussion of arthritis.

References

2000 The principles of management of congenital anomalies of the upper limb. Watson S. Arch Dis Child 83:10

1998 Pollicisation of the index finger. A 27-year follow-up study. Clark DI, Chell J, Davis TR. JBJS 80B:631

1998 Residual deformity in congenital radial club hands after previous centralization of the wrist. Ulnar lengthening and correction by the Ilizarov method. Kawabata H, et al. JBJS 80B:762

1998 Distraction lengthening of the ulna in radial club hand using the Ilizarov technique. Pickford MA, Scheker LR. J Hand Surg 23B:186

1997 Classification of ulnar deficiency according to the thumb and first web. Cole RJ, Manske PR. J Hand Surg 22A:479

1995 Pediatric hand tumors. A review of 349 cases. Colon F, Upton J. Hand Clin 11:223

1993 Overgrowth management in Klippel-Trenaunay-Weber and Proteus syndromes. Guidera KJ, et al. JPO 13:459

1991 Evaluation of joint disease in the pediatric hand. Feinstein KA, Poznanski AK. Hand Clin 7:167

1991 Anomalies of the fingers and toes associated with Klippel-Trenaunay syndrome. McGrory BJ, et al. JBJS 73A:1537

1991 Distal interphalangeal joint abnormalities in children with polyarticular juvenile rheumatoid arthritis. Zerin JM, Sullivan DB, Martel W. J Rheumatol 18:889

1990 Cleft hand. Ogino T. Hand Clin 6:661

1989 Soft-tissue tumors of the hand and wrist of children. Azouz EM, Kozlowski K, Masel J. Can Assoc Radiol J 40:251

1988 Primary bone tumours of the hand. Report of 21 cases. Kozlowski K, et al. Pediatr Radiol 18:140

1988 Dysplasia epiphysealis hemimelica at the metacarpophalangeal joint. Maylack FH, Manske PR, Strecker WB. J Hand Surg 13A:916

1980 The hand in the child with juvenile rheumatoid arthritis. Granberry WM, Mangum GL. J Hand Surg 5A:105

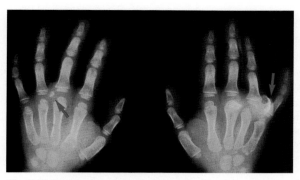

Fig. 9.61 Dysplasia epiphysialis hemimelica. Intraarticular osteochondral tumors distort joint surfaces, causing deformity and swelling (red arrows). These lesions are often confused with other disorders.

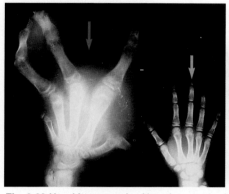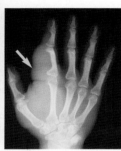

Fig. 9.62 Hand hypertrophy. Note the massive hypertrophy of the left hand (red arrow) as compared with the normal hand (green arrow). In another child hypertrophy is associated with neural hamartoma, producing soft tissue hyperplasia (yellow arrow).

Category	Disorder
Primary	Proportionate growth pattern
	Accelerated growth
Secondary	Hemangiomata
	Lymphangioma
	Neurofibromatosis
	Fibrous dysplasia
	Lipoma
	Desmoid tumor
	Fibromatous hamartoma of nerve

Fig. 9.63 Classification of macrodactyly. Secondary overgrowth may involve a variety of tissues.

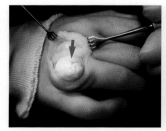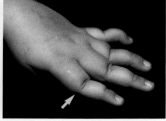

Fig. 9.64 Hand deformities in JRA. Deformity may be due to synovitis (red arrow) or muscle imbalance (yellow arrow). Most may be prevented by systemic and local treatment.

Deformity	Description
Hypoplasia	Small digits
Polydactyly	Too many digits
Syndactyly	Fusion of digits
Finger deformities	
Camptodactyly	Flexion contracture of the IP joint
Clinodactyly	Radial or ulnar angulation
Delta phalanx	Interposed delta-shaped ossicle
Kirner deformity	Progressive palmar, radial deviation of the distal phalanx of the little finger

Fig. 9.65 Classification of finger deformities. Deformities occur in the transverse or sagittal planes.

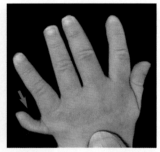

Category	Classification
Simple	Soft tissue digit
Complex	Bony duplications
Complete	Entire digit with metacarpals

Fig. 9.66 Classification of duplications. A simple method of classification is described. A simple duplication is shown (arrow).

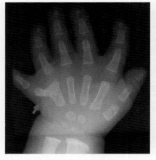

Fig. 9.67 Polydactyly. The complex polydactyly (red arrow) poses a much greater problem to repair when compared with the simple polydactyly (yellow arrow).

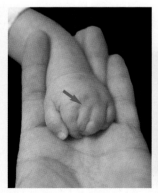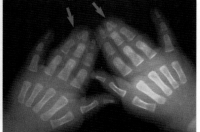

Fig. 9.68 Syndactyly. Syndactyly is readily identified. Radiographs are useful in determining the degree of bony involvement.

Fingers

Separate finger deformities into categories (Fig. 9.65). Often finger deformities are genetic, and the genes responsible for preaxial polydactyly, cleft hand and foot malformations, synpolydactyly, and types of brachydactyly have been recently identified.

Hypoplasia of Digits

Types of hypoplasia of digits are numerous and varied. This makes it necessary to individualize management with the objective of improving function, sensibility, and mobility. Digital reconstruction by toe to finger transplants or elongation of digits are examples of effective reconstructive procedures.

Polydactyly

Polydactyly is one of the most common congenital deformities (Figs. 9.66 and 9.67). Some forms of polydactyly are inherited. For example, duplications of the middle and little fingers are often inherited as autosomal dominant defects. Duplications of the index finger, central rays, and small digit each have unique characteristic features and associations. Complex anomalies such as the mirror hand and pentadactyly are also part of the polydactyly spectrum. Duplications are classified as preaxial (thumb), central, and postaxial types. Remove simple duplications in early infancy. Delay correction of complex duplications until late in the first year.

Syndactyly

Syndactyly (Fig. 9.68) is a common deformity. The syndactyly may be complete, or partial, and described as *simple,* if only the soft tissues are involved, or *complex* if bones are fused (Fig. 9.69). Syndactyly is most common between the middle and ring fingers. Syndactyly is seen in Apert, constriction band, and Poland syndromes. Correct by operative separation and full thickness skin grafting (Fig. 9.70).

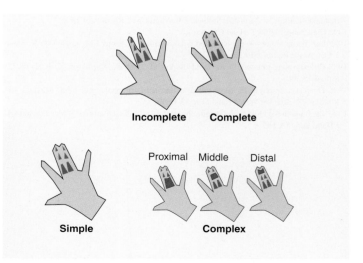

Fig. 9.69 Classification of syndactyly. Syndactyly may be complete or incomplete, simple or complex.

Bent Fingers

Bent or curved fingers occur in the frontal or sagittal planes. Except for camptodactyly, all have an underlying bony deformity. Many are associated with a variety of generalized disorders.

Camptodactyly is the common flexion deformity of the fingers (Fig. 9.71) that is divided into infantile and adolescent forms. The deformity is often progressive. Disability is usually mild. Treatment includes splinting, and rarely, operative correction.

Clinodactyly is a radial deviation of fingers, is often bilateral, and most commonly affects the little fingers (Fig. 9.72). The deformity is usually considered as a variation of normal, causes no disability, and seldom requires treatment. Rarely the deformity is severe enough to require correction. Correct by performing a wedge osteotomy of the phalanx. Delay correction until late childhood or early adolescence to reduce the risk of recurrent deformity.

Delta phalanx is an abnormal interposed triangular ossicle (Fig. 9.73 left) in the finger producing an angulatory deformity. Correct by osteotomy, or resection of the bridging physis. Following physeal resection, fill the defect with autogenous fat to prevent recurrence.

Kirner deformity This is a rare, progressive curving of the terminal phalanx of the little finger of unknown etiology. The deformity is characteristic in appearance, usually causes little disability, and seldom requires treatment. If the lesion is painful, immobilize the finger with a splint. Rarely the deformity is severe enough to require correction by a phalangeal osteotomy (Fig. 9.73 right).

Brachydactyly

Shortening of the metacarpal or fingers is often inherited as an autosomal trait or may be associated with a variety of conditions such as Poland, Holt-Oram, Cornelia de Lange, or Silver syndromes. Rarely finger lengthening procedures are appropriate.

Symphalangism

Fusions may involve the proximal or distal interphalangeal joints. The deformities are often congenital, inherited, and varied in pattern. Sometimes an osteotomy is necessary to reposition the finger in a more functional position.

Reconstructive Procedures

Finger osteotomies are often appropriate to correct deformity and position the finger in a more functional position. Fix most finger osteotomies with K wires. These procedures are commonly performed.

Toe-to-finger transfers Toe transfers are the most effective means of improving grip function of the hand in children with absent digits. Second toe transfer is usually made. Operative indications are rare.

Finger lengthening of up to 10 mm in single-stage and 30 mm by gradual distraction may be achieved. Metacarpal lengthening improves pinch function in children with either transverse deficiency or constriction band syndromes. Finger lengthening improves appearance in children with brachydactyly. These lengthening procedures are rarely indicated.

References

1998 A comparison of patients with different types of syndactyly. Kramer RC, et al. JPO 18:233

1998 Genetics of limb development and congenital hand malformations. Zguricas J, et al. Plast Reconstr Surg 101:1126

1998 Finger polydactyly. Graham TJ, Ress AM. Hand Clin 14:49

1997 Late toe-to-hand transfer for the reconstruction of congenital defects of the long fingers. Spokevicius S, Radzevicius D. Scand J Plast Reconstr Surg Hand Surg 31:345

1996 Congenital deformities of the upper extremity. Gallant GG, Bora FW. JAAOS 4:162

1994 Digital lengthening in congenital hand deformities. Ogino T, et al. J Hand Surg 19B:120

1986 Kirner's deformity: a review of the literature and case presentation. Freiberg A, Forrest C. J Hand Surg 11A:28

1970 Kirner's deformity of the little finger Carstam N, Eiken O JBJS 52A:1663

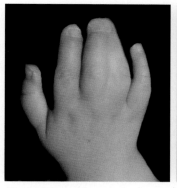
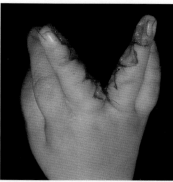

Fig. 9.70 Operative repair of syndactyly. Repair is usually effective with good functional outcomes.

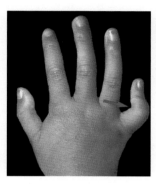

Fig. 9.71 Camptodactyly. Note the flexion deformity of the proximal interphalangeal joint (arrow).

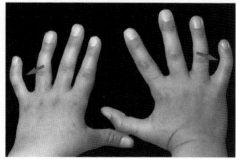

Fig. 9.72 Clinodactyly. This classic deformity involves both little fingers.

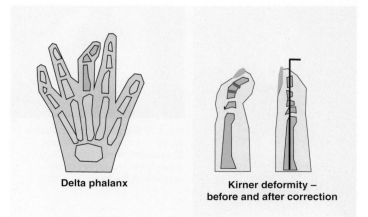

Delta phalanx

Kirner deformity – before and after correction

Fig. 9.73 Delta phalanx and Kirner deformity. The delta phalanx and Kirner deformity are caused by bony deformity that sometimes require operative correction.

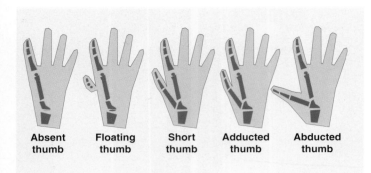

Absent thumb | **Floating thumb** | **Short thumb** | **Adducted thumb** | **Abducted thumb**

Fig. 9.74 Thumb deformities.

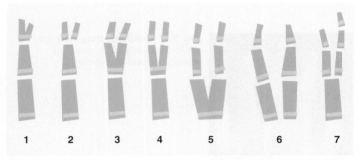

1 2 3 4 5 6 7

Fig. 9.75 Thumb polydactyly. Wassel classification. From Gallant and Bora (1996).

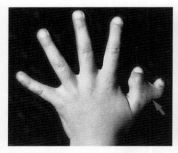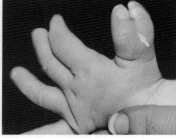

Fig. 9.76 Thumb duplication. Type 4 (red arrow) and type 3 (yellow arrow) are shown.

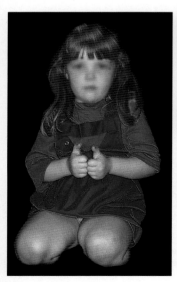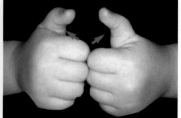

Fig. 9.77 Trigger thumbs. Bilateral trigger thumbs locked in flexion. Operative release of the pulleys allowed free movement of the tendon and the thumb to extend.

Thumb

Hypoplasia

Thumb hypoplasia accounts for about 5% of congenital hand anomalies. Management is determined by the type of displasia (Fig. 9.74).

Aplasia is treated by index pollicization.

Floating thumb, or *pouce flottant* is usually managed by amputation, and index pollicization late in the first year.

Short thumb may be associated with a variety of syndromes. If the shortening is excessive, correct by performing a lengthening osteotomy, or by deepening the web space. Tailor correction to facilitate function.

Adducted–abducted thumb deformities with shortening require tailored reconstruction that includes both soft tissue and bony reconstruction.

Polydactyly

Thumb polydactyly or *duplication,* a failure in segmentation, accounts for 5–10% of all hand deformities. Classify duplications into 7 types (Fig. 9.75). Type 4 is most common (Fig. 9.76). Types 1–6 are usually unilateral, sporatic, and most common in boys. Type 7 may be inherited, is often bilateral, and may be associated with other abnormalities. Correct late in the first year utilizing tissues from the duplicated digits to create the best possible new thumb.

Congenital Clasped Thumb

This deformity often includes a congenital absence of the flexor tendon combined with thumb hypolasia. Correct between 3 and 6 months with serial casting. If this fails, operative reconstruction is necessary.

Trigger Digits

Trigger thumbs are secondary to an acquired nodular enlargement of a segment of the flexor tendon (Fig. 9.77). Large nodules usually become wedged at the pulley, causing the digit to lock in flexion. Smaller nodules pass through the pulley, producing a snapping sensation. Initially manage by observation. If the nodule and disability persist, consider operative release of the flexor pulley. The release frees the nodule and allows the thumb to flex and extend freely.

Trigger fingers are usually due to congenital abnormalities of the flexor mechanism. Simple release of the pulley is often ineffective, and exploration and repair of the flexor mechanism is often necessary.

References

1998 Diagnosis and treatment of congenital thumb hypoplasia. Plancher KD, Kahlon RS. Hand Clin 14:101

1996 Congenital deformities of the upper extremity. Gallant GG, Bora FW. JAAOS 4:162

1996 Acquired thumb flexion contracture in children: congenital trigger thumb. Slakey JB, Hennrikus WL. JBJS 78B:481

1994 Incidence of trigger digits in newborns. Rodgers WB, Waters PM. J Hand Surg 19A:364

1994 Duplication of the thumb. A 20-year retrospective review. Naasan A, Page RE. J Hand Surg 19B:355

1992 Reconstruction of the congenitally deficient thumb. Manske PR, McCarroll HR Jr. Hand Clin 8:177

1992 Congenital trigger digit. Wood VE, Sicilia M. CO 285:205

1969 The results of surgery for polydactyly of the thumb: a review. Wassel HD. CO 64:175

Hand Infections

Hand infections (Fig. 9.78) can be serious problems in children as they are varied, often difficult to assess, and sometimes cause long-term disability.

Penetrating Injuries

Penetrating injuries may cause infections of the soft tissues, bone, or joints of the hand. The organism is usually staphylococcus aureus.

Animal Bites

Evaluate the injury by considering the animal, nature of the wound, circumstances of the attack, interval between injury and treatment, and location of the bite. Give rabies prophylaxis for bites from carnivorous wild animals, bats, and unvaccinated domestic animals. Update the child's tetanus immunizations. Administer a broad-spectrum antibiotic early. Leave deep contaminated wounds open and close secondarily.

Nail Infections

Paronychia is a localized infection of the nail base. Manage with soaks and antibiotics, or drain if suppuration has occurred (Fig. 9.79).

Subungal infections is a more extensive infection that often requires elevation and excision of the involved portion of the of the nail.

Felons

Finger tip infections may be difficult to differentiate from injury. Make this differentiation by the history, examination, systemic manifestations, and laboratory studies. Operative drainage is necessary if suppuration has occurred (Fig. 9.80).

Herpetic Hand Infections

Most herpetic hand infections occur in infants and young children who have oral lesions. Establish the diagnosis by clinical features, viral cultures, or Tzanck smears. Resolution occurs in 3–4 weeks. Antibiotic treatment is indicated only for superinfections. Cover the lesions to prevent spread.

Tenosynovitis

Inflammations or infections of tendon sheaths are not rare in children, and evaluation is more difficult because of lack of cooperation during examination. The pattern of bursa and tendon sheaths of the hand are the same in children and adults (Fig. 9.81). Ultrasound imaging may be useful in establishing the level and extent of inflammation and purulence. Manage most cases first with elevation, splinting, and antibiotics for 24 hours, then reassess. If not substantially improved consider operative drainage (Fig. 9.82).

Dactylitis

The causes of dactylitis are numerous and include tuberculosis, sickle cell disease, congenital syphilis, psoriatic arthritis, and juvenile spondyloarthropathies. Most finger infections are due to osteomyelitis (Fig. 9.83) or septic arthritis.

Hand Abscesses and Otopharyngeal Infections

Abscesses of the hand may be associated with inner ear or pharyngeal infections.

Chapter Consultant Marybeth Ezaki

References

1998 Metacarpal osteomyelitis complicating varicella-associated cellulitis of the hand. Aebi C, Ramilo O. Scand J Infect Dis 30:306

1992 Animal bites. Guidelines to current management. Anderson CR. Postgrad Med 92:134, 139, 149

1990 Pediatric herpetic hand infections. Walker LG, Simmons BP, Lovallo JL. J Hand Surg 15A:176

1989 Hand complications in children from digital sucking [see comments] Rayan GM, Turner WT. J Hand Surg 14A:933

1987 Acute suppurative tenosynovitis of the hand: diagnosis with US. Jeffrey RB Jr, et al. Radiology 162:741

1986 Abscesses of the hand associated with otopharyngeal infections in children. Pruzansky ME, Remer S. J Hand Surg 11A:844

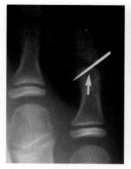
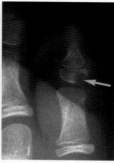
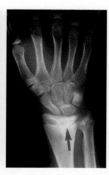

Fig. 9.78 Bacterial infections. These include cellulitis from foreign body penetration (yellow arrow), osteomyelitis (orange arrow) and rarely residual growth arrest secondary to meningococcemia (red arrow).

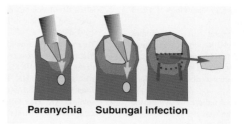

Paranychia Subungal infection

Fig. 9.79 Nail infections. These may be treated with antibiotics but if suppuration occurs surgical drainage is required.

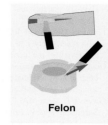

Felon

Fig. 9.80 Felon. Drain pulp abscesses through a dorsolateral incision.

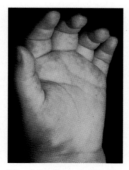

Fig. 9.81 Deep infections. These may involve the tendon sheaths of the hand and cause diffuse swelling (red arrow).

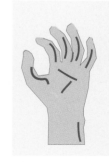

Fig. 9.82 Surgical drainage. Follows the same principles as for adults.

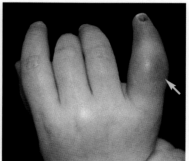
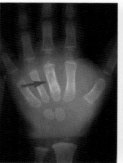

Fig. 9.83 Dactylitis. Inflammation of the the digits may occur from many causes. Metacarpal osteomyelitis (red arrow) or dacytlities associated with juvenile rheumatoid arthritis (yellow arrow) are common causes.

Almquist EE, Gordon LH, Blue AI. Congenital dislocation of the head of the radius. J Bone Joint Surg 1966;51A:1118.

Askins G, Ger E. Congenital constriction band syndrome. J Pediatr Orthop 1988;8:461.

Barot LR, Caplan HS. Early surgical intervention in Apert's syndactyly. Plast Reconstr Surg 1986;77(2):282.

Buck-Gramcko D. Radialization as a new treatment for radial club hand. J Hand Surg 1987;10A(2):964.

Burke F, Flatt AE. Clinodactyly. A review of a series of cases. Hand 1979;3:269.

Cleary JE, Omer GE. Congenital proximal radio-ulnar synostosis. Natural history and functional assessment. J Bone Joint Surg 1985;67A:539.

Dinham JM, Meggitt DF. Trigger thumbs in children. J Bone Joint Surg 1974;56B:153.

Dobyns JH, Lipscomb PR, Cooney WP. Management of thumb duplication. Clin Orthop 1985;195:26.

Dykes RG. Kirner's deformity of the little finger. J Bone Joint Surg 1978;60B:58.

Engber WM, Flatt AE. Camptodactyly: An analysis of sixty-six patients and twenty-four operations. J Hand Surg 1977;2:216.

Frykman GK, Wood VE. Peripheral nerve hamartomas with macrodactyly in the hands: Report of three cases and review of the literature. J Hand Surg 1978;3:307.

Goncalves D. Correction of disorder of the distal radioulnar joint by artificial pseudoathrosis of the ulna. J Bone Joint Surg 1974;56B:462.

Green WT, Mital MA. Congenital radio-ulnar synostosis: Surgical treatment. J Bone Joint Surg 1979;61A:738.

Ireland DCR, Takayama N, Flatt AE. Poland's syndrome: A review of forty-three cases. J Bone Joint Surg 1976;58A:52.

Jones KG, Marmor L, Lankford LL. An overview on new procedures in surgery of the hand. Clin Orthop 1974;99:154.

Mardam-Bey T, Ger E. Congenital radial head dislocation. J Hand Surg 1979;4:316.

Matev IB. Thumb reconstruction in children through metacarpal lengthening. Plast Reconstr Surg 1979;64(5):665.

May JW, Smith RJ, Peimer CA. Toe to hand free tissue transfer for thumb reconstruction with multiple digit aplasia. Plast Reconstr Surg 1981;67(2):205.

Mital MA. Congenital radioulnar synostosis and congenital dislocation of the radial head. Orthop Clin North Am 1976;7:375.

Miura T. Congenital constriction band syndrome. J Hand Surg 1984;9A:82.

Miura T, Komada T. Simple method for reconstruction of the cleft hand with an adducted thumb. Plast Reconstr Surg 1979;64:65.

Miura T, et al. Non-operative treatment of camptodactyly. J Hand Surg 1987;12A:1061.

Nielsen JB. Madelung's deformity: A follow-up study of 26 cases and a review of the literature. Acta Orthop Scand 1977;48:379.

O'Brien BMcC, Franklin JD, Morrison WA, et al. Microvascular great toe transfer for congenital absence of thumb. Hand 1978;10:113.

Ogden JA, Watson HK, Bohne W. Ulna dysmelia. J Bone Joint Surg 1976;58A:467.

Poznanski AK, Pratt GB, Manson G, et al. Clinodactyly, camptodactyly, Kirner's deformity, and other croooked fingers. Radiology 1969;93:573.

Riordan DC. Congenital absence of the radius: A 15-year follow-up. J Bone Joint Surg 1963;45A:1783.

Roberts AS. A case of deformity of the forearm and hands with an unusual history of hereditary congenital deficiency. Ann Surg 1896;3:135.

Rogala EJ, Wynne-Davies R, Littlejohn A, et al. Congenital limb anomalies. Frequency and etiological factors. J Med Genet 1974;11:221.

Smith RJ. Osteotomy for "delta-phalanx" deformity. Clin Orthop 1977;123:91.

Smith RJ, Lipke RW. Treatment of congenital deformities of the hand and forearm. N Engl J Med 1979;300:402.

Staheli LT, Clawson DK, Capps JH. Bilateral curving of the terminal phalanges of the little fingers. Report of two cases. J Bone Joint Surg 1966;48A:1171-1176.

Strauch B, Spinner M. Congenital anomaly of the thumb: absent intrinsics and flexor pollicis longus. J Bone Joint Surg 1976;58A:115.

Swanson AB. A classification for congenital limb malformations. J Hand Surg 1976;1:8.

Tada K, Yonenobu K, Tsuyuguchi Y, et al. Duplication of the thumb: A retrospective review of 237 cases. J Bone Joint Surg 1983;65A:584.

Watari S, Tsuge K. A classification of cleft hands, based on clinical findings. Plast Reconstr Surg 1979;64:381.

Watson HK, Boyes JH. Congenital angular deformity of the digits. Delta phalanx. J Bone Joint Surg 1967;49A:333.

Wood VE, Flatt AE. Congenital triangular bones in the hand. J Hand Surg 1977;2:179.

Chapter 10—Trauma

Trauma is the leading cause of death of children and second to infection as a cause of morbidity. Fractures account for about 15% of all injuries in children (Fig. 10.1).

Children's injuries not only differ from those of adults but they also vary depending on the age of the child. Infants, children, and adolescents are different. Appreciating these differences is essential to optimal management.

Statistics

Boys are injured more often than girls. Injuries increase in frequency with advancing age during childhood, and the percentage of fractures that occur through the physis increases with age (Fig. 10.2).

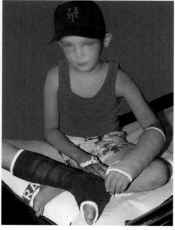

Fig.10.1 Trauma is part of a child's life. This boy sustained a fracture of his forearm and ankle during play.

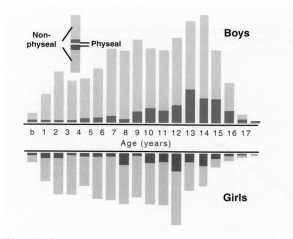

Fig. 10.2 Age distribution of physeal and nonphyseal injuries. Note the differences between boys (blue) and girls (red). From Mizuta et al. (1987).

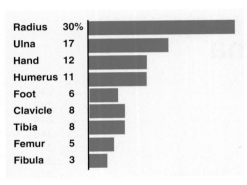

Radius	30%
Ulna	17
Hand	12
Humerus	11
Foot	6
Clavicle	8
Tibia	8
Femur	5
Fibula	3

Fig. 10.3 Fracture frequency in infants and children. Frequency of fractures in a sample of 923 children's fractures. From Mizuta (1987).

About half of boys and one-fourth of girls can expect to experience a fracture during childhood. Fractures are becoming more common as sports activities increase. The wrist is the most frequent site of injury (Fig. 10.3). Age affects the pattern of injury.

Children Prone to Injury

Low bone mineral content Children with generalized disorders such as osteogenesis imperfecta (Fig. 10.4), renal diseases, cystic fibrosis, diabetes mellitus, and growth hormone deficiencies are at risk.

Neuromuscular disorders Children with cerebral palsy, spina bifida, and arthrogryposis (Fig. 10.5) are fracture prone because of the combination of poor mineralization and joint stiffness.

Fracture personality Children in general are at greater risk due to their higher activity levels, and some children in particular who have risk-prone behaviors are at even greater risk.

References
1998 Epidemiology of children's fractures. Landin LA. JPO-b 6:70
1993 Limb fracture pattern in different pediatric age groups: a study of 3,350 children. Cheng JC, Shen WY. J Orthop Trauma 7:15
1987 Statistical analysis of the incidence of physeal injuries. Mizuta T, et al. JPO 7:518

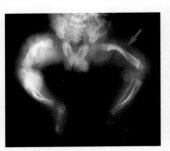

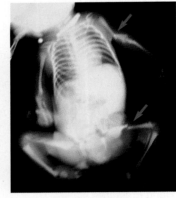

Fig. 10.4 Multiple fractures in osteogenesis imperfecta. This newborn's fragile bones resulted in paranatal fractures.

Fig. 10.5 Fractures due to joint stiffness in arthrogryposis. These birth fractures resulted from trauma at delivery due to joint contractures.

Physiology

The musculoskeletal system of children is different from that of the adult, which explains why children's fractures are different (Fig. 10.6). These differences gradually diminish with age, so that fractures in the adolescent are similar to those of the adult.

Growth Plate

The most obvious difference is that the child has a growth plate. The relative strength of the growth plate compared to adjacent bone changes with age. For example, the physis in infants is stronger than the adjacent bone so diaphyseal fractures are most common (Fig 10.6).

Helps fracture management The growth plate usually helps in managing fractures. Growth facilitates remodeling that corrects residual angulation. The potential for remodeling depends on the growth rate of the adjacent physis and on the remaining growth of the child.

Injured growth plate causes deformity Just as the physis can resolve deformity, asymmetrical physical growth causes deformity.

Bone

Higher collagen to bone ratio This lowers the modulus of elasticity and reduces the tensile strength of the bone (Fig. 10.7).

Higher cellular and porous This reduces tensile strength and reduces the tendency of fractures to propagate and explains why comminuted fractures are uncommon in children.

Bone fails in both tension and compression This explains the mechanism of the common buckle fracture in children (Fig 10.8).

Bone transitions between metaphysis and diaphysis cause a mechanical discontinuity leading to certain fracture types.

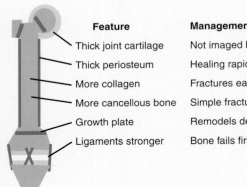

Feature	Management effect
Thick joint cartilage	Not imaged by X-ray
Thick periosteum	Healing rapid
More collagen	Fractures easily
More cancellous bone	Simple fracture patterns
Growth plate	Remodels deformity
Ligaments stronger	Bone fails first

Fig. 10.6 Bone structural features affecting management. The child's musculoskeletal system is different from the adult's in several important ways. These differences significantly affect management.

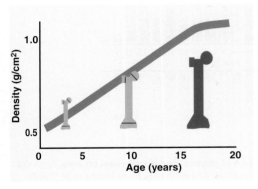

Fig. 10.7 Bone mineral density. This graph shows bone mineral density in the femoral neck in normal subjects. From Thomas (1991).

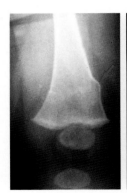
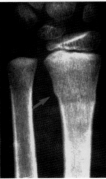

Fig. 10.8 Buckle fractures. These fractures are common in children because the bone fails in both tension and compression and because of the high collagen content.

Periosteum

Metabolically active The periosteum is more metabolically active in the child than in the adult. This explains the exuberant callus seen in the infant (Figs. 10.9 and 10.10) and the rapid union and increased potential for remodeling seen throughout childhood. Bone forms with the periosteal sleeve to create bone continuity. This active periosteum also contributes appositional bone, which facilitates remodeling.

Thickness and strength Children have increased thickness and strength of the periosteum. Fractures within the intact periosteal sleeve may have little displacement and be difficult to diagnose (Fig. 10.11). The intact periosteal hinge affects the fracture pattern (Fig. 10.12) and may be helpful in reduction of fractures.

Age-Related Fracture Patterns

These changes in bone result in changing fracture patterns throughout growth (Fig. 10.13). The infant with the diaphyseal fracture, the child with a fracture through the metaphysis, and the adolescent with an epiphyseal injury are examples of this effect.

Ligaments

Ligaments are relatively stronger than bone. Usually bone fails before ligaments, which explains various injury patterns. Avulsion injuries are common in children (Figs. 10.14 and 10.15). The distal femoral physis fails before the collateral ligaments (Fig. 10.16).

Cartilage

The increased ratio of cartilage to bone in children improves resilience but makes evaluation by radiography more difficult. The size of the articular fragment is often underestimated.

References

2000 The "muscle-bone unit" in children and adolescents: a 2000 overview. Frost HM, Schonau E. J Pediatr Endocrinol Metab 13:571

1991 Femoral neck and lumbar spine bone mineral densities in a normal population 3–20 years of age. Thomas KA, et al. JPO 11:48

1990 Growth plate physiology and pathology. Iannotti JP. Orthop Clin North Am 21:1

1989 Bone mineral content in black and white children 1 to 6 years of age: Early appearance of race and sex differences. Li JY, et al. Am J Dis Child 143:1346

1987 Statistical analysis of the incidence of physeal injuries. Mizuta T, et al. JPO 7:518

1987 Longitudinal bone growth: the growth plate and its dysfunctions. Brighton CT. AAOS Instruc Course Lect 34:3

1987 Bone structure and function. Buckwalter JA, Cooper RR. AAOS Instruc Course Lect 34:27

1987 Bone mineral content in children 1 to 6 years of age. Specker BL, et al. Am J Dis Child 141:343

1984 The growth plate. Brighton CT. Orthop Clin North Am 15:571

1983 The relationship of the periosteum to angular deformities of long bones: experimental observations of rabbits. Carvell JE. CO 173:262

1982 Collagenous architecture of the growth plate and perichondrial ossification groove. Speer D. JBJS 64A:399

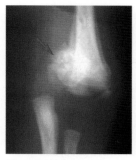
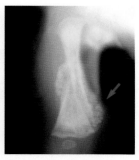

Fig. 10.9 Exuberant callus formation in the newborn fracture. This physeal separation resulted from birth trauma.

Fig. 10.10 Callus from femur fracture in an infant. Note the extensive callus formation.

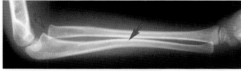

Fig. 10.11 Plastic bowing of the ulna. This child has a dislocation of the radial head with plastic bowing of the ulna.

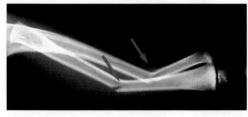

Fig. 10.12 Greenstick fracture of the forearm. Greenstick fractures are common in the forearm, as bone bends before it fractures and the periosteal sleeve maintains apposition.

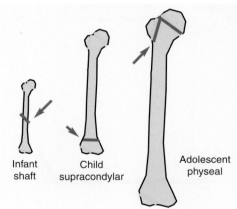

Fig. 10.13. Age-related injury types of the humerus. This injury pattern is present in other long bones with diaphyseal fractures in infants, metaphyseal fractures in children, and epiphyseal fractures in adolescents.

Infant shaft

Child supracondylar

Adolescent physeal

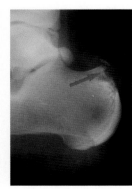

Fig. 10.14 Avulsion injury of the triceps. Avulsion of the tendo-achilles insertion is due to the greater tensile strength of the triceps tendon than calcaneal bone in the adolescent.

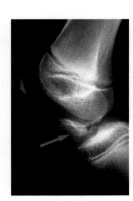

Fig. 10.15 Avulsion of the tibial spine. The bone fails before the ACL ligament, resulting in a fracture of the tibial spine.

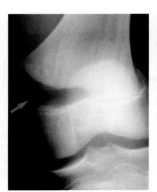

Fig. 10.16 Fracture of distal femoral epiphysis. The physis fails before the adjacent bone or collateral ligaments. This is a common injury type in adolescents.

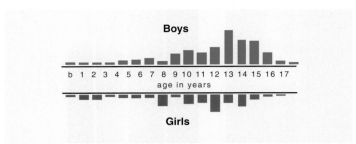

Fig. 10.17 Age distribution of physeal injuries in boys (blue) and girls (red). From Mizuta (1987).

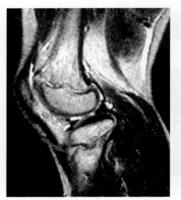

Fig. 10.18 Recurvatum deformity due to anterior tibial physeal arrest. This physis is very vulnerable to arrest.

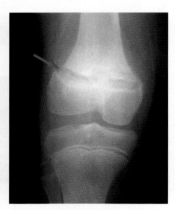

Fig. 10.19 Physeal injury in myelodysplasia. Note the physeal widening.

Physeal Injuries

Physeal injuries account for about one-fourth of all childhood fractures. They are most common in boys, in the upper limb, and in childhood (Fig. 10.17). Physeal injury may also occur from infection, tumors, or ischaemia. Physeal fractures are of great importance, as these injuries can affect subsequent growth and remodeling potential.

Anatomy

The physeal anatomy is varied but the pattern is similar. Physes can be categorized into (1) those involving long bones (femur), (2) ring epiphyses that occur in round bones (cuboid) and around secondary ossification centers, and (3) apophyses at the site of muscle or tendon insertions (greater trochanteric apophysis). Growth disturbances of long bone physes are most likely to be damaged and create the greatest deformity.

Long bone physes often show an undulating pattern with *mamallary processes.* This provides greater sheer strength but may lead to an increased risk of physeal damage from high-impact injuries. An example is the greater likelihood of growth arrest from simple physeal fractures of the distal femoral physis.

Injury

The physis usually fractures through the zone of provisional calcification, sparing the germinal cells so growth is unaffected. Less common injuries that damage the germinal zone or create a tethering bridge across the physis may slow or arrest growth.

Physeal susceptibility to arrest varies. The most sensitive long bone physis is the anterior portion of the proximal tibial epiphysis. Recurvatum deformity may occur from trivial injury (Fig. 10.18).

Stress injuries to the physis are most commonly observed in athletes and children with myelodysplasia (Fig. 10.19). The gymnast may develop a stress fracture of the distal radial physis. Such physeal injuries often cause growth arrest.

Physeal arrest is most common in injuries that allow the bone to bridge the growth plate. The location and percentage of the cross-sectional area occupied by the bony bridge determines the extent of the secondary deformity.

Classification

Several classification systems for physeal injuries exist. The most simple and widely used is that originated by Salter and Harris (SH). Fractures are divided into five categories based on pattern (Fig. 10.20). SH-5 injuries are very rare. More comprehensive classifications include ones devised by Peterson (Fig. 10.21) and by Ogden. For complex injuries, use a more comprehensive classification.

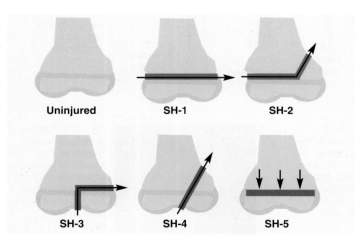

Fig. 10.20 Salter–Harris (SH) classification of growth plate injuries. These are classified as types 1 through 5 based on the fracture pattern. Types 1 and 2 (green lines) do not traverse the epiphysis and usually do not cause growth problems. Types 3 to 5 (red lines) may cause growth arrest and progressive deformity.

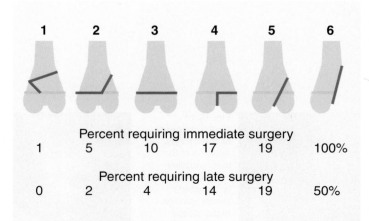

Fig. 10.21 Peterson classification. The frequency of injuries of each type requiring immediate and late surgery are shown. From Peterson (1994).

Classification of injury type is usually done by radiography. Imaging by CT scans may clarify complex fracture patterns such as those in triplane fractures of the ankle. MRI studies (Fig. 10.22) often show considerably more physeal damage than was suspected from radiographs and may change the SH category. Because our experience is based on radiographic imaging, prognosis and management based on the more sensitive MRI may lead to overtreatment.

Natural History

Most acute physeal injuries heal rapidly; any deformity remodels completely and growth proceeds normally. About 1% of physeal injuries cause physeal bridging and altered growth (Fig. 10.23). Small bridges (<10%) may lyse spontaneously. Central bridges are more likely to lyse and less likely to cause deformity than peripheral ones. Central bridges may cause a fishtail deformity, which only slows rather than arrests growth (Fig. 10.24).

Physeal Bridge Management

Physeal bridge formation usually follows SH-3, -4, or -5 injuries. The mechanism is either a crush injury to the germinal layer or a displaced fracture that allows bone to form across the physis. The prognostic significance of the type is not always consistent. For example, physeal arrest also occurs in about half of SH-1 and -2 injuries of the distal femur in the older child or adolescent (Fig. 10.25). Physeal injury may also follow fracture of the diaphysis. The mechanism is unclear.

Avoid physeal injury when placing fixation devices in children. Reaming of the upper femur for fixation of femoral shaft fractures is a common cause of physeal damage. Use alternative ways of fixation before the end of growth.

Prevention of physeal bridge formation is best achieved by an anatomic reduction of SH-3 and -4 fractures. Open reduction and internal fixation that does not traverse the physis is best. If fixation is necessary across the growth plate, use small, smooth K wires.

Monitor growth for detection of physeal bridge. If a bridge is found, make a radiograph of the involved bone and the contralateral side on the same film every 4–6 months. Note changes in relative overall length or angulation of the adjacent joint surface.

Imaging physeal bars may be done by CT scans or MRI studies. Order frontal and sagittal computer reconstruction of 1-mm CT scans. MRIs tend to show more soft tissue information but may be more difficult to interpret. Assess the location of the percentage of the cross-sectional area of the physis that the bridge occupies. See technique of physeal bar resection on page 370.

References

2000 Premature physeal closure after tibial diaphyseal fractures in adolescents. Navascues JA, et al. JPO 20:193

1999 Premature partial closure and other deformities of the growth plate: MR imaging and three-dimensional modeling. Craig JG et al. Radiology 210:835

1997 Does repetitive physical loading inhibit radial growth in female gymnasts? Caine D et al. Clin J Sport Med 7:302

1997 Local physeal widening on MR imaging: an incidental finding suggesting prior metaphyseal insult. Laor T, Hartman AL, Jaramillo D. Pediatr Radiol 27:654

1997 The use of helical computed tomographic scan to assess bony physeal bridges. Loder RT, Swinford AE, Kuhns LR. JPO 17:356

1996 MR imaging of physeal bars. Borsa JJ, Peterson HA, Ehman RL. Radiology 199:683

1996 Spontaneous resolution of an osseous bridge affecting the distal tibial epiphysis. Bostock SH, Peach BJ. JBJS 78B:662

1994 Physeal fractures: Part 3. Classification. Peterson HA. JPO 14:439

1994 Physeal fractures: Part 2. Two previously unclassified types. Peterson HA. JPO 14:431

1994 Physeal fractures: Part 1. Epidemiology in Olmsted County, Minnesota, 1979-1988. Peterson HA, et al. JPO 14:423

1993 Experimental physeal fracture-separations treated with rigid internal fixation. Gomes LS, Volpon JB. JBJS 75A:1756

1990 Premature closure of the physis following diaphyseal fractures. Beals RK. JPO 10:717

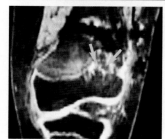
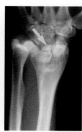
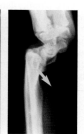
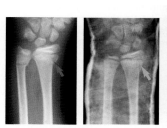

Fig. 10.22 MRI evaluation of physeal bars. The bar may appear as a bridging bone (red arrow) or as an irregularity of the physis (yellow arrow).

Fig. 10.23 Natural history of physeal injuries of the distal radius. The fracture occurred at age 10 years (red arrow). The reduction looks anatomic (orange arrow). The girl was not seen until age 20, when she complained of a wrist deformity. Note the effect of a volar bridge on the distal radius (yellow arrows).

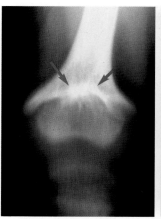
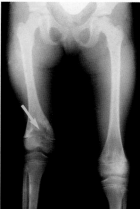

Fig. 10.24 Central bridge resection in an infant. This central bridge (red arrow) resulted from a birth fracture. The bridge was resected (yellow arrow) and growth resumed.

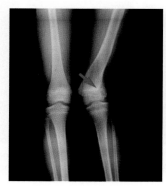

Fig. 10.25 Physeal bridge of distal femur. This bar from a SH-2 fracture caused severe valgus deformity.

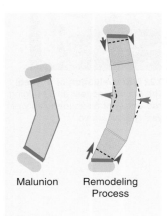

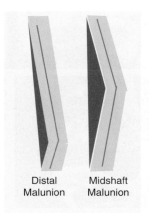

Fig. 10.26 Mechanism for remodeling. Remodeling occurs from appositional periosteal formation and resorption (blue arrows) and asymmetrical physeal growth (red arrows). Redrawn from Gasco (1997).

Fig. 10.27 Greater remodeling for midshaft deformity. For the same angular deformity, more correction (area in red) is required for midshaft than distal deformity.

Remodeling

The capacity of bone to remodel significantly influences the management of fractures in children. One of the great challenges in pediatric orthopedics is to predict accurately which fractures require reduction and which will remodel sufficiently on their own.

Mechanism

Remodeling results from a combination of appositional bone deposition on the concavity of the deformity, resorption on the convexity, and asymmetrical physeal growth (Figs. 10.26 and 10.27). Remodeling requires a functional physis and intact periosteum.

Examples of Remodeling

Remodeling is one of the most forgiving features of childhood fracture management. Examples are useful to show the potential for correction to the clinician and for reassuring families.

Proximal humerus Because the shoulder joint is multiaxial with rapid growth, remodeling is often spectacular (Figs. 10.28 and 10.30).

Distal humerus The distal humerus remodels well in flexion and extension but poorly for varus and valgus deformity (Fig. 10.29).

Wrist Note that the wrist has extensive remodeling potential (Fig. 10.31).

Femoral shaft Femoral shaft fractures in the child remodel completely (Fig. 10.32) as compared with the adolescent where remodeling is less complete (Fig. 10.33).

Proximal femur Remodeling may be complete if the fracture occurs at an early age (Fig. 10.34).

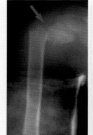
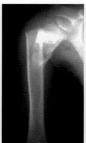
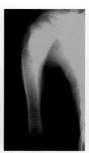
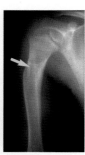

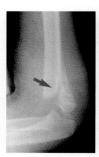
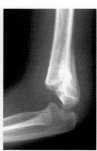
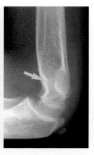

Fig. 10.28 Remodeling of the humerus. This 8-year-old boy shows a complete loss of apposition (red arrow). Note the remodeling over the next 2 years (yellow arrow).

Fig. 10.29 Remodeling of sagittal plane in a supracondylar fracture. This fracture (red arrow) remodeled over a period of 4 years (yellow arrow). Remodeling about the elbow is much slower than in the proximal humerus.

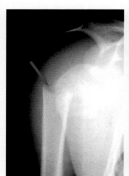
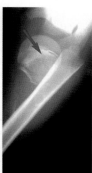
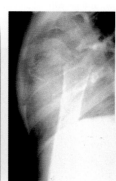
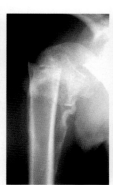
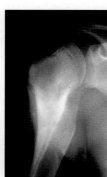
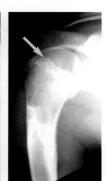

Fig. 10.30 Remodeling of the humerus. This sequence shows a fracture (red arrow) in a 12-year-old boy over a period of 2 years. The fracture was left unreduced with side-to-side apposition and shortening. Note the remodeling within the intact periosteal sheath (yellow arrow).

References

1999 Remodeling of forearm fractures in children. Johari AN, M Sinha. JPO-B 8:84

1997 Bone remodeling in malunited fractures in children. Is it reliable? Gascò J, de Pablos J. JPO-b 6:126

1997 Periosteum: its relation to pediatric fractures. Jacobsen FS. JPO-b 6:84

1996 Bone growth and remodeling after fracture. Murray DW et al. JBJS 78B:42

1996 Femoral remodeling after subtrochanteric osteotomy for developmental dysplasia of the hip. Sangavi SM, et al. JBJS 78B:917

1992 Remodeling of angular deformity after femoral shaft fractures in children. Wallace ME, Hoffman EB. JBJS 74B:765

1991 Angular remodeling of midshaft forearm fractures in children. Vittas D, Larsen E, Torp-Pedersen S. CO 265:261

1979 Remodeling after distal forearm fractures in children. III. Correction of residual angulation in fractures of the radius. Friberg KS. Acta Orthop Scand 50:741

1979 Remodeling after distal forearm fractures in children. II. The final orientation of the distal and proximal epiphyseal plates of the radius. Friberg KS. Acta Orthop Scand 50:731

1979 Remodeling after distal forearm fractures in children. I. The effect of residual angulation on the spatial orientation of the epiphyseal plates. Friberg KS. Acta Orthop Scand 50:537

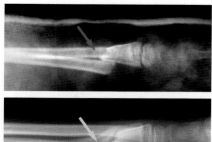
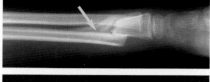
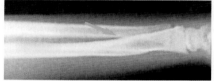

Fig. 10.31 Remodeling of forearm. The fracture fragments were in bayonette apposition (red arrow). Three months later remodeling was in progress (yellow arrow). At 2 years (orange arrow) remodeling was nearly complete.

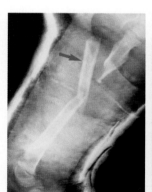
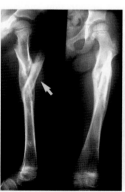
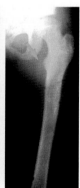

Fig. 10.32 Remodeling of femoral shaft fracture. This segmental fracture in an 8 year-old girl was managed in traction and in a cast (red arrow). Note the filling in of the periosteal sheath at 6 months (yellow arrow) and restoration of normal femoral shape at age 13 years (orange arrow).

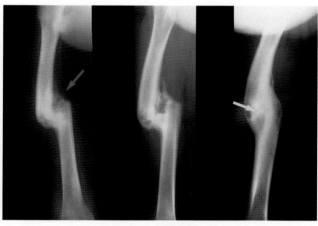

Fig. 10.33 Limited remodeling in adolescent. This transverse fracture of the midshaft of the femur (red arrow) in a 15 year-old boy healed but showed limited remodeling (yellow arrow) due to the limited remaining growth.

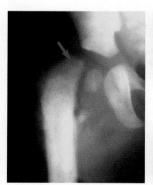
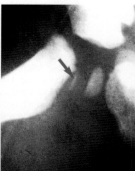
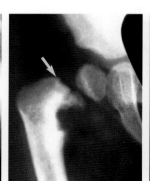
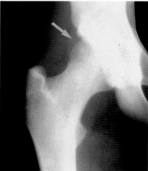

Fig. 10.34 Remodeling of proximal femoral physeal fracture in an infant. Note the remodeling of the completely displaced femoral head (red arrows) throughout childhood, yellow arrow). Normal appearance is shown at age 15 years (orange arrow). Courtesy E. Forlin.

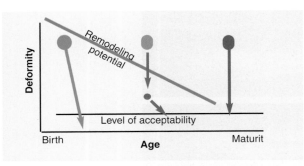

Fig. 10.35 Age-determined changes affecting reduction. With increasing age, the potential for remodeling declines (green line). For a given angulation, the age determines the required degree of reduction. In infancy (green arrow), reduction is not necessary, as remodeling is rapid and complete. The same angulation in a child (blue arrows) requires partial reduction, with remodeling correcting the remaining deformity. In the adolescent (red arrows), anatomic reduction is required.

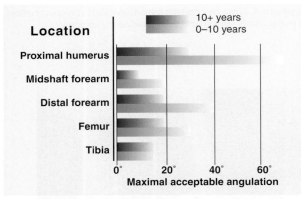

Fig. 10.36 Potential for remodeling. This graph suggests limits of acceptable, angular deformity following long-bone fractures in children. From Casco and de Pablos (1997).

Principles of Reduction

Indications for the need and accuracy of fracture reduction in children is often complex and requires good judgment. Base these decisions on underlying principles whenever possible. Unfortunately, data on which to base these principles is limited. Some generally accepted principles can be outlined for different types of fractures. A flowchart is often helpful (Fig. 10.37).

Metaphyseal–Diaphyseal Fractures

Several principles are helpful in deciding whether or not a fracture requires reduction in the child.

Age The younger the child, the greater the potential for remodeling (Figs. 10.35 and 10.39). This is possibly the most important factor. Generally children under age 10 years can be expected to remodel significant deformity.

Bone position Remodeling is greatest near the ends of bones. The amount of remodeling necessary to correct a deformity is proportional to the distance from the adjacent joint (Fig. 10.36). For example, distal forearm fractures remodel much better than midshaft deformities.

Plane of deformity Remodeling is usually greater in the sagittal than the frontal planes. Rotational or transverse plane deformity can remodel, but the amount is controversial. One reason for this controversy is the difficulty in assessing and imaging rotational remodeling.

Also, the plane of deformity is related to the axis of motion of the adjacent joints. Deformity that lies in the plane of motion of the adjacent joint will resolve or is better tolerated. For example, an anterior or posterior bow of the femur is more accepted than varus or valgus deformity.

Growth rate of adjacent physis Accept more deformity close to a physis with a great growth rate and potential. For example, the rapid growth rate of the upper humeral epiphysis contributes to its spectacular remodeling potential. In contrast, growth at the elbow is limited and varus–valgus deformities remodel poorly.

Completion of remodeling Remodeling is completed in about 5–6 years. Most occurs in the first 1 or 2 years.

Unique features Some malunions remodel poorly. The classic example is the cubitus varus deformity, resulting from malunion of supracondylar humeral fractures. Lateral condylar fractures are prone to nonunion (Fig. 10.38). The reason is unclear.

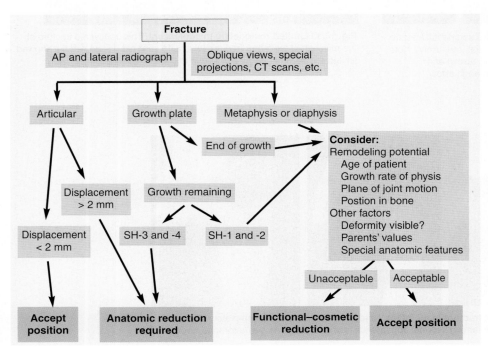

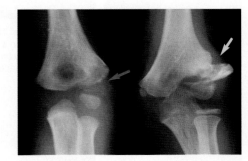

Fig. 10.38 Displaced lateral condylar fractures require anatomic reduction. This unique fracture (red arrow) is not only an articular injury but also an SH-4 fracture that is prone to nonunion. These are all indications for an anatomic reduction and internal fixation. Note that the unfixed fracture developed a nonunion (yellow arrow).

Fig. 10.37 Reduction flowchart. This may help in determining the need for reduction.

Physeal Fractures

Physeal fracture reduction is well established. SH-3 and -4 fractures should be anatomically reduced to prevent physeal bridge formation and reduce the risk of bar formation. Consider SH-1 and -2 fractures like metaphyseal injuries and apply the same principles to make decisions about management.

Articular Fractures

Articular fractures (Figs. 10.40 and 10.41) are less common in children than in adults, as the cartilage is more resilient and less readily injured. Some generalizations can be made.

Remodeling may correct some deformity Accept more articular deformity in the infant or young child than in older children or adolescents. Consider adolescents like adults.

Accept more horizontal than longitudinal displacement A step-off deformity that increases the articular loading may be less acceptable than that which widens the joint.

Apply the 2-mm rule Generally we accept displacement of less than 2 mm. This rule was established based on clinical experience. Be aware that MRI or CT studies will usually show more displacement than conventional radiographs (Fig. 10.42).

Indications for Open Reduction

Indications for open reduction change with time. These indications are affected by social, medical, and economic factors with considerable variation. Some generalizations can be made (Fig. 10.43).

Polytrauma suggests multisystem injury, not simply a child with several fractures. Many children with multiple fractures are best managed by cast immobilization, traction, or other invasive methods.

Economic indications The financial cost of management should be a factor only when deciding between options that are all medically acceptable.

References

1997 Bone remodelling in malunited fractures in children. Is it reliable? Gasco J, dePablos J. JPO-B 6:126

1996 Bone growth and remodelling after fracture. Murray DW, J Wilson-MacDonald, E Morscher, BA Rahn, M Kaslin. JBJS 78S:42

1996 Degenerative changes at the knee and ankle related to malunion of tibial fractures. 15-year follow-up of 88 patients. van der Schoot DK, et al. JBJS 78B: 722

1995 Degenerative arthritis after tibial plateau fractures. Honkonen SE. J Orthop Trauma 9: 273

1994 Long-term results of fracture of the scaphoid. A follow-up study of more than thirty years. Duppe H, et al. JBJS 76A:249

1988 Degenerative arthritis of the knee secondary to fracture malunion. Kettelkamp DB, et al. CO 234:159

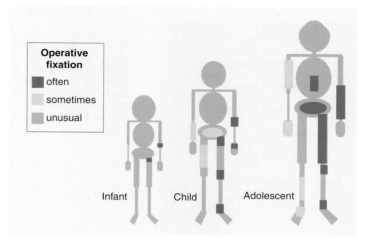

Fig. 10.39 Need for operative reduction and fixation. The need for open procedures in managing childhood fractures increases with age.

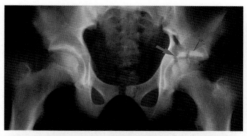
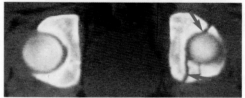

Fig. 10.40 Acetabular fractures. Anatomic reduction of most displaced acetabular fractures in adolescents is usually indicated as the hip joint poorly tolerates deformity.

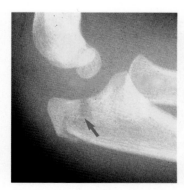

Fig. 10.41 Articular displacement >2 mm. This olecranon fracture (arrow) was reduced and fixed.

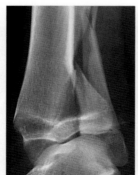

Fig. 10.42 CT imaging more accurate. The fracture is readily apparent on the lateral radiograph, but the CT scan (red arrow) best shows the extent of displacement and the need for reduction.

All Ages
  Lateral condylar fracture, humerus
  Supracondylar fracture, humerus
  SH-3 and SH-4 fractures
  Polytrauma
  Displaced articular fractures
End of growth
  Tibial triplane fractures
Age 10+ years
  Femoral shaft fractures
  Displaced midshaft forearm fractures

Fig. 10.43 Common indications for open reduction. These are also indications for internal fixation of displaced fractures.

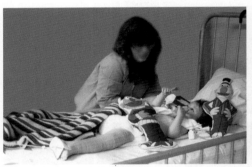

Fig. 10.44 Fixation and stability. Fixation methods provide varying degrees of stability. The ideal fixation provides adequate stability but allows the bone normal flexibility. Often combined methods of fixation are best for children.

Fixation

Reduction and internal fixation of children's fractures have become more widely practiced than in previous decades. This is due in part to increasing costs of hospitalization. The principles of internal fixation of fractures include the following:

Supplement with cast Internal fixation is often supplemented with a cast, so minimal fixation is all that is required.

Minimal fixation is adequate because bone healing is rapid and joint motion is regained quickly following injury.

Avoid transephyseal fixation except for small K wires.

Flexible fixation is usually adequate for children.

Removal of fixation devices is often optional.

Tailor fixation Be creative. Keep in mind the age of the child, the character of the fracture, the family situation, and your own skills (Fig. 10.44).

Good Choices

Cast immobilization still remains the first choice for managing childhood fractures (Fig. 10.45). Cast immobilization can be used alone or in combination with minimal internal fixation. Principles of casting in children are presented in Chapter 2, and application of spica casts is detailed on page 383.

Flexible intramedullary fixation IM rod fixation is ideal for long bone fractures in children (Fig. 10.46). Flexible rods can be easily inserted and removed. Reaming is unnecessary, reducing the risk of physeal injury. Prebending the rods adds dynamic control for reduction. Single rod fixation can be supplemented by a cast to control rotation. These devices are simpler and less expensive than rigid rods or plates. Flexible rods are especially valuable in pathologic fracture management and should be left in place to reduce the risk of refracture. These flexible rods are *load sharing* rather than *load shielding*. This maintains normal bone flexibility, making them more physiologic than plates or rigid rods.

Cross pin fixation is commonly used in fixation of humeral supracondylar and other metaphyseal fractures. Sometimes pin fixation is supplemented with a cast. Smooth pin ends are bent to prevent migration and usually left long outside the skin, making them easily removable. Use small, smooth pins when placing across the growth plate.

Bioabsorbable fixation by polyglycolic acid (PGA) or polylactide devices is ideal for children (Fig. 10.47). Such devices are small, provide adequate fixation when supplemented by a cast, do not interfere with healing, and do not require removal. They may replace metal K wires and screws in the future.

Single screw fixation is often useful to secure the metaphyseal fragment to the metaphysis (Fig. 10.48, left) or to fix a fracture through the epiphysis.

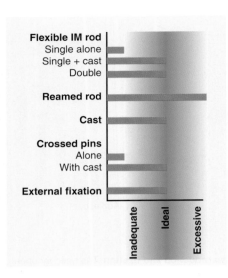

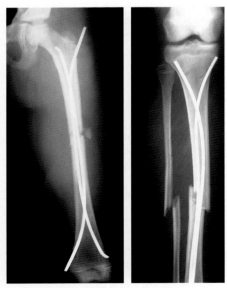

Fig. 10.45 Cast fixation. Casts are well tolerated by children. The child is often admitted for temporary traction before spica casts are applied for the femur. This boy can walk in his single hip spica cast.

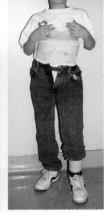

Fig. 10.46 Intramedullary fixation. This provides optimum fixation.

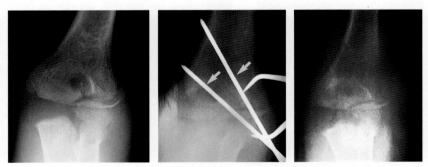

Fig. 10.47 Bioabsorbable fixation. This 6-year-old child had a displaced lateral condylar fracture (red arrows). Following reduction, the temporary fixation (yellow arrows) was replaced with polyglycolide 1.5-mm pins. These pins are not visible on the final radiograph (right).

Problems with Fixation

Plates and nail plates These may be useful for stabilizing diaphyseal fractures in children with polytrauma (Fig. 10.49). Plate application and removal requires the most extensive exposure and often leaves ugly residual surgical scars. Avoid crossing the growth plate (Fig. 10.48, right). Stress risers at the end screw increase the risk of fracture (Fig. 10.50).

External pin fixation Fixation is ideal for long bone fractures complicated by severe soft tissue injuries. This fixation allows soft tissue wound care. External pin fixation carries significant risks (Fig. 10.51, left). These include pin tract problems and fracture unions. Refractures are common following removal of the fixation after femoral shaft fractures in children. Scars for external pins are multiple, often causing dimpling, and are difficult to revise. Sometimes refracture may be prevented by applying a cast and encouraging full weight-bearing activity after fixation removal. Once the union is solid, the cast is removed.

Rigid IM fixation Reamed rodding in long bones exposes the child to the risk of physeal damage (Fig. 10.51, right) and avascular necrosis. Reamers placed through the greater trochanter or upper femur may damage appositional or enchondral bone growth and vascularity to the femoral head, causing avascular necrosis of the capital femoral epiphysis. Reserve reaming and rigid rods for fixing fractures after physeal closure.

References

1997 Osteochondritis dissecans of the patella: arthroscopic fixation with bioabsorbable pins. Matava MJ, Brown CD. Arthroscopy 13:124

1996 Flexible intramedullary nailing as fracture treatment in children. Huber RI, et al. JPO 16:602

1996 Comparison of bioabsorbable pins and Kirschner wires in the fixation of chevron osteotomies for hallux valgus. Winemaker MJ, Amendola A. Foot Ankle Int 17:623

1994 Fixation with bioabsorbable screws for the treatment of fractures of the ankle. Bucholz RW, Henry S, Henley M. JBJS 76A:319

1993 Absorbable polyglycolide pins in internal fixation of fractures in children. Böstman O, et al. JPO 13:242

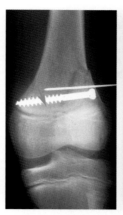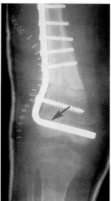

Fig. 10.48 Good and poor fixation choices. Fixation (green arrow) should not cross the growth plate. This transephyseal fixation extended across the growth plate (red arrow) and created a physeal bar.

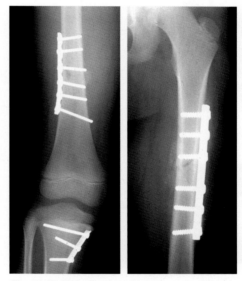

Fig. 10.49 Plate fixation. Plates are used here in a child with polytrauma as a rapid means of providing rigid fixation.

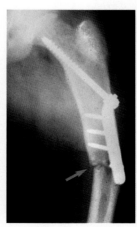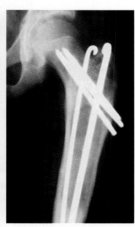

Fig. 10.50 Plate as stress riser in pathologic bone of fibrous dysplasia. Permanent IM fixation (right) is the ideal management of fibrous dysplasia.

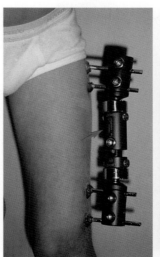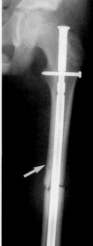

Fig. 10.51 Fixation with increased complication rates. Examples are external fixators (red arrow) and reamed IM rods (yellow arrow).

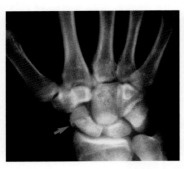

Fig. 10.52 Missed navicular fracture. This 14-year-old boy sustained polytrauma. During rehabilitation, he complained of wrist pain. A radiograph demonstrated this navicular fracture.

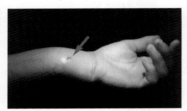

Fig. 10.53 Misleading history of trauma. This 12-year-old girl was initially seen with a history of injury to her leg. The radiographs showed periosteal new bone (yellow arrow). The pain increased gradually, and 2 months later, the lesion was larger (red arrow). A biopsy demonstrated Ewing sarcoma.

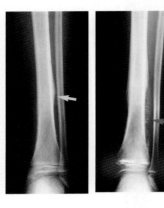

Fig. 10.54 Arm splint hiding puncture from an open fracture. The open nature of the forearm fracture was not initially appreciated because of an arm splint.

Evaluation

Establishing an accurate diagnosis in the most important step in managing childhood injuries. Most major errors of management are due to an inaccurate diagnosis. The evaluation of the injured child is difficult because injuries are sometimes multiple, the child is frequently not cooperative, and the emergency situation makes a thorough evaluation difficult.

Diagnostic errors are most significant in the child sustaining polytrauma, as subtle fractures are easily overlooked and musculoskeletal injuries are the most common cause of residual disability. In the polytraumatized child, musculoskeletal injuries seldom cause death but are a common cause of residual disability (Fig. 10.52).

Priorities

Make the first priority the evaluation of the pulmonary, cardiovascular, and neurologic status. Musculoskeletal priorities include cervical spine injury, joint dislocations (especially the hip), and unstable and open fractures.

History

The history should include the situation, velocity, mechanism, and any unique features of the accident. Be aware that a history of trauma may cloud the diagnosis of a more serious problem (Fig. 10.53).

Physical Examination

Most diagnostic errors are due to an incomplete physical examination. Perform a screening examination first. Look at the whole child. Look for obvious deformity and spontaneous movement. Pseudoparalysis in the child or infant is commonly due to trauma (Fig. 10.55).

Remove any splints (Fig. 10.54) or bandages so the examination can be complete. Look for deformity and swelling, and localize the point of maximum tenderness (PMT) (Fig. 10.56). Identifying the site of injury by physical examination is very important because much of the immature skeleton is unossified and difficult to image (see Chapter 2). Determining the PMT is one of the most important diagnostic steps in diagnosing occult injuries in children.

Evaluate the vascular status (Fig. 10.57). Be aware that the pulse is inadequate as a test of circulation. Observe the capillary refill rate and observe the child's reaction while extending the fingers or toes. Pain on passive stretching is an early sign of ischemia. Compartment syndromes may be silent in children.

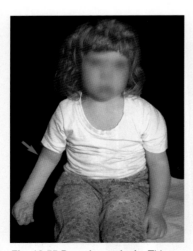

Fig. 10.55 Pseudoparalysis. This child has a pulled elbow and will not use the arm. The loss of spontaneous or volitional movement is a common sign of trauma in infants and young children.

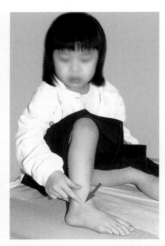

Fig. 10.56 Localization of the point of maximum tenderness. The exact PMT is a valuable finding that is sometimes diagnostic, as in this child with an anterior leaf collateral ligament sprain.

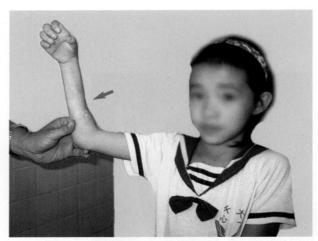

Fig. 10.57 Ischemic contracture of the forearm. This child has a contracture complicating a supracondylar fracture treated in a cast.

Imaging for Trauma

The vast majority of trauma problems can be satisfactorily imaged by conventional radiographs (Figs. 10.58 and 10.59). Comparative radiographs of the opposite side are rarely necessary in evaluating injuries in the child. Order comparative views only for special needs such as assessing ossification irregularities.

Ordering special imaging First consider additional radiographic views. Oblique radiographs may show a fracture that is suspected from the physical findings but not seen in the standard AP and lateral screening radiographs (Fig. 10.60). Displacement of articular or physeal fractures must be determined. Additional oblique projections may provide further information that may be helpful in deciding whether or not to accept the current reduction. Special imaging studies are indicated in certain situations when conventional radiographs provide insufficient information. The selection of the type of imaging is based on the physical examination findings and on a knowledge of common injury types typical in the child's age group.

Arthrography may be useful in assessing cartilagenous injuries (Fig. 10.61, left).

Bone scans are useful in screening for injuries (Fig. 10.61, right). Order a high-resolution study to pinpoint the exact location of a suspected fracture. For example, if "snuff-box" tenderness is found on physical examination and the radiographs are negative, order a high-resolution scan to determine if the scaphoid is fractured.

MRI studies require deep sedation of the infant and younger child and therefore have limited indications. Order these studies when suspecting such serious problems (Fig. 10.62) as spinal or nonaccidental injury.

Ultrasound studies are underutilized. Consider ultrasonography when evaluating such conditions as a possible physeal separation of the distal humeral epiphyseal complex in the newborn.

Arthroscopy may be helpful for evaluation of articular injuries (Fig. 10.63).

References

1999 Imaging features of avulsion injuries. Stevens MA, GY El-Khoury, MH Kathol, Brandser EA, Chow S. Radiographics 19:655

1999 Trends in pediatric emergency imaging. John SD. Radiol Clin North Am 37:995

1998 Prospective evaluation of early missed injuries and the role of tertiary trauma survey. Janjua KJ, Sugrue M, Deane SA. J Trauma 44:1000

1995 Evaluation of the role of comparison radiographs in the diagnosis of traumatic elbow injuries. Kissoon N, et al. JPO 15:449

1994 The relationships of skeletal injuries with trauma score, injury severity score, length of hospital stay, hospital charges, and mortality in children admitted to a regional pediatric trauma center. Buckley SL, et al. JPO 14:449

1994 Ultrasonographic evaluation of the elbow in infants and young children after suspected trauma. Davidson RS, et al. JBJS 76A:1804

1990 Rib fractures in children: a marker of severe trauma. Garcia VF, et al. J Trauma 30:695.

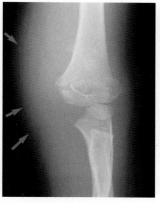
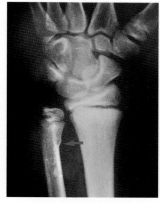

Fig. 10.58 Cortical irregularity due to a fracture. A change in contour when associated with tenderness over the same site is diagnostic of a fracture.

Fig. 10.59 Soft tissue swelling. This extensive soft tissue swelling is evidence of a fracture.

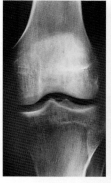
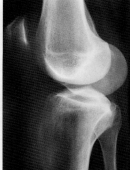
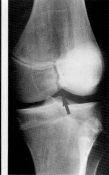

Fig. 10.60 Value of oblique radiograph. This intracondylar fracture (arrow) was not seen in the AP or lateral radiographs.

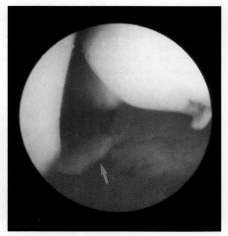

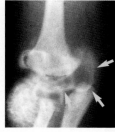
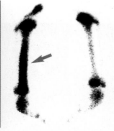

Fig. 10.61 Value of special imaging. An arthrogram (yellow arrows) shows a physeal fracture in an infant not apparent on plain radiographs. This bone scan (right) in an infant with a toddler's fracture (red arrow) shows a fracture that was not visible on conventional radiographs.

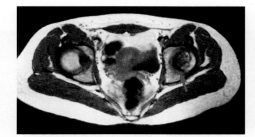

Fig. 10.62 MRI demonstration of AVN. This child had a femoral neck fracture. The MRI demonstrated the necrosis prior to radiographic changes.

Fig. 10.63 Elbow arthroscopy showing articular fracture. This fragment was not visible by radiography. Arthroscopy established the diagnosis and made removal of the fragment possible.

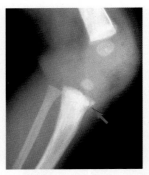

Fig. 10.64 Nonaccidental trauma. This subtle fracture of the tibial metaphysis was found to be due to child abuse.

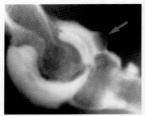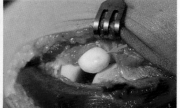

Fig. 10.65 Toddler's fractures. Subtle fractures of the tibia are sometimes seen on radiographs (yellow arrow). Cuboid fractures, another form of toddler's fractures, are typically diagnosed by bone scans (red arrow).

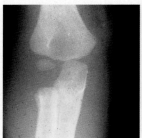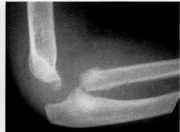

Fig. 10.66 Cartilagenous loose body. This 14-year-old boy had sustained an elbow injury. Radiographs were negative, but he later developed a clicking of the elbow. An arthrogram demonstrated a loose body (red arrow) that was removed (blue arrow).

Occult Injuries and Pitfalls in Diagnosis

Occult injuries are subtle injuries that are likely to be missed or misdiagnosed. Occult injuries are more common in infants and children because ossification is variable and incomplete and because children are difficult to examine. The child with a limp or a minor injury may have a nonlocalizing physical examination and negative radiographs. If a bone scan or MRI is performed, many subtle injuries will be detected. Are the costs and risks of the procedure worth making an exact diagnosis? Will this diagnosis change management? If the evaluation is for determining possible nonaccidental trauma, the answer to both of these questions is yes. For other problems, the answer is less clear and the decision is based on the situation.

Child Abuse

Nonaccidental trauma may be difficult to diagnose (Fig. 10.64). This is the most serious occult injury and is detailed on page 218.

Toddler's Fractures

Toddler's fractures include a variety of subtle fractures in infants and young children. They may involve the calcaneus, tibia, cuboid (Fig. 10.65), fibula, or metatarsals. The diagnosis is suspected by finding localized tenderness. Sometimes the radiograph is abnormal and diagnosis is established by a bone scan.

Cartilage Injury

Cartilage injuries are difficult to diagnose. They may first become evident by a loose body within the joint (Fig. 10.66).

Physeal Injury

Physeal injuries often pose difficulties in diagnosis, as they are poorly imaged by radiographs.

SH-1 fractures before ossification are often missed (Fig. 10.67). Other examples of such fractures include those of the lateral clavicle and medial humeral epicondyle.

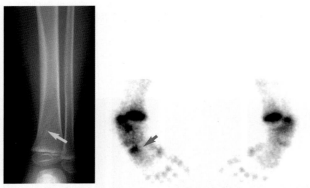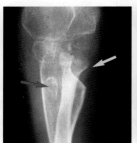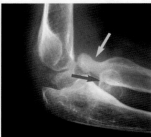

Fig. 10.67 Unrecognized fracture of the radial neck. A toddler sustained an elbow injury, and the radiographs were thought to be negative (left). He was next seen at age 7 years with a severe elbow deformity. Radiographs showed the radial head (red arrows) to be a separate fragment. The proximal radius (yellow arrows) was partly regenerated and lying anterior to the capitellum.

Physeal stress fractures of the physis are usually due to athletic injuries or neuromuscular disorders such as myelodysplasia (Fig. 10.68).

Physeal injury associated with diaphyseal fracture is not uncommon (Fig. 10.69). The physeal component is often overlooked as attention is directed to the diaphyseal fracture.

Physeal injuries of the proximal tibial epiphysis may occur with minimal trauma, immobilization, or inflammation (Fig. 10.70). This physis is very vulnerable. The reason for the vulnerability is unknown.

Undisplaced SH-1 fractures may be difficult to diagnose. Suspect the injury if tenderness is localized to the physis even when radiographs are negative.

Stress Fractures

Stress fractures are sometimes incorrectly diagnosed as something else. For example, a stress fracture of the femoral neck (Fig. 10.71) might be diagnosed as a groin pull.

Osteochondral Fractures

These fractures include a large cartilagenous component and little bone (Fig. 10.72). The bony fragment may be difficult to image or see on radiographs. Classic examples include fractures of the lateral humeral condylar and tibial spine.

References

2000 Fractures of the proximal radial head and neck in children with emphasis on those that involve the articular cartilage. Leung AG, Peterson HA. JPO 20:7

1999 The posterior fat pad sign in association with occult fracture of the elbow in children. Skaggs DL, Mirzayan R. JBJS 81A:1429

1999 Sonographic detection of occult fractures in the foot and ankle. Wang CL, et al. J Clin Ultrasound 27:421

1998 MRI of pediatric growth plate injury: correlation with plain film radiographs and clinical outcome. Carey J, et al. Skeletal Radiol 27:250

1998 Traumatic elbow effusions in pediatric patients: are occult fractures the rule? Donnelly LF, Klostermeier TT, Klosterman LA. Am J Roentgenol 171:243

1997 Neonatal transepyseal supracondylar fracture detected by ultrasound. Brown J, Eustace S. Pediatr Emerg Care 13:410

1997 Suspected scaphoid fractures in skeletally immature patients: application of MRI. Cook PA, et al. J Comput Assist Tomogr 21:511

1997 Pediatric fracture without radiographic abnormality. Description and significance. Naranja RJ Jr., et al. CO 342:141

1996 Occult fracture of the calcaneus in toddlers. Schindler A, Mason DE, Allington NJ. JPO 16:201

1993 Scintigraphy of spinal disorders in adolescents. Mandell GA, Harcke HT. Skeletal Radiol 22:393

1992 Occult fractures. Moseley CF. Instr Course Lect 41:361

1988 Occult fractures in preschool children. Oudjhane K, et al. J Trauma 28:858

1988 Early scintigraphic findings of occult femoral and tibial fractures in infants. Park HM, Kernek CB, Robb JA. Clin Nucl Med 13:271

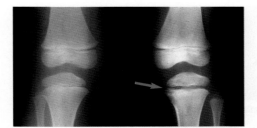

Fig. 10.68 Epiphylysis. This epiphysiolysis (arrow) due to repetitive injury of the proximal tibial physis produced swelling of the upper leg in a child with myelodysplasia.

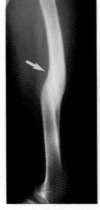
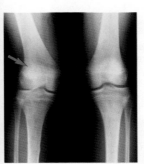

Fig. 10.69 Unrecognized physeal Injury of the femur. This 12-year-old girl sustained a femoral shaft fracture. The fracture healed and remodeled (yellow arrow), but she developed a valgus deformity of the knee. A physeal bar was identified (red arrow) and resected.

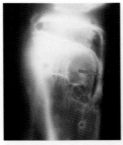
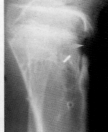

Fig. 10.70 Recurvatum deformity due to anterior physeal bar. This child was treated for a femoral fracture with a tibial traction pin. She developed a physeal bar (red arrow) that has resected (orange arrow).

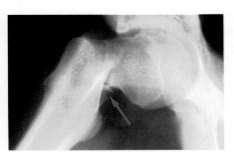

Fig. 10.71 Stress fracture misdiagnosed as a groin pull. The trainer advised this 17-year-old boy to continue sprinting. While running, he sustained this spontaneous fracture of the femoral neck.

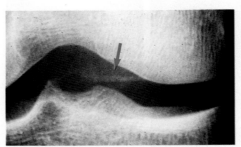

Fig. 10.72 Osteochondral fracture. This adolescent sustained an acute patellar dislocation with an osteochondral fracture. The bony rim is difficult to see on radiographs (red arrow).

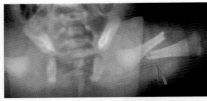

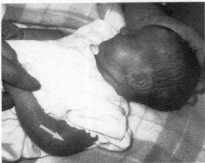

Fig. 10.73 Birth fractures. Diaphyseal fractures (red arrow) and joint injuries (yellow arrow) are examples of the spectrum of these injuries.

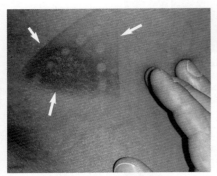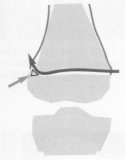

Fig. 10.74 Child abuse. This hot iron burn scar is permanent and unmistakable (white arrows). Classic fracture patterns include a metaphyseal fragment (green arrow) due to an epiphyseal fracture (red arrow).

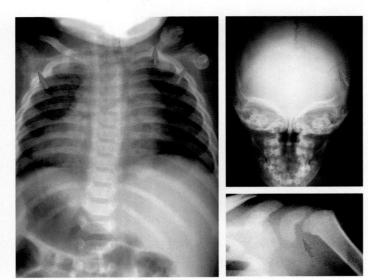

Fig. 10.75 Multiple fractures in abuse. Multiple fractures (red arrows) at varying stages of development are common in abuse.

Birth and Neonatal Injuries

Birth Injuries

Birth injuries often occur in some unusual obstetrical situations such as large birth weight, shoulder dystocia, mechanically assisted delivery, or prolonged gestational age. It also occurs in infants with some underlying problem such as osteogenesis imperfecta or arthrogryposis.

The most common injuries include brachial plexus injuries and fractures of the clavicle. Other injuries include femoral shaft fractures (Fig. 10.73) and neurologic injuries at the intracranial and spinal cord level.

Manage these fractures by simple splinting. Manage clavicular fractures by simply strapping the arm to the thorax for comfort. Manage femoral shaft fractures in a Pavlik harness. Remodeling will correct any remaining deformity.

Fractures in Early Infancy

Neonatal fractures are most common in very low birth weight premature infants who have developmental nutritional rickets. Fractures most commonly involve the ribs, radius, humerus, and femur. Manage by metabolic therapy and splinting. Avoid casts.

References

1998 Newborn clavicle fractures. McBride MT, Hennrikus WL, Mologne TS. Orthopedics 21:317

1998 Does cesarean section decrease the incidence of major birth trauma? Puza S, et al. J Perinatol 18:9

1997 Fractures in very low birth weight infants with rickets. Dabezies EJ, Warren PD. CO 335:233

1997 A retrospective analysis of Erb palsy cases and their relation to birth weight and trauma at delivery. Graham EM, Forouzan I, Morgan MA. J Matern Fetal Med 6:1

1997 Neurologic birth trauma. Intracranial, spinal cord, and brachial plexus injury. Medlock MD, Hanigan WC. Clin Perinatol 24:845

1996 Birth trauma. A five-year review of incidence and associated perinatal factors. Perlow JH, et al. J Reprod Med 41:754

1994 Ultrasound diagnosis of birth-related spinal cord trauma: neonatal diagnosis and follow-up and correlation with MRI. Fotter R, et al. Pediatr Radiol 24:241

Child Abuse

Because child abuse or nonaccidental trauma is a potentially lethal condition, consider this possibility in every infant or young child with a fracture. When the diagnosis of child abuse is missed, recurrent injuries occur in about half and it is lethal in 10% of infants and children.

Evaluation

Be suspicious of any long-bone fractures in an otherwise normal infant in the first year. Many femoral shaft fractures in early infancy are due to abuse. Be concerned if the caregiver reports only a change in behavior without a history of injury or a trivial injury. Remember that abuse can occur at any socioeconomic level.

Examination Look at the whole child. Other than the current problem, does the infant appear normal? Note any evidence of swelling, pseudoparalysis, or soft tissue trauma (Fig. 10.74, left). Bruising is more common than fractures.

Imaging If you are suspicious, order an AP radiograph of the chest, all four limbs, and a lateral of the skull. Order a bone scan to show recent fractures if further evaluation is indicated.

Fracture patterns in abuse Fractures that have a high degree of specificity for abuse are metaphyseal fractures (Fig. 10.74, right) and fractures of the humeral shaft, ribs (Fig. 10.75), scapula, outer end of the clavicle, and vertebra. Bilateral fractures, complex skull fractures, and those of different ages are suspect. Fractures of varying ages occur in only about 13% of cases. Try to date the fractures by radiographic appearance (Fig. 10.76).

If Abuse Is a Possibility

Personally call a social worker or case worker. Communicate your concern and index of suspicion. Consult your pediatric colleagues for their opinion. Carefully document your findings and efforts. Parents of infants with accidental injuries usually accept consultations with a simple explanation of the reason. Objection should raise suspicion.

References

2000 Femur shaft fractures in toddlers and young children: rarely from child abuse. Schwend RM, Werth C, Johnston A. JPO 20:475

1998 A regional approach to the classic metaphyseal lesion in abused infants: the distal femur. Kleinman PK, Marks SC Jr. Am J Roentgenol 170:43

1996 Circumferential growth plate fracture of the thoracolumbar spine from child abuse. Carrion WV, et al. JPO 16:210

1995 Relationship of the subperiosteal bone collar to metaphyseal lesions in abused infants. Kleinman PK, Marks SC Jr. JBJS 77A:1471

1994 The relationship of skeletal injuries with trauma score, injury severity score, length of hospital stay, hospital charges, and mortality in children admitted to a regional pediatric trauma center. Buckley SL, et al. JPO 14:449

1993 Fractures in young children. Distinguishing child abuse from unintentional injuries. Leventhal JM, et al. Am J Dis Child 147:87

1993 Metaphyseal extensions of hypertrophied chondrocytes in abused infants indicate healing fractures. Osier LK, Marks SC Jr., Kleinman PK. JPO 13:249

1991 Fracture patterns in battered children. Loder RT, Bookout C. J Orthop Trauma 5:428

1991 Long-bone fractures in young children: distinguishing accidental injuries from child abuse. Thomas SA, et al. Pediatrics 88:471

1988 Analysis of 429 fractures in 189 battered children. King J, et al. JPO 8:585

Polytrauma

Multiple injuries (Fig. 10.77) occur in about 10% of children admitted to hospitals for trauma. Trauma center management provides the best outcome. Trauma prevention remains our greatest challenge.

Injury severity is greater for fractures involving the spine, pelvis, clavicle, and scapula (Fig. 10.78).

Possible neck injury in infants requires transport with a pad under the shoulders to maintain the neck in a neutral position.

Polytrauma requires multidisciplinary care and ideally in a trauma center. Keep priorities in mind, which are airway (Fig. 10.79), circulation, neurologic, gastrointestinal, genitourinary, and then musculoskeletal. Consider the age of the patient when planning management. Managing an infant (Fig. 10.80) is often very different from managing the same injuries in an older child or adolescent.

Conditions Requiring Early Orthopedic Care

Include orthopedic management in the initial management plan.

Femoral shaft fracture and head injury Fix the femur by whatever method is most practical. In some centers, this is done by plating, external fixators, or flexible IM rodding.

Compartment syndromes Vascular injury or findings suggestive of a compartment syndrome requires early evaluation.

Floating knee often requires internal fixation. This fixation may be applied to one or both bones. Stabilizing one fracture may allow the other fracture to be managed in a cast.

Look for occult fractures Keep in mind that injuries that initially are not life threatening can cause the greatest problems in the future.

Firearm Injury

Gunshot injuries often cause polytrauma. These injuries constitute the third most common cause of death in children during the second decade and are a major public health problem.

References

1997 Pediatric polytrauma: short-term and long-term outcomes. van der Sluis CK, et al. J Trauma 43:501

1995 The pediatric polytrauma patient. Cramer KE. CO 318:125

1995 A population-based study of severe firearm injury among children and youth. Zavoski RW, et al. Pediatrics 96:278

1994 Firearm injuries in children and adolescents: epidemiology and preventive approaches. Christoffel KK, Naureckas SM. Curr Opin Pediatr 6:519

1987 Pediatric polytrauma: orthopedic care and hospital course. Loder RT. J Orthop Trauma 1:48

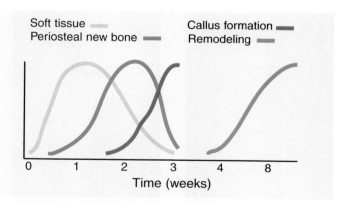

Fig. 10.76 Age of fractures in infants. Radiographs can be used to determine the age of fractures based on X-ray features.

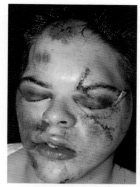

Fig. 10.77 Polytrauma. This requires multidiciplinary care. This child had extensive facial injuries in addition to a femur fracture.

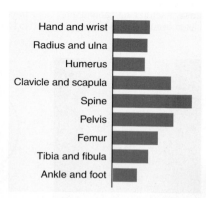

Fig. 10.78 Injury severity score by fracture type. From Buckley (1994).

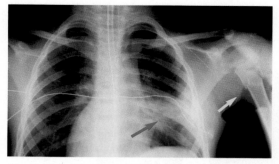

Fig. 10.79 Polytrauma priorities. The pulmonary contusion with atelectasis (red arrow) takes priority over the humeral fracture (yellow arrow).

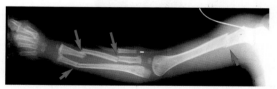

Fig. 10.80 Multiple fractures. These multiple fractures alone constitute polytrauma, but in the infant, these fractures may only require immobilization in a long-arm cast.

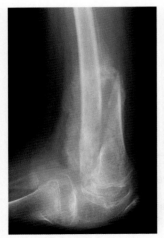

Fig. 10.81 Fracture in child with cerebral palsy. The bone easily fractures and abundant callus occurs during healing.

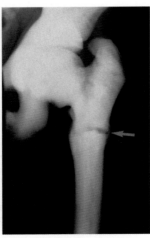

Fig. 10.82 Fracture in osteopetrosis. These bones fracture easily and are difficult to fix internally.

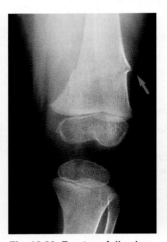

Fig. 10.83 Fracture following DDH treatment in a spica cast.

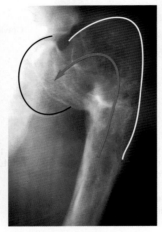

Fig. 10.84 Multiple fractures in fibrous dysplasia. The child has developed a *shepherd crook deformity* from repeated fractures.

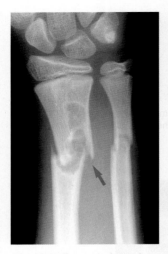

Fig. 10.85 Fracture through a nonossifying fibroma.

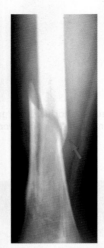

Fig. 10.86 Fracture through malignant asteogenic sarcoma. This is the most worrisome fracture to miss.

Pathologic Fractures

Pathologic fractures are relatively common in children. Fractures frequently occur through osteopenic bone in children with neuromuscular disorders and through bone weakened by tumors.

Evaluation

Be concerned if the trauma required for fracture is less than normal. Normal infants and young children's bone can fracture with simple falls. Usually a history and screening examination will separate normal children from those with underlying osteopenic problems.

Management

Generalized disorders include those that decrease or increase bone density. Manage fractures through osteopenic bone in children with conditions such as cerebral palsy (Fig. 10.81), spina bifida, and osteogenesis imperfecta with a minimum period of immobilization because mobilization increases deossification and increases the risk of additional fractures. Dysplasias increase bone density and may also be prone to fracture (Fig. 10.82).

Cast treatment for conditions such as developmental hip dysplasia increase the risk of fracture. The period of greatest vulnerability is shortly after cast removal, as joints are stiff and bone is weakened by immobilization (Fig. 10.83).

Benign bone lesions are often the sites of fracture.

Small localized tumors If the lesion is small and the trauma significant, immobilize in a cast until union has occurred. Usually it is best to allow the fracture to heal and then deal with the lesion. For larger lesions, especially those involving the upper femur, stabilization and bone grafting may be necessary.

Fibrous dysplasia Consider early augmentation with a flexible intramedullary rod (Fig. 10.84) to increase bone strength and reduce the risk of fracture. This treatment usually shortens the period of convalescence.

Unicameral bone cysts Most cysts should be allowed to heal and then be managed as described in Chapter 13. Those of the upper femur require special consideration. Most require internal fixation to prevent malunion. Graft and fix during the same operative session. Avoid threaded or large fixation across any the growth plate in the child under age 8–10 years. Smooth K wires may be applied across the proximal femoral physis. Bend over the pins to avoid migration.

Nonossifying fibromas are a common site of fracture (Fig. 10.85). If they involve more than 50% of the transverse bone area, they may require grafting.

Malignant tumors Be most concerned about missing a fracture through a malignant tumor such as an osteogenic sarcoma (Fig. 10.86). Ask if the child or adolescent had night pain before the fracture. Night pain is often an indicator of a malignant tumor. Carefully review the radiograph with attention to the character of the bone. Early identification of the pathologic aspect of the fracture is the primary concern.

References

1996 The surgical treatment and outcome of pathological fractures in localised osteosarcoma. Abudu A, et al. JBJS 78B:694

1996 Pathological fractures in patients with cerebral palsy. Brunner R, Doderlein L. JPO-b 5:232

1990 Pathologic fractures in severely handicapped children and young adults. Lee JJ, Lyne ED. JPO 10:497

1984 Surgical treatment of pathological subtrochanteric fractures due to benign lesions in children and adolescents. Malkawi H, Shannak A, Amr S. JPO 4:63

Open Fractures

Open fractures in children most commonly involve the tibia, but they may also complicate supracondylar fractures and fractures of the fore-arm, femur, and other bones.

Classification

The classification of open injuries is basically the same as for adults (Fig. 10.87). Overall the prognosis for a given grade is better in children, especially infants and young children. Adolescents behave more like adults.

Management

Sequence Manage acute injuries in the same sequence as done for adults. This involves antibiotic prophylaxis, tetanus update, debridement (Figs. 10.88 and 10.89), and immobilization. Limb salvage is usually feasible. Open fractures in younger children can be managed less aggressively than those of the adolescent.

Different management for the child Managing the child differs from managing the adult in several ways: (1) soft tissue healing is much more rapid and complete, (2) devitalized bone that is not contaminated can be left in place and will incorporate, (3) the periosteum will gener-ate new bone when bone is lost (Fig. 10.90), (4) delayed or nonunion is uncommon, and (5) external fixators may be left in place for prolonged periods to be certain bony union is solid.

References

2000 Effect of delay of surgical treatment on rate of infection in open fractures in children. Skaggs DL, et al. JPO 20:19

2000 Open femur fractures in children: treatment, complications, and results. Hutchins CM, PD Sponseller, Sturm P, Mosquero R. JPO 20:183

1997 Treatment of type II and type III open tibia fractures in children. Bartlett CS, Weiner LS, Yang EC. J Orthop Trauma 11:357

1997 The orthopedic and social outcome of open tibia fractures in children. Levy AS, et al. Orthopedics 20:593

1996 Age as a prognostic factor in open tibial fractures in children. Blasier RD, Barnes CL. CO 331:261

1996 Severe (type III) open fractures of the tibia in children. Buckley SL, et al. JPO 16:627

1996 Open fracture of the tibia in children. Cullen MC, et al. JBJS 78A:1039

1996 Open fractures of the tibia and femur in children. Robertson P, Karol LA, Rab GT. JPO 16:621

1996 Open fractures of the tibia in children. Song KM, et al. JPO 16:635

1992 Open fractures of the diaphysis of the lower extremity in children. Treatment, results, and complications. Cramer KE, Limbird TJ, Green NE. JBJS 74A:218

Gustilo classification of open fractures		
Type	Soft tissue	Bone
Type 1	Clean wound	< 1 cm laceration
Type 2	Soft tissue injury not extensive	> 1 cm laceration
Type 3	Extensive soft tissue injury	Includes segmental fractures

Fig. 10.87 Classification of open fractures in children.

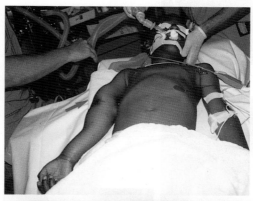
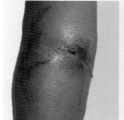
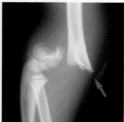

Fig. 10.88 Open supracondylar fracture. This type 1 open fracture (arrows) produced only a puncture wound above the elbow. The wound was irrigated and edges debrided.

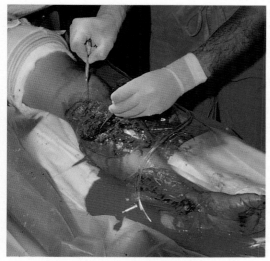

Fig. 10.89 Fracture debridement. While swimming, this boy sustained an open tibial fracture from a boat propeller. This debridement was carefully performed to remove all devitalized and foreign material. An external fixator was placed, and the bone healed without infection.

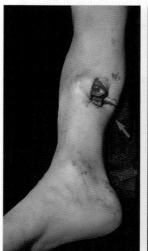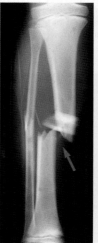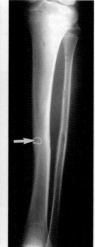

Fig. 10.90 Open segmental fracture of the tibia. This fracture (red arrow) was managed by debridement and removal of the loose contaminated segment. Note that the bone regenerated within the periosteum (yellow arrow).

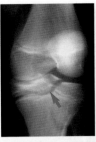
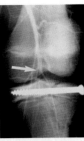
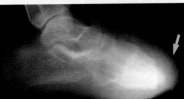

Fig. 10.91 Unrecognized vascular injury. This proximal tibial fracture (red arrow) was reduced and fixed with a screw. Loss of perfusion prompted an arteriogram that showed an arterial injury (yellow arrow). The delayed diagnosis resulted in the need for a transmetatarsal amputation (orange arrow).

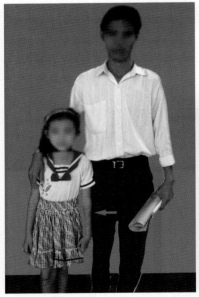
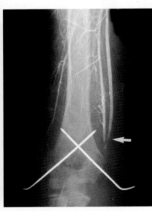

Fig. 10.92 Volkmann contracture following a supracondylar fracture. This girl has an ischemic forearm contracture (red arrow) following cast management of a supracondylar fracture. Vascular compromise is seen in this pinned fracture (yellow arrow).

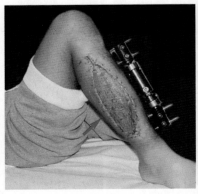
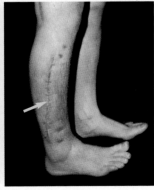

Fig. 10.93 Compartment syndrome successfully managed. These patients developed compartment syndromes which were managed by compartmental release and external fixation. The wounds were primarily grafted (red arrow) in one and closed secondarily (yellow arrow) in the other. In both, muscle function was preserved.

Complications

The major challenge in managing trauma is avoiding complications. Children's fractures generally heal quickly. Vascular complications (Fig. 10.91) are uncommon, nerve injuries usually recover with time, and joint motion recovers spontaneously. In general, outcomes are excellent, unless problems develop. Most complications are due to the injury, while a few result from mismanagement. A good strategy in managing trauma is to consider what complications are most likely to occur from that injury and to take active measures to avoid them.

Misdiagnosis

It has been estimated that about 15% of children's fractures are misdiagnosed. Being aware of occult injuries and pitfalls and performing a careful evaluation will reduce this risk.

Problem Fractures

Be aware that certain fractures carry a high rate of complications.

Supracondylar fractures The risks include forearm ischemic contracture (Fig. 10.92), nerve injuries, and malunion causing cubitus varus.

Lateral condylar fractures This injury has the potential for nonunion and displacement.

Radial neck fractures For severely displaced fractures, avascular necrosis, overgrowth, and rotational stiffness are risks.

Midshaft forearm fractures in older children and adolescents may be complicated by malunion that limits forearm rotation, causes refracture, and rarely cross union.

Femoral neck fracture may develop avascular necrosis and coxa vara.

Distal femoral physeal fracture often develops growth arrest.

Proximal tibial metaphyseal fracture may result in overgrowth causing genu valgum.

Nonpreventable Complications from Injuries

Some complications are due to irreparable damage at the time of injury.

Avascular necrosis of the proximal femur or radial head can be caused by vascular injuries to the epiphysis vessels. Even with joint decompression and anatomic reduction, this complication may occur.

Physeal injuries that damage the germinal layer of the growth plate often cause shortening and angulatory deformity.

Preventable Complications

Some complications can be avoided by skillful management.

Compartment syndromes may result from vascular injury, prolonged operative procedures, cannulation of arteries, catheterization procedures, intravenous fluid infiltration, osteomyelitis, and necrotizing fascitis. Prevent or manage effectively by early recognition and treatment before muscle necrosis occurs.

Malunion due to inadequate reduction or loss of position are most common in older children and adolescents.

Physeal bar formation results from fractures that simply traverse rather than damage the germinal layer. Anatomic reduction reduces the risk of a physeal bar forming across the growth plate.

Deformity from small physeal bars can be prevented by identifying and resectioning bars (less than 50% of physis) before significant deformity occurs.

Most fixation complications are preventable by proper selection and application that is age appropriate. Fixation complications include placement that damages the physis, a type that is inadequate, a position that leads to stress risers, and premature removal that results in secondary fracture.

Cast complications are common and usually due to excessive pressure that causes limb ischemia or pressure sores. Poor cast technique may result in cast failure and loss of correction. Failure to mold the cast may result in loss of reduction while being immobilized.

Avoiding Complications

Before treatment consider what serious complications are possible and take steps to avoid them. These suggestions have been made earlier, but they are worth restating here for emphasis.

1. Avoid tibial traction pins Femoral pins are equally effective and pose less risk.

2. Avoid intravenous narcotics In the postreduction period, these may mask a compartment syndrome or other serious problem.

3. Assume the child will be unreliable Make the cast extra thick, and immobilize with the knee flexed to prevent walking.

4. Split casts for fractures Do this where swelling is common, such as in tibial and forearm fractures (Fig. 10.94).

5. Avoid high-risk treatment methods For example, avoid Bryant's overhead traction for femur fractures in infants and external pin fixation (Fig. 10.96) for closed noncomminuted fractures.

6. Inform families about risks Do this in advance for deformities from physeal injuries, avascular necrosis, and compartment syndromes.

7. Provide follow-up See patients with fractures after 1 week for radiographs to identify any loss of reduction while rereduction is still feasible. Follow physeal injuries for 1 year to be certain that growth is proceeding normally.

8. Respect the physis Avoid any injury from fixation such as reaming for IM fixation in the growing child (Fig. 10.96) and large devices across the physis.

9. Communication problems Be concerned about the fussing infant or young child or the child with a communication problem because they cannot identify or describe a site of pain or other problem (Fig. 10.97).

10. Allow stiffness to resolve spontaneously Forceful ranging of the joint may increase stiffness or fracture the adjacent bone (Fig. 10.98).

11. Compartment syndromes Be aware that compartment syndromes are often silent in the child.

12. Avoid prolonged immobilization In osteopenic children, avoid casts in conditions such as osteogenesis imperfecta and myelodysplasia.

References

2000 Open femur fractures in children: treatment, complications, and results. Hutchins CM, Set al. JPO 20:183

1998 Complications of intramedullary fixation of pediatric forearm fractures. Cullen MC, et al. JPO 18:14

1997 Primary epineural repair of the median nerve in children. Hudson DA, Bolitho DG, Hodgetts K. J Hand Surg [Br] 22:54

1997 Ulnar nerve injury following midshaft forearm fractures in children. Stahl S, Rozen N, Michaelson M. J Hand Surg [Br] 22:788

1995 Acute neurovascular complications with supracondylar humerus fractures in children. Dormans JP, Squillante R, Sharf H. J Hand Surg [Am] 20:1

1995 Clinical assessment of primary digital nerve repair. Efstathopoulos D, et al. Acta Orthop Scand Suppl 264:45

1993 Incidence of anterior interosseous nerve palsy in supracondylar humerus fractures in children. Cramer KE, Green NE, Devito DP. JPO 13:502

1993 Distal forearm fractures in children. Complications and surgical indications. Dicke TE, Nunley JA. Orthop Clin North Am 24:333

1992 Complications associated with fracture of the neck of the femur in children. Forlin E, et al. JPO 12:503

1990 Compartment syndrome following forearm fracture in children. Royle SG. Injury 21:73

1989 Results of median nerve repair in children. Tajima T, Imai H. Microsurgery 10:145

1986 Upper limb motor and sensory recovery after multiple proximal nerve injury in children: a long term review in five patients. Stevenson JH, Zuker RM. Br J Plast Surg 39:109

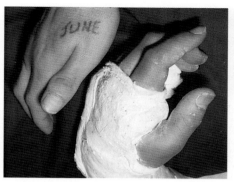

Fig. 10.94 Ischemia due to a tight cast. This patient had a forearm fracture immobilized in a cast. Note the swelling and congestion. The cast was split and the problem resolved.

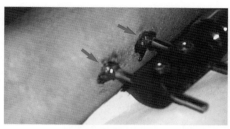

Fig. 10.95 External pin fixation complications. External pins carry a high rate of complications, including pin tract infections (arrows).

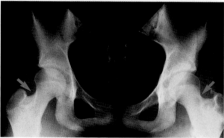

Fig. 10.96 Growth damage from femoral reaming. At age 11 years, this patient was treated with reamed rods for bilateral femoral fractures. Growth of the upper femoral was damaged, causing narrowing of the femoral necks.

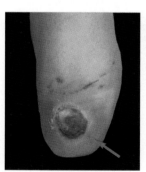

Fig. 10.97 Cast pressure sores. Patients with poor sensation or inability to communicate are at extra risk. This heel ulcer occurred in a child with cerebral palsy and was not diagnosed until the cast was removed.

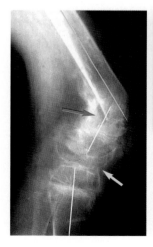
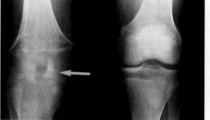

Fig. 10.98 Damage from overtreatment of postoperative stiffness. This girl with a tibial spine fracture had forceful physical therapy and a manipulation under anesthesia. She sustained a manipulation fracture (red arrow), joint damage (yellow arrow), and eventually a knee fusion (orange arrow).

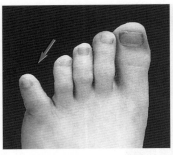

Fig. 10.99 Toe fractures. This displaced fracture of the proximal phalanx required closed reduction.

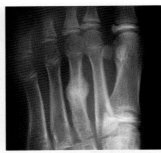

Fig. 10.100 Metatarsal stress fracture. These fractures are most common in adolescence.

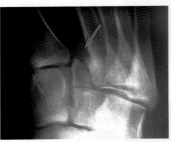

Fig. 10.101 Tarsal–metatarsal fracture dislocation. This adolescent sustained this fracture dislocation. It was anatomically reduced and fixed with temporary screw fixation.

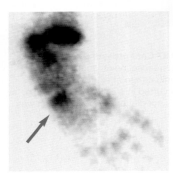

Fig. 10.102 Occult cuboid fracture. This 3-year-old child walked with a limp, and slight swelling over the lateral aspect of the foot was seen. Radiographs were negative, but this bone scan demonstrated a fracture (arrow).

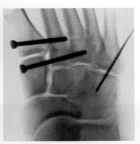

Fig. 10.103 Navicular fracture. This adolescent sustained this displaced articular fracture (arrow). The fracture was reduced open and fixed with a screw.

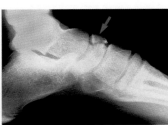

Foot Injuries

Foot fractures account for about 6% of all children's fractures and about half involve the metatarsals. Soft tissue injuries are relatively common because the child's foot is vulnerable to injury.

Fractures

Toe fractures sometimes require reduction (Fig. 10.99) and can often be immobilized by taping the toe to the adjacent digit.

Metatarsal fractures most commonly affect the fifth MT and are most common in the second decade of life. In early childhood, the first MT is most commonly fractured. These fractures remodel well, and closed management is usually satisfactory. Stress fractures become more common during adolescence (Fig. 10.100).

Tarsal–metatarsal fractures are most common in older children. Unstable injuries may require internal fixation (Fig. 10.101).

Cuboid fractures make up about 5% of foot fractures.

Acute fractures may be caused by direct trauma or forced abduction of the foot. These are uncommon fractures. Suspect this fracture if tenderness and swelling over the cuboid is present. Make oblique radiographs if necessary to establish the diagnosis. An anatomic or near anatomic reduction is necessary in the older child if the articular surface is deformed.

Stress fractures are most common in early childhood (Fig. 10.102) and are frequently missed unless identified by a bone scan Consider this diagnosis in the child with an undiagnosed limp. Manage with a short-leg walking cast for 2 weeks.

Navicular fractures are rare injuries and, if displaced, may require open reduction and fixation (Figs. 10.103 and 10.104).

Talus fractures are rare injuries (Fig. 10.105). Manage nondisplaced fractures by cast immobilization. Reduce articular fractures and fix anatomically. Outcomes are generally good. AVN and degenerative changes are rare complications.

Calcaneal fractures can be divided into acute or stress fractures.

Acute fractures can be classified like adult fractures. About 60% are extraarticular (Fig. 10.106). Comminution is less common in children. Manage most with a short-leg cast. Avulsion of the tendo achilles can be managed closed if displacement is minimal (Fig. 10.107). The prognosis is usually good. Anatomically reduce and fix displaced articular fractures.

Stress fractures cause limping in infants and children. The diagnosis can often be established by finding tenderness over the heel. Treat with a short leg cast for 2–3 weeks. If the diagnosis is unclear, a bone scan is diagnostic (Fig. 10.109). Follow-up radiographs taken at 2–3 weeks will often show the arc of sclerosis across the calcaneal tuberosity.

Lawn Mower Injuries to the Foot

These devastating injuries are usually due to falls from riding mowers. Most serious injuries involve the plantar–medial aspect of the foot. Microvascular repairs, composite, cross-leg, and free grafts are often necessary for management. Attempts at preservation are justified because of the child's great potential for healing.

Child Abuse

Include high-resolution radiographs of the feet in the skeletal survey performed for suspected child abuse. Torus and other subtle fractures are typical findings.

Burns of the Feet

Burns of the feet often result in severe contracture formation. Management may require releases and grafting or gradual correction with an Ilizarov frame.

Bicycle Spoke Injuries

These accidents often cause soft tissue injuries and occasionally fractures. They usually occur while riding with an adult.

Soft Tissue Injuries

Compartment syndromes Swelling, pain with passive motion, and elevated compartment pressure establish the diagnosis. Treat with multicompartment releases and delayed skin closure.

Severe soft tissue injuries may result in necrosis (Fig. 10.108), skin loss, or neurovascular complications. The greater healing potential of the child may result in less of a disability compared to an equivalent injury in an adult.

References

2000 Acute traumatic compartment syndrome of the foot in children. Bibbo C, Lin SS, Cunningham FJ. Pediatr Emerg Care 16:244

2000 Calcaneal fractures in children. Long-term results of treatment. Brunet JA. JBJS 82B:211

1999 Sonographic detection of occult fractures in the foot and ankle. Wang CL, et al. J Clin Ultrasound 27:421

1998 Tendon transfer with a microvascular free flap for injured feet in children. Hahn SB, Lee JW, Jeong JH. JBJS 80B:86

1998 Fracture of the cuboid in children: case report and review of the literature. Holbein O, Bauer G, Kinzl L. JPO 18:466

1998 Calcaneal fractures in children. Inokuchi S, et al. JPO 18:469

1998 Motorbike toe: a toddler sporting injury. Kane S. J Accid Emerg Med 15:22

1996 The bicycle spoke injury: an avoidable accident? D'Souza LG, et al. Foot Ankle Int 17:170

1996 Occult fracture of the calcaneus in toddlers. Schindler A, Mason DE, Allington NJ. JPO 16:201

1995 A study of metatarsal fractures in children. Owen RJ, Hickey FG, Finlay DB. Injury 26:537

1995 Compartment syndrome of the foot in children. Silas SI, et al. JBJS 77A:356

1995 Fractures of the cuboid in children: a source of leg symptoms. Simonian PT, et al. JBJS 77B:104

1995 Lawn mower injuries of the pediatric foot and ankle: observations on prevention and management. Vosburgh CL, et al. JPO 15:504

1994 Prognosis of fracture of the talus in children. 21 year follow-up of 14 cases. Jensen I, et al. Acta Orthop Scand 65:398

1994 Open physeal fractures of the distal phalanx of the great toe. A case report. Noonan KJ, Saltzman CL, Dietz FR. JBJS 76A:122

1993 Reconstruction of foot burn contractures in children. Alison WE Jr., et al. J Burn Care Rehabil 14:34

1993 Stubbed great toe injury: a unique clinical entity. Rathore MH, Tolymat A, Paryani SG. Pediatr Infect Dis J 12:1034

1988 Post-traumatic bony regeneration in a toe. Neumann L. J Trauma 28:717

1984 Fractures of the tarsus and metatarsus in children--diagnosis, treatment, results. Hahn M, Stock HJ. Zentralbl Chir 109:23

1981 Pediatric Lisfranc injury: "bunk bed" fracture. Johnson GF. Am J Roentgenol 137:1041

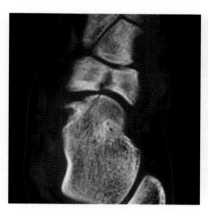

Fig. 10.104 CT scan of tarsal fractures. The character of this displaced navicular fracture was difficult to assess by conventional radiographs.

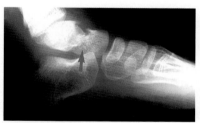

Fig. 10.105 Displaced talar neck fracture. This fracture was managed in a short-leg cast. The fracture healed and full motion was restored.

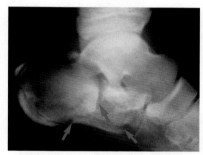

Fig. 10.106 Comminuted fracture of the calcaneus. This fracture resulted from a fall. It was managed in a cast with a good outcome.

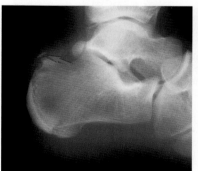

Fig. 10.107 Avulsion fracture of the tendo achilles. Note the small fragment of bone avulsed with the tendon. Because the displacement is minimal, the fracture was managed by immobilization in a short-leg cast.

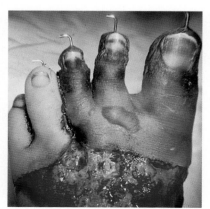

Fig. 10.108 Severe crush injury. An attempt was made to save as much of the foot as possible. With time the level of viability became well defined.

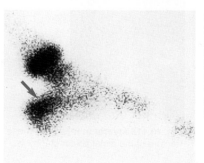

Fig. 10.109 Occult calcaneal fracture. This 5-year-old boy had a limp and initially negative radiographs of the foot. The bone scan confirmed the fracture. Radiographs at 3 weeks demonstrated changes consistent with an undisplaced fracture.

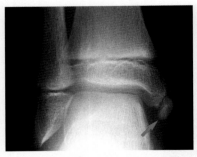

Fig. 10.110 Medial malleolar ossicle.
This ossicle was found incidentally.

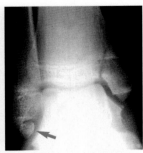

Fig. 10.111 Os subfibulare.
This ossicle was seen in a
patient with a medial
malleolar fracture. It was an
incidental finding. Note the
rounded edges.

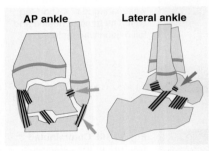
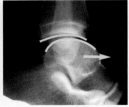

Fig. 10.112 Ankle ligaments. The lateral ligaments of the ankle are most
vulnerable to injury (green arrows). Of these ligaments, the anterior
ligament is the least strong and most vulnerable (red arrows).

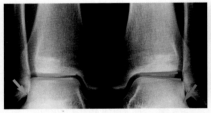

Fig. 10.113 Chronic ankle instability. With inversion stress of both ankles,
instability is noted on the left side (red) as compared to the stable right
(green). Anterior stress demonstrates AP instability as well (yellow).

Early childhood
   Metaphyseal fractures
Middle childhood
   Adduction
   Abduction
   Plantar flexion
Transitional
   Tillaux
   Triplane
     Lateral
     Medial

**Fig. 10.114 Classification of
ankle fractures in children.**

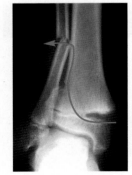
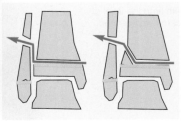

Fig. 10.115 Inversion injuries. These injuries often result in
fracture of the distal fibular diaphysis.

Ankle Injuries

Accessory Ossicles

Accessory ossification centers occur in both the medial (Fig. 10.110)
and lateral malleoli. In some cases, this ossification center fails to fuse
with the epiphysis and an accessory ossicle develops. Fracture of the
synchrondrosis between the ossicle and the malleolus may occur and
cause pain. The tenderness is exactly localized over the tip of the malleolus. This unique localization is often diagnostic.

   Os subfibulare This ossicle of the lateral malleolus may be trauma-
tically separated and painful (Fig. 10.111). Manage acute separation as
a fracture. Immobilize in a short-leg cast for 4 weeks. Rarely healing
fails, and excision or grafting of the painful ossicle may be required.

Ankle Sprains

Ankle sprains become increasingly common with advancing age.
Sprains are common in adolescents. Lateral sprains that involve the cal-
caneocuboid ligament and lateral collateral ligaments are most common
(Fig. 10.112). The site of sprain can usually be determined by the PMT.
If bone tenderness is found or clinical findings are atypical, make AP,
oblique, and lateral radiographs of the ankle.

   Mild sprains Sprains of the anterior talofibular and calcanocuboid
ligament are managed with an elastic bandage, elevation, and cold application. Limit activity until tenderness is no longer present.

   Moderate to severe sprains Manage in a short-leg walking cast for
3–4 weeks.

   Recurrent sprains Order stress radiographs to access stability (Fig.
10.113). Unstable and symptomatic ankles may require repair as in
adults.

Ankle Fractures

Ankle fractures are varied and complex. These fractures result from a
complex interplay of the mechanism of injury and the changing physiology of the immature ankle. Management of ankle fractures is presented on page 371.

   Age Fracture patterns change with age (Fig. 10.114).

   Early childhood During infancy and childhood, the weakest part of
the bone is often the metaphysis. These injuries may spare the physis
and ligaments.

   Middle to late childhood Later in childhood, physis becomes relative
weaker and failure may occur at that level. Disruption of the distal fibular epiphysis may be difficult to diagnose.

   Adolescence Complex fracture patterns in teens are due to asymmetrical closure of the physis. Such fractures are often categorized as
transitional. Tears of the collateral ligaments become more common.

   Inversion and eversion fractures Lateral failure may occur through
the ligaments, the epiphysis, or the physis (Figs. 10.115 and 10.116).
Often the physis fails. This may be difficult to recognize by examination
or conventional imaging. MRI studies of ankles demonstrate physeal
failure to be quite common. Manage these injuries by immobilization in
a short-leg cast for 4 weeks.

Plantar–flexion fracture Failure may occur in the distal tibia or growth plate (Fig. 10.117).

Tibial physeal fracture Evaluate by AP, lateral, and both oblique radiographs. If the extent of displacement is uncertain, CT evaluation may be necessary (Fig. 10.121). Displacement of >2 mm requires reduction. Fix with metalic or absorbable fixation devices. Supplement fixation in a long-leg cast for 4 weeks.

Triplane fractures These are transitional fractures of the distal tibia. Fracture patterns at the end of growth are based on relative strength of the bone and physis and also on the sequence of closure of the physis. They are classified as medial or lateral types (Fig. 10.118). Each type has subtypes with two, three, four, or more fragments. Numerous classification schemes have been devised because the patterns are so diverse as to defy easy categorization.

Evaluation Study AP, mortise, and lateral radiographs of the ankle. If the pattern is unclear, order a CT scan. Often the CT scan shows more displacement than conventional radiographs. If still uncertain, a 3D reconstruction may be necessary. Whenever possible, try to understand the fracture pattern and plan the reduction before undertaking the procedure.

Management The major objective is to restore the articular surfaces to prevent degenerative arthritis. Apply the 2-mm rule. Vertical displacement is more significant than simple horizontal separation of the fragments. Following reduction, fix with screws and immobilize in a long-leg cast for 4 weeks followed by a short-leg cast for an additional 2 weeks.

Tillaux fracture This fracture pattern results from asymmetrical closure of the distal tibial epiphysis (Fig. 10.119) because the anterolateral aspect of the growth plate may remain open when the remainder is fused. Avulsion of this unfused portion of the epiphysis produces this unique fracture (Fig. 10.120). CT imaging may be useful to evaluate the true displacement of this fracture (Fig. 10.121).

References

2000 Distal tibial and fibular epiphyseal fractures in children: prognostic criteria and long-term results in 158 patients. de Sanctis N, Della S, Pempinello C. JPO-b 9:40

1997 The triplane fracture: four years of follow-up of 21 cases and review of the literature. Karrholm J. JPO-b 6:91

1996 Distal tibial triplane fractures: long-term follow-up. Rapariz JM, et al. JPO 16:113

1989 Sports injuries in school-aged children. An epidemiologic study. Backx FJ, et al. Am J Sports Med 17:234

1988 Triplane fracture of the distal tibial epiphysis. Long-term follow-up. Ertl JP, et al. JBJS 70A:967

1987 Symptomatic ossicles of the lateral malleolus in children. Griffiths JD, Menelaus MB. JBJS 69B:317

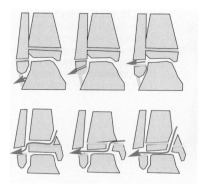

Fig. 10.116 Inversion and supination injuries. Failure may occur through the lateral structures only (blue arrows) or through the whole ankle (red arrows).

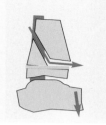

Fig. 10.117 Plantar–flexion injury. The bone fails in tension, producing a sagittal plane deformity.

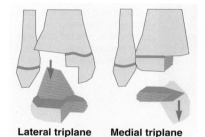

Lateral triplane   Medial triplane

Fig. 10.118 Simple classification of triplane fractures. These fractures can be divided into medial and lateral, but these simple categories have many subtypes.

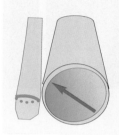

Fig. 10.119 Asymmetrical closure of distal tibial epiphysis. Fusion starts on the posteromedial quadrant and ends in the anterolateral quadrant.

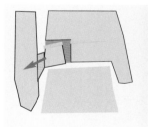
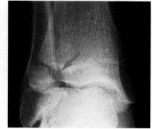

Fig. 10.120 Tillaux fracture. This is a transitional fracture. Because the anterolateral portion of the physis closes last, tension from the attached tibiofibular ligament may avulse an anterolateral segment of the epiphysis (red arrows), producing this characteristic fracture.

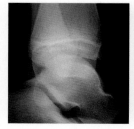
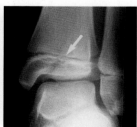
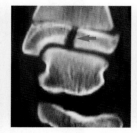
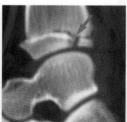
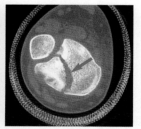

Fig. 10.121 Tillaux fracture. This fracture, not visible on the lateral view, shows little displacement on the AP projection (yellow arrow). The CT scan demonstrates the extent and displacement well (red arrows).

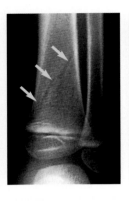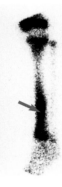

Fig. 10.122 Toddler fracture. Note the oblique metaphyseal location (yellow arrows). A bone scan in a case without radiographic changes shows the typical increased uptake (red arrow) in the distal tibia.

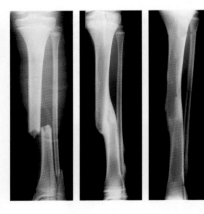

Fig. 10.123 Distal fracture of the tibia and fibula. These fractures (red arrow) were reduced and placed in a cast. The reduction was incomplete, and the cast was then wedged (yellow arrow) to correct residual angulation.

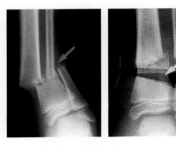

Fig. 10.124 Remodeling of side-to-side apposition. This 8-year-old child sustained this fracture, which was aligned but not reduced. Over a period of 2 years, tibia remodeling resulted in a good outcome.

Tibial Fractures

Tibial fractures account for about 8% of children's fractures. Because the tibia has little softtissue cover and the leg is exposed to view with normal clothing, malunion is more obvious than for most longbone fractures. Overgrowth following fracture is less for the tibia than for the femur.

Toddler Fracture

Toddler fractures typically occur in children 1–4 years old from minimal trauma. A faint fracture line extends obliquely across the distal metaphysis to terminate medially (Fig. 10.122). Sometimes the fracture line cannot be seen on radiographs. The diagnosis can be established by imaging with a bone scan. Midshaft fractures should raise suspicion of child abuse. Manage by immobilization in a walking cast for 2–3 weeks.

Closed Tibial Shaft Fractures

Isolated tibial fractures are most common in the distal one-third. Manage by reduction and long-leg cast immobilization with the knee flexed about 30°. Make certain rotation is correct. Because of the intact fibula, a varus drift is common. Follow with weekly radiographs for 3 weeks, and wedge the cast to correct deformities exceeding about 5°.

Both bone fractures are often easier to manage than fracutres of the tibia alone. Avoid excessive shortening. Be aware that varus angulation corrects better than valgus deformity. Wedge the cast to correct deformities exceeding 5°–10° (Fig. 10.123). Side-to-side apposition is acceptable for children (Fig. 10.124). Rotational deformities correct poorly, especially in the older child.

Operative fixation of tibial fractures may be necessary in the adolescent if length or alignment cannot be satisfactorily managed by cast immobilization. Flexible intramedullary fixation (Fig. 10.125) is a good cosmetic choice, as the scars are minimal and fixation adequate. In contrast, the scars from external pin fixation or plating are less acceptable.

Polytrauma often involves the tibia. Operative fixation may be necessary; the urgency mandates the mode of fixation. Especially in the older child or adolescent, the "floating knee" may require internal fixation of one or both bones.

Pathologic fractures are most common through nonossifying fibromas (Fig. 10.126). These lesions usually occur in the distal lateral aspect of the tibia and have a characteristic appearance. Most fractures occur in very large lesions or secondary to a significant injury. Manage by cast immobilization until union has occurred. Because the natural history is of spontaneous resolution, curettage and bone grafting are seldom necessary.

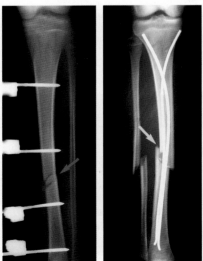

Fig. 10.125 External fixation. The external fixator (red arrow) was applied for a child with polytrauma. IM fixation (yellow arrow) was done for an adolescent with an unstable fracture.

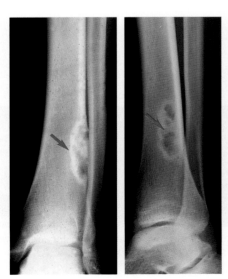

Fig. 10.126 Nonossifying fibroma of the tibia. This classic lesion (arrow), as seen in AP and lateral projections, requires no treatment because the diagnosis is obvious and the chance for fracture is small.

Dysplastic tibia is a rare cause of fracture. Dysplastic features include cortical tapering, sclerosis, and medullary cysts. This may represent a mild form of pseudoarthrosis tibiae and can be seen in the child with neurofibromatosis. Manage with flexible intramedullary rod fixation that is not removed (Fig. 10.127).

Open Tibial Fractures

Open fractures of the tibia (Fig. 10.128) may be associated with severe trauma and have a significant mortality and amputation rate. Most fractures are less severe and are managed like other open fractures.

Severity Severe open fractures are likely to be associated with other very serious injuries and can cause significant mortality and limb loss. Because of the greater potential for healing, attempt limb salvaging whenever a possibility of success exists.

Age is a significant factor in prognosis and influences management. Children can be managed less aggressively than adolescents. Complications in adolescents are similar to those seen in adults. Manage children over age 12 years as adults.

Manage with intravenous antibiotics, repeated debridement, and appropriate fixation. In young children, a windowed cast may be adequate. Apply external pin fixation for older children with significant soft tissue injury. Intramedullary fixation is an alternative in the adolescent.

Stress Fractures

Stress fractures are not rare in children. About half occur with sports. They are becoming more common in girls. The proximal tibia (Fig. 10.129) and distal fibula are common sites. Girls show greater variation in location than boys. Suspect when pain and localized tenderness is found in the very active child. Initial radiographs may be negative. Bone scans show focal uptake. MRI studies are seldom indicated but show an inflammatory reaction. Manage by immobilization or limitation of activity. Monitor healing by a loss in tenderness and pain. Consider healed when asymptomatic and when the callus is mature. Displacement or nonunion occurs rarely.

Proximal Tibial Metaphyseal Fracture

Undisplaced fractures of the metaphyseal in the young child are often complicated by the development of a valgus deformity. The cause of the progressive deformity is most likely due to relative overgrowth of the tibia. This asymmetrical growth is sometimes demonstrated by obliquity of the Harris line or growth arrest line (Fig. 10.130).

Manage with this complication in mind. Advise the family that a knee deformity may develop in the months after the injury even if the fracture is anatomically reduced. Immobilize the extremity in a long-leg cast with the knee flexed at about 20°. Apply varus stress during cast application. Remove the cast at 6 weeks. Follow for 6–12 months. If the deformity occurs, resist the temptation to correct by osteotomy because the deformity will likely recur. Near the end of growth, if the deformity has not resolved, correct with a hemistapling of the proximal medial tibial physis.

References

1999 Posttraumatic valga in children. Tuten RH, et al. JBJS 81A:799

1997 Pathologic fractures through nonossifying fibromas: is prophylactic treatment warranted? Easley ME, Kneisl JS. JPO 17:808

1997 Isolated fractures of the tibia with intact fibula in children: a review of 95 patients. Yang JP, Letts RM. JPO 17:347

1996 Open fractures of the tibia in children. Song KM, et al. JPO 16:635

1996 Stress fractures in skeletally immature patients. Walker RN, Green NE, Spindler KP. JPO 16:578

1993 Late-onset pseudarthrosis of the dysplastic tibia. Roach JW, Shindell R, Green NE. JBJS 75A:1593

1992 Isolated tibial fractures in children. Briggs TW, Orr MM, Lightowler CD. Injury 23:308

1991 Stress fracture of the fibula in the first decade of life. Report of eight cases. Kozlowski K, Azouz M, Hoff D. Pediatr Radiol 21:381

1991 The toddler fracture revisited. Tenenbein M, Reed MH, Black GB. Am J Emerg Med 9:99

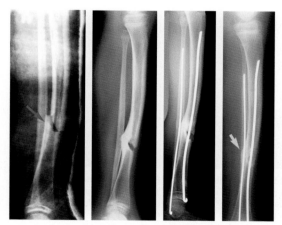

Fig. 10.127 Fracture in a dysplastic tibia. This 11-year-old boy with neurofibromatosis sustained a tibial fracture (red arrow) that was managed with a cast. Healing was incomplete, so permanent flexible IM rods were placed to augment the defective tibia. The fracture healed (yellow arrow).

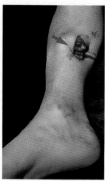 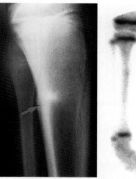

Fig. 10.128 Grade 3 open tibial fracture. This fracture was segmental.

Fig. 10.129 Stress fracture of the upper tibia. This posteromedial position of the fracture callus and the isotope uptake is typical of a tibial stress fracture.

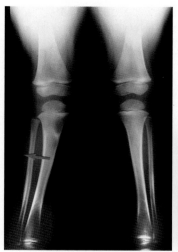 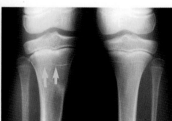

Fig. 10.130 Valgus following tibial metaphyseal fracture. A 5-year-old girl sustained an undisplaced proximal tibial fracture. After 20 months, this valgus deformity developed (red arrow). Note the oblique Harris line (yellow arrows) demonstrating asymmetrical tibial growth.

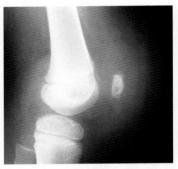

Fig. 10.131 Soft tissue swelling. This infant has a severe knee injury with only extensive soft tissue swelling seen on radiographs.

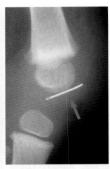

Fig. 10.132 Penetrating injury. This infant has a needle fragment imbedded in the knee (arrow).

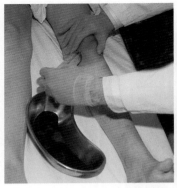

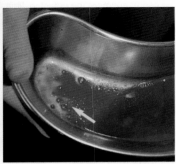

Fig. 10.133 Hemarthrosis aspiration. Aspiration of a hemarthrosis provides relief of pain and may be useful diagnostically. The finding of fat in the aspirate (arrow) suggests the presence of an osteochondral fracture.

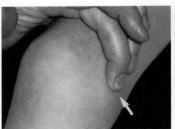

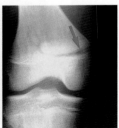

Fig. 10.134 Localization of tenderness. This child has localized tenderness over the medial collateral ligament (yellow arrow). For physeal injuries (red arrow), swelling is greater and tenderness is localized more proximally.

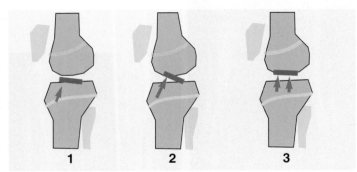

Fig. 10.135 Classification of tibial spine fractures. These fractures are classified as type 1 with minimal displacement, type 2 with elevation but posterior attachment, and type 3 with separation of the fragment from the tibia.

Knee Injuries

Evaluation

Severe soft tissue injury suggests the possibility of occult bone, cartilage, or ligamentous injury (Fig. 10.131). An MRI may be necessary to access the extent of injury.

Imaging should include AP and lateral radiographs. Add special views and MRI studies if ligament or meniscal injury is suspected. MRI is less reliable in the young child because congenital abnormalities are more common. When multiple injuries are present, MRI is also less reliable.

Foreign bodies may be imbedded when the child falls. The body may be readily imaged (Fig. 10.132) or require special imaging by ultrasound or MRI to demonstrate radiolucent objects. Remove all foreign material from within the joint

Diaphyseal femoral or tibial fractures may be associated with ligamentous injuries of the knee or physeal injury. Examine the knee as part of the evaluation of shaft fractures.

Hemarthrosis is often an indication of a significant knee injury. The presence of fat in the aspirate is consistent with a fracture (Fig. 10.133). A hemarthrosis or severe knee injury may be an indication for an arthroscopic evaluation. Its routine use for all hemarthrosis is controversial.

Arthroscopy is indicated when following a hemarthrosis if knee symptoms persist. Common arthrographic findings include meniscal and ligament injury, evidence of patellar dislocation, and osteochondral fractures.

Meniscal Injuries

Meniscal injuries are becoming more common as more children participate in sports. Also, demonstration of these injuries is more likely now because of improved diagnostic skills and expanded use of arthroscopy and MRI. Meniscal injuries increase with increasing age. In young children, tears are usually associated with discoid meniscus. (Management of meniscal injuries is detailed in Chapter 6.)

Collateral Ligament Injuries

Localized tenderness and swelling over the medial collateral ligament and instability suggests this diagnosis. Rule out a physeal fracture as the cause of the instability. A stress radiograph is usually diagnostic (Fig. 10.134). Other imaging studies are less reliable than for meniscal or ACL injuries. MCL, ACL, and meniscal injuries may occur together.

Manage acute grade 1 and 2 injuries by immobilization. Management of grade 3 injuries in the adolescent is controversial. Consider repair of the ligament when injuries are multiple, when very severe, and if a return to demanding activities is planned.

Cruciate Injuries

Cruciate injuries in the immature athlete are becoming more common, especially among girls. Suspect this injury if symptoms persist and physical signs are consistent. Be aware that coexisting meniscal injuries are common. Conservative management is often unsuccessful and reconstruction is often necessary if the patient is to return to preinjury activities (for more details, see Chapter 6).

Anterior Tibial Spine Fracture

This injury is most common in late childhood, and a fall from a bicycle is a typical history. The anterior cruciate ligament may stretch and finally fail through the bone, causing the avulsion fracture.

Evaluation From the lateral radiograph, classify by severity to guide management (Fig. 10.135).

Management Manage type 1 injuries by cast immobilization in slight flexion for 4 weeks to allow healing. Start isometric quadriceps exercises in the cast. Allow a return to full activities after full rehabilitation.

Manage type 2 injuries with the knee in extension if required to reduce the fragment (Fig. 10.136). If reduction is incomplete, consider open repair.

Manage type 3 injuries by reduction and fixation. This may be performed open or by arthroscopy. Make certain that reduction is complete to avoid a residual step-off and add to the anterior cruciate ligament laxity. Fix the fragment with suture, pins, or screws. Avoid traversing the physis. Consider fixation with heavy absorbable sutures through the fragment and into the epiphysis. Manage postoperatively as with type 1 and 2 injuries.

Prognosis About 80–90% of cases do well. About 40% will show abnormal ACL laxity.

Patellar Dislocation

Acute dislocation of the patella occurs in adolescents with valgus flexion injuries and are more common in individuals with anatomic features that make the patella less stable. These features include shallow sulcus, knee valgus, or rotational malalignment. Individuals with ligamentous laxity may be more likely to dislocate but less likely to sustain osteochondral fractures.

Evaluate Osteochondral fractures (Fig. 10.137) occur in about 40% of acute dislocations of the patella. The site of fracture varies (Fig. 10.138). AP, lateral, and sulcus views often show the lesions. MRI usually shows an effusion, bone bruising of the femoral condyle, and medial retinacular tears. Arthroscopy will demonstrate lesions and make early treatment possible.

Risk of recurrence About one-third to half of patellar dislocations will recur. Recurrence is most likely in those cases that dislocated with minimal trauma, reduced spontaneously, and were associated with minimal swelling.

Management Options include early arthroscopy, aspiration, or immobilization.

Arthroscopy is most invasive, but appropriate if an osteochondral fragment is seen or suspected. Remove small osteochondral fragments. Replace and fix large fragments.

Aspiration provides pain relief. The finding of fat in the bloody aspirate suggests a fracture. Effusions often recur rapidly.

Immobilization is the final option. Apply a knee immobilizer for 7–10 days. Start isometric exercises early. If symptoms persist, consider additional studies.

Advise the family of the risks of recurrence. Reestablish range of motion and quadriceps strength before allowing return to full activity.

References

2000 Anterior cruciate ligament reconstruction in adolescents with open physes. Aronowitz ER, et al. Am J Sports Med 28:168

1999 Anterior cruciate ligament tears: MR imaging-based diagnosis in a pediatric population. Lee K, et al. Radiology 213:697

1998 Articular cartilage injury with acute patellar dislocation in adolescents. Arthroscopic and radiographic correlation. Stanitski CL, Paletta GA. Jr. Am J Sports Med 26:52

1997 Recurrence after patellar dislocation. Redislocation in 37/75 patients followed for 6-24 years. Maenpaa H, Huhtala H, Lehto MU. Acta Orthop Scand 68:424

1996 Anterior cruciate ligament injuries in skeletally immature patients. Janarv PM, et al. JPO 16:673

1996 Magnetic resonance imaging of knee injuries in children. King SJ, Carty HM. Pediatr Radiol 26:287

1996 Meniscal and nonosseous ACL injuries in children and adolescents. Williams JS Jr., et al. Am J Knee Surg 9:22

1995 Long-term follow-up of anterior tibial spine fractures in children. Janarv PM, et al. JPO 15:63

1995 Medial collateral ligament injuries: evaluation of multiple signs, prevalence and location of associated bone bruises, and assessment with MR imaging. Schweitzer ME, et al. Radiology 194:825

1995 Articular hypermobility and chondral injury in patients with acute patellar dislocation. Stanitski CL. Am J Sports Med 23:146

1994 Acute patellar dislocation in children: incidence and associated osteochondral fractures. Nietosvaara Y, Aalto K, Kallio PE. JPO 14:513

1993 Observations on acute knee hemarthrosis in children and adolescents. Stanitski CL, Harvell JC, Fu F. JPO 13:506

1993 Acute dislocation of the patella: MR findings. Virolainen H, Visuri T, Kuusela T. Radiology 189:243

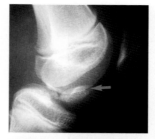
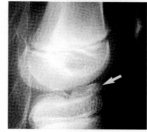
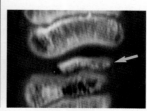

Fig. 10.136 Tibial spine fractures. This type 2 fracture involved a large fragment of bone and cartilage. The bony portion may be large (red arrow) and the position may be improved in extension (yellow arrow), but a CT scan shows the fragment still significantly elevated (orange arrow). This position was accepted, a controversial decision for this older boy.

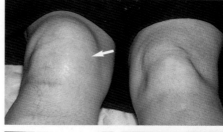
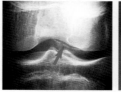
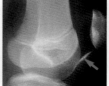
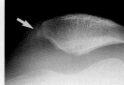

Fig. 10.137 Osteochondral fractures. These fractures are often associated with a tense hemarthrosis (white arrow). On conventional radiographs, the fracture may be obvious (red arrows) or subtle (yellow arrow).

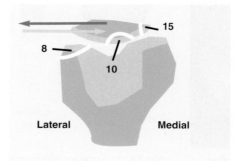

Fig. 10.138 Distribution of osteochondral fractures in children. Trauma dislocates the patella laterally (red arrow) then spontaneously reduces (yellow arrow). The number and distribution of articular fractures secondary to 72 acute patellar dislocations is shown. Based on Nietosvaara et al. (1994).

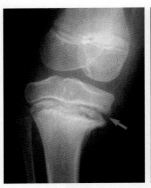
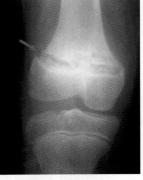

Fig. 10.139 Physeal stress injuries in myelodysplasia. Note the localized widening of the physes (arrows).

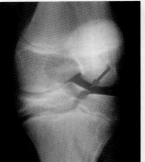
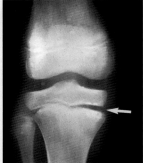

Fig. 10.140 Proximal tibial physeal fractures. The displaced SH-3 fracture (red arrow) was associated with a popliteal artery injury. The SH-1 fracture (yellow arrow) caused a valgus deformity.

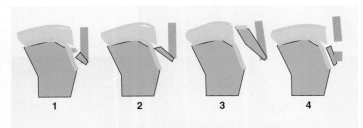

Fig. 10.141 Classification of tibial avulsion injuries. Grade 4, which involves tears of the patellar ligament, is often not included in the classification.

Knee Fractures

Stress Physeal Injuries

These injuries are most common in myelodysplasia (Fig. 10.139). Manage by prolonged immobilization with weight-bearing activities.

Proximal Tibial Physeal Fractures

If these rare injuries extend posteriorly, they may damage the popliteal artery. They are often classified with tibial tubercle fractures. This separation is useful to alert one to the risk of this injury (Fig. 10.140). These injuries can be associated with severe polytrauma.

Tibial Tubercle Fractures

Tibial tubercle fractures occur at the end of growth when the physis is unable to withstand the tensile loading imposed by the adolescent. Classification includes the traditional types 1–3 with the addition of a fourth category—rupture of the patellar tendon (Fig. 10.141). Manage most type 1 and 2 fractures with cast immobilization with the knee in extension. Severely displaced fractures may require reduction and fixation to prevent a disabling residual prominence. Type 3 fractures require open reduction and internal fixation. Type 4 may require tendon repair.

Patellar Fractures

Patellar fractures take a variety of forms.

Transverse fractures If these fractures are displaced (Fig. 10.142), reduce anatomically and fix with tension-band wires as done in adults.

Marginal fractures may occur from the medial, superior (Fig. 10.143), or lateral side of the patella. Often only a small rim of bone is displaced, but the cartilage fragment is often large. Manage most by cast immobilization.

Sleeve fractures are characterized by avulsions of the patellar ligament from the distal pole of the patella (Fig. 10.144). Because the fragment includes cartilage, it is usually considerably larger than the radiographic defect. Sometimes MRI is necessary to show the extent of the injury. Reduce widely displaced sleeve fractures and fix by suture repair.

Femoral Physeal Fracture

The distal femoral epiphysis may fail before the medial collateral ligament. This differentiation between the physeal fracture and ligament tear can usually be made by physical examination. Occasionally, stress radiographs may be necessary to show the site of instability (Fig. 10.145). These must be done gently and with the patient completely relaxed.

Fracture patterns The fracture patterns are variable. Most are SH-1 and SH-2. SH-3 fractures may be difficult to demonstrate without a notch view.

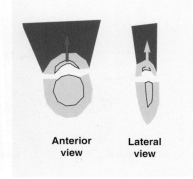

Fig. 10.142 Transverse patellar fracture. This displaced fracture required open reduction and tension band wire fixation.

Fig. 10.143 Superior margin patellar fracture. Marginal fractures may occur on any surface. This shows a superior margin fracture that includes a small rim of bone. Based on Grogan et al. (1990).

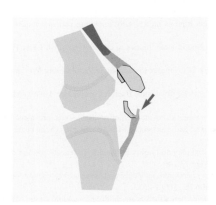

Fig. 10.144 Sleeve fracture. This classic childhood fracture is primarily an avulsion of cartilage. The bone fragment may be small (arrow), making the fracture more difficult to identify.

Management Most femoral physeal fractures require anatomic reduction and internal fixation. Without fixation, displacement in the cast often occurs. For SH-2 types, fix the metaphyseal fragment with a transverse screw. Supplement with a long-leg cast. SH-1 fractures can be fixed with two smooth crossed pins (Fig. 10.146). SH-3 fractures may require metaphyseal screw fixation, which avoids injury to the physis. Sometimes this is supplemented with a second screw or pin (Fig. 10.147).

Prognosis These physeal fractures are different from most physeal injuries. About half of these fractures develop physeal bars, causing deformity and shortening. Inform the family of this risk when first consulted. Follow carefully for signs of femoral shortening or changes in knee angle. Identify and resect small bridges early before significant deformity develops. Extensive bridges (Fig. 10.149) may cause serious shortening, requiring femoral lengthening or shortening procedures.

Distal Femoral Metaphyseal Fractures

This is a common site for pathologic fractures seen in neuromuscular disorders or following cast immobilization for management of conditions such as DDH (Fig. 10.148). These fractures may also occur from therapeutic manipulations of stiff knees.

Manage most cases by splinting until pain subsides and by early mobilization to prevent further deossfication. For displaced fractures, fix with long flexible IM rod(s) and mobilize early.

References

1999 Fractures of the patella in children. Dai LY, Zhang WM. Knee Surg Sports Traumatol Arthrosc 7:243

1999 Transverse stress fracture of the patella in a child. Garcia Mata S, et al. JPO-b 8:208

1997 Totally absorbable fixation in the treatment of fractures of the distal femoral epiphysis. A prospective clinical study. Partio EK, et al. Arch Orthop Trauma Surg 116:213

1997 Chronic physeal fractures in myelodysplasia: magnetic resonance analysis, histologic description, treatment, and outcome. Rodgers WB, et al. JPO 17:615

1995 Fractures of the distal femoral epiphyseal plate. Thomson JD, Stricker SJ, Williams MM. JPO 15:474

1994 Patellar sleeve fracture: demonstration with MR imaging. Bates DG, Hresko MT, Jaramillo D. Radiology 193:825

1994 Fractures about the knee: growth disturbances and problems of stability at long-term follow-up. Buess-Watson E, Exner GU, Illi OE. Eur J Pediatr Surg 4:218

1993 Fractures of the patella in children and adolescents. Maguire JK, Canale ST. JPO 13:567

1990 Fracture of the tibial tubercle in the adolescent. Chow SP, Lam JJ, Leong JC. JBJS 72B:231

1990 Avulsion fracture of the tibial tubercle with avulsion of the patellar ligament. Report of two cases. Frankl U, Wasilewski SA, Healy WL. JBJS 72A:1411

1990 Avulsion fractures of the patella. Grogan DP, et al. JPO 10:721

1985 Fracture of an unossified tibial tubercle. Driessnack RP, Marcus NW. JPO 5:728

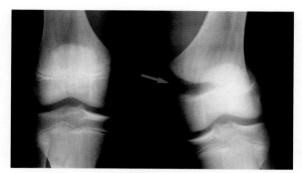

Fig. 10.145 Stress radiographs. These were necessary to demonstrate the unstable physeal fracture (arrow).

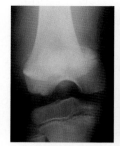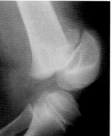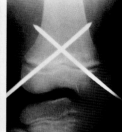

Fig. 10.146 Displaced epiphyseal fracture. This fracture required closed reduction and percutaneous fixation with crossed smooth pins. Growth arrest is likely.

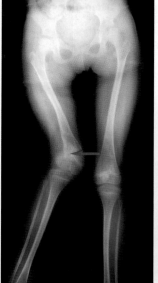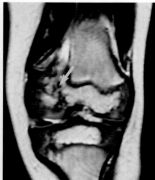

Fig. 10.149 Physeal injury. This child sustained an injury to the lateral distal femoral physis (red arrow) with progressive valgus deformity. Note the disruption of the physis shown on the MRI (yellow arrow).

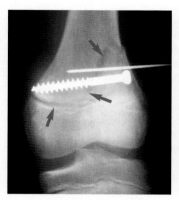

Fig. 10.147 Metaphyseal fixation. This SH-2 fracture (arrows) was fixed with a transmetaphyseal screw.

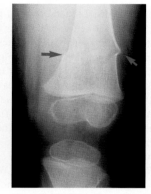

Fig. 10.148 Metaphyseal buckle fracture. This fracture occurred following removal of a cast used in DDH treatment.

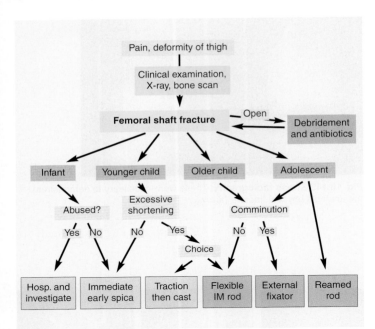

Fig. **Fig. 10.150 Management of femoral shaft fractures.** Tailor management to the age of the child, type of injury, and risks inherent in the procedure.

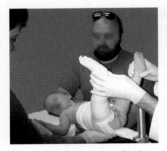

Fig. 10.151 Spica cast. Apply most with the hips flexed and abducted as done for DDH.

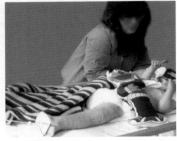

Fig. 10.152 Overnight simple traction. This is applied for comfort while waiting for the spica cast application.

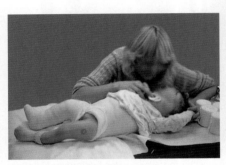

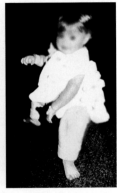

Fig. 10.153 Make certain cast is comfortable before discharge. Instruct the parents on cast care.

Fig. 10.154 Be prepared for the toddler to stand in the cast.

Femoral Shaft Fractures

Principles

Some generalizations can be made about femoral shaft fractures. The femur heals spontaneously even with widely displaced fragments. Nonunion is rare. The healing rate is age dependent, and the relationship between time of union and age is nearly linear. Overgrowth is greatest during early and middle childhood and is related to the degree of osseous and soft tissue disruption. Because of this overgrowth, childhood femoral fractures should be allowed to override by 1–1.5 cm to compensate for the overgrowth. Overgrowth averages 1 cm for femoral fractures in childhood. As compared to adults, blood loss seldom reaches a level that requires replacement. Most femoral fractures heal without disability if complications are avoided. Select management with the least risks. Tailor management based on the patient's age, family situation, and management options available. A general flowchart is useful to guide management decisions (Fig. 10.150).

Infant Management

Consider and rule out nonaccidental trauma.

Early infancy Consider management in a Pavlik harness or in a spica cast (Fig. 10.151). Apply the spica cast under either sedation or anesthesia. Immobilize in the human position as done in DDH management. Flex the hips and knees to about 80°. Abduct the hips to allow easy diapering. See again at about 4 weeks for cast removal. Avoid burdening the family by suggesting they restrict the infant's activities following cast removal.

Toddler Manage in an early spica cast. Immobilize in the spica cast with the hips flexed to about 45°. Leave the feet free. If the fracture is stable, a single hip spica is adequate. Immobilize for about 5 weeks.

Early Childhood Management—Spica Casts

Management in early childhood can be provided by early spica cast immobilization with or without initial traction.

Overgrowth corrects shortening, and the immobilization is well tolerated. Although the cast may be applied in the emergency room and the child discharged home (immediate spica), an overnight admission is usually more practical (Fig. 10.152). This allows arranging a convenient time for applying the spica cast, instruction of the family in cast care, and being certain the child is comfortable in the cast before discharge (Fig. 10.153).

Initial traction Apply about 2–3 pounds of longitudinal skin traction during the overnight stay. This provides adequate immobilization and alignment.

Sedation Provide sedation or a light general anesthetic when applying the cast.

Leg position Position the extremity based on the level of the fracture. The objective is to align, not reduce the fracture. Position the limb to align the distal to the proximal fragment. The position of the proximal fragment is determined by the level of the fracture. This position is due to the attachment of the muscles about the femur. Proximal fractures should be immobilized with the hip in about 45° flexion, 45° abduction and 20° lateral rotation (45-45-20°). Position midshaft fractures in about 30-30-10°. Position distal fractures in a more neutral position, about 20-20-10°. The young child may stand in the cast (Fig. 10.154).

Avoid excessive shortening The major risk of early spica immobilization is excessive shortening. The amount of acceptable shortening is controversial but falls between 1.5 and 3 cm. Consider several methods of avoiding this complication.

Resting radiograph of femur Without traction applied, measure the amount of shortening. If the shortening exceeds about 20–25 mm, consider traction treatment.

Fracture mechanism Transverse midshaft fractures secondary to high-velocity injuries are most likely to shorten excessively. Periosteal stripping and hemorrhage may cause swelling. This swelling may hold the fracture out to length. When the swelling subsides, the femur may shorten excessively (Fig. 10.155).

Follow-up radiographs Make radiographs at 1–2 weeks following injury to assess length. If excessive shortening occurs, remove the cast and place the child in skin traction until union has occurred.

Duration of cast immobilization Continue immobilization for a total of 6 weeks in the child under 5 years of age and 8 weeks for children 5–10 years of age.

Post-cast care Allow spontaneous restoration of activity and mobility. Physical therapy is not necessary. Limit vigorous play for 1 month. Reevaluate the child after 6–12 months for range of motion, length, and any residual deformity.

Early Childhood Management—Traction

Traction remains an effective method of managing femoral shaft fractures. For children, traction treatment is safe and complications are uncommon. Because hospitalization is prolonged, however, traction has become less commonly used today. Increased cost is given as a reason for avoiding this treatment. When all expenses are considered, traction is about the same as for other forms of management. Prolonged inpatient management is easier for some families and more difficult for others. Tailor traction to the age and level of the fracture.

Skin traction is suitable for most children under age 8 years with most fracture patterns (Figs. 10.156 and 10.157) (see page 368).

Skeletal traction is most useful for the older child (Fig. 10.158) and those with subtrochanteric fractures that require 90°–90° positioning. Apply pin traction through a distal femur pin placed at the level of the superior pole of the patella. Inset the pin with the knee flexed to 90° to avoid binding of the iliotibial band (see page 369).

Length Adjust traction weights to allow about 1 cm of shortening. Be aware that the major risk of 90°–90° traction treatment is excessive length of the fractured limb due to insufficient shortening at the time of union. Overgrowth then lengthens the limb beyond its normal length.

Duration Continue traction until early union has occurred. The callus should be nontender, and moving the leg should not be uncomfortable for the child. The duration may vary from 2 weeks in early childhood, to 3 weeks in middle childhood, and 4 weeks in late childhood. Up to 6–8 weeks is appropriate for the adolescent. Avoid the common error of discontinuing traction too soon. Premature cast application may result in the fracture angulating and shortening in the cast. This complication is usually not diagnosed early enough to correct by reinstituting traction treatment. Correction may require mobilizing the fragments, restoring length, and applying internal or external fixation.

Acceptable alignment Side-to-side apposition is best. Avoid end-to-end reduction, as union is slower and the femur is likely to be longer than the other side.

Frontal plane Align to within about 10°–20°. More deformity is acceptable in the younger patient and with more proximal fractures.

Sagittal plane Accept alignment to within 20°–30°. Because the deformity is in the plane of joint motion, more deformity can be accepted. More procurvatum and recurvatum is acceptable.

Transverse plane This is difficult to measure. Position the limb in about 10°–15° of lateral rotation in traction and the cast.

Align fractures Adjust the position of the controllable distal fragment to be in alignment with the proximal fragment (Fig. 10.159).

Bryant traction This type of traction should be avoided or used with caution. Catastrophic vascular complications are a risk with this treatment.

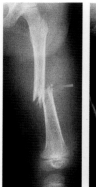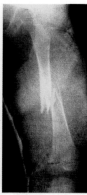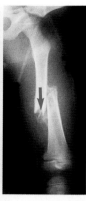

Fig. 10.155 Excessive shortening. This 5-year-old child sustained a high-energy fracture with extensive swelling (green arrow). A spica cast was applied the next day (yellow arrow). At 10 days, shortening was unacceptable (red arrow). The patient was readmitted and placed in traction; the lost length was regained. Once stable, a spica cast was applied.

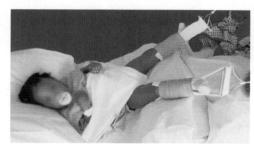

Fig. 10.156 Infant traction. Apply about 2 pounds of traction to each leg. Let the legs rest on a pillow.

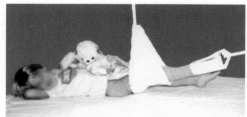

Fig. 10.157 Young child traction. This skin traction provides longitudinal traction and support for the knee.

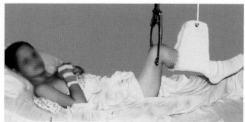

Fig. 10.158 Skeletal traction at 90°–90°. This traction is best for older children and adolescents. It may also be used for proximal fractures in younger children.

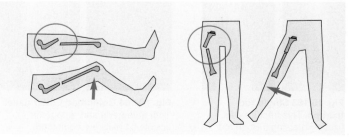

Fig. 10.159 Aligning proximal femoral fractures. To align the distal to the proximal fragments, flex (red arrow) and abduct (blue arrow) the leg.

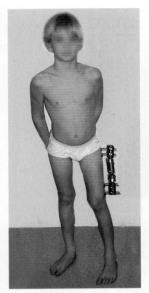

Fig. 10.160 External fixator. Note that the boy holds his leg in abduction. This was the position of the leg when the fixator was applied.

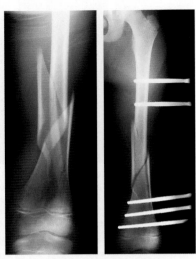

Fig. 10.161 Comminuted fracture management. The external fixator provides optimum management. Length, alignment, and stability are achieved.

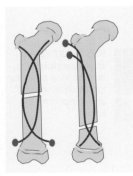

Fig. 10.162 Flexible IM rod fixation. Flexible rods are an excellent method of fixing the femur in the child. The physis is not disturbed and adequate fixation is achieved. The rods may be inserted from proximal or distal ends (red dots). Redrawn from Huber et al. (1996).

External Fixation

External fixation (Fig. 10.160) is an overused method of fixing femoral fractures, and complications with this fixation are frequent.

Indications for use of external fixation are limited.

Open fractures Open fractures and concurrent soft tissue injuries are managed effectively by external fixation because this method allows access to the soft tissue injury.

Comminuted fractures Unstable segmental fractures (Fig. 10.161) that would shorten excessively if managed by flexible rods provide an indication for external fixation.

Polytrauma Use external fixation when devices can be rapidly applied.

Complications with this method of management are common.

Pin tract infections are common due to the high activity level of children and their lack of attention to pin care.

Delayed union is often slow, as the fracture may be reduced or distracted.

Refracture is common following removal of the fixator.

Suggestions Limit use of fixators. Instead, use techniques that cause fewer complications such as flexible IM rods. Allow fractures to override to enhance union rate and avoid distraction. Dynamize to provide loading to enhance callus formation. Consider applying a single-hip walking spica cast after removal of fixation if the union is tenuous or the patient is uncooperative.

Flexible IM Rod Fixation

Flexible IM rods are an excellent method of fixing femoral shaft fractures in children (Figs. 10.162–10.165). This fixation is adequate, safe, relatively easy to apply and remove, and associated with few complication. Its use is gaining enthusiasts.

Indications for flexible IM rod fixation are quite broad.

Fractures in older children This is the most appropriate fixation method for children 8 years of age to maturity.

Polytrauma Complicating problems necessitate fracture stabilization at any age.

Floating knee This method provides fixation of at least one fracture.

Complications Few complications are reported with this technique. Some children complain of discomfort over the ends of the pins if they are left prominent.

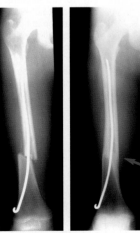

Fig. 10.163 Single rod fixation. This fracture was fixed with a single Rush rod supplemented with a single hip walking spica cast. Healing was rapid (arrow).

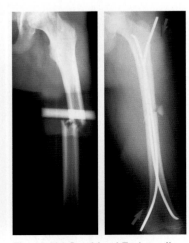

Fig. 10.164 Combined Ender nails. Both antegrade and retrograde flexible IM nails are combined.

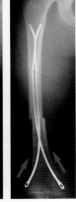

Fig. 10.165 Retrograde flexible IM fixation. This is the most common placement of flexible IM fixation.

Reamed Rod Fixation

Indications Reamed rods are useful only *after* physeal closure.

Complications Before physeal closure, reaming causes an unacceptably large number of complications.

Avascular necrosis (AVN) This complication is more common when the piriformis fossa entry point is utilized. Estimated likelihood of the complication is about 1% (Fig. 10.166).

Altered growth Physeal damage is common (Fig. 10.167). The physis of the upper femur extends across the greater trochanter and the upper femoral neck. Reaming in the pyriformis fossa or through the greater trochanter may alter growth. Hypoplasia of the greater trochanter and femoral neck (Fig. 10.168) are serious problems. These complications may lead to abductor insufficiency and cervical fractures in adult life.

Nerve injury Sciatic nerve injury is not uncommon. Fortunately, most recover spontaneously.

Plates

Indications Plates have few indications. They have been used to provide rapid and secure fixation of children with polytrauma (Fig. 10.169).

Complications

Refracture There are several causes of refracture. Stress risers through the distal screw hole may cause fracture. Stress shielding of bone under the plate fails to hypertrophy, making it more likely to refracture following plate removal.

Difficult removal may require excessive bone removal to expose plate. The weakened bone is susceptible to refracture.

General operative risks are greater than applying and removing other fixation devices due to the greater magnitude of the procedure. In addition, the residual scar is longer.

Consultant Jim Beaty, e-mail: jbeaty@campbellclinic.com

References

2000 Ender rod fixation of femoral shaft fractures in children. Cramer KE, et al. CO 119

2000 Immediate hip spica casting for femur fractures in pediatric patients. A review of 175 patients. Infante AF, et al. CO 106

2000 Accidental and nonaccidental femur fractures in children. Scherl SA, et al, CO 96

1999 Femoral shaft fracture treatment in patients age 6 to 16 years. Stans AA, Morrissy RT, Renwick SE. JPO 19:222

1998 Displaced fractures of the femoral shaft in children. Unique features and therapeutic options. Greene WB. CO 353:86

1998 Femur fractures in children; treatment with early sitting spica casting. Illgren R, et al. JPO 18:481

1997 Fracture of the femur in children. Macnicol MF. JBJS 79B:891

1996 Flexible intramedullary nail fixation of pediatric femoral fractures. Carey TP, Galpin RD. CO 332:110

1996 Flexible intramedullary nailing as fracture treatment in children. Huber RI, et al. JPO 16:602

1996 Neurologic complications of pediatric femoral nailing. Riew KD, et al. JPO 16:606

1995 Femoral shaft fractures in children and adolescents. Beaty JH. JAAOS 3:207

1995 Intramedullary nailing of the femur in children. Effects on its proximal end. Gonzalez-Herranz PJ, et al. JBJS 77B:262

1995 Limb length after fracture of the femoral shaft in children. Corry IS, Nicol RO. JPO 15:217

1994 Rotational deformity and remodeling after fracture of the femur in children. Davids JR. CO 302:27

1993 Pediatric femur fractures: an overview of treatment. Levy J, Ward WT. Orthopedics 16(2):183

1993 Kuntscher nailing of femoral shaft fractures in children and adolescents. Maruenda-Paulino JI, et al. Int Orthop 17:158

1993 Premature greater trochanteric epiphysiodesis secondary to intramedullary femoral rodding. Raney EM, et al. JPO 13:516

1992 Femoral stress fractures in children. Meaney JE, Carty H. Skeletal Radiol 21:173

1992 Remodeling of angular deformity after femoral shaft fractures in children. Wallace ME, Hoffman EB. JBJS 74B:765

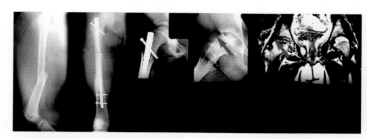

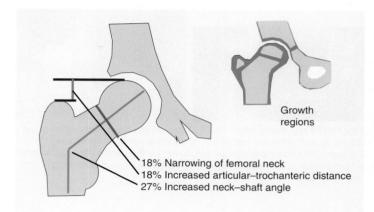

Fig. 10.166 AVN complication of reamed rod. Reamed rod fixation was used in this patient. She developed avascular necrosis. From Beaty (1995).

Growth regions

18% Narrowing of femoral neck
18% Increased articular–trochanteric distance
27% Increased neck–shaft angle

Fig. 10.167 Effect of reaming on proximal femoral growth. This shows the percentage of upper femora showing abnormalities following reamed rodding during childhood. The vulnerable growth plates are shown in the upper right. From Gonzáles-Herranz et al. (1995).

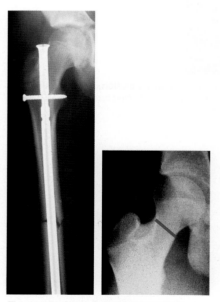

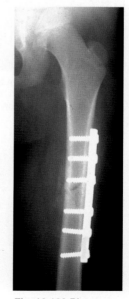

Fig. 10.168 Growth disturbance. This patient had a reamed rodding at age 11 years. Note the reduction in neck width and coxa valga.

Fig. 10.169 Plate fixation. This child sustained polytrauma.

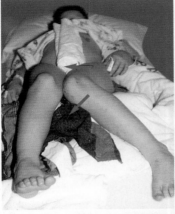

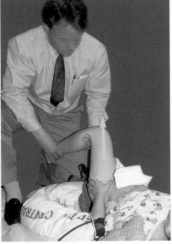

Fig. 10.170 Hip dislocation. This 10-year-old boy has a dislocation of the left hip. Note the flexion, adduction, and medial rotation (red arrows). Radiographs show the posterior dislocation (orange arrow). Reduction was accomplished in the emergency room by gradual traction on the leg (yellow arrow).

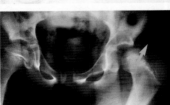

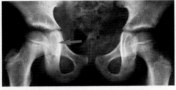

Fig. 10.171 Ligamentum teres avulsion interposition. Note that after reduction of a dislocation, the joint space is wide (red arrow). The MRI shows interposition (yellow arrow).

Hip Dislocations

Dislocations of the hip are uncommon in children. Fracture dislocations are most common in the adolescent.

Simple Dislocations

Manage most by early closed reduction (Fig. 10.170). With sedation and the hip flexed to 90°, apply gentle traction to the limb. After reduction, check stability and concentricity of reduction. If the joint space is asymmetrical, evaluate with CT or MRI for evidence of ligamentous or labral interposition (Fig. 10.171). For younger children, immobilize in a panty spica cast for 4 weeks. Redislocations are uncommon. Overall about 10% develop AVN. This complication is more likely if reduction is delayed beyond 6–8 hours after injury.

Fracture Dislocations

These fractures in children may be more difficult to diagnose than in adults, as the fragment may be largely cartilage. Image carefully. If unstable after reduction, operative reduction and fixation are required.

Pathologic Dislocations (Recurrent)

Children with underlying connective tissue disorders may have recurrent dislocations. The dislocations may occur with play and may reduce spontaneously. Establish the diagnosis by performing an arthrogram under anesthesia. Stress the joint to establish instability. Manage by spica cast immobilization for 8–10 weeks. Rarely, operative procedures are necessary to enhance bony stability and correct excessive capsular laxity.

Proximal Femur Fractures

Fractures of the upper femur are serious injuries with many complications. They are classified by the Delbet–Colonna system (Fig. 10.172).

Type I—Transepiphyseal Fractures

These fractures are most common in infancy and early childhood (Fig. 10.173). They are often associated with child abuse. Manage undisplaced fractures in a spica cast in the human position as with DDH management. Displaced fractures usually require reduction. Decompress the joint. Place two or three smooth parallel K wires across the physis. Avoid joint penetration. Bend over the ends outside the femoral metaphysis to prevent migration. Advise the family of the risks of AVN and growth problems.

Type 2—Transcervical Fractures

Manage undisplaced fractures in a spica cast. Displaced fractures should be reduced, decompressed, and internally fixed (Fig. 10.174). Fix with two cannulated screws if enough proximal bone is available. Otherwise fix with three smooth parallel K wires that traverse the growth plate. Supplement fixation with a spica cast. Plan 8 weeks of immobilization. Advise the family of the risk of AVN.

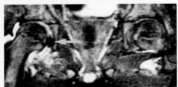

Type	1	2	3	4
Frequency	15%	35%	35%	15%
AVN	75%	50%	25%	0%

Fig. 10.172 Delbet–Colonna classification of hip fractures. The approximate incidence (in percent) of avascular necrosis complicating management are shown.

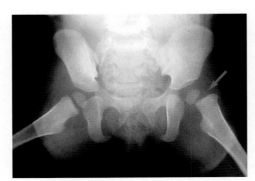

Fig. 10.173 Type 1 fracture. This is an SH-1 fracture with moderate displacement.

Type 3—Cervicotrochanteric Fractures

Manage as a type 2 injury (Fig. 10.175). Decompress and fix with screws. Supplement with a spica cast unless fixation is very secure to avoid coxa vara. Advise family of risk of AVN.

Type 4—Intertrochanteric Fractures

Provide secure internal fixation to avoid residual varus deformity.

Complications

Avascular necrosis This complication occurs in about one-third to half of hip fractures. This complication is due to the tenuous vascularity of the femoral head. The vascular supply may be interrupted at several levels (Figs. 10.176 and 10.177) causing varied patterns of necrosis. Early capsular decompression appears to reduce the risk of AVN. Follow hips at risk every month or two with a hip rotation test. With loss of motion or guarding, suspect this complication.

Growth disturbance This complication occurs when physeal damage occurs. It is more common in type 1 injuries. It is probably not preventable.

Coxa vara This complication is usually preventable by providing internal fixation of unstable fractures.

Nerve injury This complication is more common than often recognized. Fortunately, most recover spontaneously in 3–6 months.

Stress Fractures

Stress fractures of the femoral neck are rare in children. These fractures often cause pain. Radiographs may show sclerosis of the inferior portion of the neck (Fig. 10.178). Bone scans are diagnostic. Manage by limiting activity or possible immobilization in a single-hip fiberglass walking spica cast to ensure compliance.

References

2000 The Scottish incidence of traumatic dislocation of the hip in childhood. Macnicol MF. JPOB 9:122

2000 Traumatic dislocation of the hip in children. Salisbury RD, Eastwood DM. CO 377:106

1996 Effect of early hip decompression on the frequency of avascular necrosis in children with fractures of the neck of the femur. Ng GP, Cole WG. Injury 27:419

1994 Interlocking intramedullary nailing of femoral-shaft fractures in adolescents: preliminary results and complications. Beaty JH, et al. JPO 14:178

1994 Fractures of the head and neck of the femur in children. Hughes LO, Beaty JH. JBJS 76A:283

1992 Hip fractures in children: a long-term follow-up study. Davison BL, Weinstein SL. JPO 12:355

1990 Fractures of the hip in children and adolescents. Canale ST. Orthop Clin North Am 21:341

1962 Fractures of the neck of the femur in children. Ratliff AHC. JBJS 44B:528

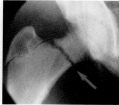
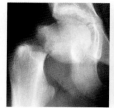
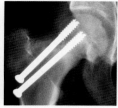

Fig. 10.174 Type 2 low transcervical fracture. This 13-year-old girl sustained this injury while skiing. It was reduced with traction, decompressed, and pinned with cannulated screws. The fracture healed without complications.

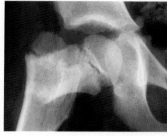
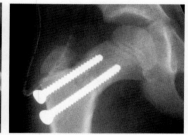

Fig. 10.175 Type 3 cervicotrochanteric fracture. This fracture was sustained in an auto accident. The capsule was opened and screw fixation and a cast were applied. Healing was uncomplicated.

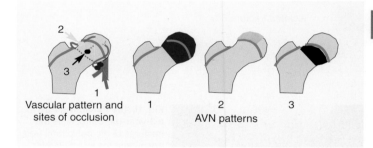

Vascular pattern and sites of occlusion 1 2 3 AVN patterns

Fig. 10.176 Patterns of avascular necrosis. Location and extent of AVN after femoral neck fractures depend on the site of vascular occlusion. Type I (blue) is most common and results from obstruction of both medial and lateral vascularity. Type 2 (orange) involves the lateral physeal vessel, causing variable necrosis of the epiphysis. Type 3 (black) involves the distal femoral neck only and is due to obstruction of the posterior ascending vessels. Based on Ratliff (1962).

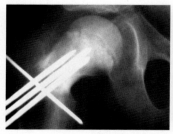
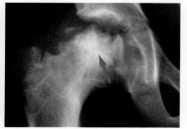

Fig. 10.177 Type 1 AVN. This fracture was fixed with multiple pins and developed avascular necrosis (arrow) of the entire proximal fragment.

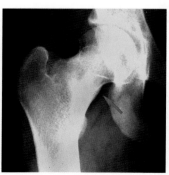

Fig. 10.178 Stress fracture of the femoral neck. Note the sclerosis in the region of the calcar of this 15-year-old boy with hip pain.

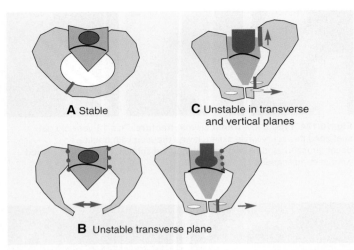

Fig. 10.179 Pelvic fracture classification. Fractures can be classified as A, stable; B, unstable in the horizontal plane; or C, unstable in horizontal and vertical planes. From Tile (1988).

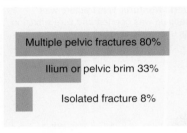

Fig. 10.180 Relationship between pelvic fracture pattern and concurrent abdominal or GU injuries. From data by Bond et al. (1991).

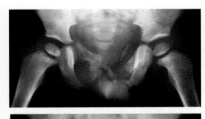

Fig. 10.181 Pelvic fracture in a 3-year-old child. Note the fractures of the pubic rami (red arrow) and the intact bladder (yellow arrow).

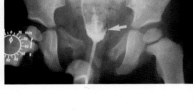

Fig. 10.182 Pelvic fracture with bladder injury. Note the extravasation of dye during the cystogram.

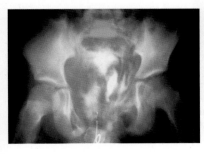

Pelvic Fractures

Pelvic fractures are often associated with other serious injuries.

Pelvic Ring Fractures

Tile classification This classification is used for both child and adult fractures (Fig. 10.179).

Class A These fractures are inherently stable. They may include avulsion injuries; other injuries are uncommon.

Class B This includes fractures that are unstable in the transverse (horizontal) plane.

Class C These fractures show instability in both transverse and vertical planes.

Torode and Zieg classification This classification includes four groups of pelvic fractures.

Type I avulsion Occur at sites of bone or tendon attachment.

Type II iliac wing These are relatively common and typical of childhood pelvic fractures.

Type III simple ring These usually involve the pubic rami or symphysis.

Type IV ring disruption In these fractures, the pelvis is unstable.

Evaluate by careful examination and imaging. Order a CT scan if the fracture pattern is unclear. Type III and IV fractures suggest the possibility of additional injuries (Fig. 10.180). Evaluate the abdomen, gastrointestinal, and gastrourinary systems (Figs. 10.181 and 10.182). Keep in mind that a pelvic fracture is a marker for other injuries that pose more threat than the fracture.

Manage most pelvic fractures conservatively. Stabilize type IV ring disruptions by external fixators or internal fixation (Fig. 10.183). Most late musculoskeletal disability results from pelvic malunion, causing persisting pelvic asymmetry and malunited acetabular fractures. Nonunions may remain silent (Fig. 10.184). Overall mortality is about 10–15% due to associated injuries. Need for transfusions is only about 15–20%, considerably less than for adults.

Avulsion Fractures

Avulsion fractures are relatively common injuries. They occur at a variety of sites (Fig. 10.185). Avusions are most common in the anterior inferior spine, lessor trochanter, and anterior superior spine. Avulsions of the ischael tuberosity and greater trochanter are less common but more serious. These injuries may be acute with an injury or due to repetitive trauma.

Diagnosis With chronic lesions, the differential diagnosis includes tumors and infection. The localization of tenderness, radiographic features, and improvement following limited activities are usually diagnostic.

Management Manage most by rest. Ischael avulsions with displacement exceeding 1 cm may be considered for replacement to prevent asymmetry for sitting or nonunion. Reduce and fix avulsion fractures of the greater trochanter.

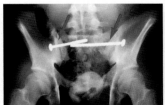

Fig. 10.183 Sacraliliac disruption. This fracture (arrows) was reduced and fixed with long screws.

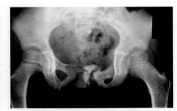

Fig. 10.184 Nonunion of pubis. This nonunion remained silent and was not repaired.

Acetabular Fractures

Classification Acetabular fractures are classified based on location, displacement, and stability (Fig. 10.186).

Diagnosis A diagnosis of osteochondral or chondral fractures is most difficult to make. Be suspicious if joint space widening is seen following reduction. Bony injury pattern can be evaluated by 3D CT reconstructions.

Management Openly reduce and fix unstable posterior fracture dislocations and irreducible central fracture dislocations of the hip (Fig. 10.187). Apply the 2-mm rule as with other articular fractures.

Prognosis Osteoarthritis may complicate unreduced or comminuted fractures.

Triradiate Injuries

Triradiate cartilage injuries are rare but serious because they may result in physeal closure and progressively increasing acetabular dysplasia (Fig. 10.188).

Diagnosis Evaluate by radiographs and CT scans. Three-dimensional reconstructions may be helpful in assessing the injury. Later, the fusion may be visible by plane radiographs. Often the diagnosis is made late when fusion is obvious and acetabular deficiency develops.

Management Physeal bridge resection is difficult and its outcomes are uncertain. Acetabular insufficiency may require correction by acetabular augmention or Chiari osteotomy.

References

2000 Early functional outcome in children with pelvic fractures. Upperman JS, et al.. J Pediatr Surg 35:1002

2000 Disruption of the pelvic ring in pediatric patients. Blasier RD, et al. CO 87

2000 Acetabular fractures in children and adolescents. Heeg M, et al.. CO 80

1998 Long-term results of unstable pelvic ring fractures in children. Schwarz N, et al. Injury 29:431

1997 Acute and chronic avulsive injuries. el-Khoury GY, et al. Radiol Clin North Am 35:747

1997 Fractures of the pelvis in children. Rieger H, Brug E. CO 336:226

1995 Traumatic loosening of apophyses in the pelvic area and the proximal femur. Hosli P, von Laer L. Orthopade 24:429

1994 Avulsion fractures of the pelvis in children: a report of 32 fractures and their outcome. Sundar M, Carty H. Skeletal Radiol 23:85

1994 Posttraumatic acetabular dysplasia. Trousdale RT, Ganz R. CO 305:124

1993 Pediatric pelvic fractures combined with an additional skeletal injury is an indicator of significant injury. Vazquez WD, Garcia VF. Surg Gynecol Obstet 177:468

1991 Predictors of abdominal injury in children with pelvic fracture. Bond SJ, et al. J Trauma 31:1169

1988 Injuries of the acetabular triradiate cartilage and sacroiliac joint. Heeg MJ, et al. JBJS 70B:34

1988 Pelvic ring fractures: should they be fixed? Tile M. JBJS 70b:1

1985 Pelvic fractures in children. Torode I, Zieg D. JPO 5:76

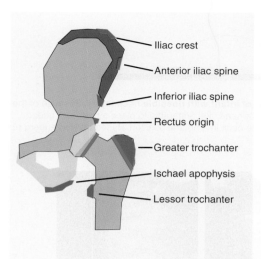

Fig. 10.185 Avulsion fractures of the hip.

- Iliac crest
- Anterior iliac spine
- Inferior iliac spine
- Rectus origin
- Greater trochanter
- Ischael apophysis
- Lessor trochanter

Classification of Acetabular Fractures

Undisplaced fractures
Osteochondral–chondral fractures
Triradiate cartilage fractures
Central fracture dislocations
  Stable postreduction
  Unstable postreduction
Posterior fracture dislocations
  Stable postreduction
  Unstable postreduction

Fig. 10.186 Classification of acetabular fractures. This classification is useful to facilitate management.

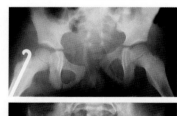

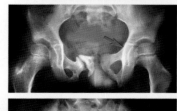

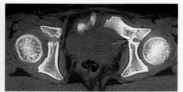

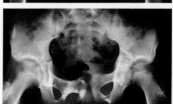

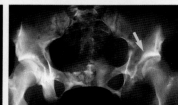

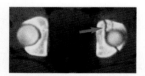

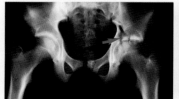

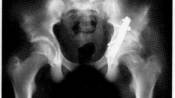

Fig. 10.187 Acetabular fracture. This displaced acetabular fracture (arrows) in a 16-year-old boy was managed by open reduction and plate fixation.

Fig. 10.188 Triradiate cartilage injury causing acetabular insufficiency. This 5-year-old boy sustained multiple pelvic fractures and a fracture of the left femur (upper left). The fractures healed, but a fusion of the triradiate cartilage was demonstrated by AP radiographs and CT (red arrows). Note the development of acetabular dysplasia between ages 12 and 17 years (yellow arrows).

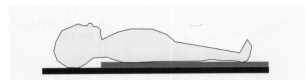

Fig. 10.189 Transport of infant with possible neck injury. Because of the larger size of the infant's head, it is preferable to place a pad (red) under the body to maintain the neck in a neutral position. Based on Herzenberg et al. (1989).

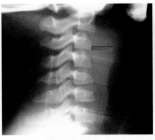
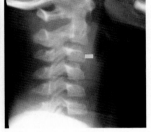

Fig. 10.190 Effect of crying on retropharyngeal space. Crying causes venous engorgement, increasing the retropharyngeal soft tissue space anterior to C3 (red line). These changes may be confused with cervical spine trauma. In this infant, a second radiograph taken while the infant was quiet shows a normal space (yellow line).

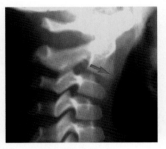
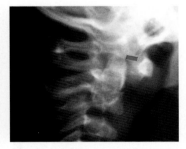

Fig. 10.191 Pseudo-subluxation of C2–3. Forward displacement of C2 (arrow) on C3 is a common normal variation seen in children.

Fig. 10.192 Atlanto-dens interval (ADI). This interval is normally 3–5 mm in children.

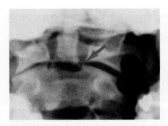

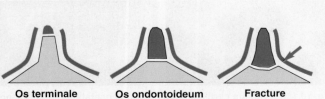

Fig. 10.193 Odontoid discontinuity. This shows differentiate growth centers as seen in the os terminale and os ondontoideum from fracture. Fractures (arrow) usually extend through the base of the odontoid.

Spine Injuries

Spine injuries are relative uncommon in children, accounting for only about 2–3% of spinal trauma cases. Trauma may result from falls, auto accidents, sporting activities, and nonaccidental injury.

Mechanism

Most injuries involve the cervical spine because of greater mobility in the child and a relatively large head and less muscular support. Most injuries cause hyperflexion with compression injuries. Other injuries result from restraints in vehicular accidents such as seat belt fractures. The flexibility of the child's spine accounts for cord injury without apparent skeletal trauma. It has been estimated that the child's spine can be distracted as much as 2 inches without apparent cord injury.

Evaluation

A careful neurologic examination is essential. Spinal shock with flaccid paralysis and total loss of all reflexes may follow severe spine trauma. This may cloud the examination.

AP and lateral radiographs are made on the stretcher. Be aware that transport and lateral radiographs should be made with compensation for the relatively larger head of the child (Fig. 10.189). Place a pad under the trunk to neutralize the position of the neck. Include the entire spine, as multiple fracture sites are not uncommon.

CT scans, MRI and other studies can be done as necessary. Carefully image the upper cervical spine, especially if the child has a head injury, neck pain, or muscle spasm.

Anatomic variations are relative common and may cause confusion.

Pseudosubluxation of C2–C3 level Up to 4 mm of pseudosubluxation is within the normal range for the child (Fig. 10.191).

Retropharyngeal swelling may result from venous encouragement due to crying (Fig. 10.190). In the quiet child, the retropharyngeal space is normally less than 7 mm and the retrotracheal space less than 14 mm.

Atlanto-dens interval (ADI) The normal range is 3–5 mm, which is 1 mm greater than in adults (Fig. 10.192).

Odontoid discontinuity may be due to a growth plate rather than a fracture (Fig. 10.193).

Anterior wedging of the cervical vertebra is often seen in normal infants and younger children.

Spinal Cord Injury without Radiographic Abnormality

Spinal cord injury without radiographic abnormality (SCIWORA) is one of the unique spinal injuries of childhood (Fig. 10.194). SCIWORA is due to the elasticity of the musculoskeletal system, which allows the spinal column to elongate as much as 2 inches without disruption—far greater than the inelastic spinal cord. The condition occurs in children under age 8 years. Recurrent injury may occur because of instability. Evaluate with MRI.

Spinal Injuries Unique to Children

Unique odontoid injuries
Spinal cord injury without radiographic abnormality (SCIWORA)
Varied seat belt fractures
Vertebral apophyseal fractures
Child abuse
Rotatory subluxation
Pathologic fractures associated with tumors
   Eosinophilic granuloma
     Compression fractures associated with leukemia, etc.

Fig. 10.194 Unique features of childhood spine injuries.

Lap-Belt Injuries

Lap-belt injuries are due to a flexion distraction mechanism causing compression fractures of the lumbar vertebrae thought to be due to the elasticity of the posterior ligamentous structure present in children (Fig. 10.195). Suspect this mechanism if contusions are present over the abdominal wall. These fractures vary widely in pattern. Often CT scans are necessary to establish the fracture pattern. Half will have associated abdominal injuries.

Apophyseal Injuries

These injuries are through the vertebral end plate and can take many forms. Posterior physeal fracture with displacement may simulate disc herniation (Fig. 10.196).

Child Abuse

Because these injuries usually occur in infants and show varied patterns of injury, they may require CT or MRI studies for adequate evaluation.

Acute Rotatory Subluxation

Rotatory atlanto-axial subluxation may result from mild trauma, infection, or surgical procedures. The child shows acute torticollis (Fig. 10.197). Early diagnosis is important. Evaluate by plane radiographs and CT scans with head maximally rotated in each direction. These CT scans show fixation of the first and second cervical vertebrae. If the duration is less than 1 week since onset, manage with a cervical collar and bed rest for a week. If not improved, hospitalize for traction. See details on page 188.

Pathologic Fractures

Pathologic fractures occur in children with generalized osteopenia or with lesions such as eosinophilic granuloma (Fig. 10.198).

Injuries with Neurologic Deficit

Children generally do better than adults. Most have only incomplete lesions, and about 20% of those with complete lesions show improvement. Manage with assessment by MRI and treatment with steroids.

References

2000 Pediatric cervical spine injuries: report of 102 cases and review of the literature. Eleraky MA, et al. J Neurosurg 92:12

2000 Pediatric spinal injury. Reynolds R. Curr Opin Pediatr 12:67

2000 Post-traumatic findings of the spine after earlier vertebral fracture in young patients: clinical and MRI study. Kerttula LI, et al. Spine 25:1104

2000 Spectrum of occipitoatlantoaxial injury in young children. Sun PP, et al. J Neurosurg 93:28

1996 Circumferential growth plate fracture of the thoracolumbar spine from child abuse. Carrion WV, et al. JPO 16:210

1993 Wedging of C-3 in infants and children: usually a normal finding and not a fracture. Swischuk LE, Swischuk PN, John SD. Radiology 188:523

1992 Seat-belt injuries of the spine in young children. Rumball K, Jarvis J. JBJS 74B:571

1990 Operative treatment of spine fractures in children. Crawford AH. Orthop Clin North Am 21:325

1990 The diagnosis and treatment of pediatric lumbar spine injuries caused by rear seat lap belts. Johnson DL, Falci S. Neurosurgery 26:434

1989 Emergency transport and positioning of young children who have an injury of the cervical spine. Herzenberg JE, et al. JBJS 71A:15

1989 Spinal cord injury without radiographic abnormality in children--the SCIWORA syndrome. Pang D, Pollack IF. J Trauma 29:654

1989 The management of rotatory atlanto-axial subluxation in children. Phillips WA, Hensinger RN. JBJS 71A:664

1988 Pediatric spinal trauma. Review of 122 cases of spinal cord and vertebral column injuries. Hadley MN, et al. J Neurosurg 68:18

1988 Spinal cord injury without osseous spine fracture. Yngve DA, et al. JPO 8:153

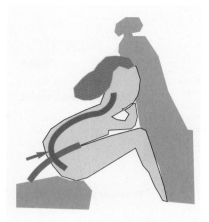

Fig. 10.195 Seat belt injuries in children. The constraining seat belt creates tension posteriorly and compression anteriorly on the lumbar spine. Based on Johnson (1990).

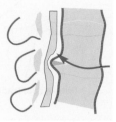

Fig. 10.196 Apophyseal fractures. The fracture line may extend through the apophysis.

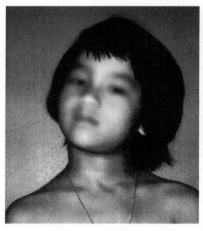

Fig. 10.197 Acute rotatory subluxation. This child had rotatory subluxation from slight trauma.

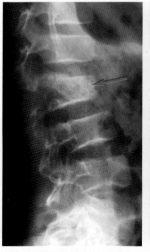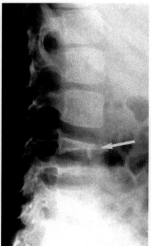

Fig. 10.198 Pathologic fractures. These may be associated with generalized osteopenia (red arrow) or a focal lesion such as an eosinophilic granuloma (yellow arrow).

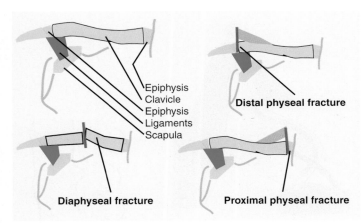

Fig. 10.199 Clavicular fracture types. Fractures may occur at numerous sites along the clavicle. Fractures through the proximal and distal physis can be easily confused with dislocations.

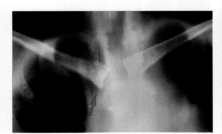

Fig. 10.200 Immobilizing shoulder injuries. These simple slings are usually adequate for managing most shoulder injuries in children.

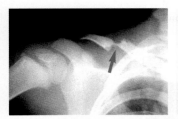
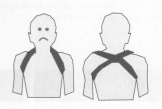

Fig. 10.201 Clavicular fracture. Traditionally, these fractures (arrow) were managed by figure-eight splints (right). These splints do little more than make the child uncomfortable.

Shoulder Injuries

Clavicle Fractures

Clavicle fractures may occur through bone or through proximal or distal growth plates (Fig. 10.199).

Diaphyseal fractures are most common in the mid clavicle. Unless open or with neurovascular compromise, manage closed. Less is best. Place the affected arm in a sling (Fig. 10.200) until the pain has subsided. The common figure-eight strapping is uncomfortable and unnecessary (Fig. 10.201). Shortening and malunion are rarely problems.

Physeal fractures are sometimes difficult to differentiate from dislocation of the of the sternoclavicular or acromioclavicular joints. Physeal fractures usually occur in younger children and show tenderness over the physis rather than the joint. Physeal fractures are less serious, requiring only sling mobilization and no reduction. Remodeling and recovery of normal function occur with time.

Sternoclavicular Dislocations

These injuries are rare but do occur in children (Fig. 10.202). The dislocation may be anterior or posterior. To differentiate from physeal fractures and to plan management, order a CT scan. Reduce by shoulder retraction or by traction on the medial clavicle with a towel-clip.

A-C Separation

Separations usually occur after age 13 years. Sometimes the separation is minimal, with slight swelling and tenderness over the joint. Manage separations as done for adults. The challenge is to differentiate A-C separation from physeal fracture. Order comparative spot radiographs of the the A-C joint using soft tissue technique.

Scapular Fractures

Scapular fractures are rare in children. Manage closed except for those of the glenoid fossa that have significant displacement.

Shoulder Dislocations

Shoulder dislocations are rare in children, and recurrence occurs in the vast majority. Reduce dislocations and immobilize in a sling until comfortable. Inform the family that recurrent dislocation is probable and that operative correction is likely. Posterior dislocation is sometimes associated with brachial plexus palsy in infancy and joint laxity in adolescence (Fig. 10.203).

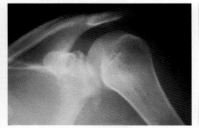

Fig. 10.202 Sternoclavicular separation. These fractures (arrow) may be difficult to visualize by conventional radiographs.

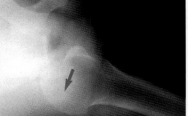

Fig. 10.203 Posterior shoulder dislocation. This dislocation occurred in an adolescent with joint laxity. The dislocation is best shown on an axillary view (arrow).

Humeral Fractures

Humeral fractures may occur at any location. Proximal humeral fracture management is influenced by the extraordinary remodeling potential of the upper humerus (Fig. 10.204). This remodeling is due to the great growth potential of the proximal humeral epiphysis and the forgiving effect of the mobile shoulder joint.

Proximal epiphyseal fractures occur in infants as well as later in childhood.

Infants Consider the possibility of child abuse if these fractures are seen (Fig. 10.205). Unlike the femur, avascular necrosis of the proximal epiphysis is very rare.

Children and adolescents Considerable displacement is common. Manage by immobilizing the arm in a sling for 2–3 weeks. Accept side-to-side alignment and considerable angulation, as remodeling will correct the deformity.

Adolescents at end of growth Reduction at this age is sometimes difficult because of button-holing of the metaphysis into the deltoid or interposition of the biceps tendon between the fragments. If angulation exceeds 60°, attempt a closed reduction. Often the reduction is unstable and the deformity recurs.

Sometimes it is possible to prevent this loss of reduction by placing one or more K wires percutaneously across the fragments. Pin tract inflammation is common. Remove the wires in 2 weeks. Sometimes the postion can be maintained with a shoulder spica cast or brace. Be aware that if the fracture is opened and internally fixed, the surgical scar is usually more unsightly than the slight shoulder asymmetry from malunion.

Pathologic fractures are common (Fig. 10.206). Most are due to unicameral bone cysts (see Chapter 13, page 310).

Humeral Shaft Fractures These are uncommon injuries in children. Look for radial and ulnar nerve and arterial injury. Nearly all nerve injuries recover spontaneously. Operative fixation is necessary only for polytrauma, open injuries, and other unusual situations.

Infants Consider child abuse if these fractures are seen.

Children Manage young children by simple immobilization in a sling and swath. In older children, immobilize with the elbow flexed to a right angle in a soft dressing. Place pads to align fragments. Overwrap with fiberglass. Usually healing is sufficient at 3 weeks to convert to a sling.

Adolescents Be concerned about residual midshaft angulation exceeding 20°–30° in the patient nearing maturity. Because remodeling may be incomplete, operative fixation may be necessary (Fig. 10.207).

References
1998 Severely displaced proximal humeral epiphyseal fractures: a follow-up study. Beringer DC, et al. JPO 18:31
1997 Open reduction and internal fixation of a glenoid fossa fracture in a child: a case report and review of the literature. Lee SJ, et al. Orthop Trauma 11:452
1997 Shortening of clavicle after fracture. Incidence and clinical significance, a 5-year follow-up of 85 patients. Nordqvist A, et al. Acta Orthop Scand 68:349
1997 Humerus shaft fractures in young children: accident or abuse? Shaw BA, et al. JPO 17:293
1996 Diagnosis and treatment of posterior sternoclavicular joint dislocations in children. Yang J, al-Etani H, Letts M. Am J Orthop 25:565
1993 Humeral shaft fracture in childhood. Machan FG, Vinz H. Unfallchirurgie 19:166
1992 The fate of traumatic anterior dislocation of the shoulder in children. Marans HJ, et al. JBJS 74A:1242
1990 Operative management of children's fractures of the shoulder region. Curtis RJ Jr. CO 21:315
1990 Fractures of the proximal humerus in children. Nine-year follow-up of 64 unoperated on cases. Larsen CF, Kiaer T, Lindequist S. Acta Orthop Scand 61:255
1989 Posterior dislocation of the shoulder associated with obstetric brachial plexus palsy. Dunkerton MC. JBJS 71B:764
1984 Distal clavicular physeal injury. Ogden JA. CO 188:68
1981 Clavicle fractures. Eidman DK, Siff SJ, Tullos HS. Am J Sports Med 9:150

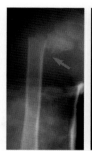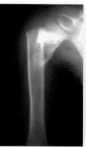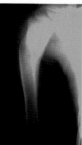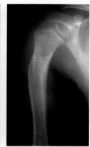

Fig. 10.204 Proximal humeral fracture. The remodeling potential of the proximal humerus is excellent. Few fractures in children require reduction. This fracture (arrow) in a 8-year-old child remodeled well over 2 years.

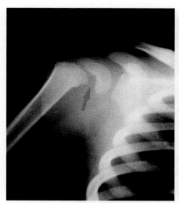

Fig. 10.205 Proximal humeral physeal fracture. Consider child abuse for this type of fracture.

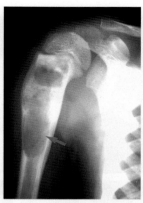

Fig. 10.206 Pathologic humeral fracture. Fractures through bone cysts are common in the upper humerus.

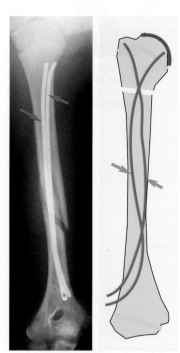

Fig. 10.207 Flexible IM fixation. Ender nail fixation (red arrows) and Metaizeau fixation (green arrows) are effective methods of fixing humeral fractures.

Elbow Fractures in Children

Supracondylar	55 %	7.4 years
Radial neck	14	9.8
Lateral condyle	12	8.7
Medial epicondyle	8	12
Olecranon	7	10
Combinations	1.7	11
Radial head	1.6	14
T or Y fractures	0.7	8
Intracondylar	0.5	14

Fig. 10.208 Elbow fractures in children. The percentage and mean age are shown. Based on 589 elbow fractures in Swedish children. From Landin (1986).

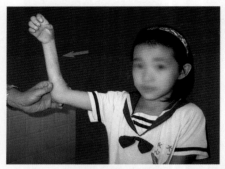

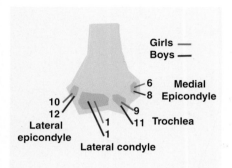

Fig. 10.209 Vascular compromise. The outcome of elbow injuries may be Volkmann contracture (red arrow). Be concerned if ischaemia of the hand is present (bottom left). This may indicate the need for vascular exploration. In this elbow (bottom right), the brachial artery was caught between the fracture fragments (yellow arrow).

Elbow Injuries

Elbow fractures are common, complex, and frequently complicated. Supracondylar fractures are most common (Fig. 10.208). Fracture combinations sometimes occur. The most common combinations involve the olecranon and medial epicondyle and the olecranon and radial neck.

Evaluation

Physical examination Note the location and extent of soft tissue swelling. Lateral condylar fractures produce unilateral swelling that may prompt additional views should the standard radiographs show no fracture. Evaluate nerve function, including the anterior interosseous nerve and circulation. These fractures can be complicated by compromised circulation (Fig. 10.209) and compartment syndromes.

Imaging In every significant injury, an accurate diagnosis is essential. Order radiographs specifically to best show the suspected site of injury. Often the elbow cannot be fully extended for an anteroposterior view. Order either a distal humeral or proximal radial view (Fig. 10.210). Recall the ossification sequence (Fig. 10.211) about the elbow. Observe the alignment of the elbow on the distal humeral AP radiograph (Fig. 10.212), as this will often differentiate the common types of injuries. If conventional radiographs are nondiagnostic, consider MRI, arthrography, or ultrasound. Avoid *diagnostic* arthroscopy. Special studies are most likely to be necessary in early childhood, when ossification is limited.

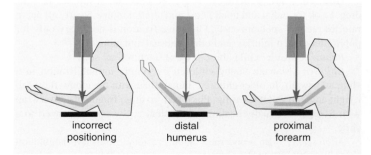

Fig. 10.210 Positioning for radiographs of the elbow. For radiographs of the distal humerus and proximal forearm, these bones should be parallel to the film.

incorrect positioning — distal humerus — proximal forearm

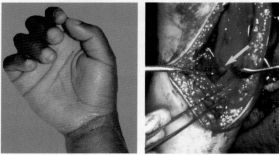

Fig. 10.211 Ossification of distal humerus. Average age in years of ossification is given for girls (red) and boys (blue).

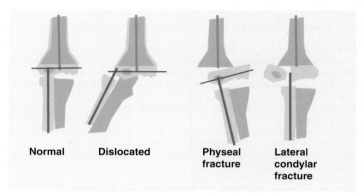

Normal — Dislocated — Physeal fracture — Lateral condylar fracture

Fig. 10.212 Alignment as a guide to assessment. Note that the axis of the radius falls lateral to the capitellar center for dislocated elbows but not for physeal fractures. Based on Hansen et al. (1982).

Pulled Elbow

Pulled elbow, or nursemaids elbow, occurs in about 1% of children each year. Half have no history of a pull. Whether or not it is more common in hypermobile children is controversial. Girls are more commonly affected. The pathology is uncertain, although capsular interposition is the most favored theory (Fig. 10.213).

Clinical Features The arm is held in slight flexion and the forearm pronated; the child resists moving the elbow or extremity (Fig. 10.214). Swelling and tenderness are absent. The diagnosis is clinical, and radiographs are necessary only if the situation or findings are atypical.

Management Unless there is a history of a prior pulled elbow, consider taking a prereduction radiograph to rule out an accult injury. Rotate the forearm through 180° to free the interposed soft tissue. Often a snap is felt. Repeat in 15 minutes if the first attempt is unsuccessful. Return of function is usually immediate but may be delayed, especially in infants. Recurrence is not uncommon. Inability to free the interposition with manipulation does occur. In such cases, place the arm in a sling and see the child the next day and repeat the manipulation.

Physeal Separation Distal Humerus

These uncommon injuries usually occur in infants and young children and may be due to child abuse. The fracture may be misdiagnosed as an elbow dislocation. Suspect this diagnosis by the young age and posteromedial displacement of the proximal radius and ulna relative to the humeral shaft (Fig. 10.215). If necessary, confirm the diagnosis by ultrasound or arthrography. Manage similar to a supracondylar fracture. Because cubitus varus deformity is a common complication, consider fixation with percutaneous pins.

References

2000 The treatment of pulled elbow: a prospective randomized study. Taha AM. Arch Orthop Trauma Surg 120:336

1998 Comparison of supination/flexion to hyperpronation in the reduction of radial head subluxations. Macias CG, Bothner J, Wiebe RA. Pediatrics 102:10

1995 Epiphyseal separation of the distal end of the humeral epiphysis: a follow-up note. Abe M. et al. JPO 15:426

1995 Pulled elbow--not the effect of hypermobility of joints. Hagroo GA, et al. Injury 26:687

1995 Acute annular ligament interposition into the radiocapitellar joint in children (nursemaid's elbow). Choung W, Heinrich SD. JPO 15:454

1991 Fracture-separation of the distal humeral epiphysis. de Jager LT, Hoffman EB. JBJS 73B:143

1990 Radial head subluxation: epidemiology and treatment of 87 episodes. Schunk JE. Ann Emerg Med 19:1019

1986 Elbow fractures in children. An epidemiological analysis of 589 cases. Landin LA, Danielsson LG. Acta Orthop Scand 57:309

1982 Arthrographic diagnosis of an injury pattern in the distal humerus of an infant. Hansen PE, Barnes DA, Tullos HS. JPO 2:569

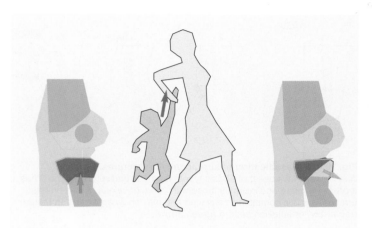

Fig. 10.213 Pulled elbow pathology. The annular ligament (red) normally extends around the radial head (green arrow). With a pull on the elbow (blue arrow), the radial head may subluxate partially out from under the ligament (orange arrow). With forearm rotation or normal use, the head slips back to its orginal position.

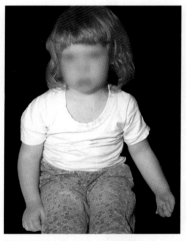

Fig. 10.214 Pulled elbow. This 3-year-old girl shows unwillingness to use the left elbow due to a pulled elbow.

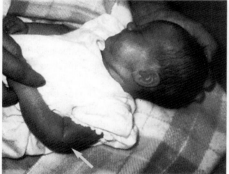
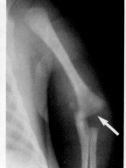
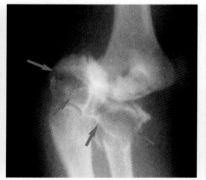
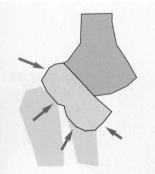

Fig. 10.215 Birth trauma. This newborn sustained trauma during delivery. Note the swollen elbow (yellow arrow) and radiographs showing medial displacement of the radius and ulna relative to the humerus (white arrow). The arthrogram shows the displaced unossified epiphysis (red arrows).

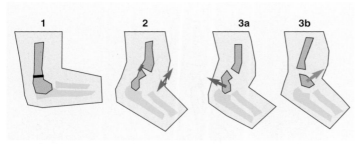

Fig. 10.216 Classification of supracondylar fractures. Gartland classification includes three basic types. Type 1 is undisplaced. Type 2 has a posterior hinge and includes those with varus or valgus impaction (blue arrow). Type 3 is completely displaced and may show an extension pattern (red arrow) or a flexion pattern (green arrow).

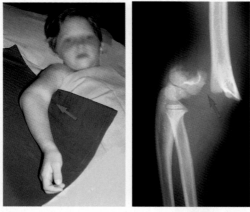

Fig. 10.217 Type 3 fracture. This extension fracture is the most common serious type.

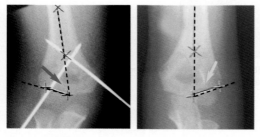

Fig. 10.218 Measuring Baumann angle. Assess the angle on the fracture side (red arrow) and compare the value with the normal side (yellow arrow).

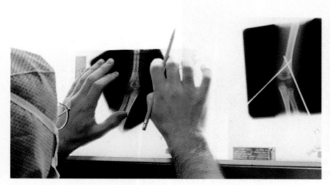

Fig. 10.219 Assessing alignment. Compare the radiographic measures with the clinical appearance of the arm.

Supracondylar Fractures

Supracondylar fractures are the most common elbow injuries. Serious neurovascular injuries and residual cubitus varus deformities are common. This is one of most challenging pediatric fractures. It results mainly from falls at home in children 4 years of age or less and on the playground after 4 years of age. It occurs mostly in girls and in the left arm.

Classification

These fractures are classified into three major categories (Fig. 10.216).

Type 1—Undisplaced fractures These are usually stable and can be managed in a splint for 3 weeks.

Type 2—Extension injuries with posterior hinge These are usually stable with the elbow flexed to a right angle. The difficult types are those with impaction. Impaction may occur in varus or valgus. Impaction fractures with varus deformity of >5° and valgus deformity of >10° should be reduced and percutaneously pinned.

Type 3—Complete and displaced fractures These fractures (Fig. 10.217) are most at risk for associated vascular injury. The majority are the extension type. The flexion type are less common but may be difficult to reduce because of a medial metaphyseal spike.

Assessment

Examine carefully, as problems are common with this fracture.

Skin Check the skin to be sure there is no laceration over the metaphyseal spike, making it an open fracture.

Vascular status Check pulses, capillary filling in nail-beds, and discomfort on finger extension. Vascular injuries occur in 2–3% of type 3 fractures. Be aware that a simple loss of radial pulse is not a definite sign of vascular impairment.

Neurologic status Nerve injuries occur in about 10% of type 3 injuries. Nerve injuries most commonly affect the anterior interosseous, radial, median, and ulnar nerves, in that order.

Carrying angle In type 1 and 2 injuries, gently extend the elbow and observe the carrying angle. Varus or valgus deformities are not uncommon in type 2 injuries and are better diagnosed on physical examination than by radiographs. Following fixation of type 4 injury gently extended the elbow to assess the carrying angle.

Baumann angle is sometimes used (Fig. 10.218) to assess the carrying angle by radiographs. This is an angle between the axis of the humerus and capitellar epiphysis. Assess on both sides. The normal range is usually from 87° to 93°. Make certain the radiographic and clinical findings agree (Fig. 10.219).

Management

Keep in mind vascular compromise and cubitus varus—the major complications of this fracture. Most fractures are managed by cast immobilization or percutaneous pinning. Traction treatment is rarely used (Fig. 10.220).

Type 1 Manage with the elbow flexed to a right angle and immobilized in a posterior splint for 2–3 weeks. Allow motion to recover naturally.

Type 2 Look for evidence of varus or valgus impaction. If deformity exceeds about 5° of varus or 10° of valgus, reduce under anesthesia and fix with percutaneous pins. Otherwise, manage as with type 1 fractures with the elbow flexed.

Type 3 Determine whether it is the extension or flexion type.

Extension fractures are much more common. Manage most with closed reduction and percutaneous pinning. See page 373.

Flexion fractures account for about 10% of these injuries. The posterior angulation is less pronounced, and a medial metaphyseal spike is often present. This spike makes reduction more difficult. The reduction may be facilitated by applying a towel clip through the olecranon and applying traction to the distal fragment. Sometimes open reduction is necessary. Once reduced, fix with percutaneous pins. An alternative in the young child is to immobilize the arm in extension.

Open reduction Indications for open reduction are vascular injuries and fractures that cannot be reduced adequately for placement of percutaneous pins.

Vascular compromise Vascular injuries pose an urgent problem. If detected upon arrival, attempt to position the arm in a neutral alignment with about 30° of flexion. Plan early reduction under anesthesia. Be prepared to perform an open reduction. A simple loss of the radial pulse and good capillary filling is not an indication for arterial exploration. If, after reduction in the operating room, vascularity is not restored, then brachial artery exploration is indicated. Avoid delays. Consider alerting a vascular surgeon of the problem. Avoid arteriography. Explore the artery. Usually the artery is compressed by the fracture fragments, and once freed, circulation is restored. Rarely, arterial repair or bypass grafting is necessary.

Nerve injury Nearly all nerve injuries recover spontaneously in 2 weeks to 4 months. Exploration is not indicated before 6 months. See the patient frequently, as the family may need ongoing reassurance during the period of recovery. EMG, nerve conduction, and other studies are not necessary.

Postoperative management Immobilize for about 3 weeks. Then place the arm in a sling for an additional 1 to 2 weeks. Motion recovers spontaneously. Avoid stretching. Physical therapy is not helpful. Recovery of motion usually requires several months. Allow return to full activities in about 3 months.

Complications

Hyperextension is common. This deformity tends to improve with time (Fig. 10.221). Always compare with the opposite elbow, as hyperextension is common in loose-jointed children. This deformity alone is not an indication for operative correction. The deformity is commonly associated with the cubitus varus deformity. Both components are corrected by osteotomy.

Cubitus varus This complication is common with traction and uncommon with pin fixation treatment. The normal carrying angle is about 5°–10° of valgus. A cubitus varus deformity causes a cosmetic and some functional disability (Figs. 10.222 and 10.223). The deformity is due to malunion and can usually be avoided by careful management. The deformity becomes apparent once the elbow can be fully extended. It is seldom improved by remodeling. Operative correction by osteotomy may be necessary (Fig. 10.224).

References

2000 Displaced supracondylar fractures of the humerus in children. Audit changes practice. O'Hara LJ, Barlow JW, Clarke NM. JBJS 82B:204

2000 Neurovascular injuries in type III humeral supracondylar fractures in children. Lyons ST, Quinn M, Stanitski CL. CO 62

1998 Cosmetic results of supracondylar osteotomy for correction of cubitus varus. Barrett IR, Bellemore MC, Kwon YM. JPO 18:445

1998 Etiology of supracondylar humerus fractures. Farnsworth CL, Silva PD, Mubarak. SJ. JPO 18:38

1996 Vascular injuries and their sequelae in pediatric supracondylar humeral fractures: toward a goal of prevention. Copley LA, Dormans JP, Davidson RS. JPO 16:99

1996 Variation of Baumann's angle with age, sex, and side: implications for its use in radiological monitoring of supracondylar fracture of the humerus in children. Keenan WN, Clegg J. JPO 16:97

1996 Treatment of posttraumatic cubitus varus in the pediatric population with humeral osteotomy and external fixation. Levine MJ, Horn DB, Pizzutillo PD. JPO 16:597

1995 Acute neurovascular complications with supracondylar humerus fractures in children. Dormans JP, Squillante R, Sharf H. J Hand Surg Am 20:1

1995 The "floating elbow" in children. Simultaneous supracondylar fractures of the humerus and of the forearm in the same upper limb. Templeton PA, Graham HK. JBJS 77B:791

1995 Clinical evaluation of crossed-pin versus lateral-pin fixation in displaced supracondylar humerus fractures. Topping RE, Blanco JS, Davis TJ. JPO 15:435

1993 Incidence of anterior interosseous nerve palsy in supracondylar humerus fractures in children. Cramer KE, Green NE, Devito DP. JPO 13:502

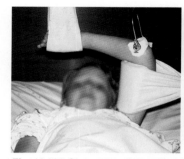
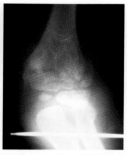

Fig. 10.220 Olecranon pin traction. This is an option in managing difficult fractures. This fracture was comminuted, making pin fixation more difficult.

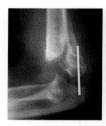
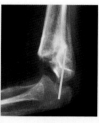
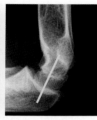

Fig. 10.221 Remodeling in sagittal plane. This sagittal plane deformity (yellow lines) gradually improved over a period of 3 years.

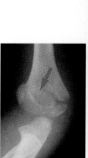
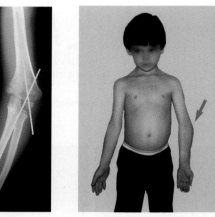

Fig. 10.222 Impacted type 2 varus. This minimally displaced fracture at age 3 years (red arrow) resulted in a cubitus varus, as shown at age 5 years (yellow lines).

Fig. 10.223 Cubitus varus. This deformity (arrow) was the outcome of malunion following supracondylar fracture.

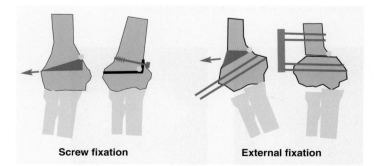

Screw fixation　　**External fixation**

Fig. 10.224 Correction of cubitus varus. There are numerous techniques using screw, external fixator, and other fixation devices. It is important to translate the distal fragment laterally (yellow dots) to avoid a lateral prominence of the distal fragment.

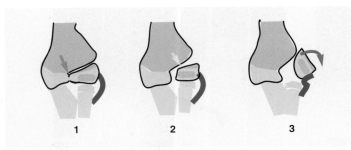

Fig. 10.225 Classification of lateral condylar fractures. In type 1, the articular cartilage remains intact, creating a hinge (green arrow); the fracture is stable. In type 2, the fragment is completely separated but not rotated (yellow arrow). In type 3, the fragment is widely separated and rotated, sometimes 90° or more (red arrow). From Jakob et al. (1975).

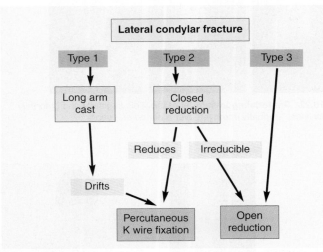

Fig. 10.226 Management flowchart for lateral condylar fractures.

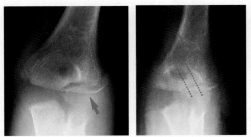

Fig. 10.227 Type 2 lateral condylar fracture. This fracture (arrow) was reduced and fixed with two absorbable pins (dotted lines).

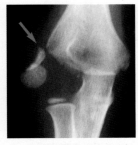

Fig. 10.228 Type 3 lateral condylar fracture (arrow).

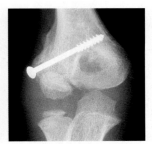

Fig. 10.229 Delayed union fixed with metaphyseal screw.

Lateral Condylar Fractures

These fractures account for about 12% of elbow fractures in children. They result from a violent force with the elbow in extension. These fractures are unique for the risk of nonunion.

Diagnosis

Children show swelling and pain on the lateral aspect of the elbow. Order AP, lateral, and oblique radiographs of the distal humerus. Sometimes the displacement is absent or minimal, and the diagnosis is established by localized soft tissue swelling over the lateral condyle.

Classification

The classic classification (Fig. 10.225) is based on the extent of displacement. The fracture line may extend through the lateral condylar ossification center, between the capitellum and trochlea, or through the trochlear cartilage. Assess minor degrees of displacement in millimeters. Type 1 shows less than 2 mm of displacement.

Management

Management is based on the degree of displacement (Fig. 10.226).

Type 1 Manage with a long-arm cast with the the elbow flexed to 80° and the forearm in neutral rotation. Use fiberglass or limit the amount of plaster about the elbow to facilitate radiographic assessment. Repeat an AP radiograph of the distal humerus in 1, 2, and 3 weeks to ensure that the fracture is stable. For stable fractures, continue immobilization for 6 weeks. Should the fracture displace, closed or open reduction and pin fixation will be necessary.

Type 2 Manage fractures with displacements of 2–4 mm by closed reduction and percutaneous pinning. If the fracture cannot be reduced closed to <2 mm, open reduction is required.

Type 3 This type (Fig. 10.228) is managed by open reduction and pin fixation. Fix two smooth K wires or absorbable pins (Fig. 10.227) that securely fix the condyle and metaphysis. Leave pins protruding outside the skin to allow removal in the clinic in 4–6 weeks. Splint for comfort and to reduce irritation of pin sites.

For detailed operative reduction and pinning procedures, see page 374.

Complications

Nonunion is uniquely common for this fracture, possibly because of the intraarticular position and limited blood supply. Manage based on duration. Early nonunions (less than 6 months) can be reduced and fixed like an acute fracture (Fig. 10.229). Late nonunions should be stabilized to the metaphysis *in situ*, as they remodel and will not fit if replaced. Attempt to fuse the metaphyseal fragment of the fracture to the metaphysis. Screw fixation is optimal.

Malunion Early malunions (less than about 2 months) may be revised for anatomic reduction. Leave most malunions.

Avascular necrosis This complication may result from excessive stripping of the soft tissue attachments to the fragment during reduction.

References

2000 The posterolateral approach to the distal humerus for open reduction and internal fixation of fractures of the lateral condyle in children. Mohan N, Hunter JB, Colton CL. JBJS 82B:643

1998 Nonoperative treatment for minimally and nondisplaced lateral humeral condyle fractures in children. Bast SC, Hoffer MM, Aval S. JPO 18:448

1997 Lateral condyle fractures in children: evaluation of classification and treatment. Mirsky EC, Karas EH, Weiner LS. J Orthop Trauma 11:117

1997 Osteosynthesis for the treatment of non-union of the lateral humeral condyle in children. Shimada K, et al. JBJS 79A:234

1995 Lateral condylar fractures of the humerus in children: fixation with partially threaded 4.0-mm AO cancellous screws. Sharma JC, et al. J Trauma 39:1129

1995 Nondisplaced and minimally displaced fractures of the lateral humeral condyle in children: a prospective radiographic investigation of fracture stability. Finnbogason T, et al. JPO 15:422

1994 Percutaneous pinning in the treatment of displaced lateral condyle fractures. Mintzer CM, et al. JPO 14:462

1991 Biodegradable pin fixation of elbow fractures in children. A randomised trial. Hope PG, et al. JBJS 73B:965

Medial Epicondylar Fractures

This is a relatively common fracture in late childhood and adolescence. The epicondyle is avulsed as a SH-1 or SH-2 type fracture (Fig. 10.230). Because the fragment is not articular and the epicondyle does not contribute to the longitudinal growth of the humerus, residual serious problems are rare.

Management

Manage most by simple immobilization for the acute painful period, followed by early motion. Operative exploration, reduction, and fixation are essential if the fragment is entrapped in the joint (Fig. 10.231) or if a significant ulnar nerve injury is present. If the fracture occurs in the dominant arm of a throwing athlete or gymnast, consider operative reduction and fixation with a lag screw to provide elbow stability (Fig. 10.232).

Prognosis

Minor problems are common. These include hyper- or hypoplasia of the epicondyle and pseudoarthrosis. Of those without fixation, about half develop pseudoarthrosis. Rarely is the pseudoarthrosis symptomatic. Occasionally, mild ulnar nerve symptoms are present. Elbow motion is unaffected. In other cases, the medial epicondyle may be prominent.

Elbow Dislocations

Elbow dislocations in children are important because about two-thirds are associated with fractures about the elbow.

Dislocation without Fracture

The diagnosis is usually obvious (Fig. 10.233, left). Manage by gentle closed reduction. Immobilize in a posterior splint for about 2–3 weeks, then in a sling for another 1 to 2 weeks. Allow spontaneous return of motion. Complications from simple dislocations are rare.

Dislocation with Osteochondral Fracture

Identify the fragment (Fig. 10.233, right) and remove by arthroscopy or arthrotomy.

Dislocation with Avulsion of Medial Epicondyle

Suspect this pattern to be certain that the diagnosis is made. The epicondyle can nearly always be seen on conventional radiographs (Fig. 10.234). Be suspicious of this diagnosis if, after reduction, the joint space is wide and motion is irregular or restricted. If the epicondyle is trapped in the joint following reduction, attempt to free it by extending the elbow while supinating the forearm. If this is unsuccessful, operative reduction and pin fixation are required.

Complicating Features

Divergent dislocation is a rare injury, due to disruption of the superior radio-ulnar joint. Closed reduction is usually successful.

Recurrent dislocations are very rare and require operative repair.

Associated with birth palsy usually require operative repair.

Intrapment of median nerve requires open reduction.

Associated radial neck fractures may be complicated by radio-ulnar synostosis.

References

2000 Using sonography to diagnose an unossified medial epicondyle avulsion in a child. May DA, et al. AJR Am J Roentgenol 174:1115

1996 Infantile dislocation of the elbow complicating obstetric palsy. Cummings RJ, et al. JPO 16:589

1994 Deformity after internal fixation of fracture separation of the medial epicondyle of the humerus. Skak SV, Grossmann E, Wagn P. JBJS 76B:297

1991 Recurrent dislocation of the elbow in a child: case report and review of the literature. Beaty JH Donati NL. JPO 11:392

1990 Elbow dislocation with avulsion of the medial humeral epicondyle. Fowles JV, Slimane N, Kassab MT. JBJS 72B:102

1987 Intra-articular entrapment of the median nerve after elbow dislocation in children. Floyd WE 3d, Gebhardt MC, Emans JB. J Hand Surg Am 12:704

1986 Epicondylar elbow fracture in children. 35-year follow-up of 56 unreduced cases. Josefsson PO, Danielsson LG. Acta Orthop Scand 57:313

1986 Divergent dislocation of the elbow in a child. Sovio OM, Tredwell SJ. JPO 6:96

1984 Posterior dislocation of the elbow in children. Carlioz H, Abols Y. JPO 4:8

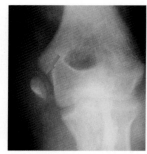
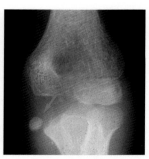

Fig. 10.230 Mild displacement of medial epicondyle. Displacement is minimal.

Fig. 10.231 Epicondyle in joint. This entrapment (arrow) required operative reduction.

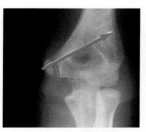

Fig. 10.232 Rigid fixation. To provide elbow stability, consider fixation with a lag screw (site shown by red arrow).

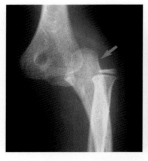
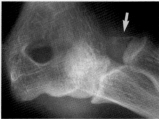

Fig. 10.233 Elbow dislocation. Most are simple dislocations without fracture (red arrow). Rarely, the dislocation is complicated by an osteochondral fracture, which can be seen as a faint radiolucent linear lesion (yellow arrow).

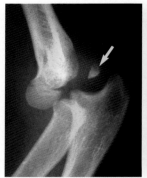
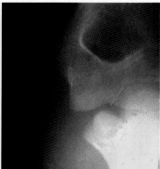

Fig. 10.234 Elbow dislocation with medial epicondyle entrapped in the joint. Note the epicondyle before (yellow arrow) and after (red arrow) reduction.

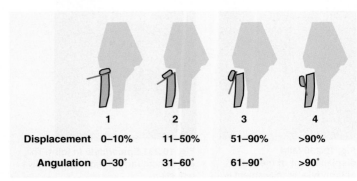

Fig. 10.235 Grading of radial neck fractures. This grading is done by displacement and angulation. From Steele and Graham (1992).

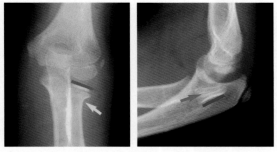

Fig. 10.236 Grade 1 and 4 radial neck fractures. The fracture sites and tilt of the radial head (blue lines) are shown for a type 1 fracture (yellow arrow), and the complete displacement in a grade 4 fracture (red arrow).

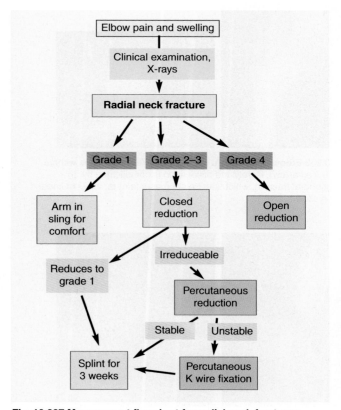

Fig. 10.237 Management flowchart for radial neck fractures.

Radial Head and Neck Fractures

Radial neck fractures occur most often from the ages of 4 to 14 years and are often associated with other elbow injuries. Together these injuries often cause outcomes that are less satisfactory than most pediatric fractures. This is due to the vulnerability of vascularity, the growth plate, and the intraarticular position of the fracture.

Diagnosis

The child will show swelling and tenderness over the proximal radius. Radiographs usually show the fracture. Be aware that to grade the severity accurately, the radiograph should show the fracture displacement in profile. Often the grade is higher than expected from routine views. Undisplaced fractures can be imaged by ultrasound or MRI.

Classification

Classify the severity based on both displacement and angulation (Figs. 10.235 and 10.236). Grade 4 injuries include those with the radial head displaced to a position anterior or posterior to the proximal radius.

Management

Manage based on severity.

Grade 1 These fractures require only resting in an arm sling until the pain has subsided.

Grades 2 and 3 These fractures may reduce with manipulation. With satisfactory anesthesia, rotate the forearm until the displaced radial head is most prominent. Apply thumb pressure while rotating the forearm to reduce the radial head. If reduction to a grade 1 level is not achieved, then percutaneous reduction is indicated. See details of this procedure on page 375.

Grade 4 This type of fracture requires open reduction. Internal fixation with a suture or pins (Fig. 10.238) may be necessary.

Complications

Complications include stiffness, avascular necrosis, growth arrest, overgrowth, malunion, nonunion, cross union, posterior interosseous nerve injury, and compartment syndromes.

References

2000 Fractures of the proximal radial head and neck in children with emphasis on those that involve the articular cartilage. Leung AG, Peterson HA. JPO 20:7

1999 Radial neck fractures in children: a management algorithm. Evans MC, Graham HK. JPOB 8:93

1998 The use of ultrasonography in the diagnosis of occult fracture of the radial neck. A case report. Lazar RD, Waters PM, Jaramillo D. JBJS 80A:1361

1997 Reliability of fat-pad sign in radial head/neck fractures of the elbow. Irshad F, Shaw NJ, Gregory RJ. Injury 28:433

1995 Compartment syndrome in the forearm following fractures of the radial head or neck in children. Peters CL, Scott SM. JBJS 77A:1070

1991 Dislocation of the elbow joint associated with fracture of the radial neck in children. Papavasiliou VA, Kirkos JM. Injury 22:49

1990 Fractures of the olecranon and radial neck in children. Dormans JP, Rang M. Orthop Clin North Am 21:257

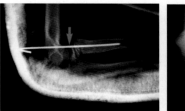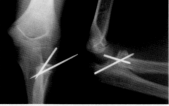

Fig. 10.238 Fixation of radial neck fractures. Transcapitellar fixation is often complicated by breakage of the K wire at the joint level (red arrow). Oblique single or double pin fixation is preferable (right).

Olecranon Fractures

Olecranon fractures are uncommon injuries and may be associated with radial neck fractures. Be aware that the displacement may exceed that seen on the lateral radiograph.

Management

Minimal displaced fractures Manage fractures with less than 2–3 mm of displacement with immobilization in a long-arm cast with the elbow flexed to about 30°.

Displaced fractures Reduce and fix fractures in children with non-parallel smooth K wires (Fig. 10.239) and in adolescents with tension band wiring (Fig. 10.240). Immobilize for about 3–4 weeks in a long-arm cast. Allow natural recovery of range of motion.

Other Fracture Types

Olecranon physeal separation Manage this rare injury with reduction and K wire fixation.

Stress physeal fractures This type may occur in the gymnast.

Monteggia Fracture Dislocations

These injuries are serious and sometimes overlooked. If unreduced, they are likely to cause long-term disability because of the radial head dislocation.

Diagnosis

Be suspicious that an isolated ulnar fracture may be associated with a radial head dislocation. Be aware that associated injuries are common. Nerve injuries may involve the posterior interosseous and radial nerves.

Classification

Classify into one of Bado four types (Fig. 10.241). Equivalent lesions include the following: (1) dislocation of the radial head with plastic bowing of the ulna (Fig. 10.242), (2) fractures of the neck of the radius and midshaft ulna, and (3) dislocation of the radial head with midshaft ulna and olecranon fractures.

Management

Manage most by closed reduction and long-arm cast immobilization with the elbow flexed to a right angle and the forearm supinated.

Open reduction This is necessary if the reduction is unstable. A flexible IM transolecranon rod is best. This fixation is easily placed and removed and is adequate for children.

Chronic lesions Manage by operative reduction and fixation up to about 6 years following the initial injury. Perform an osteotomy of the ulna. Reconstruct the annular ligament if the reduction is unstable.

References

1998 Corrective ulnar osteotomy for malunited anterior Monteggia lesions in children. 12 patients followed for 1-12 years. Inoue G, Shionoya K. Acta Orthop Scand 69:73

1997 Surgical treatment of displaced olecranon fractures in children. Gaddy BC, et al. JPO 17:321

1996 Chronic Monteggia lesions in children. Complications and results of reconstruction. Rodgers WB, Waters PM, Hall JE. JBJS 78A:1322

1994 Management of old unreduced Monteggia fracture dislocations of the elbow in children. Best TN. JPO 14:193

1994 Monteggia fracture-dislocation in children. Gleeson AP, Beattie TF. J Accid Emerg Med 11:192

1993 Fractures of the olecranon in children: long-term follow-up. Graves SC, Canale ST. JPO 13:239

1989 Monteggia and equivalent lesions in childhood. Olney BW, Menelaus MB. JPO 9:219

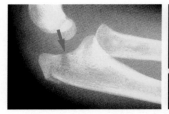
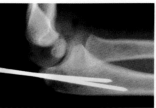

Fig. 10.239 K wire fixation. This olecranon fracture (arrow) in a 5-year-old child with moderate displacement was fixed with two smooth K wires (right).

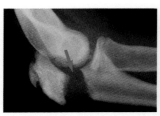
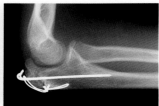

Fig. 10.240 Tension band fixation. This olecranon fracture (arrow) in a 14-year-old child with wide displacement tension was stabilized with tension band fixation (right).

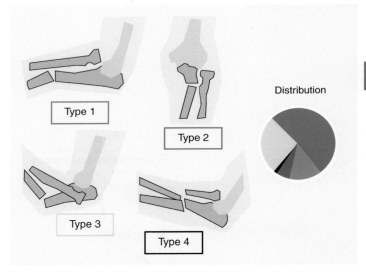

Fig. 10.241 Classification and distribution. Bado classifies Monteggia fractures into four types. Distribution of the injuries based on type are shown by colors on the pie chart. Equivalent lesions are shown in green. From Olney and Menelaus (1989).

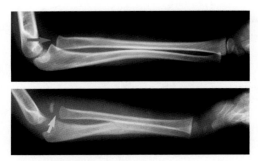

Fig. 10.242 Monteggia equivalents. A variant is the dislocation of the radial head (red arrow) with plastic deformation of the ulna. A chronic lesion is present in a 5-year-old child (bottom). The ulna fracture was treated with a cast, but the dislocated radial head (yellow arrow) was not diagnosed for 6 months.

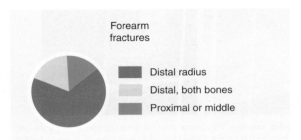

Forearm
fractures

Distal radius
Distal, both bones
Proximal or middle

Fig. 10.243 Distribution of forearm fractures. The vast majority are fractures of the distal radius. From Czerny (1994).

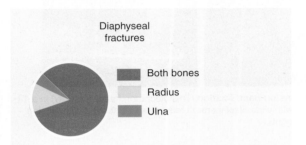

Diaphyseal
fractures

Both bones
Radius
Ulna

Fig. 10.244 Distribution of diaphyseal fractures. Both bones fracture in most. From Wurfel (1995).

Forearm Fractures

Distal forearm fractures are most common (Fig. 10.243), and those involving the metaphysis usually involve both bones (Fig. 10.244). Diaphyseal fractures are most common in girls ages 10 to 12 years and in boys ages 12 to 14 years.

Evaluation

Consider the possible complicating factors. Look for concurrent nerve injuries, vascular compromise, and compartment syndromes

Open fractures significantly increase the risk of complications, with about 10% of cases having nerve injuries or compartment syndromes. Delayed or nonunion, malunion, and refracture are frequent in type 2 and 3 fractures. Nerve injuries recover spontaneously, but compartment syndromes require urgent release.

Ulnar styloid fractures are usually not solitary injuries. Look for other associated fractures.

Angulation Conventional AP and lateral radiographs may not show the greatest degree of angulation. Oblique views or fluoroscopy are helpful.

Diaphyseal Fractures

Management of diaphyseal fractures can be guided by a flowchart (Fig. 10.245). It is often helpful to use finger traps and gravity (Fig. 10.246) to support and aid in maintaining reduction following manipulation. Immobilize most by flexible IM fixation (see page 377). Open reduction becomes increasingly likely with increasing age. Accurate reduction is necessary at the end of growth to avoid malunion and limited forearm rotation.

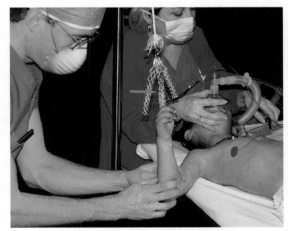

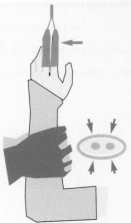

Fig. 10.246 Finger traction. Finger traction (green arrows) is useful to align the fracture and determine the position or rotation for immobilization. Be certain to mold the cast (red arrows) to reduce the likelihood of drift in the cast or splint.

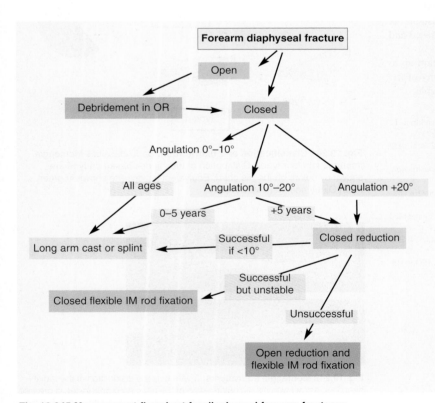

Fig. 10.245 Management flowchart for diaphyseal forearm fractures.

Anesthesia Options include general, local, regional, or even no anesthesia. The no anesthetic option is appropriate for fractures that can with absolute certainty be reduced with one deft manipulation. The child is given the choice of this option. The other methods require several injections and prolonged emergency department or hospital stays. The child usually accepts and later appreciates this choice.

Greenstick fractures are contained within the periosteum (Fig. 10.247). Complete the fracture, place in finger traction, and immobilize in a long-arm cast with the forearm in a position assumed naturally with traction.

Plastic deformation often involves the ulna. Look for a dislocation of the radial head, making it a Monteggia equivalent. Most simple deformation occurs in early childhood when remodeling will correct malunion. Immobilize for 3 weeks. For more severe angulation, gradual but forceful manipulation may be necessary to correct the deformity.

Complete fractures Manage most by performing a manipulative reduction and then applying finger traction during cast application. Immobilize in the position of rotation naturally assumed by the forearm when traction is applied. Diaphyseal fractures in late childhood and adolescence often require operative reduction and internal fixation (Figs. 10.248 and 10.249) (see pages 376 and 377).

Radius fractures Isolated injuries may be difficult to align, as the proximal fragment is uncontrollable. Rotate the forearm to align the forearm with the free proximal radius fragment. Use fluoroscopy to make this match.

Preventing reduction loss Molding the cast to provide a snug fit will help. Repeat radiographs at weekly intervals for 3 weeks. Union of these diaphyseal fractures can take several weeks.

Acceptable alignment Side-to-side alignment is acceptable for children under age 8 years. In children over 10 years, do not accept malalignment greater than 10°. Malposition in the older child is an indication for operative reduction and internal fixation.

Refracture This occurs in about 10% of fractures (Fig. 10.250). Try to prevent it by a good reduction and immobilization until bridging callus is seen on both sides of the fracture.

Malunion Remodeling will correct nearly any degree of malunion in the child under age 5 years. Malunions of greater than 10° in the older child or adolescent cause limitation of forearm rotation. This loss of motion is readily apparent on physical examination but is rarely noticed by the patient. This disparity between motion loss and disability is a source of confusion when assessing outcomes of forearm fractures.

References

2000 Intramedullary Steinmann pin fixation of forearm fractures in children. Long-term results. Pugh DM, Galpin RD, Carey TP. CO 39

1999 The management of forearm fractures in children: a plea for conservatism. Jones K, Weiner DS. JPO 19:811

1997 Remanipulation of forearm fractures in children. Chan CF, et al. N Z Med J 110:249

1996 Refracture of the forearm in children. Schwarz N, et al. JBJS 78B:740

1995 Open fractures of the arm in children. Haasbeek JF, Cole WG. JBJS 77B:576

1995 Forearm fractures in children: avoiding redisplacement. Haddad FS, Williams RL. Injury 26:691

1995 Compartment syndrome in the forearm following fractures of the radial head or neck in children. Peters CL, Scott SM. JBJS 77A:1070

1995 New aspects in the treatment of complete and isolated diaphyseal fracture of the forearm in childhood. Wurfel AM, et al. Unfallchirurgie 21:70

1994 Forearm fractures in children. Czerny F, et al. Unfallchirurgie 20:203

1993 Distal forearm fractures in children. Complications and surgical indications. Dicke TE, Nunley JA. Orthop Clin North Am 24:333

1992 Both-bone forearm fractures in children. Carey PJ, et al. Orthopedics 15:1015

1990 Compartment syndrome following forearm fracture in children. Royle SG. Injury 21:73

1990 Significance of ulnar styloid fractures in childhood. Stansberry SD, et al. Pediatr Emerg Care 6:99

1988 Epidemiology of distal forearm fractures in Danish children. Kramhoft M, Bodtker S. Acta Orthop Scand 59:557

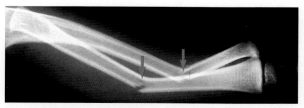

Fig. 10.247 Greenstick fracture. Note that the fractures (arrows) are at different levels, indicating a rotational component to the injury.

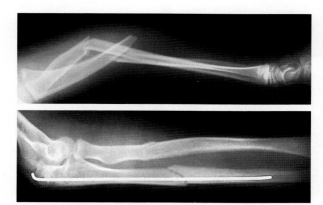

Fig. 10.248 Single bone fixation. This fixation was selected for a 12-year-old boy with this fracture. Because the fractures are aligned and considerable growth remains, this fixation is adequate.

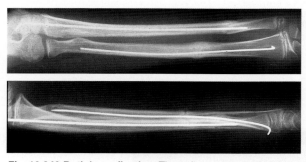

Fig. 10.249 Both bone fixation. These fine rods provide adequate fixation for fractures.

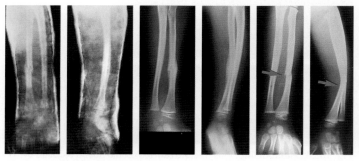

Fig. 10.250 Refracture. Refractures (arrows) are not uncommon and are sometimes difficult to prevent.

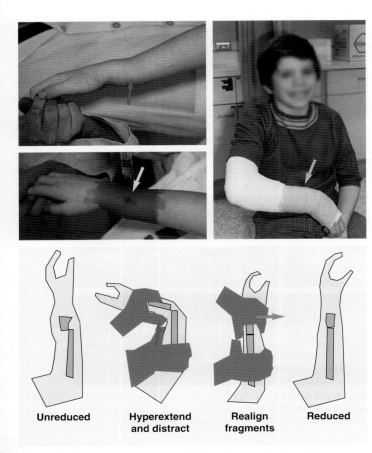

Fig. 10.251 Reduction of displaced distal forearm fracture. The fractures (red arrow, top) can be reduced with a hematoma block (yellow arrow). Manipulate by hyperextension and distraction (blue arrow), realigning the fragments (green arrow), and immobilizing the arm in a cast or cast-splint (orange arrow).

Unreduced — Hyperextend and distract — Realign fragments — Reduced

Distal Radius Fractures

Manage most distal forearm fractures with significant displacement by closed reduction (Fig. 10.251). Generally, if a deformity is visible, reduction is appropriate.

Anesthesia In addition to the options available for diaphyseal fractures, hematoma block is available. Its simplicity, effectiveness, and safety make it a good choice.

Manipulation This requires considerable force. The fracture is accentuated, the ends approximated with traction, and the bones then repositioned. See page 376.

Acceptable reduction The amount depends on the child's age. Side-to-side position is acceptable in a child (Fig. 10.252). The potential for remodeling of malunions of the distal radius is great. Seldom are malunions not remodeled to an acceptable position.

Unstable reduction At the end of growth, unstable reduction may require internal fixation for stabilization. A single smooth K wire is usually adequate.

Immobilization Apply a long-arm cast with the wrist flexed in the degree achieved by gravity alone. Mold the cast to produce an oval shape in cross-section and provide slight pressure over the apex of the original deformity.

Complications These include compartment syndromes, displacement in the cast (drift), and malunion.

Compartment syndromes are uncommon complications. See page 222.

Displacement in the cast Drift is most likely when reduction is incomplete. Make a radiograph at about 1 week postreduction (Fig. 10.253). If uncertain about the need for re-reduction, remove the cast and show the parents. If drift has caused a deformity that is unacceptable, re-reduce the fracture. If the fracture is drifting, follow closely with radiographs twice weekly. Try to identify excessive drift before union.

Malunion This often creates considerable initial concern, but over several months, the deformity remodels and seldom is it a problem beyond a year. During this period of remodeling, the family and physician may become stressed.

Buckle fractures These are usually stable (Fig. 10.254); however, if one cortex is completely fractured, the fracture may be unstable and can drift. Repeat the radiograph at 1 week. Immobilize in a short-arm cast for about 3 weeks.

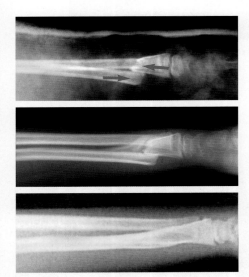

Fig. 10.252 Remodeling. This fracture (arrows) could not be reduced by manipulation and was left with side-to-side alignment. Remodeling corrected the deformity in 18 months (bottom).

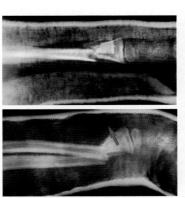

Fig. 10.253 Displacement in the cast. Note the loss of position that occurred during the first week of casting (arrow).

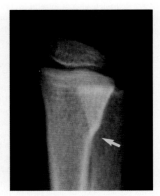

Fig. 10.254 Buckle fracture. Note the change in contour of the distal radius (arrow) consistent with a buckle fracture.

Galeazzi fractures The childhood equivalent of a Galeazzi fracture is distal radial and ulnar SH-2 epiphyseal fractures. Variations of this pattern can occur (Fig. 10.255). This very rare fracture may be difficult to recognize. Sometimes open reduction and K wire fixation are necessary. Growth disturbance is uncommon.

Distal radial physeal fractures These fractures are usually SH-1 or -2 types (Fig. 10.256). These fractures can usually be reduced by manipulation. SH-3 fractures require anatomic reduction (Fig. 10.257). Growth arrest following these fractures is common (Fig. 10.258). Repeat an AP radiograph of the wrist in about 6 months to identify any arrest early on. Early identification allows bridge resection before signification angulation or shortening develops.

References
1997 Remanipulation of forearm fractures in children. Chan CF, Meads BM, Nicol RO. N Z Med J 110:249

1996 Refracture of the forearm in children. Schwarz N, et al. JBJS 78B:740

1995 Percutaneous Kirschner-wire pinning for severely displaced distal radial fractures in children. A report of 157 cases. Choi KY, et al. JBJS 77B:797

1995 Open fractures of the arm in children. Haasbeek JF, Cole WG. JBJS 77B:576

1995 Forearm fractures in children: avoiding redisplacement. Haddad FS, Williams RL. Injury 26:691

1995 Compartment syndrome in the forearm following fractures of the radial head or neck in children. Peters CL, Scott SM. JBJS 77A:1070

1995 New aspects in the treatment of complete and isolated diaphyseal fracture of the forearm in childhood. Wurfel AM, et al. Unfallchirurgie 21:70

1994 Forearm fractures in children. Czerny F, et al. Unfallchirurgie 20:203

1993 Distal forearm fractures in children. Complications and surgical indications. Dicke TE, Nunley JA. Orthop Clin North Am 24:333

1993 Galeazzi-equivalent injuries of the wrist in children. Letts M, Rowhani N. JPO 13:561

1992 Both-bone forearm fractures in children. Carey PJ, et al. Orthopedics 15:1015

1991 Variant of Galeazzi fracture-dislocation in children. Landfried MJ, Stenclik M, Susi JG. JPO 11:332

1990 Significance of ulnar styloid fractures in childhood. Stansberry SD, et al. Pediatr Emerg Care 6:99

1990 Compartment syndrome following forearm fracture in children. Royle SG. Injury 21:73

1988 Epidemiology of distal forearm fractures in Danish children. Kramhoft M, Bodtker S. Acta Orthop Scand 59:557

1987 Cross-union complicating fracture of the forearm. Part II: children. Vince KG, Miller JE. JBJS 69A:654

1982 Malunited fractures of the forearm in children. Fuller D, McCullough CJ. JBJS 64B:364

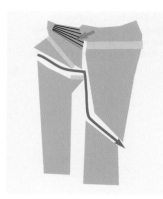

Fig. 10.255 Childhood Galeazzi variant. This fracture includes ulnar SH-2 and radial metaphyseal fractures (red arrow). The triangular fibrocartilagenous complex (green arrow) remains intact. Based on Landfried et al. (1991).

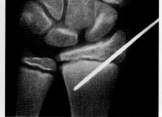
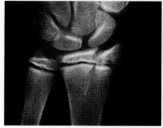

Fig. 10.256 Complex wrist fracture. This is an SH-2 fracture of the distal radius and a metaphyseal fracture of the distal ulna. This high-energy injury is likely to cause a growth arrest.

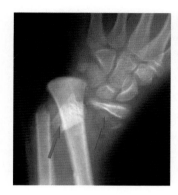

Fig. 10.257 SH-3 distal radius fracture. Because this fracture was articular and physeal, anatomic reduction was necessary. This was fixed with a single, smooth K wire. Growth arrest is a risk with this injury.

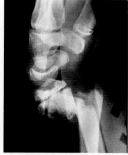
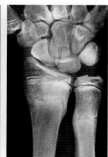
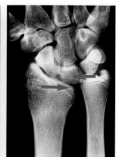
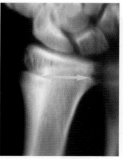

Fig. 10.258 Growth arrest distal radius. This 13-year-old girl sustained this distal metaphyseal fracture of both bones without apparent physeal injury. Soon after union, the radioulnar relationship is normal (orange arrows). One year later, shortening of the radius is present (red arrows). Note the large physeal bridge (yellow arrow). This bridge was too large for resection.

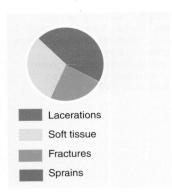

Fig. 10.259 Hand injuries in children. The incidence of these injuries is shown in this pie chart. From data of Bhende et al. (1993).

- Lacerations
- Soft tissue
- Fractures
- Sprains

Hand Injuries

Most hand injuries in children involve soft tissue (Fig. 10.259). Often these soft tissue injuries are most difficult to evaluate.

Soft Tissue Injuries

Nerve injuries Nerve transection of the hand should be repaired. Sharp transection of the nerves repaired by group fascicular techniques yields nearly consistently excellent results. Outcomes are better in children than in adults.

Fingertip crush injuries These injuries can occur at any age (Fig. 10.260), but are especially common in the toddler.

Fingertip amputation These are common injuries (Figs. 10.261 and 10.262). Manage most by leaving the wound open and allow closure and healing be secondary intention. When the tip is available, it can be sutured back in place as a composite graft. This repair should not be delayed, as results before 5 hours are good and after that are poor.

Tendon lacerations Primarily repair tendon lacerations (Figs. 10.263 and 10.264) at all levels and immobilize for 3–4 weeks. Some improvement in motion will occur over a period of several years. Outcomes are usually excellent in children.

Replantation Replantation should be undertaken when feasible in children. About two-thirds of replanted digits survive. Best results occur in clean-cut injuries, vascular repairs, bone shortening, and interosseous bone fixation. Results are better when the body weight is over about 25 pounds. Results are usually excellent. Function and sensation recover well. About one-third will have cold intolerance and another one-third fingertip atrophy. Growth is slightly retarded, but the length generally is acceptable.

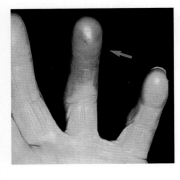

Fig. 10.260 Finger crush injury. Note the extensive discoloration and swelling.

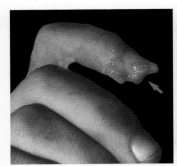
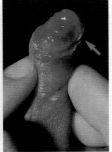

Fig. 10.261 Fingertip amputation. Note the loss of the fingertip in this 12-year-old boy.

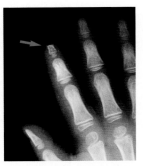

Fig. 10.262 Fingertip amputation. The terminal portion of the index finger is missing.

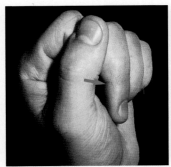
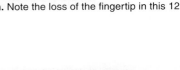

Fig. 10.263 Profundus tendon laceration. This injury was not initially appreciated. Note the loss of terminal flexion of the long finger (arrows).

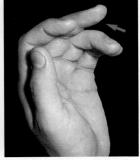
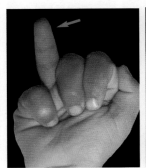
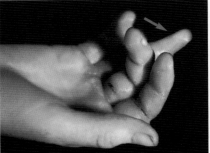

Fig. 10.264 Flexor tendon laceration. Laceration of both tendons produces this characteristic deformity (arrows).

Joint Injuries

Metacarpophalangeal joint dislocations These dislocations usually involve the index finger (Fig. 10.265) or little finger. They usually require open reduction. This should be done early to avoid vascular compromise.

Thumb dislocations Manage by closed reduction (Fig. 10.266). Splint for 2–3 weeks, then allow active motion. Return to full activity in 6 weeks.

Interphalangeal joint dislocations Manage most with closed reduction. Open reduction may be necessary if articular fracture is present.

Interphalangeal joint sprains These injuries are common and resolve slowly (Fig. 10.267).

Carpal Fractures

Navicular fractures These are uncommon injuries in children. In most, the diagnosis is not difficult. Tenderness is localized to the anatomic sniff-box, and radiographs nearly always show the lesion. Order a navicular view in addition to AP and lateral studies. Two-thirds of these fractures occur in the distal third (Fig. 10.268). Manage by immobilization in a thumb spica cast for about 7 weeks. Nonunions in children are rare. For children with tenderness but without radiographic changes, immobilize for 2 weeks and repeat the radiographs.

Other carpal fractures The capitate, triquetrum, hamate, and trapezoid are very rare injuries in children. Most can be managed by cast immobilization.

Burns Most burns occur on the hand and are common in children. Fortunately, most are minor, requiring only a nonadherent dressing. More serious burns (Fig. 10.269) require intensive treatment, including debridement and skin grafts.

References

2000 Injuries to the hand from dog bites. Grant I, Belche H Jr. J Hand Surg [Br] 25:26

1998 Carpal fractures in children. Wulff RN, Schmidt TL. JPO 18:462

1997 Composite graft replacement of digital tips. 2. A study in children. Moiemen NS, Elliot D. J Hand Surg 22B:346

1997 Replantation in childhood and adolescence. Long-term outcome. Schwabegger AH, et al. Unfallchirurg 100:652

1995 Microsurgery in children. Beris AE, Soucacos PN, Malizos KN. CO 314:112

1995 Bone growth after replantation in children. Demiri E, et al. J Reconstr Microsurg 11:113

1994 Digit replantation in infants and young children: determinants of survival. Baker GL, Kleinert JM. Plast Reconstr Surg 94:139

1994 Flexor tendon injuries in children. Grobbelaar AO, Hudson DA. J Hand Surg 19B:696

1994 Results of zone I and zone II flexor tendon repairs in children. O'Connell SJ, et al. J Hand Surg 19 A:48

1993 Hand injuries in children presenting to a pediatric emergency department. Bhende MS, Dandrea LA, Davis HW. Ann Emerg Med 22:1519

1991 Finger tip amputations in children. Rosslein R, Simmen BR. Handchir Mikrochir Plast Chir 23:312

1990 Operative treatment of fractures and dislocations of the hand and wrist region in children. Campbell RM Jr. Orthop Clin North Am 21:217

1989 Results of median nerve repair in children. Tajima T, Imai H. Microsurgery 10:145

1988 Complex dislocation of the index metacarpophalangeal joint in children. Light TR, Ogden JA. JPO 8:300

1987 Burns of the upper extremity in children: long-term evaluation of function following treatment. Melhorn JM, Horner RL. JPO 7:563

1986 Hand injuries in children. Almquist EE. Pediatr Clin North Am 33:1511

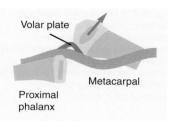

Fig. 10.265 Complex dislocation of index finger. This drawing demonstrates the pathology of dorsal displacement of the volar plate and proximal phalanx. This injury requires open reduction. Based on Light and Ogden (1988).

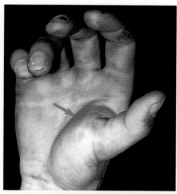
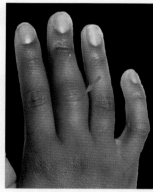

Fig. 10.266 Dislocation of thumb. This dislocation was reduced by manipulation.

Fig. 10.167 Finger sprain. This boy sustained this injury from a ball strike on the end of the finger.

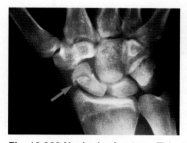

Fig. 10.268 Navicular fracture. This 15-year-old boy sustained this injury in an auto accident.

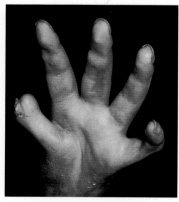

Fig. 10.269 Burned hand. This severe injury resulted from an open flame.

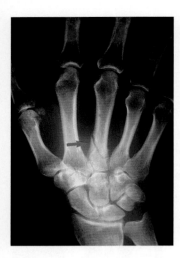

Fig. 10.270 Metacarpal diaphyseal fracture. Order a true lateral radiograph of the metacarpal to be sure that this satisfactory alignment is present in the sagittal plane. This fracture (arrow) was managed in a short-arm cast with a long finger extension for 3 weeks.

Hand Fractures

Hand and wrist fractures in children are common and potentially serious because minor deformities can cause disability.

Management

Most hand injuries are not difficult to diagnose. Deformity is usually obvious, and tenderness is well localized.

Child abuse The presence of finger fractures in the infant should bring to mind the possibility of abuse. Order high-resolution radiographs of the hands and feet in suspected abuse cases as part of the skeletal survey.

Fracture displacement This is most common in the thumb, index, and little fingers. Fracture displacement within a given digit is common in the metacarpal, the proximal phalanx, and distal phalanges, in that order. The middle phalanx is least likely to be malaligned.

Avoid malunion This can be avoided by taking several steps.

Make AP and true lateral radiographs of the individual digits to accurately determine the extent of malalignment.

Evaluate rotational correction by assessing the postreduction alignment with the finger in full finger flexion.

Accurately reduce displaced articular fractures, which requires anatomic reduction and fixation.

Avoid overestimating remodeling potential, especially near the end of growth.

Be aware of problem fractures such as displaced intraarticular fractures, SH-1 distal phalangeal fractures due to crushing injuries, displaced subcondylar fractures, and open fractures.

Indications for open reduction Perform open reduction on irreducible dislocations and articular fractures of the small joints. Align angulated fractures of the middle and proximal phalanx in the region of the neck or distal shaft because of the poor remodeling capacity in these regions.

Fixation Fix most fractures with small transcutaneous smooth K wires. Consider absorbable fixation as an alternative.

Metacarpal Fractures

Diaphyseal fracture Obtain true lateral radiographs to assess the degree of angulation. Assess the rotational status with fingers in flexion. Reduce to align fracture. If reduction is unstable, transfix fracture with a smooth K wire. Immobilize with a finger-to-forearm cast with finger extensions in a functional position for 3 weeks (Fig. 10.270).

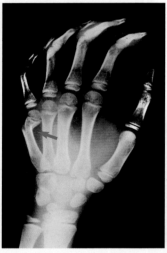

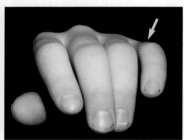

Fig. 10.271 Boxer's fracture. Assess this fracture (red arrow) with a true lateral radiograph to determine the full extent of angulation. Make certain the finger is aligned in flexion. Some depression of the metatarsal contour is apparent on physical exam (yellow arrow). This fracture was managed with an ulnar nerve block, reduction, and immobilization in a short-arm cast with a well-padded extension around the flexed little finger.

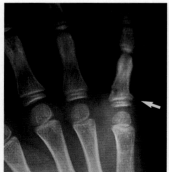

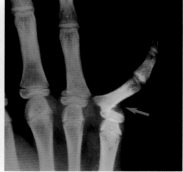

Fig. 10.272 Physeal fractures of the first phalanx. These common injuries include those with minimal displacement (yellow arrow) and those with severe angulation (red arrow) that require reduction. Place an ulnar nerve block, manipulate, and fix if unstable.

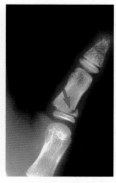

Fig. 10.273 Thumb physeal injury. Align and immobilize in a thumb spica cast if the position is satisfactory and reduction stable.

Distal metacarpal fracture This fracture, also called boxer's fracture (Fig. 10.271), is a pure flexion fracture that will remodel with spontaneous return of range of motion. If the angulation is >45°, reduce with an ulnar nerve block with the finger flexed to 90°. Immobilize for about 3 weeks with the finger flexed to control rotation. Anatomically reduce intraarticular fractures.

Base of thumb metacarpal fracture This fracture, also called Bennett fracture, extends through the proximal thumb metacarpal. It requires reduction. Be certain that rotational alignment is correct. If unstable, fix with a transcutaneous K wire and supplement with a thumb spica cast.

Phalangeal Fractures

Proximal phalanx physeal fractures These are common injuries (Figs. 10.272 and 10.273). Reduce closed or open if SH-3 (Fig. 10.276) or SH-4. Assess rotation in flexion. Use internal fixation if unstable.

Mid and distal phalanx physeal fractures These injuries are uncommon but may cause growth arrest and deformity (Fig. 10.275).

Diaphyseal fractures Assess with true AP and lateral radiographs (Fig. 10.274). Align and fix internally if unstable.

Mallet finger This may involve an SH-1 fracture in the young child or often an SH-3 fracture in the adolescent (Fig. 10.277). Reduce in hyperextension. Stabilize in a finger splint. SH-3 fractures require anatomic reduction.

Tuft fracture These fractures are commonly associated with crush injuries (Fig. 10.278). As these are open fractures, manage with antibiotics, soft tissue care, and follow-up. Complications include osteomyelitis and nail damage.

Chapter Consultant Kaye Wilkins, e-mail: drkwilkins@aol.com

References

1999 Salter-Harris types III and IV epiphyseal fractures in the hand treated with tension-band wiring. Stahl S, Jupiter JB. JPO 19:233

1997 Fractures of the hands and feet in child abuse: imaging and pathologic features. Nimkin K, Spevak MR, Kleinman PK. Radiology 203:233

1996 Finger fractures in children treated with absorbable pins. Vandenberk P, De Smet L, Fabry G. JPO-b 5:27

1995 Stress fracture of index metacarpal in an adolescent tennis player. Waninger KN, Lombardo JA. Clin J Sport Med 5:63

1994 Physeal and periphyseal injuries of the hand. Patterns of injury and results of treatment. Fischer MD, McElfresh EC. Hand Clin 10:287

1990 Operative treatment of fractures and dislocations of the hand and wrist region in children. Campbell RM Jr. Orthop Clin North Am 21:217

1988 Epiphyseal injuries in the small joints of the hand. Torre BA. Hand Clin 4:411

1987 Fractures about the interphalangeal joints in children. Crick JC, Franco RS, Conners JJ. J Orthop Trauma 4:318

1984 Hand fractures in children. A statistical analysis. Hastings H 2d, Simmons BP. CO 188:120

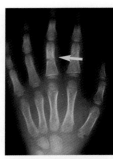
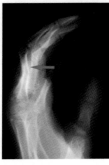
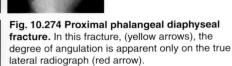

Fig. 10.274 Proximal phalangeal diaphyseal fracture. In this fracture, (yellow arrows), the degree of angulation is apparent only on the true lateral radiograph (red arrow).

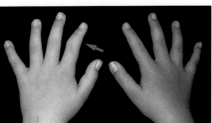

Fig. 10.275 Growth disturbance. This child sustained an epiphyseal injury to the midphalanx. It was not anatomically reduced. This outcome is rare.

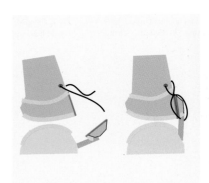

Fig. 10.276 Figure-eight tension band wiring. Use this for fixation of avulsed epiphyseal fractures. Based on Stahl and Jupiter (1999).

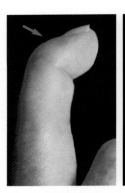

Fig. 10.277 Mallet finger. This fracture requires anatomic reduction and fixation.

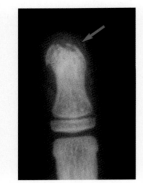

Fig. 10.278 Tuft fracture. This open injury is more serious than often appreciated.

Akbania BA, Silberstein MJ, Rende RJ, et al. Arthography in the diagnosis of fractures of the distal end of the humerus in infants. J Bone Joint Surg 1986;68A:599-602.

Allen BL Jr, Kant AP, Emery FE. Displaced fractures of the femoral diaphysis in children: Definitive treatment in a double spica cast. J Trauma 1977;17:8-19.

Amir J, Katz K, Grunebaum M, et al. Fractures in premature infants. J Pediatr Orthop 1988;8:41-44.

Aronson DD, Singer RM, Higgins RF. Skeletal traction for fractures of the femoral shaft in children: A long-term study. J Bone Joint Surg 1987;69A:1435-1439.

Bailey DA, Wedge JH, McCulloch RG, et al. Epidemiology of fractures of the distal end of the radius in children as associated with growth. J Bone Joint Surg 1989;71A:1225-1231.

Balthazar DA, Pappas AM. Acquired valgus deformity of the tibia in children. J Pediatr Orthop 1984;4:538-541.

Barquet A. Natural history of avascular necrosis following traumatic hip dislocation in childhood: A review of 45 cases. Acta Orthop Scand 1982;53:815-820.

Beals RK. The normal carrying angle of the elbow: A radiographic study of 422 patients. Clin Orthop 1976;119:194-196.

Bernstein SM, King JD, Sanderson RA. Fractures of the medial epicondyle of the humerus. Contemp Orthop 1981;637-641.

Brouwer KJ, Molenaar JC, van Linge B. Rotational deformities after femoral shaft fractures in childhood: A retrospective study 27-32 years after the accident. Acta Orthop Scand 1981;52:81-89.

Bryan WJ, Tullos HS. Pediatric pelvic fractures: Review of 52 patients. Trauma 1979;19:799-805.

Burke SW, Jameson VP, Roberts JM, et al. Birth fractures in spinal muscular atrophy. J Pediatr Orthop 1986;6:34-36.

Currey JD, Butler G. The mechanical properties of bone tissue in children. J Bone Joint Surg 1975;57A:810-814.

Davis DR, Green DP. Forearm fractures in children: Pitfalls and complications. Clin Orthop 1976;120:172-183.

Eidman DK, Siff SJ, Tullos HS. Acromioclavicular lesions in children. Am J Sports Med 1981;9:150-154.

Ertl JP, Barrack RL, Alexander AH, et al. Triplane fracture of the distal tibial epiphysis: Long-term follow-up. J Bone Joint Surg 1988;70A:967-976.

Fiddian NJ, Grace DL. Traumatic dislocation of the hip in adolescence with separation of the capital epiphysis: Two case reports. J Bone Joint Surg 1983;65B:148-149.

Flynn JC. Nonunion of slightly displaced fractures of the lateral humeral condyle in children: An update. J Pediatr Orthop 1989;9:691-696.

Fowles JV, Kassab MT. Displaced fractures of the medial humeral condyle in children. J Bone Joint Surg 1980;62A:1159-1163.

Fuller DJ, McCullough CJ. Malunited fractures of the forearm in children. J Bone Joint Surg 1982;64B:364-367.

Herndon WA, Mahnken RF, Yngve DA, et al. Management of femoral shaft fractures in the adolescent. J Pediatr Orthop 1989;9:29-32.

Herzenberg JE, Hensinger RN, Dedrick DK, et al. Emergency transport and positioning of young children who have an injury of the cervical spine. J Bone Joint Surg 1989;71A:15-22.

Holda ME, Manoli A II, La Mont RI. Epiphyseal separation of the distal end of the humerus with medial displacement. J Bone Joint Surg 1980;62A:52-57.

Hresko MT, Kasser JR. Physeal arrest about the knee associated with non-physeal fractures in the lower extremity. J Bone Joint Surg 1989;71A:698-703.

King J, Diefendorf D, Apthorp J, et al. Analysis of 429 fractures in 189 battered children. J Pediatr Orthop 1988;8:585-589.

Kohler R, Trillaud JM. Fracture and fracture separation of the proximal humerus in children: Report of 136 cases. J Pediatr Orthop 1983;3:326-332.

Koo WWK, Sherman R, Succop P, et al. Fractures and rickets in very low birth weight infants: Conservative management and outcome. J Pediatr Orthop 1989;9:326-330.

Labelle H, Bunnell WP, Duhaime M, et al. Cubitus varus deformity following supracnodylar fractures of the humerus in children. J Pediatr Orthop 1982;2:539-546.

Lancourt JE, Dickson JH, Carter RE. Paralytic spinal deformity following traumatic spinal-cord injury in children and adolescents. J Bone Joint Surg 1981;63A:47-53.

Landin L, Nilsson BE. Bone mineral content in children with fractures. Clin Orthop 1983;178:292-296.

Langenskiöld A. Surgical treatment of partial closure of the growth plate. J Pediatr Orthop 1981;1:3-11.

Larsen E, Vittas D, Torp-Pedersen S. Remodeling of annulated distal forearm fractures in children. Clin Orthop 1988;237:190-195.

Lawson JP, Ogden JA, Bucholz RW, et al. Physeal injuries of the cervical spine. J Pediatr Orthop 1987;7:428-435.

Letts RM, Gibeault D. Fractures of the neck of the talus in children. Foot Ankle 1980;1:74-77.

Light TR, Ogden DA, Ogden JA. The anatomy of metaphyseal torus fractures. Clin Orthop 1984;188:103-111.

Mabrey JD, Fitch RD. Plastic deformation in pediatric fractures: Mechanism and treatment. J Pediatr Orthop 1989;9:310-314.

Malkawi H, Shannak A, Amr S. Surgical treatment of pathological subtrochanteric fractures due to benign lesions in children and adolescents. J Pediatr Orthop 1984;4:63-69.

McDonald GA. Pelvic disruptions in children. Clin Orthop 1980;151:130-134.

Nimityongskul P, Anderson LD. The likelihood of injuries when children fall out of bed. J Pediatr Orthop 1987;7:184-186.

Offierski CM. Traumatic dislocation of the hip in children. J Bone Joint Surg 1981;63B:194-197.

Ogden JA. Growth slowdown and arrest lines. J Pediatr Orthop 1984;4:409-415.

Ogden JA, Tross RB, Murphy MJ. Fractures of the tibial tuberosity in adolescents. J Bone Joint Surg 1980;62A:205-215.

Olney BW, Lugg PC, Turner PL, et al. Outpatient treatment of upper extremeity injuries in childhood using intravenous regional anaesthesia. J Pediatr Orthop 1988;8:576-579.

Oppenheim WL, Clader TJ, Smith C, et al. Supracondylar humeral osteotomy for traumatic childhood cubitus varus deformity. Clin Orthop 1984;188:34-39.

Pirone AM, Graham HK, Krajbich JI. Management of displaced extension-type supracondylar fractures of the humerus in children. J Bone Joint Surg 1988;70A:641-650

Riseborough EJ, Barrett IR, Shapiro F. Growth disturbances following distal femoral physeal fracture-separations. J Bone Joint Surg 1983;65A:885-893.

Rockwood CA Jr. Fracture of the outer clavicle in children and adults, abstract. J Bone Joint Surg 1982;64B:642.

Salter RB, Zaltz C. Anatomic investigations of the mechanism of injury and pathologic anatomy of "pulled elbow" in young children. Clin Orthop 1971;77:134-143.

Sanders WE, Heckman JD. Traumatic plastic deformation of the radius and ulna: A closed method of correction of deformity. Clin Orthop 1984;188:58-67.

Schmidt TL, Weiner DS. Calcaneal fractures in children: An evaluation of the nature of the injury in 56 children. Clin Orthop 1982;171:150-155.

Silberstein MJ, Brodeur AE, Graviss EMERGENCY ROOM . Some vagaries of the lateral epicondyle. J Bone Joint Surg 1982;64A:444-448.

Spiegel PG, Cooperman DR, Laros GS. Epiphyseal fractures of the distal ends of the tibia and fibula: Bone Joint Surg. 1978;60A:1046-1050.

Spiegel PG, Mast JW, Cooperman DR, et al. Triplane fractures of the distal tibial epiphysis. Clin Orthop 1984;188:74-89.

Steinberg EL, Golomb D, Salama R, et al. Radial head and neck fractures in children. J Pediatr Orthop 1988;8:35-40.

Theodorou SD, Ierodiaconou MN, Mitsou A. Obstetrical fracture-separation of the upper femoral epiphysis. Acta Orthop Scand 1982;53:239-243.

Tredwell SJ, Van Peteghem K, Clough M. Pattern of forearm fractures in children. J Pediatr Orthop 1984;4:604-608.

Vahvanen V, Westerlund M. Fracture of the carpal scaphoid in children: A clinical and roentgenological study of 108 cases. Acta Orthop Scand 1980;51:909-913.

Viljanto J, Kiviluoto H, Paananen M. Remodeling after femoral shaft fracture in children. Acta Chir Scand 1975;141:360-365.

Vince KG, Miller JE. Cross-union complicating fracture of the forearm: Part II. J Bone Joint Surg 1987;69A:654-661.

Wagner KT Jr, Lyne ED. Adolescent traumatic dislocations of the shoulder with open epiphysis. J Pediatr Orthop 1983;3:61-62.

Wiley JJ. Tarso-metatarsal joint injuries in children. J Pediatr Orthop 1981;1:255-260.

Yngve DA, Harris WP, Herndon WA, et al. Spinal cord injury without osseous spine fracture. J Pediatr Orthop 1988;8:153-159.

Ziv I, Blackburn N, Rang M. Femoral intramedullary nailing in the growing child. J Trauma 1984;24:432-434.

Ziv I, Rang M. Treatment of femoral fracture in the child with head injury. J Bone Joint Surg 1983;65B:276-278.

Chapter 11 – Sports

Introduction

Involvement in sports is increasing. It is estimated that about half of boys and one-fourth of girls participate in sports in the United States, which amounts to about 20 million children in athletic activities outside school and 25 million in school activities. Children are beginning competitive sports at an increasingly younger age.

Sports participation (Fig. 11.1) and natural play are important to the health of children (Fig. 11.2). Childhood obesity levels are increasing at an alarming rate (Fig. 11.3). Sports provide a valuable diversion from the TV–refrigerator complex. Sports teaches the child discipline, interpersonal skills, and problem-solving techniques. Participation should be fun, providing the child with opportunities to be creative and to become proficient in a sport that best fits the child's native ability. Ideally, a sports activity can be continued throughout adult life. Experts believe that sports activities prepare both boys and girls for success in the competitive world.

On the downside, the value of the child's sports experience is often diminished by pushy parents, aggressive coaches, and artificially limited options. The child may be pressured into a sport for which he or she has little ability. The child performs poorly, is embarrassed, and ends up with a damaged self-image.

When the major emphasis is on winning, the chances of a child continuing long term on the team diminishes with time. Most kids eventually get "cut" from the varsity team. Those who "make it" may find a conflict between the demands of the sport, their social life, and their education. Those who really succeed and become elite athletes may become narrowly focused. This limited focus has some short-term advantages and some long-term problems. Parents and children, as well as most physicians, have little information on the long-term risks of contact sports (Fig. 11.4).

This chapter describes the principles of managing sports problems in children and adolescents. Acute injuries that occur in sports are covered in Chapter 10. Overuse injuries are common in sports. Certain types of injuries that commonly occur in the sporting environment are covered in this chapter.

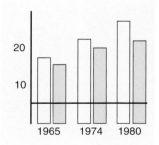

Fig. 11.1 Sports participation a priority. Even in densely populated areas, providing room for sports is an important community priority (Hong Kong).

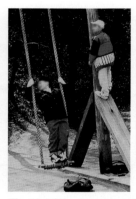

Fig. 11.2 Play, the occupation of the child. Play, whether individual or in teams, is a vital part of a child's life.

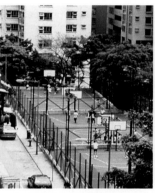

Fig. 11.3 Percentage of obese children in United States. Percentage of obese children ages 6–11 years (light yellow); 12–17 years (dark yellow), by year. From Gortmaker (1987).

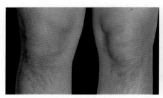
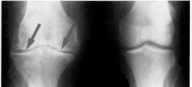

Fig. 11.4 Effect of menisectomy during childhood. At age 13, this patient sustained a torn medial meniscus while playing football. An arthroscopic menisectomy was performed. At age 29, the man has disabling pain and significant disability. The radiograph shows severe osteoarthritis (arrows).

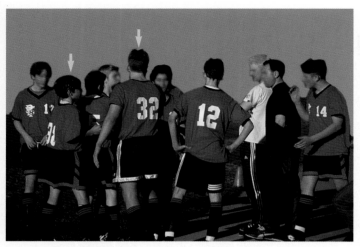

Fig. 11.5 Size differences in same age children. The largest boy is nearly double the weight of the smallest boy on the team (yellow arrows).

Physiology

A child is not a small adult. The child's physiology and psychology are different. These differences are important in sports medicine.

Size Differences

Children of the same age differ greatly in body size, which can place smaller individuals at greater risk for injury or failure (Fig. 11.5). In competitive contact sports, such as American football, matching children by size, not age, can reduce injuries.

Gender Differences

Significant differences in the genders include the following features:

Effect of sports on maturation has little effect on boys but may delay menarche in girls involved in highly aerobic sports.

Running performance tends to plateau at puberty in girls but continues to increase in boys (Fig. 11.6).

Muscle strength gains during teen years accelerate in boys but taper off in girls (Fig. 11.7). Strength increases most rapidly about 1 year after the adolescent growth spurt. Maximum strength for girls develops during the growth spurt. Muscle fiber size peaks at a higher level in men than in women and declines later in life (Fig. 11.8). In an athletic male, muscle makes up 40% of his weight compared to 23% in women. This contributes to a disadvantage in sports competition between adolescent boys and girls.

Body fat is more equivalent in young girls and boys, but during the adolescent growth spurt, girls acquire substantially more fat than boys. In adult women, about 15% of body weight is from fat as compared to about 5% in men.

Heat Regulation

Children sweat less than adults, making them more susceptible to overheating. Avoid hyperthermia by providing abundant fluid intake. Cool environments are best for sports activities.

Effects of Strength Training

Intensive strength training may lead to a *fatigue syndrom,* which increases susceptibility to viral infections.

Joint Hypermobility

Hypermobility syndromes increase risk for sprains and dislocations but may decrease the risk of such injuries as articular fractures, which often occur with acute patellar dislocations.

Ventilatory Capacity

Children are less efficient in pulmonary function than adolescents (Fig. 11.9).

Psychology

Aggressiveness, self-confidence, and tactical abilities learned in sports participation are characteristics useful in achieving success in the competitive world for both boys and girls.

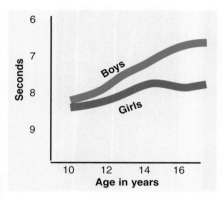

Fig.11.6 Performance. The 50-yard dash in seconds related to age and sex. From Hunsicker (1976).

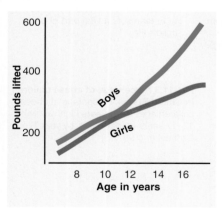

Fig. 11.7 Quadriceps strength by age. Shows increasing strength of the quadriceps. From Parker (1990).

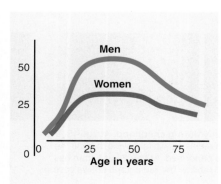

Fig. 11.8 Biceps fiber size by age. From Kukulas and Adams (1985).

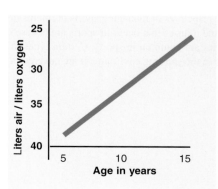

Fig. 11.9 Ventilatory efficiency. Shows liters of air ventilated per liter of oxygen utilized. From Maffulli (1995).

Injury Statistics

Parents and children are often unaware of the potential of injury from sports. It is useful to educate them with data. Fortunately, most sports injuries are minor and heal rapidly, but some are serious. Injuries (from all causes) are the leading cause of childhood death. Significant injuries can cause long-term disability. Most deaths in sports are due to cardiovascular disease or head injuries. Most trauma deaths are the result of high-speed injuries beyond the velocities of childhood sports. Few injuries lead to permanent disability. The most common serious injuries occur in American football (Fig. 11.10), causing ligamentous or meniscal tears in the knee.

Sport

Injury rates vary considerably among sports (Fig. 11.11). Football and wrestling cause acute injuries, whereas running and field events tend to produce overuse problems.

Age

Injury rates and severity increase with age (Fig. 11.12). The small child simply does not have the speed or mass to cause serious injury. In young children, fractures occur more commonly through bone and less commonly through growth plates, reducing the risk of altering growth.

Gender

Boys are injured more frequently than girls (Fig. 11.12) because they play the highest risk games, American football and wrestling. When these two sports are removed from the injury profile, overall injury rates between boys and girls are comparable, except for the 2–3 times greater incidence of ACL injuries in girls playing basketball and soccer.

Disability

Disability may occur early from the acute injury or appear later from osteoarthritis due to articular damage.

Short-term disability from injuries is usually temporary because the majority of injuries are minor (Fig. 11.13) and are disabling only during the period required for healing and rehabilitation.

Long-term disability is most serious and usually due to osteoarthritis in a site that has sustained more than one injury. Twenty years after playing high school football, radiographic changes showed osteoarthritis of the knee (Fig. 11.14). In midadult life, osteoarthritis of the hip severe enough to require total hip replacement is quadrupled in men who had moderate to high exposure to sports (Fig. 11.15). When these men had physically demanding work, their risk increased eightfold above the control group. The majority of college football players who sustained major knee injuries had previously sustained injury to the same knee during high school. Whether or not modern techniques of meniscal and ACL repair will alter these statistics remains to be determined. These studies suggest that injuries from high-impact sports during adolescence are likely to have significant adverse consequences in adult life. These risks should be balanced against the substantial benefits of high school team sports participation.

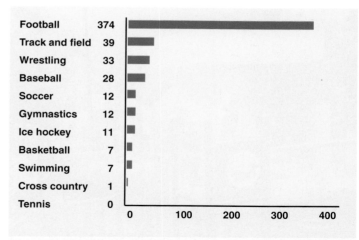

Fig. 11.10 Fatal and catastrophic injuries in high school sports. Based on rates per 100,000 participants. From Cantu and Mueller (1999).

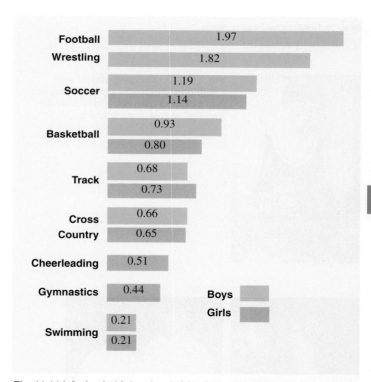

Fig. 11.11 Injuries in high school althletics per athlete per year in the United States. From Beachy et al. (1997).

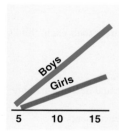

Fig. 11.12 Injuries by age groups in years. From Beachy et al. (1997).

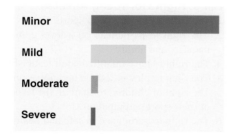

Fig. 11.13 Injury severity. Percentage of injuries by severity. From Beachy et al. (1997).

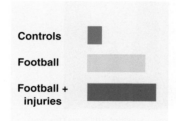

Fig. 11.14 Percentage with osteoarthritis 20 years after high school football. From Moretz (1984).

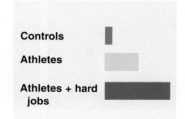

Fig. 11.15 Frequency of total hip replacement by history of activity. From Vingard (1993).

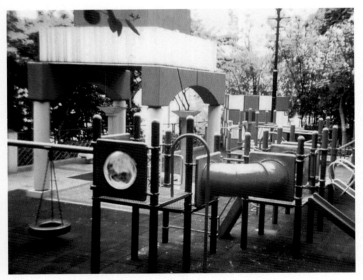

Fig. 11.16 Hard surface. This attractive play area for children has a serious flaw: a concrete surface. The children may stay cleaner but are much more likely to sustain injuries with falls.

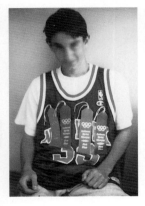

Fig. 11.17 Outstanding athlete with childhood orthopedic problem. This boy had a clubfoot deformity and became an excellent athlete in many sports.

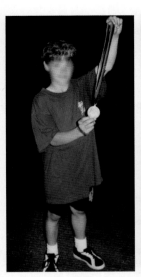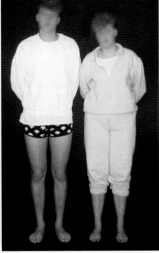

Fig. 11.18 Elite athletes. These patients are excellent athletes. The boy (left) had DDH as an infant and underwent a pelvic osteotomy for correction of residual acetabular dysplasia. He is an outstanding soccer player. The brother and sister (right) have contracture of the heel-cords and secondary overuse syndromes but are still outstanding runners.

Prevention

It is estimated that about half of sports injuries are preventable. As sports injuries account for about one-third of all childhood injuries, the potential impact on childhood is enormous. Environmental and personal factors are both important.

Environmental Factors

Thermal regulation is of critical importance in children. Select a cool environment when possible. Avoid excessive clothing and prolonged exposure to sunlight. Insist on adequate fluid intake.

Playing surface should be as shock absorbing as possible (Fig. 11.16). Avoid running on hard surfaces. Insist on padded surfaces for playgrounds and for field events where falls are common.

Motor vehicles are dangerous in areas of play, especially for sledding and biking.

Encourage adults to focus more on safety than winning (good luck!).

Maintain equipment in good working condition and be certain the equipment is size appropriate.

Provide medical care for preparticipation evaluation and ongoing management.

Individual Factors

Wear protective devices such as helmets, face and mouth guards, and body protection in vulnerable sites.

Properly condition to improve strength, flexibility, and endurance.

Limit rate of increase in loading or repetitions to about 10% per week (10% rule).

Proper footwear provides good shock absorption and traction.

Psychological factors Early excessive grooming of competitive and elite athletes exposes children to external pressure to perform inappropriate training regimes, sometimes at the expense of their health and psychological well-being. It is essential for the physician to balance the benefits of appropriate participation in sports and exercise with the risks of physical and psychological injury.

Sporting environment control

Preseason medical evaluation should identify which conditions could be worsened by sports participation and identify musculoskeletal problems that could be improved by rehabilitation before returning to sports.

Provide medical coverage at high-risk events to provide prompt profession diagnostic and management.

Improved coaching skill is an important factor. Coaches should advance progression in sports participation appropriately to avoid placing the young athlete at risk. Too rapid advancement increases risk of injury.

Special Children

Children at both ends of the spectrum of ability have special needs. They are vulnerable to over- or underparticipation. Each has its unique problems. These children are in special need of the Bill of Rights from the book *The Pediatric Athlete* (Sullivan, 1988):

Bill of Rights for Young Athletes

1. The right to participate in sports.
2. The right to participate on a level commensurate with each child's maturity and ability.
3. The right to have qualified adult leadership.
4. The right to play as a child and not as an adult.
5. The right of children to share in the leadership and decision-making of their sport participation.
6. The right to participate in safe and healthy environments.
7. The right to proper preparation for participation in sport.
8. The right to an equal opportunity to strive for success.
9. The right to be treated with dignity.
10. The right to have fun in sports.

Children with Orthopedic Disabilities

Children with hip dysplasia, clubfeet, and other orthopedic deformities (Fig. 11.17) may become outstanding athletes. This is important information to give parents while treating these children.

Elite Athletes

Elite or outstanding athletes can have musculoskeletal problems (Fig. 11.18). It is commonly believed that to become an elite athlete, children must start training during their first decade; however, this has not been documented. Studies have demonstrated that the injury rate in elite juvenile athletes is lower than that of average-ability athletes. Elite athletes are stronger and more flexible than their peers. As many will progress on to participate in impact sports in late adolescence and adulthood, they risk long-term disability from osteoarthritis later in life.

Focused juvenile athletes are preoccupied with their sport. This is beneficial in enhancing self-esteem; promoting a healthy lifestyle by discouraging the use of drugs, smoking, and obesity; and possibly providing scholarships or other sport-generated income. On the downside, academic achievement, socialization, interpersonal skills, and other broadening experiences may be limited. The cost to girls may be greater. Menstrual irregularities, possibly shortened stature, and eating disorders may occur. The preoccupation with thinness in gymnasts and dancers creates special problems for girls.

Children with Disabilities

Children with disabilities need physical activity as much as or more than other children. An objective of management is the normalization of these children's lives (Fig. 11.19). This often requires special efforts by the family, sponsoring organizations, and medical providers.

Skiing programs are useful for children with limb deficiencies and mild cerebral palsy.

Wheelchair sports such as basketball and racing (Fig. 11.20) are excellent choices for providing exercise with little risk.

Organized sports participation requires a supportive system both by the adults as well as other children to succeed. An integrated play environment is healthy not only for the disabled child but also for the teammates. The teammates gain understanding and are more likely to befriend the child with a disability.

Special summer camps are effective in providing supervised programs (Fig. 11.21) with medical support.

Horseback riding programs are popular but they require close adult supervision to prevent falls. They may be expensive. Horseback riding is not more therapeutic than other outdoor activities.

Family programs are most important. Encourage the family to include the special child in their normal activities (Fig. 11.22). Unfortunately, families often overprotect the child, limiting the child's experiences and thereby harming the child. Encourage families to go ahead with the travel and physical activities that they would normally undertake and include the whole family.

References

1998 The medical demands of the special athlete. Batts KB, Glorioso JE Jr, Williams MS. Clin J Sport Med 8:22

1998 Prevention of sports injuries. Hergenroeder AC. Pediatrics 101:1057

1996 Considerations in child and adolescent athletes. Emery HM. Rheum Dis Clin North Am 22:499

1993 Pediatric wheelchair athletics: sports injuries and prevention. Wilson PE, Washington RL. Paraplegia 31:330

1992 The injury experience and training history of the competitive skier with a disability. Ferrara MS, et al. Am J Sports Med 20:55

1991 Snow skiing for the physically disabled. Laskowski ER. Mayo Clin Proc 66:160

1990 Self-concepts of disabled youth athletes. Sherrill C, et al. Percept Mot Skills 70:1093

1988 Sports medicine and the wheelchair athlete. Shephard RJ. Sports Med 5:226

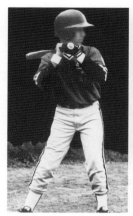
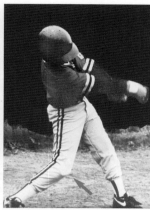

Fig. 11.19 Limb deficient child. This child with a right lower limb amputation is an excellent baseball player. The only sign is the upper rim of the prosthesis visible in unusual positions (arrow).

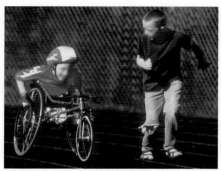

Fig. 11.20 Wheelchair sports. This child has paraplegia and is an outstanding athlete.

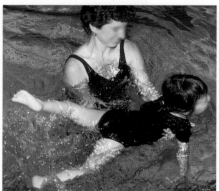

Fig. 11.21 Swimming. This child with arthrogryposis is learning to swim. This can be a lifetime sport.

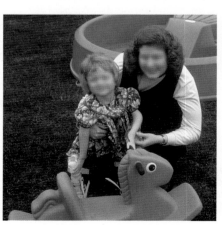

Fig. 11.22 Playing. Selecting play equipment that is stable, rounded. and lightweight increases safety.

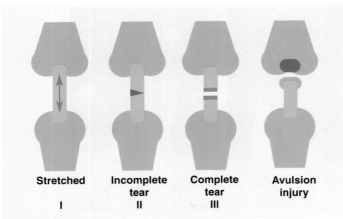

Fig. 11.23 Grading of ligamentous injury. These may be graded into three categories. Avulsion with a bone fragment (right) is common in children and does not fall into the numerical classification.

| Stretched | Incomplete tear | Complete tear | Avulsion injury |
| I | II | III | |

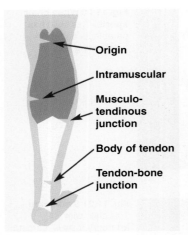

Fig. 11.24 Musculotendon injuries. Injuries of this complex may occur at different locations.

Origin
Intramuscular
Musculo-tendinous junction
Body of tendon
Tendon-bone junction

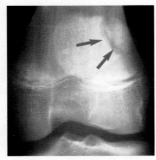

Fig. 11.25 Bipartite patella. Stress injuries can disrupt the chondral junction between the patella and the ossicle causing a synchondrosis disruption.

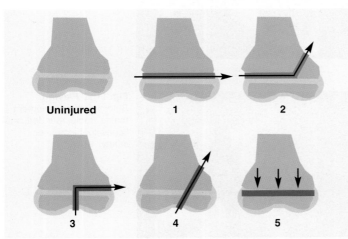

Uninjured 1 2
3 4 5

Fig. 11.26 Salter-Harris classification of growth plate injuries. These are classified as types 1 through 5 based on the fracture pattern. Types 1 and 2 (green lines) do not traverse the epiphysis and usually do not cause growth problems. Types 3 to 5 (red lines) may cause growth arrest and progressive deformity.

Injury Types

Injury types from athletic participation include acute and stress injuries. *Acute injuries* are the same as those that occur in nonsporting accidents. *Stress injuries* result from repetitive microtrauma and are unique to sports medicine. These injuries are the focus of this chapter.

Acute Injuries

Contusions are common injuries and usually heal quickly and completely. Secondary hematomas are less common in children, presumably due to enhanced hemostatic control in children. Rarely do contusions lead to formation of myositis ossificans. This is most common in the quadriceps. Avoid prolonged immobilization. These lesions mature over time. They may be confused with osteogenic sarcoma.

Ligament injuries Because ligaments are two to three times stronger than bone in children, avulsion fractures are common during growth. Ligamentous injuries can be graded (Fig.11.23) as follows:

Grade I represent stretch injuries without disruption of fibers that cause tenderness and swelling but without detectable instability.

Grade II are partial tears that allow greater mobility but with a definite endpoint.

Grade III are complete tears involving greater soft tissue injury and instability.

Ligament injuries are most common around the ankle and knee, and when associated with capsular disruption cause joint instability. They may coexist with bony injuries as seen in tibial spine fractures. When the tibial spine is avulsed, the anterior cruciate ligament is stretched, leading to residual laxity following bony union.

Bone injuries Acute bony injuries can fall into the same patterns as those occurring from accidental trauma in nonathletic situations (they are covered in Chapter 10).

Muscle tendon injuries can occur at many sites (Fig. 11.24). Complete separations are rare, and healing usually occurs spontaneously as no discontinuity occurs.

Synchondrosis disruptions Accessory ossification centers may become separated from their parent bone. The classic examples are the bipartite patella (Fig. 11.25), accessory tarsal navicular, and accessory ossicles below the ankle malleoli.

Physeal injuries are classified by the fracture patterns (Fig. 11.26). Repetitive stress injury may damage the growth plate in a unique fashion. These stress-induced physeal injuries are most common about the wrist and upper humerus in the child. Stress results in a disruption of the growth plate as seen in type 5 injuries. Unlike the usual simple physeal fracture, the growth plate, becomes widened, irregular, and tender but not grossly unstable. Such injuries may result in physeal damage and altered growth. Type 5 injuries occur in the distal radial epiphysis in gymnasts and in the proximal humeral epiphysis in pitchers.

Common Sites	Sport
Medial epicondyle	Throwing sports, especially baseball
Iliac apophysis	Running and dancing
Inferior pole patella	Basketball, jumping sports, running
Tibial tubercle	Football, running, soccer, basketball
Calcaneal apophysis	Soccer, hockey, basketball, running

Fig. 11.27 Sites of traction injuries. These are common sites and causes of traction injuries.

Traction and compression bone injuries Traction injuries may be acute or chronic and cause bony failure or inflammation at the tendon-bone junction (Fig. 11.27). Compression injuries are usually chronic with the classic example being the lateral compartment of the elbow in "little league elbow." Throwing causes compression of both the capitellum and radial head, which may cause vascular damage and bone necrosis.

Juvenile Osteochondroses

This is a term describing a heterogenous group of conditions that are characterized by sclerosis and fragmentation of the epiphysis or apophysis in the immature. Irregular ossification may be a normal variation of ossification or represent a disorder. Classic descriptions include many sites (Fig. 11.28).

Osteochondritis Dissecans

Osteochondritis dissecans (OCD) is a segmental avascular necrosis of articular subchondral bone. These OCD lesions are most common at the end of growth and during early adult life and are more common in joints subjected to repetitive microtrauma. OCD lesions may be familial and may occur in several locations in the same individual.

These are lesions that affect the subchondral bone and cartilage of a joint. These lesions are discussed in chapters on their various anatomic locations but some general features are appropriately discussed under sports as the lesions are often seen in the immature athlete and pose questions in management and athletic participation.

Etiology The causes are probably multiple. The predisposing factors include marginal vascularity, possible constitutional factors such as a coagulopathy, and repetitive micro-trauma.

Classification Lesions may be classified anatomically (Fig. 11.29) and based on radiographic or MR imaging. Assess activity and healing potential by dynamic bone scan in younger patients.

Location of lesions Lesions occur in the knee (Figs. 11.30 and 11.31), talus, capitellum, patella, radial head, and femoral head. Femoral head OCD may be idiopathic but usually complicates LCP disease and avascular necrosis secondary to trauma and infection.

Natural history OCD has the potential to cause permanent disability (Fig. 11.32) and is one of the more serious sports-related problems for the young athlete. The prognosis is better for smaller lesions, early onset, and a favorable location. Disability is more likely for large lesions in load-bearing areas of joints that progress to separation.

References

1999 Osteochondritis dissecans: a multicenter study of the European Pediatric Orthopedic Society. Hefti F, et al. JPO-b 8:231

1998 Osteochondritis dissecans of the talus during childhood and adolescence. Higuera J, et al. JPO 18:328

1997 Osteochondral lesions in the radiocapitellar joint in the skeletally immature: radiographic, MRI, and arthroscopic findings in 13 consecutive cases. Janarv PM, Hesser U, Hirsch G. JPO 17:311

1995 Osteochondritis dissecans of the femoral head in children and adolescents: a report of 17 cases. Wood JB, Klassen RA, Peterson HA. JPO 15:313

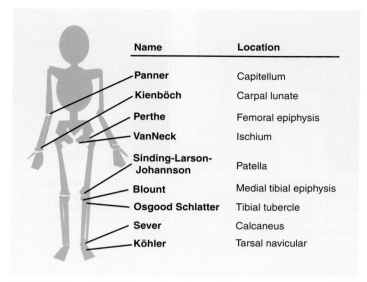

Fig. 11.28 Classic list of osteochondroses. Name and location are shown.

Name	Location
Panner	Capitellum
Kienböch	Carpal lunate
Perthe	Femoral epiphysis
VanNeck	Ischium
Sinding-Larson-Johannson	Patella
Blount	Medial tibial epiphysis
Osgood Schlatter	Tibial tubercle
Sever	Calcaneus
Köhler	Tarsal navicular

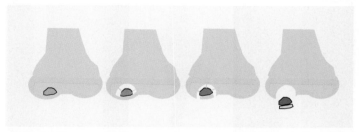

Fig. 11.29 Osteochondritis dissecans. These are the stages of this disease. Over time the lesion may become unstable and finally separate into the joint and become a loose body.

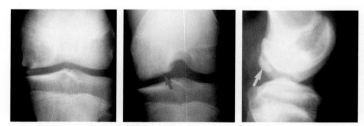

Fig. 11.30 Osteochondritis dissecans. Lesion not seen on AP radiograph, shown on notch (red arrow) and lateral (yellow arrow) views.

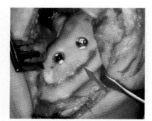

Fig. 11.31 Replaced large ostochondritic fragment. This large lesion was replaced and fixed with two screws.

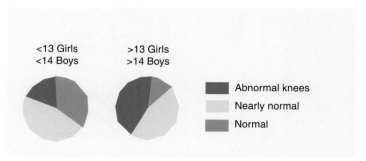

Fig. 11.32 Age and outcome for OCD lesion of the knee. Based on 509 OCD lesions from Hefti (1999).

<13 Girls <14 Boys   >13 Girls >14 Boys

Abnormal knees
Nearly normal
Normal

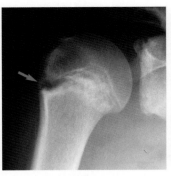

Fig. 11.33 Physeal stress injuries. This adolescent pitcher developed a stress reaction causing widening of the proximal humeral physis (red arrow).

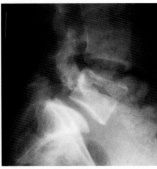

Fib. 11.34 Spondylolithesis. This gymnast had back pain and a grade I spondylolithesis. This is due to a stress fracture through the pars.

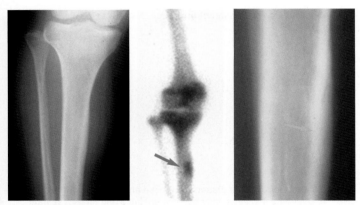

Fig. 11.35 Tibial stress fracture. A 17-year-old female cross country runner has had "shin splints" for 3 months. The proximal tibia is tender. Radiograph (left) is negative, the bone scan (red arrow) shows an area of increased uptake over upper tibia (red arrow), and the CT scan shows sclerosis (orange arrow).

Overuse Injuries

Between 30–50% of injuries of immature athletes are due to overuse. This varies from about 15% in soccer to 60% in swimmers. Sports that require repetitive acts are most likely to cause overuse problems. As compared with acute injuries, overuse injuries take longer to heal and result in more time away from competition.

Overuse injury seldom occurs in the normal play of children. The protective mechanism of pain limits overuse and promotes recovery. This protective mechanism is often repressed during regimented childhood sports. A large portion of sports medicine in children deals with care of these overuse conditions.

Mechanism

Overuse injuries result from repetitive submaximal loading. These injuries from this *microtrauma* are usually reversed by rest. Repetitive microtrauma without intervals of rest is cumulative and causes stress injuries.

Stress injury to bone creates a progression of inflammation, periosteal swelling, and endosteal and cortical disruption. Stress injuries in children include fractures through the growth plate (Fig. 11.33) or bone (Fig. 11.34) and disruption of bone to tendon or muscle junctions. They may also affect the vascularity of bone resulting in bone necrosis as seen in osteochondritis dissecans. Before an overt fracture occurs, the injuries are referred to as *stress reactions*.

Sites of Overuse Injuries

The location of the injury depends upon the stresses created during specific activities of each sport. For example, wrist and back pain from overuse are common among gymnasts, Swimmers have shoulder pain whereas running injuries occur in the lower limbs (Fig. 11.35).

Diagnosis

Make an accurate diagnosis to be certain that some more serious problem is not the cause of pain.

History should include the type of sporting activity associated with the onset, training including frequency and duration, previous injuries, new techniques or equipment, and if the patient is in a period of rapid growth. Detail the onset, character, location, and pain relationships with activity and time of day. Beware of night pain as this can be a sign of a tumor.

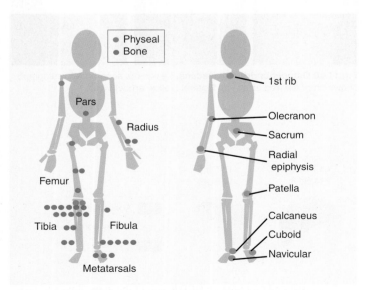

Fig. 11.36 Common and rare sites of stress fractures in children. Common sites (red and blue dotes) include both physeal and bony fractures. Rare sites of stress fractures (green dots) are shown. Each dot represents a case in the series. From Walker (1996).

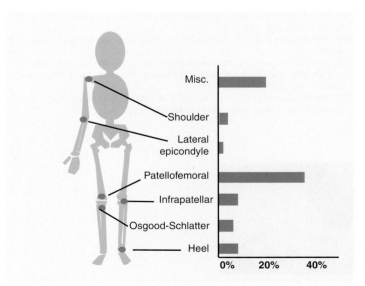

Fig. 11.37 Sites of overuse injuries. Based on 139 athletes ages 9–16 years, from Dalton (1992).

Examination Localize the pain and determine the site of maximum tenderness. This will often help establish the diagnosis (Figs. 11.36 and 11.37). Localized tenderness to the tibial tubercle is classic for Osgood-Schlatter disease, and tenderness over the origin of the plantar fascia and insertion of the Achilles tendon are classic findings for the common heel-pain in children. Look for evidence of malalignment problems in lower limbs such as the combination of femoral antetorsion and external tibial torsion or malalignment of the quadriceps mechanism.

Assess the interaction of the parent(s) and patient. Overzealous and controlling parents may aggravate the problem. Attempt to assess the patients attitude regarding physical education– is participation a positive or negative experience for the patient? Does the patient exaggerate the disability in an attempt to get a *PE excuse,* or is the injury being minimized to reduce the risk of being *benched,* or is the injury overplayed to avoid unwanted participation forced on them in the first place?

Differentiating stress fractures from neoplasm or infection This is usually not difficult. Stress fractures occur in specific locations and show typical clinical and imaging features (Figs. 11.38 and 11.39). Assess the effect of rest. *With rest, the pain and tenderness of stress fractures resolve or improve over a period of days.* If the clinical features are atypical and the early differentiation important, image with CT scans to show the fracture line, bone scan to exactly localize the lesion, and laboratory studies of CRP and ESR to aid in differentiating infections. Rarely are MRI or biopsy necessary to make the differentiation.

Management

Management of stress injuries is simple–rest. The challenge is in preventing recurrence. This requires an understanding of the cause.

Rest the part by modifying activities. If necessary immobilize with a cast or splint.

Modify factors contributing to stress injuries These are commonly categorized as *extrinsic* or *intrinsic* (Fig. 11.40). Identify and modify these factors, provide pain control, and rehabilitate before returning the patient to activity.

Return to sports should be carefully supervised and gradual.

Prognosis Most stress injuries and fractures heal with rest and cause no long-term disability. Stress injuries are rarely serious.

Displaced stress fractures are rare but may occur if the activity continues even when pain occurs. The most serious fractures include the femoral neck and tibia.

Spondylolithesis is common in gymnasts. Displacement progresses to the severity that fusion becomes necessary.

Growth plate injuries such as the distal radius in gymnasts and proximal tibia in runners may lead to growth arrest and bone shortening.

Osteochondritis dissecans commonly causes permanent joint damage with premature degenerative arthritis and long-term disability.

Bony overgrowth such as a permanent prominence of the tibial tubercle or radial head may cause mild long-term disability.

References

1999 Overuse injuries in children and adolescents. DiFiori JP. Phy and Sportsman 27:75
1996 Stress fractures in skeletally immature patients. Walker RN, Green NE, Spindler KP. JPO 16:578
1995 Femoral neck stress fractures in children and adolescents. St Pierre P, Staheli LT, Smith JB, Green NE. JPO 15:470
1993 Knee overuse disorders in the pediatric and adolescent athlete. Stanitski CL. Inst Lectures Am Acad Ortho Surg 42:483
1992 Overuse injuries in adolescent athletes. Dalton SE. Sports Med 13:58
1992 Femoral stress fractures in children. Meaney JE, Carty H. Skeletal Radiol 21:173
1963 Stress fractures in children Devas MB. JBJS 45B:528

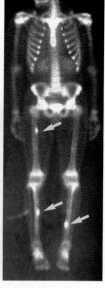
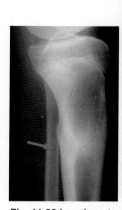

Fig. 11.38 Imaging stress fractures. Often the location and radiographic appearance of stress fractures is diagnostic on plain radiographs such as the proximal tibia (red arrow). Stress fractures may be multiple as shown by a bone scan (yellow arrows).

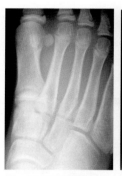
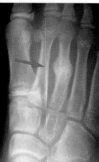

Fig. 11.39 Metatarsal stress fracture. This 14-year-old runner complained of foot pain and demonstrated localized tenderness over the third metatarsal. Initial radiographs (left) were negative. Radiographs 3 weeks later show the fracture and callus (arrow).

Factors contributing to overuse injuries

Extrinsic factors that contribute include:
   Adult or peer pressures
   Incorrect sport technique
   Hard or rough surfaces
   Excessively rapid progression of training
   Too little rest
   Inappropriate equipment
Intrinsic factors
   Anatomic malalignment
   Psychological factors
   Inadequate conditioning
   Prior injury
   Growth

Fig. 11.40 Factors contributing to overuse injuries in children. Modified from DiFioni (1999).

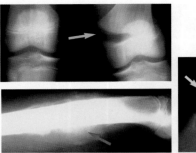
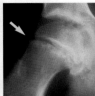

Fig. 11.41 Pitfalls in diagnosis. Epiphyseal fractures (orange arrow) can be confused with ligament injury. Malignant tumors (red arrow) may be confused with intrinsic knee problems. Slipped capital femoral epiphysis (yellow arrow) may be confused with anterior knee pain.

More Significant	Less Significant
Night pain	Long duration
Unilateral	Bilateral
Onset with significant trauma	Poorly localized
History of feeling a "pop"	No localized tenderness
Inability to walk or run	Pain lasting only seconds
Local signs of swelling	Stable joint
Short duration	
Localized tenderness	
Instability	
Joint effusion	

Fig. 11.42 Features and significance. Features that suggest the problem is more serious (left) versus less serious (right).

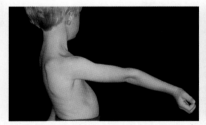
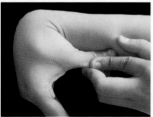

Fig. 11.43 Joint laxity. Individuals with excessive joint laxity show excessive wrist flexion, finger extension, and hyperextension of the elbows and knees.

Evaluation

Be prepared for difficulty in evaluating the injured athlete. Some players fearful of being pulled from the game or letting down teammates may understate the significance of their injury. The parents may have their own agenda and overstate or understate the problem. The coach may push for the player to return to the game.

History

Keep in mind the pitfalls in management (Fig. 11.41). A common mistake is to attribute the problem to trauma based on a history of an injury. Injuries are a normal part of a child's daily activity. Many serious tumors and infections have been missed because the problem was erroneously attributed to an injury. Some features of the history are more significant than others (Fig. 11.42). A report of feeling or hearing a "pop" is significant. Be suspicious of a history of night pain (for a tumor).

Physical Examination

Assess joint laxity to help establish what is normal for the child (Fig. 11.43). Joint laxity is more common in the younger child and in girls. Excessive laxity occurs in about 5% of adolescents and predisposes them to sprains and joint dislocations. Examine the uninjured side and consider the child's joint laxity when assessing possible ligamentous injury.

Localize tenderness and pain to help in pinpointing the site of injury. *Knee pain* should prompt a check of the hips. Perform the hip rotation test to rule out the hip as the source of the pain.

Assess active motion during screening. Unguarded full movement usually means the part is not injured.

Determine instability by applying the appropriate test.

Ankle stability is assessed by stressing the ligaments between the leg and foot. Stabilize the leg and attempt to move the foot forward (Fig. 11.44). Note any instability.

Lachman test is performed with the knee flexed to 20°. One hand stabilizes the thigh while the other applies an anterior and posterior force to the upper leg (Fig. 11.45). Instability of the anterior crucitate ligament is determined.

Collateral ligament stability should be assessed with the knee flexed to 30° with varus and valgus stress applied (Fig. 11.46). Consider the patient's joint laxity evaluation in assessing the significance of laxity of the knee. Grade the findings.

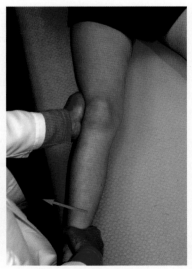

Fig. 11.46 Medial collateral ligament stability testing. Flex the knee 20°–30° and apply a valgus stress to the knee (arrow). Note any instability.

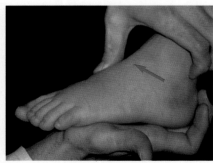

Fig. 11.44 Ankle stability assessment. Stabilize the foot against a flat surface or by hand. Attempt to displace the ankle (talus) forward (arrow) to demonstrate ankle instability.

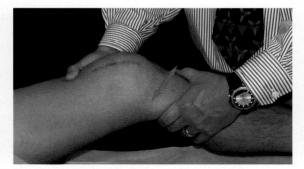

Fig. 11.45 Lachman test. Flex the knee to an angle of about 20° and apply anterior and posterior forces (arrow). Note any instability.

Assess flexibility by manipulating the joint or checking mobility. Stiffness is often a sign of an injury, while limited motion is often indicative of disease (Fig. 11.47). The loss of mobility may be either a cause or an effect of the disease. Order imaging studies thoughtfully.

Imaging

Request plain radiographs first. Radiographs are most available, least likely to be misread, and least expensive. Each study has special indications (Fig. 11.48).

Arthroscopy

Few arthroscopic studies are necessary in children as compared to adults. Arthroscopy is useful for the knee, ankle, elbow, shoulder, and hip (Fig. 11.49), but it is most commonly used for evaluating knee problems. Because hip arthroscopy requires distracting the joint, it is less commonly used.

Arthroscopy is useful when noninvasive methods do not provide a diagnosis or when treatment can be part of the arthroscopic procedure. Knee arthroscopy is appropriate for the traumatic hemarthrosis associated with instability. Arthroscopy is helpful in evaluating osteochondritis dissecans of the ankle, knee, hip, and elbow. Arthroscopy is useful for removal of loose bodies in joints, meniscal repairs, reconstruction of cruciate tears or avulsions, and replacement and fixation of osteochondral fractures and osteochondral lesions from osteochondritis dissecans.

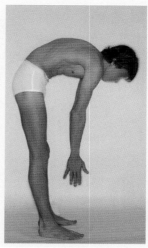

Limited motion	Problem
Forward bending	Spine problem
Backward bending	Spondylolysis (listhesis)
Straight leg raising	Spondylolysis (listhesis)
Hamstring–quad	Osgood-Schlatter disease
Quadriceps	Patellofemoral disorders
Medial hip rotation	Hip injuries and inflammation
Subtalar motion	Tarsal coalition
Elbow motion	Little league elbow

Fig. 11.47 Significance of limited motion. Limited motion is often associated with specific disorders. A child should be able to reach to mid-tibial level on forward bending (above).

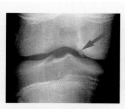

Conventional radiographs
Order before any other imaging study
Osteochondritis dissecans (arrow)

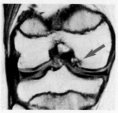

Magnetic resonance imaging
Mensical injuries
Herniated intervertebral disc
Early stress injuries
Physeal bridges
Loose bodies in joints
Osteochondritis dissecans (arrow)

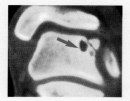

Bone scans
Stress injuries (arrows)
Occult fractures
Spondylolysis
Osteomyelitis

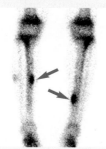

Computer tomography
Complex fractures
Bony lesions
Osteochondritis dissecans (arrow)

Fig. 11.48 Imaging choices. This table shows the studies most likely to establish a diagnosis.

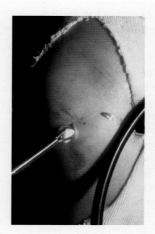

Diagnosis
Acute instability
Loose bodies
Osteochondritis dissecans
Meniscal injuries
Impingement problems

Treatment
Removal of loose bodies
ACL reconstruction
Repair of meniscus
Repair of OD lesions

Fig. 11.49 Indications for arthroscopy. Some of the diagnostic and therapeutic indications are listed.

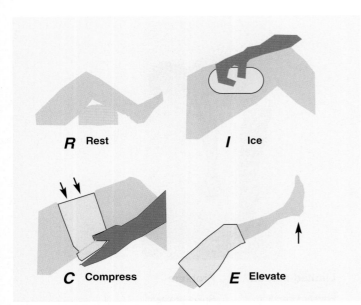

Fig. 11.50 RICE management for acute injuries. R for rest, I for ice, C for compression, and E for elevation.

Management Plan

1. Acute management: RICE
2. Identify causative factors:
   Training factors (most common)
   Anatomic factors
   Environmental factors
3. Establish plan to modify these factors before child returns to activity
4. Provide adequate period of rest to heal injury
5. Maintain strength, endurance, and flexibility during healing period
6. Reintroduce activity in progressive fashion

Fig. 11.51 Management plan. Include each step in the overall plan. Discuss plan with coach, trainer, and parents.

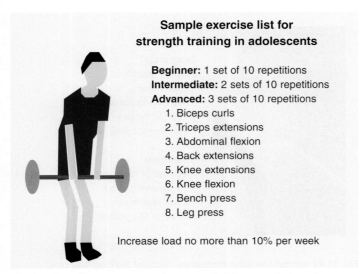

Sample exercise list for strength training in adolescents

Beginner: 1 set of 10 repetitions
Intermediate: 2 sets of 10 repetitions
Advanced: 3 sets of 10 repetitions
1. Biceps curls
2. Triceps extensions
3. Abdominal flexion
4. Back extensions
5. Knee extensions
6. Knee flexion
7. Bench press
8. Leg press

Increase load no more than 10% per week

Fig. 11.52 Strength training program. This program is the type often prescribed for adolescents. Weekly increases should be limited to 10%.

Management Principles

Management of sports injuries is unique, because these injuries are sometimes predictable and often preventable. Management is complicated by pressures to return the child to sports before healing is complete. Being the child's advocate and protector is important and sometimes difficult.

Acute Injury

Manage the acute injury using the RICE sequence (Fig. 11.50). Ice in a plastic bag or plastic cup works well. The ice minimizes pain. Advise the family to discontinue the cold if the skin becomes numb. This initial management is designed to minimize swelling and is continued for the first 24 hours, then tapered.

Nonsteroidal antiinflammatory drugs (NSAIDs) are useful in reducing pain and inflammation. Tolmetin, naproxen, and ibuprofen are acceptable drugs for children and adolescents. Ibuprofen is widely used because it is inexpensive and available without a prescription.

Establish a Diagnosis

Be certain the diagnosis is accurate. Make radiographs of sites of tenderness over bones or joints. Follow with additional imaging studies or seek consultation. Be very careful in managing injuries around joints such as the elbow and knee.

Preparing Family and Coach

Patients, family, and coach need to be advised in advance of the predicted healing time.

Establish a Management Plan

Develop a plan to manage the acute problem and the rehabilitation (Fig. 11.51). The child should not return until the acute effects of the trauma and the secondary effects on muscle strength, endurance, and joint stiffness have resolved.

Identify causative factors that may have contributed to the current problem.

Training regimens are the most common cause of overuse syndrome. These regimens should not add more than about 10% per week of additional load (Fig. 11.52). Discourage excessive pressure from the trainer or family.

Anatomic features may predispose the child to injury. Such problems include rotational malalignment (femoral and tibial torsion), ligamentous joint laxity, tarsal coalitions, and tight heel cords.

Environmental problems contributing to the injury should be identified. The factors include surfaces, equipment size, and condition.

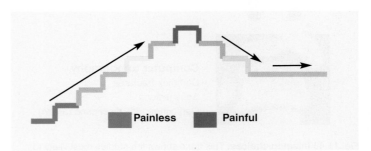

Fig. 11.53 Activity staircase. Activities are gradually increased (left, green), and if overuse symptoms develop (red line), the activity is reduced to the maximum level at which the child remains entirely pain free (green).

Modify causative factors while the child is recovering to prevent recurrence of the problem.

Provide adequate time for healing of the bone, collagen, or muscle tissue because time, not treatment, is the principal factor in healing. The secondary effect of muscle atrophy and joint stiffness can be prevented by an exercise program. Do not underestimate the seriousness of soft tissue injuries, as they also require considerable time for recovery.

Prevent muscle atrophy during convalescence. Rest the injured part but plan an exercise program to maintain strength in nonaffected muscle groups. Isometric exercises may be used around an injured part. Avoid exercises that cause pain.

Reintroduce activities progressively after healing is complete. Healing requires a minimum of 6 weeks (and sometimes longer) for bone, cartilage, ligaments, and tendons. Reintroduce activities using the step model (Fig. 11.53). Break down sports into components and add progressively to the repetitions. If the new level of activity is performed without pain, then progress to the next level. If pain recurs, then move to the next lower level of activity.

Return to sports participation gradually Add sport-specific tasks with progressively increasing speeds prior to returning the patient to sports. Then start with practice sessions.

Return to competition Allow only after healing and rehabilitation are complete. Make certain the initial causative factors are corrected to avoid repeating this cycle.

Strength Training

Exercise programs for children and adolescents can increase strength and should be undertaken to overcome muscle weakness that may contribute to further injuries. Make the programs fun and varied. Children become bored quickly. Avoid many repetitions. Strictly adhere to the 10% rule and decrease the load promptly if symptoms develop (Fig. 11.53).

Exercises for Rehabilitation

Exercises should be tailored to the child (Fig. 11.54). Exercises help in maintaining or restoring strength following injury and in preparing the individual for demands of certain sports.

Braces and Splints

Providing immobilization and protection is useful following sprains and fractures. A splint is often used in place of a cast when only protection is required. Commercial splints (Fig. 11.55) can be more expensive than casts but less expensive than custom braces from an orthotist.

References

1998 Correlation of arthroscopic and clinical examinations with magnetic resonance imaging findings of injured knees in children and adolescents. Stanitski CL. Am J Sports Med 26:2

1997 Pediatric and adolescent sports injuries. Stanitski CL. Clin Sports Med 16:613

1996 Paediatric sports injuries in Hong Kong: a seven year survey. Maffulli N, et al. Br J Sports Med 30:218

1996 Sports injuries in children and adolescents treated at a sports injury clinic. Watkins J, Peabody P. J Sports Med Phys Fitness 36:43

1995 Issues in the pediatric athlete. Cook PC, Leit ME. Orthop Clin North Am 26:453

1988 Management of sports injuries in children and adolescents. Stanitski CL. Orthop Clin North Am 19:689

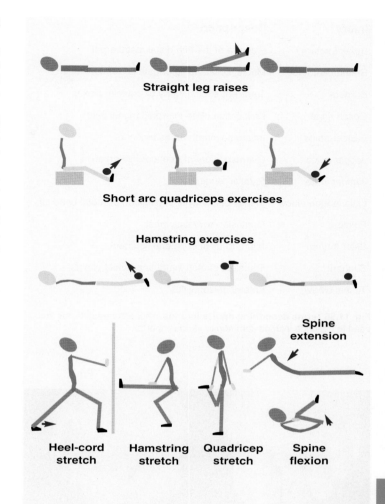

Straight leg raises

Short arc quadriceps exercises

Hamstring exercises

Spine extension

Heel-cord stretch   Hamstring stretch   Quadricep stretch   Spine flexion

Fig. 11.54 Exercise programs. An exercise program should be tailored to the needs of the child or adolescent. Shown here are some types of exercises frequently prescribed.

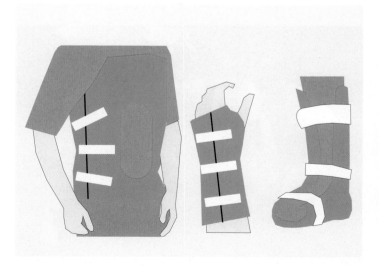

Fig. 11.55 Brace types. Prefabricated splints and braces are often adequate. Their advantages are lower cost and immediate availability.

Injury	Description
Boxer fracture	Fracture of the fifth distal metacarpal
Breastroker knee	Medial collateral lig.or patellar tendon inflam.
Burners	Transient stretch injury to brachial plexus
Coach finger	Dislocation of an interphalangeal joint
Dancer ankle	Inflammation of the os trigonum
Jogger ankle	Overuse injury of heel-cord insertion
Jumper knee	Patellar tendinitis
Little league elbow	Medial epicondyle, capitellum, or radial head inj.
Pointers	Contusion over iliac crest
Skier thumb	Injury to ulnar collateral ligament
Stingers	Transient stretch injury to brachial plexus
Tennis elbow	Lateral epicondylitis

Fig. 11.56 Terms describing sports injuries. These common terms are used to describe injuries common to various sports.

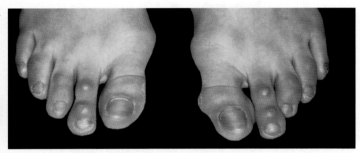

Fig. 11.57 Dancer toes. These are the toes of a ballerina. Note the callosities over the second toe.

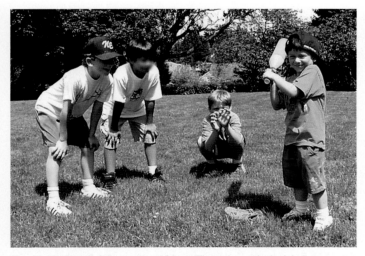

Fig. 11.58 Baseball in young chidren. These low-velocity injuries are seldom serious. Being struck with the bat is the most serious risk.

Sport Specific Problems

Knowledge of a sport's demands, lore, and jargon aids in understanding the athlete's problems (Fig. 11.56).

Ballet Dancing

Moderate risk. Reports of specific injuries, which include stress fractures of the pars, distal fibula, base of second metatarsal, achilles tendonitis, cuboid subluxation, os trigonum impingement syndrome, and trigger toes. Toes are severely stressed (Fig. 11.57). Delay in puberty and emphasis on slenderness is a problem for girls and can lead to eating disorders.

Baseball

Moderate risk depending upon the child's age (Fig. 11.58). Most acute injuries are associated with sliding, collisions, and ball or bat strikes. Most deaths occur from ball strikes to the head, neck, or chest. Overuse injuries, such as little league elbow, are preventable but potentially serious problems. Unusual injuries include apophysitis of the acromion, distal humeral epiphyseal separation, persistence of the olecranon physis, and avulsion of the iliac crest apophysis while swinging a bat.

Basketball

Moderate risk. Injuries as compared with other sports often but usually mild. Injuries in children under 12 usually mild with mainly contusions, sprains, lacerations, and rarely a fracture. Seldom serious injury. Adolescent injuries are more common and more likely to be serious, such as contusions, sprains, and sometimes fractures. Ankle and knee are affected most. Most serious are ACL injuries. Ankle injuries require rehabilitation to prevent recurrence.

Cycling

High risk (Fig. 11.59). Most serious accidents are due to collision with motor vehicles. Prevention is essential through education of children, use of helmets, and avoidance of congested roadways. Potential long-term disability from head injury is significant.

Diving

High-risk (Fig. 11.60). There is a risk of head and cervical spine injury with quadriplegia. Attention to diving height, water depth, and technique are essential in prevention.

American Football

High risk. Most injuries are due to collisions in this most risky sport. Catastrophic head and neck injuries can be reduced by using a well-fitting helmet and by avoiding spearing (initial head contact in blocking and tackling). A quarter of the players are obese. Injury rates increase with maturation. Long-term osteoarthritis of knee and hip are possible sequela from major injuries of the hip or knee. Most problems result from acute injury and are due to joint and neurological damage. Try to control pushy coaches and educate parents.

Gymnastics

Moderate risk. Overuse injuries commonly produce spondylolysis (Fig. 11.61) and wrist problems. Wrist pain occurs in about 75%, and radiographic changes of the distal radial physis were found in 25%. Long-term problems may result from growth arrest of distal radial epiphysis and spondylolisthesis. Great focus on slimness may cause eating disorders and menstrual and growth problems in girls. Stress injuries of the elbow in 19 adolescent elite gymnasts are reported.

Elbow changes include avascular necrosis of the capitellar epiphysis, distortion of the articular surface, and osteochondritis of the radial head. Olecranon changes are common with fragmentation of the epiphysis to chronic Salter Type I stress fractures of the growth plate.

Specifically, rapid periods of growth and advanced levels of training and competition appeared to be related to injury proneness.

Ice Hockey

Moderate to high risk. Facial lacerations and shoulder injuries are common from collision and puck and stick strikes. Protective gear is essential. Head injuries and joint damage may lead to long-term problems.

Horseback Riding

Moderate to high risk. Injuries are due to horse handling and falls. Serious falls with head and neck injuries and fractures are common. Protective helmets and special training for handling horses can reduce risks. Horseback riding is proposed as therapeutic for children with cerebral palsy, scoliosis, and other conditions but proof of effectiveness is lacking.

Playground

The playground is a dangerous place for children (Fig. 11.62). Soft surfaces and reduced height of playground equipment are important design features.

Referemces

Ballet

1997 Intensive dance practice. Repercussions on growth and puberty. Pigeon P, et al. Am J Sports Med 25:243

1989 Injuries to dancers: prevalence, treatment, and perceptions of causes. Bowling A. BMJ 298:731

Baseball

1998 Little Leaguer's shoulder. A report of 23 cases. Carson WG Jr, Gasser SI. Am J Sports Med 26:575

1998 Early detection of osteochondritis dissecans of the capitellum in young baseball players. Report of three cases. Takahara M, et al. JBJS 80A:892

Basketball

1998 Sports members' participation in assessment of incidence rate of injuries in five sports from records of hospital-based clinical treatment. Kingma J, ten Duis HJ. Percept Mot Skills 86:675

1996 Incidence of injury in Texas girls' high school basketball. Gomez E, De Lee JC, Farney WC. Am J Sports Med 24:684

1991 Safety of a preadolescent basketball program. Gutgesell ME. Am J Dis Child 145:1023

Cycling

1997 Bicycle-spoke injuries: a prospective study. Segers MJ, Wink D, Clevers GJ. Injury 28:267

1997 Bicycle-related injuries among preschool children. Powell EC, Tanz RR, Di Scala C. Ann Emerg Med 30:260

1995 Cycling to school--a significant health risk? Kopjar B, Wickizer TM. Inj Prev 1:238

1993 Bicycle accidents often cause disability--an analysis of medical and social consequences of nonfatal bicycle accidents. Olkkonen S, et al. Scand J Soc Med 21:98

Diving

1993 Injuries of the cervical spine in children and adolescents. Schwarz N, et al. Unfallchirurg 96:235

1990 Diving injuries of the cervical spine. Bailes JE, et al. Surg Neurol 34:155

Football

1995 Incidence of adolescent injuries in junior high school football and its relationship to sexual maturity. Linder MM, et al. Clin J Sport Med 5:167

1995 Effect of obesity on injury risk in high school football players. Kaplan TA, et al. Clin J Sport Med 5:43

Gymnastics

1997 Distal radial growth plate injury and positive ulnar variance in nonelite gymnasts. Di Fiori JP, et al. Am J Sports Med 25:763

1996 Factors associated with wrist pain in the young gymnast. Di Fiori JP, et al. Am J Sports Med 24:9

1991 Chronic stress injuries of the elbow in young gymnasts. Chan D, et al. Br J Radiol 64:1113

1992 Derangement of the articular surfaces of the elbow in young gymnasts. Maffulli N, Chan D, Aldridge MJ. JPO 12:344

1989 An epidemiologic investigation of injuries affecting young competitive female gymnasts. Caine D, et al. Am J Sports Med 17:811

Ice Hockey

1995 Injuries in youth ice hockey: a pilot surveillance strategy. Stuart MJ, et al. Clin Proc 70:350

1992 Children's ice hockey injuries. Brust JD, Leonard BJ, Pheley A, Roberts WO. Am J Dis Child 146:741

Horseback riding

1990 Common injuries in horseback riding. A review. Bixby-Hammett D, Brooks WH. Sports Med 9:36

Playground

1997 Safety of surfaces and equipment for children in playgrounds. Mott A, et al. Lancet 349:1874

1997 Playground injuries in children. Lillis KA, Jaffe DM. Pediatr Emerg Care 13:149

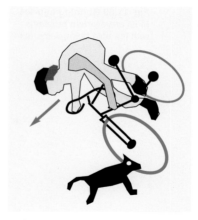

Fig. 11.59 Bicycling. Striking objects or collisions with cars pose serious risks.

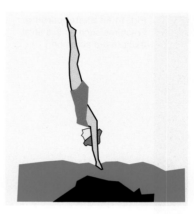

Fig. 11.60 Diving. Greatest risk is striking an underwater object.

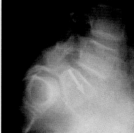
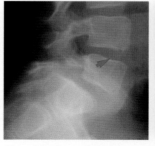

Fig. 11.61 Spondylolisthesis. Grade 1 (red arrow) and grade 3 (yellow arrow) displacement are shown.

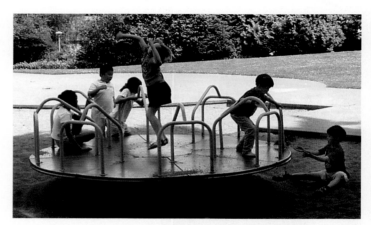

Fig. 11.62 Playground equipment. Reduce risk by providing soft surfaces (sand) and playground equipment of limited height to reduce fall distance.

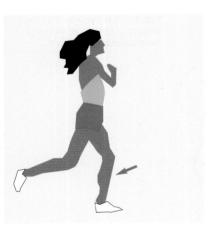

Fig. 11.63 Running injuries. Most are overuse problems with the tibia being vulnerable.

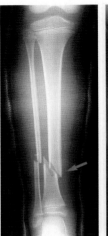

Fig. 11.64 Skateboarding. Fractures such as this tibial fracture are common.

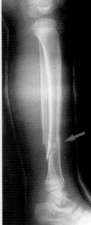

Fig. 11.65 Ski racing. These activities increase the risk of serious injury.

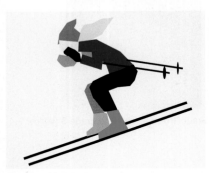

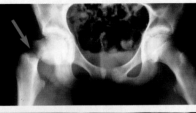

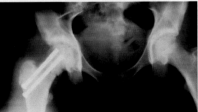

Fig. 11.66 Skiing collision fracture. This 12-year-old girl was struck by an airborne adolescent skier. She sustained this displaced femoral neck fracture. The fracture was reduced, fixed with two screws, and healed. Avascular necrosis of the femoral head occurs in a third of femoral neck fractures.

Running

Low to moderate risk. Overuse injury rates are high (Fig. 11.63), but serious injuries are uncommon. Most injuries are preventable by appropriate training, shoes, and selection of proper running surface. Long-term sequelae are unlikely.

Skateboarding

High risk (Fig. 11.64). Children 10 to 14 years old were injured with greatest frequency. Nontrivial injuries were more common among children younger than 5 years old, reflecting a larger proportion of head and neck injuries. Boys sustained more frequent and more severe skateboard-related injuries. Observed injury patterns include head and neck injuries in younger children, extremity injuries in older children, and more severe head and neck injuries in older children. Acute injury is common and is related to boards being difficult to control and being used on hard surfaces, unsupervised, with potential for collision. Use protective gear and avoid obstacles and high speed. Long-term sequelae risk is moderate and primarily results from head injury.

Skating (Inline)

Low to moderate risk. Collisions and falls cause forearm fractures and contusions. Use protective gear. Long-term sequelae are unlikely.

Skiing

Moderate to high risk. Jumping and racing (Fig. 11.65) injuries pose the greatest risks. Tibial fractures, medial collateral ligament injuries, and thumb and shoulder injuries are common. Collision injuries are the most serious, as head, spine, and extremity injuries (Fig. 11.66) may have long-term sequelae. The most common injuries were a contusion of the knee in children, and a sprain of the ulnar collateral ligament of the thumb in adolescents. With increasing age, lower extremity injuries decrease but upper extremity injuries increase.

Snowboarding

Moderate to high risk. Injuries are due to impact. More ankle and upper extremity injuries occur than in skiing, but there are fewer torsional, knee, and thumb injuries. Snowboarders were younger, predominantly male, and were more often beginners than were skiers. They most commonly sustained ligament strains, dislocations, and fractures, with the hand, forearm, and shoulder most affected.

Soccer

Moderate risk (Figs. 11.67 and 11.68). Overuse and injuries involving the ankle and knee are common. ACL injuries are 2–3 times greater in girls. Long-term disability risk is low to moderate. The incidence increased with age, and injuries are more common in girls. Seventy percent of the injuries were located in the lower extremities, particularly the knee (26%) and ankle (23%). Back pain occurred in 14% of players. Fractures, which accounted for 4% of injuries, were more often in the upper extremities. Indoor most risky.

Swimming

Low risk. Overuse injuries of shoulder, back, and knee are common, but long-term disability risk is low. Good training and modification of swimming strokes are important in preventing and managing these problems. Shoulder pain is due to impingement or instability. Preparedness for swimming is optimal between ages 5 and 6 years.

Tennis

Low risk (Fig. 11.69). Acute injuries involving the lower limbs with sprains are the most common injuries. Upper extremity injuries, often due to overuse, are preventable with appropriate training, stroke technique, and equipment. Long-term disability risk is low.

Trampoline

Very high risk. Most injuries occur from falls on hard surfaces to the side of the device. Head and cervical spine injuries are relatively common and the potential for long-term disability is great. Discourage families from allowing children to play on trampolines.

Strength Training

Low to moderate risk. With proper supervision and low weights, this sport is relatively safe. Overuse injury is most common. Fractures of the distal radius and ulna and avulsion of the iliac apophysis occur. Long-term sequelae are low. It appears that a training frequency of twice per week is sufficient to induce strength gains in children.

Wrestling

High risk. More injuries occur in large adolescents and during competition than in practice. The upper limb and knee are the most common site of injury, and dislocations are more common than fractures (Fig. 11.70). Most injuries are acute sprains. Medial epicondyle fractures, olecranon epiphyseal stress fractures, scapular avulsion fractures, and unusual injury patterns are common. Long-term disability risk is low to moderate.

References

Running

1990 Risks in distance running for children. American Academy of Pediatrics Committee on Sports Medicine. Pediatrics 86:799

1985 Adolescent runners. Apple DF Jr. Clin Sports Med 4:641

1984 Adolescent running injuries. Paty JG Jr; Swafford D. J Adolesc Health Care 5:87

Skateboard

1995 Skateboard injuries. American Academy of Pediatrics Committee on Injury and Poison Prevention. Pediatrics 95:611

1991 Skateboarding injuries in children. A second wave. Retsky J, Jaffe D, Christoffel K. Am J Dis Child 145:188

Skiing

1998 Skiing injuries in children, adolescents, and adults. Deibert MC, et al. JBJS 80A:25

1996 Skiing injuries in children and adolescents. Shorter NA, et al. J Trauma 40:997

Snowboard

1996 Differing injury patterns in snowboarding and alpine skiing. Sutherland AG, Holmes JD, Myers S. Injury 27:423

Soccer

1993 Injuries in adolescent and preadolescent soccer players. Kibler WB. Med Sci Sports Exerc 25:1330

1991 Injuries among young soccer players. Schmidt-Olsen S, et al. Am J Sports Med 19:273

Swimming

1997 Clinical findings in competitive swimmers with shoulder pain. Bak K, Faunl P. Am J Sports Med 25:254

1997 Starting age and aquatic skill learning in young children: mastery of prerequisite water confidence and basic aquatic locomotion skills. Parker HE, Blanksby BA. Aust J Sci Med Sport 29:83

Tennis

1995 Injury surveillance at the USTA Boys' Tennis Championships: a 6-yr study. Hutchinson MR, et al. Med Sci Sports Exerc 27:826

Trampoline

1998 Injuries to children in the United States related to trampolines, 1990-1995: a national epidemic. Smith GA. Pediatrics 101:406

Weight training

1996 The effectiveness of resistance training in children. A meta-analysis. Falk B, Tenenbaum G. Sports Med 22:176

1986 Strength training for children. Sewall L, Micheli LJ. JPO 6:143

Wrestling

1992 Injuries in adolescent and preadolescent boys at two large wrestling tournaments. Lorish TR, et al. Am J Sports Med 20:199

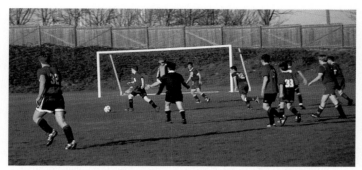

Fig. 11.67 Soccer. These high school soccer players have greater risk than those of younger age.

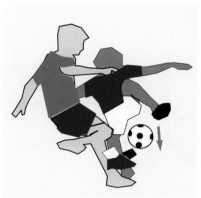

Fig. 11.68 Soccer. Soccer (football) injuries are most common in the lower limbs.

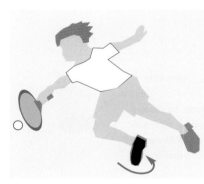

Fig. 11.69 Tennis. Ankle injuries and overuse injuries are most common.

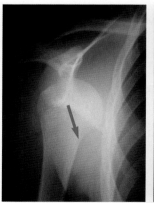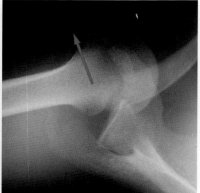

Fig. 11.70 Anterior shoulder dislocation. Shoulder dislocations are common injuries in wrestling.

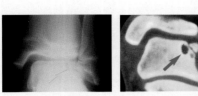

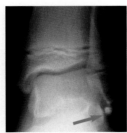

Fig. 11.71 Osteochondritis dissecans of the talus. This 15-year-old runner complained of ankle pain. Radiographs showed an indistinct lesion of the lateral talus (yellow arrow). CT scan shows the lesion well (red arrow).

Fig. 11.72 Os subfibulare. This ossicle lies just below the tip of the fibula (green arrow). Once the synchondrosis has fractured, it becomes painful.

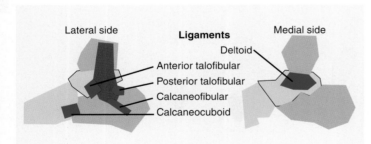

Stress fracture
Insertion Achilles tendon
Apophysis
Insertion plantar fascia

Fig. 11.73 Sites of heel pain. The common sites of heel pain include the point of insertion of the heel-cord, the apophysis of the calcaneus, and insertion of the plantar fascia. Stress fractures may occur through the calcaneus.

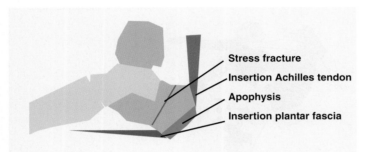

Lateral side   **Ligaments**   Medial side
Deltoid
Anterior talofibular
Posterior talofibular
Calcaneofibular
Calcaneocuboid

Fig. 11.74 Ankle ligaments. These ligaments may be sprained anterior talofibular, calcaneofibular, posterior talofibular, calcaneocuboid, and deltoid.

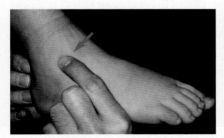

Fig. 11.75 Classic grade 1 ankle sprain. This 15-year-old basketball player twisted his ankle during play. He had mild swelling and well-localized tenderness just anterior to the distal fibular, the site of the anterior talofibular ligament.

Foot and Ankle Problems

Foot and ankle problems are common in nearly all sports (Figs. 11.71 and 11.72). Most problems are generic and occur during play or athletic participation. Sports add intensity to normal activity and may bring out problems that might otherwise remain unnoticed. For example, a congenital tarsal coalition may remain silent only to become painful during adolescence. Some problems cause pain in adolescence then subside in early adult life once activity is reduced. The girl may have anterior knee pain playing sports during her teens, but this resolves once she starts college and physical activity diminishes. Tight heel-cords may cause added stress on the tendon-bone interfaces around the calcaneus and cause pain in the 10-year-old soccer player. The two most common problems are detailed here.

Heel Pain

Heel pain is common during late childhood and adolescence and may occur at one of several levels (Fig. 11.73). Pain may occur at the insertion of the Achilles tendon into the calcaneus or at the origin of the plantar fascia as it attaches to the calcaneus. Irregular ossification of the calcaneal apophysis is often seen in asymptomatic children and is not a cause of pain. Stress fracture of the calcaneus is a rare cause of heel pain. If the condition is at all unusual or unilateral, make a radiograph of the calcaneus to rule out other problems.

Manage most heel problems by elevating and padding the heel and modifying activities. Do the least that controls the pain. Unlike some other overuse problems, resolution occurs with time and no disability follows. Start with modifying the activity if the family concurs. Next recommend shoes with a slightly elevated heel and a cushioned sole. If necessary, add a foam wedge of compressed felt, 3/4 inch in maximum thickness, in the heel of a high top shoe. Some recommend flexibility exercises of the triceps.

Ankle Sprains

Ankle sprains are the most common injury in sports. They occur in classic locations. Most involve the lateral collateral ligament complex (Fig. 11.74). Sprains are common in children and often involve avulsion of fragments of bone or cartilage. Sprains may become chronic and pose disability as in adults. Sprains are usually classified into three grades (Fig. 11.76).

Evaluation Mild sprains damage only the anterior leaf of the lateral collateral ligament (Fig. 11.75). Moderate sprains involve the middle (calcaneofibular ligament), and severe sprains damage the whole complex. Except for mild sprains with classic findings, order AP and lateral radiographs of the ankle to rule out other problems. Be aware that SH–1 epiphyseal injuries of the distal fibular (tenderness over mid-distal fibula), tears of the peroneal retinaculum (localized tenderness just behind the distal fibula), and tenderness inferior to the tip of the malleolus (os subfibulare, Fig. 11.72), may suggest a different diagnosis.

Less common locations for sprains include the medial collateral ligaments (much stronger than laterals) and the calcaneocuboid ligaments. These sprains are usually managed as mild sprains because they produce no late instability.

Manage sprains with RICE overnight and exercises to maintain muscle strength about the foot and ankle during convalescence.

Mild sprains are those with minimal swelling and tenderness. The classic example is the anterior talofibular ligament with localized tenderness just anterior to the distal fibula. Manage by rehabilitation to prevent recurrence. Sometimes an air-stirrup splint improves comfort.

Moderate sprains have more swelling and a wider area of tenderness with little or no instability. Manage by resting the ankle with a plastic splint or a cast for 2–3 weeks. Allow return to activities once muscle strength is regained, tenderness resolved, and range of motion restored.

Severe sprains produce severe swelling and instability may be demonstrated. Management of ankle instability for sprains is controversial but repairs of chronic instability may be necessary. Most may be managed by cast immobilization (Fig. 11.77) for 6 weeks.

Tibia Problems

The common problems include fractures (covered in Chapter 10), stress fractures, and shin splints. Because leg pain and shin splints are common and sometimes perplexing, the subject is detailed here.

Leg Pain

Leg pain is caused by a variety of disorders that include periostitis, compartment syndromes, stress fractures, and muscle herniation. The most common cause is a periostitis at the origin of the soleus muscle on the posteromedial aspect of the lower leg.

Evaluate by localizing the tenderness (Fig. 11.78), palpate for swelling and muscle hernia, and image with AP and lateral radiographs of the tibia. Consider other possibilities such as tumors or infection.

Periostitis is most common. It occurs in the older adolescent and is often bilateral. Tenderness covers a broader area than a stress fracture. The tenderness is localized to the posteromedial aspect of the distal tibia, and radiographs are negative.

Stress fractures cause localized tenderness over bone (Fig. 11.79).

Chronic compartment syndromes are less common and characterized by a history of pain with activity, relief with rest, and rarely tenderness and swelling over the involved compartment.

Muscle herniation is identified by palpating a protruding muscle, usually over the distal lateral leg.

Manage by applying the standard management principles of RICE, gradual conditioning, appropriate shoes, and NSAIDs.

Determine the underlying cause(s) of the initial pain and make modifications before returning the adolescent back to full activity to prevent recurrence. Rarely is operative correction such as periosteal release indicated.

References

2000 Pediatric stress fractures. de la Cuadra P, Albinana J. Int Orthop 24:47

1999 Double-stress fracture of the tibia in a ten-year-old child. Mitchell AD, Grimer RJ, Davies AM. JPOB 8:67

1997 Shin splints: MR appearance in a preliminary study. Anderson MW, et al. Radiology 204:177

1996 Chronic, painful ankle instability in skeletally immature athletes. Ununited osteochondral fractures of the distal fibula. Busconi BD, Pappas AM. Am J Sports Med 24:647

1995 Shin splints--a review of terminology. Batt ME. Clin J Sport Med 5:53

1995 Treatment of acute ankle sprain. Comparison of a semi-rigid ankle brace and compression bandage in 73 patients. Leanderson J, Wredmark T. Acta Orthop Scand 66:529

1994 An epidemiological survey on ankle sprain. Yeung MS, et al. Br J Sports Med 28:112

1989 Surgical treatment of chronic upper ankle joint instability in childhood. Zwipp H, Tscherne H, Hoffmann R. Z Kinderchir 44:97

1983 Sprained ankle in children. A clinical follow-up study of 90 children treated conservatively and by surgery. Vahvanen V, Westerlund M, Kajanti M. Ann Chir Gynaecol 72:71

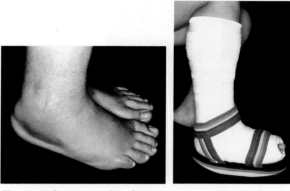

Grading of ankle sprains		
1	**Attenuation**	Mild swelling and tenderness
2	**Partial tears**	Moderate swelling, unable to bear weight
3	**Complete tears**	Marked swelling, bleeding, instability, and disability

Fig. 11.76 Classic grading of ankle sprains.

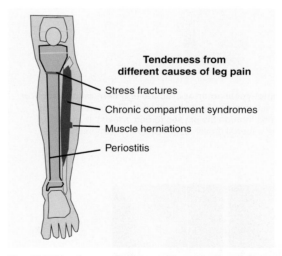

Fig. 11.77 Severe sprains. Severe swelling, ankle discoloration. and broad areas of tenderness are often associated with osteochondral injuries and are best managed by immobilization.

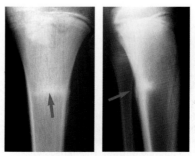

Tenderness from different causes of leg pain

Stress fractures

Chronic compartment syndromes

Muscle herniations

Periostitis

Fig. 11.78 Tenderness in types of leg pain. Localizing tenderness is helpful in separating the different types of midleg pain.

Fig. 11.79 Tibial stress fractures. The classic location for tibial stress fractures is in the proximal posterior tibia (red arrows). When stress fractures occur over the tibial shaft they are more likely to be included in the differential diagnosis of shin splints. This boy had multiple stress fractures involving the right femur and both tibiae.

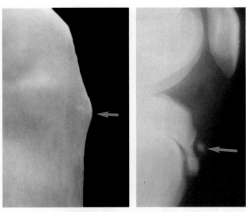

Fig. 11.80 Osgood-Schlatter disease. This 14-year-old boy has the typical swelling over the tibial tubercle, and the radiograph shows an ossicle at the site of tenderness.

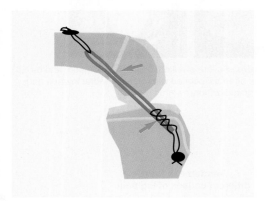

Fig. 11.81 Transepiphyseal anterior cruciate ligament reconstruction. This repair utilizes a hamstring tendon graft (red). The repair is mostly anatomic but extends through the physes (green arrows). It should be performed after the pubertal growth spurt. Based on Simonian (1999).

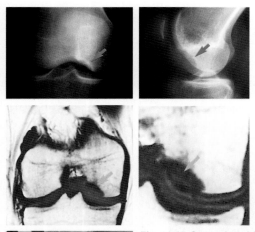

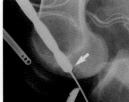

Fig. 11.82 Osteochondritis in 16-year-old girl. Note the typical location of the lesion (red arrows). The MRI shows the cartilage to be intact (orange arrows). The transcondylar approach to drilling lesion (yellow arrow) is shown.

Knee and Thigh Problems

Knee problems are common. Perform the hip rotation test to be certain the problem has its origin in the knee and not from the hip. The most common problems are Osgood-Schlatter disease and anterior knee pain.

Osgood-Schlatter Disease (OSD)

OSD is a traction apophysitis of the tibial tubercle due to repetitive microtrauma. It occurs between ages 10 and 15 years with the onset in girls about 2 years before that in boys. OSD is usually unilateral and occurs in 10–20% of children participating in sports. Without treatment, OSD resolves with time in most children. In about 10% of knees, some residual prominence of the tibial tubercle or persisting pain from an ossicle may cause problems.

Physical examination will demonstrate swelling and localized tenderness over the tibial tubercle and no other abnormalities. Order a radiograph if the condition is unilateral or atypical. Radiographs usually show soft tissue swelling and a separate ossicle over the tubercle (Fig. 11.80).

Manage by ordering modifications of activities, use of NSAIDs, and a knee pad to control discomfort. If OSD is severe or persists, apply a knee immobilizer for a week or two to relieve inflammation. Injection of steroids is not recommended. Complete resolution may be slow, often requiring 12–18 months. Persisting pain after closure of the growth plate indicates the presence of a residual ossicle. Excision of this ossicle solves the problem. See page 118.

Anterior Knee Pain

Anterior knee pain includes a variety of often ill-defined overuse problems. Make certain the pain is not referred from the hip. Identify any underlying problems such as rotational malalignment (medial tibial and lateral femoral torsion) or patellofemoral malalignment. Even if these problems exist, the condition is most likely benign and resolvable by simple measures. See page 118.

Manage by giving reassurance, NSAIDs, isometric quadriceps exercises and stretching, and modification of activities. Apply the "staircase" approach to finding the appropriate level of activity. Apply the 10% rule to avoid too much activity too soon.

Anterior Cruciate Ligament Insufficiency

Anterior cruciate ligament tears are becoming more common in adolescents, especially among girls playing basketball or soccer. Management is controversial. The natural history of instability and return to competitive sports is unsatisfactory as many have repeated injuries including meniscal damage.

Manage first with exercises, activity modification, and possibly bracing. Bracing clearly communicates that the problem is legitimate but hinders performance and doubtfully protects the knee. Once rehabilitation is complete, activity modification has gone to the acceptable limit, the adolescent is near the end of growth, and if disability is unacceptable, then repair is justified. Assess bone age and Tanner staging to assess level of maturation. When possible, delay repair until the patient is pubescent, or about 15 years of age for boys and 13 years for girls. Repair any meniscal tears with the ACL reconstruction.

Extraarticular repairs are not anatomic, leading to stretching with time. Furthermore, the dissection for placement may damage the physis.

Intraarticular repair may be physeal sparing, partial transphyseal through the central tibia, or completely transphyseal through the central femur and tibia. Repairs through the physis should be performed as late as feasible (Fig. 11.81) with care taken to make transphyseal penetrations as central and small as possible to minimize the risk of physeal arrest. Use autogenous hamstring or central patellar tendon grafts. If performed in the prepubescent patient, follow limb lengths and knee angles frequently to diagnosis any growth disturbance promptly.

Osteochondritis Dissecans

May involve the medial (Fig. 11.82) or lateral condyle or patella. The lateral side of the medial condyle is the classic location. Symptoms include pain, a mild effusion, or later mechanical symptoms. See page 119.

Thigh Problems

The thigh is heavily muscled and more protected than the tibia. It is also more difficult to examine because localization of tenderness is less exact. A variety of problems may occur, including fractures, stress fractures, and contusions. Contusions of the quadriceps may cause myositis ossificans.

Myositis Ossificans

Blunt trauma to the front of the thigh may cause the accumulation of a hematoma, which may lead to myositis ossificans. Treat the acute injury by applying RICE. Some recommend immobilization in flexion. Immobilize for 5–7 days, then encourage active knee flexion. Ossification in the damaged muscle progresses in a sequence of changes (Fig. 11.83) that are sometimes difficult to distinguish from that of osteogenic sarcoma. The lesions of myositis ossificans tend to be better localized, are often mid-anterior thigh in location, and arise in the muscle rather than the bone. Consider excision in the rare case when the mass is troublesome.

Hip Problems

Varied sport-related problems occur about the hip. The usual injuries such as avulsion fractures, dislocations, and acute slipping of the proximal femoral epiphysis are common in sports.

Overuse Injuries

Overuse injury of muscle attachments can occur in the same location as avulsion injuries (Fig. 11.84).

Bursitis

Bursitis may involve the greater trochanteric bursa and the iliopectineal bursa located anterior to the hip joint. Manage bursitis with NSAIDs and rest.

Snapping Hip

This condition is due to friction of the iliotibial band over the greater trochanter or subluxation of the psoas tendon. Irritation from overuse may cause swelling and aggravate the problem.

Iliotibial band snapping The diagnosis is established by palpating a snap over the greater trochanter. While palpating the trochanter, ask the patient to voluntarily produce the snap. If this is not helpful, ask the patient to walk in place. Sometimes the snap cannot be felt and only a presumptive diagnosis is made by the history. Patients are often erroneously told that they have a *dislocating hip*.

Iliopsoas tendon subluxation may be demonstrated by ultrasound evaluation (Fig. 11.85).

Manage by NSAIDs and activity modification. Resolution is often slow.

References

1999 Osteochondritis dissecans: a multicenter study of the European Pediatric Orthopedic Society. Hefti F, et al. JPO-b 8:231

1999 Anterior cruciate ligament injuries in the skeletally immature patient. Simonian PT, Metcalf MH, Larson RV. Am J Sport Med 99:624

1998 Anterior cruciate ligament injury in the skeletally immature athlete. Stanitsky CL. Operative Techniques in Sports Medicine 6:228

1997 Radiologic study of patellar height in Osgood-Schlatter disease. Aparicio G, et al. JPO 17:63

1997 Anterior cruciate ligament tears in children: an analysis of operative versus nonoperative treatment. Pressman AE, Letts RM, Jarvis JG. JPO 17:505

1995 Tibial tuberosity excision for symptomatic Osgood-Schlatter disease. Flowers MJ, Bhadreshwar DR. JPO 15:292

1991 Tibia recurvatum as a complication of Osgood-Schlatter's disease: a report of two cases. Lynch MC, Walsh HP. JPO 11:543

1991 Osteochondritis dissecans of the knee. A long-term study. Twyman RS, Desai K, Aichroth PM. JBJS 73B:461

1990 Natural history of Osgood-Schlatter disease. Krause BL, Williams JP, Catterall A. JPO 10:65

1990 Patellofemoral pain in children. Yates CK, Grana WA. CO 225:36

1985 The natural history of anterior knee pain in adolescents. Sandow MJ, Goodfellow JW. JBJS 67B:36

1981 Functional versus organic knee pain in adolescents. A pilot study. Fritz GK, Bleck EE, Dahl IS. Am J Sports Med 9:247

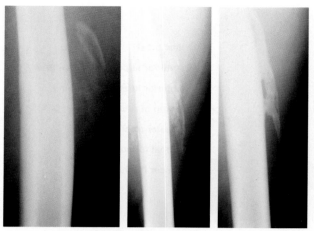

Fig. 11.83 Myositis ossificans. Serial radiographs show the evolution of the lesion at 3 weeks, 6 weeks, and 6 months following injury.

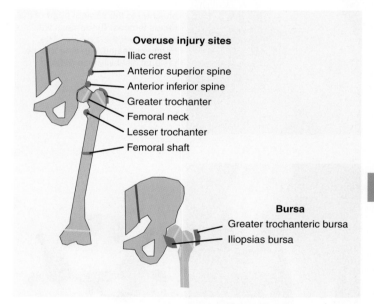

Overuse injury sites
- Iliac crest
- Anterior superior spine
- Anterior inferior spine
- Greater trochanter
- Femoral neck
- Lesser trochanter
- Femoral shaft

Bursa
- Greater trochanteric bursa
- Iliopsias bursa

Fig. 11.84 Overuse problems about the hip. These probelms include fractures, apophysitis, or bursitis.

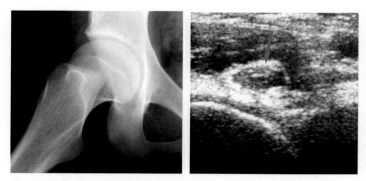

Fig. 11.85 Snapping iliopsoas tendon. Note the normal radiograph and the iliopsoas tendon (arrow) shown by ultrasound. Subluxation of the tendon was demonstrated.

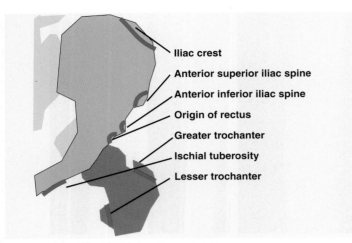

Fig. 11.86 Sites of avulsion injuries about the hip.

- Iliac crest
- Anterior superior iliac spine
- Anterior inferior iliac spine
- Origin of rectus
- Greater trochanter
- Ischial tuberosity
- Lesser trochanter

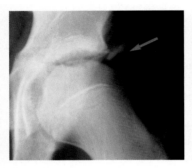

Fig. 11.87 Avulsion of the origin of rectus. The fleck of bone is attached to the straight head of the rectus femoris. Tenderness was present over the avulsion. The fragment healed with time and no residual disability was present.

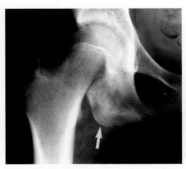
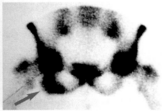

Fig. 11.88 Ischael avulsion. This 16-year-old runner sustained an avulsion of the hamstring origin on the ischium. Note the prominence (yellow arrow) and increased uptake (red arrow) on the bone scan. The bone scan was unnecessary.

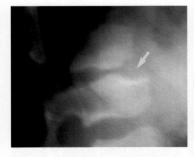
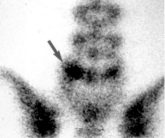

Fig. 11.89 Back pain in the athlete. Herniation of the nucleus pulposus into the vertebral body causes narrowing of the disc space (yellow arrow). The lesions may be painful. The radiographic defect is sometimes called a lumbar *Schmorl node*. Bone scans in spondylolysis show increased uptake. The condition may be unilateral (red arrow).

Pelvis Problems

Avulsion Injuries

Avulsion injuries occur in a variety of locations about the hip and pelvis (Figs. 11.86–11.88). Most of these injuries are managed by rest because healing of the fracture occurs spontaneously. Some surgeons recommend replacing displaced large avulsion fractures of the ischium, but this is controversial.

Hip Pointers

Hip pointer is a contusion over the iliac rim seen in American football and other contact sports. These injuries are usually managed by RICE and NSAIDs, but may be slow to recover.

Stress Injuries

Osteitis pubis is an overuse syndrome that occurs in the adolescent. Tenderness is localized over the symphysis. Lower extremity malalignment may contribute to the problem. Manage by rest and NSAIDs.

Pubic ramus stress fractures may occur. The diagnosis is suspected by the location of the tenderness and confirmed by a positive bone scan.

Spine Problems

Spine injuries and back pain (Fig. 11.89) are common sport injuries that are discussed in Chapters 8 and 10.

Neck Problems

Some of the most catastrophic injuries in sports involve the cervical spine. Fortunately, such injuries are rare. They have reduced in frequency since the ban of "spearing" (deliberate use of the head for primary contact) and with improved football helmet design. Most cervical spine injuries occur in diving, trampoline, and American football. Quadriplegia and death are potential consequences of such injuries.

Stingers and Burners

These are injuries resulting in burning pain in the arm that may be transient (stingers) or persist for several hours (burners). These injuries result from nerve root traction from sport-induced trauma. They are most common in American football and in individuals who have congenital narrowing of the cervical canal. These injuries resolve, but they are a warning to be careful.

Sports in Children with Down Syndrome

Physicians are frequently asked to assess the child with trisomy-21 who wishes to participate in sports. These children are at risk due to instability of C1– C2 caused by stretching of the apical ligament. Down syndrome children have extreme joint laxity, and C1– C2 instability is one of the more serious outcomes of this underlying defect. Be concerned if the measure is >5 mm. Discourage participation in contact sports. Follow yearly with examination and every several years with radiographs. Some recommend fusion with ADI >10 mm.

Upper Limb Problems

Shoulder

A variety of lesions occur about the shoulder. Swimmers commonly develop impingement syndrome. American football players often injure the medial or lateral aspects of the clavicle (Fig. 11.90), and wrestlers dislocate their shoulders. Overuse injuries of the upper humeral epiphysis occur in pitchers.

Elbow

Elbow injuries are common in sports. The elbow is vulnerable because of its anatomic complexity and its position in the upper limb where it is subjected to excessive loads.

Little League Elbow

The elbow is easily overloaded during the act of overhand throwing or during serves in racket sports. This is aggravated by poor throwing mechanics when pitching is done with more enthusiasm than skill. This causes excessive valgus loading of the joint. This overloading causes traction on the medial side and compression on the lateral side of the elbow joint (Fig. 11.91) . The most common injury is the traction injury to the medial epicondyle, the common origin of the forearm flexors and pronators. Less common but more serious are the compression injuries on the capitellum and radial head. Compression injuries usually occur in the adolescent.

Medial epicondylar injuries may result in an inflammation or frank separation from the humerus. As the medial epicondyle is extraarticular, this injury is less serious.

Capitellar osteochondritis is more serious because it can lead to damage to the joint. Compressive loading causes osteochondritic lesions that may separate and create loose bodies in the joint.

Radial head osteochondritis more commonly leads to overgrowth and joint incongruity.

Diagnosis is usually not difficult. The child is often a baseball pitcher, tenderness is localized over the site of the problem, and radiographs often show changes. Range of motion of the elbow is usually reduced.

Manage the acute problem with the usual RICE and NSAIDs. Insist that any throwing be avoided for 4–6 weeks. Encourage the child to bike or run as a diversion. Evaluate and correct poor throwing mechanics. Reintroduce throwing gradually. Initially limit throwing to 20–30 feet. Use the 10% rule. To prevent recurrence, limit pitching to a specific number of throws or innings per game (Fig. 11.92). The number depends upon the age and condition of the child. If the joint is damaged, the adolescent should switch to another sport.

Forearm and Wrist

The forearm is frequently fractured in falls (see Chapter 10). The wrist may be injured by overuse in gymnastics. Gymnastic injuries may damage the distal radial physis and cause impingement from hyperextension and fractures.

Hand

Boxer fracture results from a fracture of the distal end of the fourth or fifth metacarpal, reducing the prominence of the knuckle.

Skier thumb results from falls that damage the ulnar collateral ligament or fracture the proximal phalanx of the thumb, producing instability or deformity.

Coach finger results from an axial loading of the proximal interphalangeal joint of a finger, causing a dislocation of the joint. The coach may "snap" the finger back into position. Always take a radiograph to rule out a fracture. Articular fractures should always be referred to an orthopedist.

Baseball finger (jammed finger) is a sprain of the proximal interphalangeal joint resulting from ball strikes to the end of the digit. Radiographs are negative and the joint is stable. Healing may take several weeks.

Mallet finger results from a forced flexion of the distal finger joint causing rupture or fracture of the insertion of the extensor tendon.

Chapter Consultant Carl Stanitski, email: stanitsc@musc.edu

References

1999 Osteochondritis dissecans of the elbow. Hall TL, Galae AM. Phy and Sportsmed 27:75

1998 Early detection of osteochondritis dissecans of the capitellum in young baseball players. Report of three cases. Takahara M, et al. JBJS 80A:892

1997 Osteochondral lesions in the radiocapitellar joint in the skeletally immature: radiographic, MRI, and arthroscopic findings in 13 consecutive cases. Janarv PM, Hesser U, Hirsch G. JPO 17:311

1996 Development of a distance-based interval throwing program for Little League-aged athletes. Axe MJ, et al. Am J Sports Med 24:594

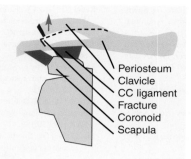

Fig. 11.90 Fracture of distal clavicle. This type of fracture through the growth plate of the distal clavicle may be confused with an AC separation. The clavicle is often displaced upward through a tear in the periosteum. The coracoclavicular (CC) ligament remains intact. Reduction is not necessary, as remodeling rapidly corrects the deformity.

Periosteum
Clavicle
CC ligament
Fracture
Coronoid
Scapula

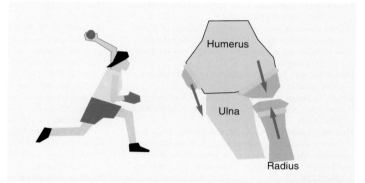

Humerus

Ulna

Radius

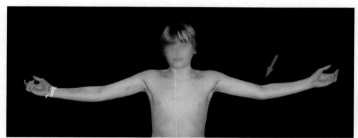

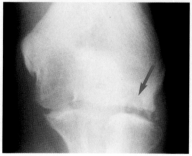

Fig. 11.91 Little league elbow. The adolescent above has osteochondritis of the capitellum (red arrows) that causes limited extension of the left elbow. The act of throwing causes medial traction (blue arrow–upper drawing), which tends to avulse the medial epicondyle. Throwing also causes lateral compression of the capitellum and radial head (red arrows).

Pitching Guidelines

Age
  Before 8 yrs – throwing only
  After 8 yrs – allow pitching
  After 14 yrs – allow curve balls

Games per week
  About 2

Pitches per game
  Progress from about
    Age 8 – 50 pitches to
    Age 17 – 100 pitches

Fig. 11.92 Pitching guidelines This is a rough guide. Tailor to fit child. Based on Whiteside (1999).

American Academy of Pediatrics. Committee on Sports Medicine. Atlantoaxial instability in Down syndrome. Pediatrics 1984;74(1):152-4.

Arendt EA, Dick R. Knee injury patterns among men and women in collegiate basketball and soccer: NCAA data and review of literature. Am J Sports Med 1995;23:694-701.

Backs FJG, et al, Sports injuries in school-aged children. Am J Sports Med 1989;17:234.

Beachy G. et al, High school sports injuries. Am J Sports Med 1997;25:675.

Caine D, et al. Stress changes of the distal radial growth plate. Am J Sports Med 1992;20:290.

Cantu RC, Mueller FO. Fatalities and catastrophic injuries in high school and college sports, 1982–1997. Phy and Sportsmedicine 1999;27:35.

Cook PC; Leit ME, Issues in the pediatric athlete. Orthop Clin North Am 1995;26(3):453-64.

Current comment from the American College of Sports Medicine. August 1993 "The prevention of sport injuries of children and adolescents" Med Sci Sports Exerc 1993;25(8 Suppl):1-7.

DiFiori JP, et al, Factors associated with wrist pain in the young gymnast. AOSPM 1996;24:9.

Gomez E, DeLee JC, Farney WC. Incidence of injury in texas girls' high school basketball. Am J Sports Med 1996;24:684.

Graf BK, Lange RH, Fujisaki K, Landry GL, Saluja RK. Anterior cruciate ligament tears in skeletally immature patients: Meniscal pathology at presentation and after attempted conservative treatment. Arthroscopy 1992;8:229-233.

Guzzanti V, Falciglia F, Gigante A, Fabbriciani C. The effect of intra-articular ACL reconstruction on the growth plates of rabbits. J Bone Joint Surg 1994;76B:960-963.

Indelicato PA. Isolated medial collateral ligament injuries in the knee. J Am Acad Orthop Surg 1995;3:9-14.

Janarv P, Wesblad P, Johansson C, et al. Long-term follow-up of anterior tibial spine fractures in children. J Ped Orthop 1995;15:63-68.

Kadel NJ, Teitz CC, Kronmal RA. Stress fractures in ballet dancers. Am J Sports Med 1992;20:445.

Kakulas BA, Adams RD, Disease of Muscle, Pathological Foundation of Clinical Myology (4th ed) 1985 Harper and Row.

Kraus JF, Conroy C. Mortality and morbidity from injuries in sports and recreation. Annu Rev Public Health 1984;5:163-92.

Lorish TR, et al. Injuries in adolescent and preadolescent boys at two large wrestling tournaments. Am J Sports Med 1992;20:199.

MacDonald GL. Sports injuries in children. Necessary consequence of competition? Postgrad Med 1985;78(1):279-81.

Maffulli N. Sports medicine in childhood and adolescence. 1995 Mosby-Wolfe.

Maffulli N. The growing child in sport. Br Med Bull 1992;48(3):561-8.

McCarroll JR, Shelbourne KB, Rettig AC, et al. Patellar tendon graft reconstruction for midsubstance anterior cruciate ligament rupture in junior high school athletes: an algorithm for management. Am J Sports Med 1994;22:478-484.

McCoy RL 2nd, Dec KL, McKeag, DB, Honing EW. Common injuries in the child or adolescent athlete. Prim Care 1995;22(1):117-44.

McKeag DB, The role of exercise in children and adolescents. Clin Sports Med 1991;10(1):117-30.

Moretz JA, et al, Long-term followup of knee injuries in high shcool football players. Am J Sports Med 1984;12(4):298.

Nyska et al, Avulsion fracture of the medial epicondyle caused by arm wrestling. Am J Sports Med 1992;20:347.

Parker DF, et al. A cross-sectional survey of upper and lower limb strength in boys and girls during childhood and adolescence. Ann. Human Biol 1990;17:199-211.

Sahlin Y. Sport accidents in childhood. Br J Sports Med. 1990;24(1):40-44.

Schutz RW, Smoll FL, Wood TM. Physical activity and sport: attitudes and perceptions of young Canadian athletes. Can J Appl Sport Sci 1981;6(1):32-39.

Stanitski CL. Articular hypermobility and chondral injury in patients with acute patellar dislocations. Am J Sports Med 1995;23:146.

Stanitski CL. Common injuries in preadolescent and adolescent athletes. Recommendations for prevention. Sports Med 1989;7(1):32-41.

Stanitski CL. Knee overuse disorders in the pediatric and adolescent athlete. Inst Lectures Am Acad Ortho Surg 1993;42:483.

Stanitski CL. Management of sports injuries in children and adolescents. Orthop Clin North Am 1988;19(4):689-98.

Stanitski CL. Pediatric and Adolescent Sports Medicine. 1994 WB Saunders.

Stanitski CL, Harvell JC, Fu F. Observations on acute knee hemarthrosis in children and adolescents. J Ped Orthop 1993;3:506-510

Stuart MJ, Smith A. Injuries in junior A ice hockey. Am J Sports Med 1996;23:458.

Sullivan A, The Pediatric Athlete. 1988 Am Acad Ortho Surg.

Teitz CC. Sports medicine concerns in dance and gymnastics. Pediatr Clin North Am 1982;29(6):1399-421.

Thabit G, Micheli LJ. Patelloemoral pain in the pediatric patient. OrthoClin North Am 1992;23:567.

Tursz A; Crost M. Sports-related injuries in children. A study of their characteristics, frequency, and severity, with comparison to other types of accidental injuries. Am J Sports Med 1986;14(4):294-9.

Vingard E, et al. Sports and osteoarthrosis of the hip. An epidemiologic study. Am J Sports Med 1993;21(2):195.

Warme WJ, et al, Ski injury statistics, 1982 to 1993, Jackson Hole ski resort. Am J Sports Med 1996;23:597.

Willis R, Blocker C, Stoll T, et al. Long-term follow-up on anterior tibial eminence fractures. J Ped Orthop 1993;13:361-364

Zaricznyj B, et al, Sports-related injuries in school-aged children. Am J Sports Med 1980;8(5):318-24.

287

Chapter 12 – Infection

Infections involving the musculoskeletal system are common (Fig. 12.1) and can cause severe disability. With optimum management, practically all infections may be cured, and deformity and disability prevented.

The prevalence of osteomyelitis is declining and changing character. Long-bone infections caused by staphylococcus aureus and septic arthritis caused by *h. influenza* have declined most. Osteomyelitis has changed forms with more complex and unusual patterns (Fig. 12.2). Infection with resistant strains is increasing.

Infections are still important and often challenging, but improved management makes poor outcomes less common and less acceptable.

Pathogenesis
An understanding of the pathogenesis of musculoskeletal infections facilitates management.

Portals of Entry
Most infections are hematogenous with the primary site of entry in the in the ear, oropharynx, respiratory, GI or GU tracts (Fig. 12.3). Skin infections as occur after chicken pox and penetrating injuries such as nails in the sole of the foot or infections from surgical procedures are less common (Fig. 12.4). Extension of contiguous infections are least common, although adjacent joint infections are relatively commonly associated with adjacent osteomyelitis (Fig. 12.2).

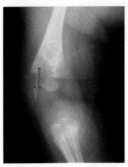

Fig. 12.1 Infection causes systemic illness. This infant has septic arthritis of the elbow and is systemically ill.

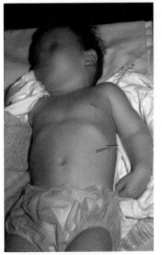

Fig. 12.2 Local spread. Infection from metaphyseal osteomyelitis may spread into adjacent joints in the infant.

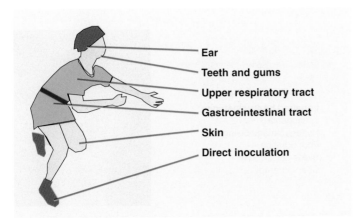

Fig. 12.3 Portals of bacterial entry.

Ear
Teeth and gums
Upper respiratory tract
Gastrointestinal tract
Skin
Direct inoculation

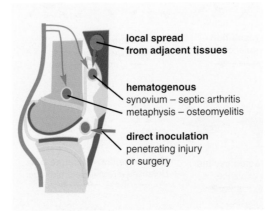

local spread
from adjacent tissues

hematogenous
synovium – septic arthritis
metaphysis – osteomyelitis

direct inoculation
penetrating injury
or surgery

Fig. 12.4 Spread to bone and joints. Infection is commonly hematogenous but may be by local spread or from direct inoculation.

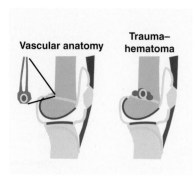

Fig. 12.5 Vascular anatomy of the metaphysis. Bacteria may accumulate in vascular loops in the metaphysis. Trauma with hematoma formation provide good environment for bacterial proliferation.

Vascular anatomy

Trauma–hematoma

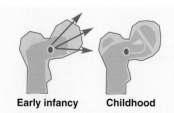

Fig. 12.6 Transphyseal spread. Transepiphyseal vessels allow spread of infection from the metaphysis into the joint (red arrows). The presence of a physis blocks this spread (yellow arrow).

Early infancy

Childhood

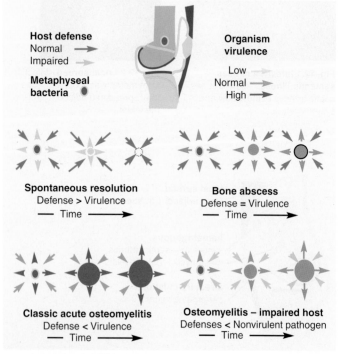

Fig. 12.7 Neonatal septic arthritis of the hip. Note the widening of the joint space. This is a late finding.

Initial Deposition

Bacteremia is a common event that rarely causes bone and joint infections. Why bone and joints are more vulnerable than other tissues is unknown.

Bone is usually infected in the metaphysis. Bacteria are deposited in capillary loops adjacent to the physeal plate. Nearly always these bacteria are quickly destroyed by phagocytosis. Trauma is a factor that reduces resistance by causing the formation of a hematoma (Fig. 12.5). Bacterial proliferation is enhanced by the elaboration of *biofilm,* which enhances bacterial adhesion to bone and provides protection from phagocytosis or antibiotics.

Joints may be infected by hematogenous spread via the synovium, penetrating injury of joints, by direct spread from a contiguous infection, or by bacterial transport by way of transphyseal vessels. Transphyseal vessels are present in early infancy before the formation of the growth plate (Fig. 12.6). This may account for the frequency of septic arthritis of the hip in the neonate (Fig. 12.7). In children about a third of long-bone osteomyelitis is associated with septic arthritis of the adjacent joint.

Natural History of Infection

It is probable that the vast majority of bacterial colonies are destroyed by systemic and local mechanisms. The likelihood of progression is based on the balance between organism virulence and host resistance (Fig. 12.8).

Spontaneous resolution is common. Host resistance exceeds the virulence of the organism.

Subacute osteomyelitis is less common. Host resistance and virulence are about equal. A bone abscess forms reactive sclerotic bone walls off the abscess. No equivalent of this subacute form exists for septic arthritis.

Classic acute osteomyelitis or septic arthritis results from a virulent organism and a normal host. The patient becomes systemically ill, and untreated may develop septicemia and die. In others, extensive local bone necrosis occurs and chronic osteomyelitis follows.

Impaired host may allow development of a bone or joint infection from organisms of relatively low virulence as seen in conditions such as sickle cell disease (Fig. 12.9).

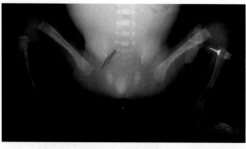

Host defense
Normal
Impaired

Metaphyseal bacteria

Organism virulence
Low
Normal
High

Spontaneous resolution
Defense > Virulence
— Time —

Bone abscess
Defense = Virulence
— Time —

Classic acute osteomyelitis
Defense < Virulence
— Time —

Osteomyelitis – impaired host
Defenses < Nonvirulent pathogen
— Time —

Fig. 12.8 Natural history of osteomyelitis determined by host resistance and organism virulence.

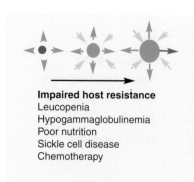
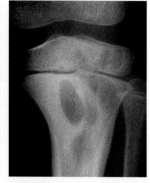

Impaired host resistance
Leucopenia
Hypogammaglobulinemia
Poor nutrition
Sickle cell disease
Chemotherapy

Fig. 12.9 Impaired host resistance. Organisms of low virulence may cause infections when host resistance is impaired.

Organisms

The organisms that infect the musculoskeletal system are numerous, varied, continually changing, and have predilection for site, tissue, and age of host (Fig. 12.10).

Staphylococci

Gram positive organisms are the most common cause of infections. The incidence is declining. *Staphlyococcus aureus* includes a variety of pathogenic strains. New strains are methicillin resistant. *Staphlyococcus epidermidis* may cause infection in impaired hosts.

Streptococci

Streptococcal infections cause soft tissue and bony infections. *b-hemolytic streptococci* are common pathogens. *Streptococcus pneumonia* may cause septic arthritis. *Streptococcus agalactiae* is a common cause of neonatal osteomyelitis. *Streptococcus pyogenese* is a less common pathogen.

Neisseria Meningitidis

Meningococcal septicemia causes acute and chronic orthopedic problems. The disseminated intravascular coagulation and focal infections acutely cause necrotizing fascitis and damage physeal circulation, causing physeal arrest and limb deformities (Fig. 12.11).

Pseudomonas Aeroginosa

This is a gram negative rod, chondrophilic, common cause of joint infections of the foot from penetrating injuries.

Escherichia Coli

This is a gram negative rod and a rare cause of musculoskeletal infections.

Salmonella

This is a gram negative rod most likely to be encountered in sickle cell osteomyelitis.

Mycobacteria Tuberculosis

This is an acidfast organism with resurgence of worrisome drug resistant strains. It causes bone and joint infections in children. Tuberculous spondylitis with kyphosis is a common and serious deformity (Fig. 12.12).

Kingella kingae

This is a gram negative coccobacillus common in the respiratory system, slow growing, aerobic, and fastidious. It is difficult to culture. Only recently has it been found to cause musculoskeletal infections. It remains susceptible to most antibiotics.

Haemophilus influenzae

This was previously a common cause of septic arthritis in infants. Now it is rare because of immunization programs.

References

2000 The incidence of joint involvement with adjacent osteomyelitis in pediatric patients. Perlman MH, et al. JPO 20:40.

1998 Increasing prevalence of Kingella kingae in osteoarticular infections in young children. Lundy DW, Kehl DK. JPO 18:262

1992 The changing epidemiology of osteomyelitis in children. Craigen MA, Watters J, Hackett JS. JBJS 74B:541

1991 Changing pattern of bone and joint infections due to Staphylococcus aureus: study of cases of bacteremia in Denmark, 1959-1988. Espersen F, et al. Rev Infect Dis 13:347

1989 Chondro-osseous growth abnormalities after meningococcemia. A clinical and histopathological study. Grogan DP, et al. JBJS 71A:920

1959 The three types of acute haematogenous osteomyelitis. A clinical and vascular study. Trueta J. JBJS 41B:671.

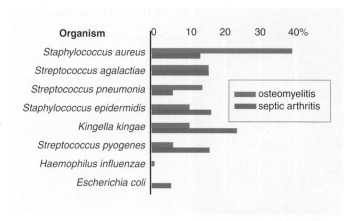

Fig. 12.10 Infecting organism in bone and joint infections in children under 36 months of age. The percentage of 30 cases of osteomyelitis (blue bars) and 30 cases of septic arthritis (red bars) caused by different organisms. From data of Lundy and Kehl (1998).

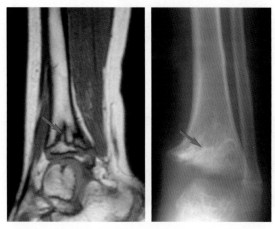

Fig.12.11 Septic physeal fusion. This child with meningococcemia developed a fusion of the distal tibial growth plate (arrows).

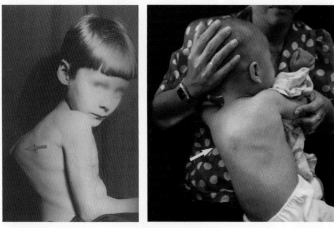

Fig.12.12 Tuberculous spondylitis with kyphosis. This was a common condition in the past (red arrow) in North America, and it is still prevalent in developing countries (yellow arrow).

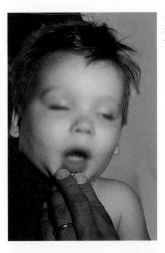

Fig. 12.13 Ill Child. This child is systemically ill from septic arthritis. Note the lethargy and dehydration.

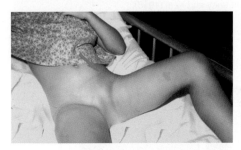

Fig. 12.14 Cellulitis involving the hip. This child has a cellulitis about the left hip (arrow). The limb is held in a position of flexion and abduction that reduces soft tissue pressure and minimizes discomfort.

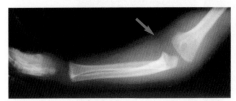

Fig. 12.15 Soft tissue swelling. Soft tissue swelling is present in this infant with septic arthritis of the elbow.

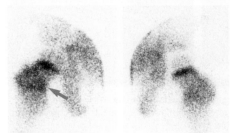

Fig. 12.16 Delay in radiographic appearance of osteomyelitis. This original film at the onset of the disease was normal (left). At 2 weeks (right), the lytic lesion is seen in the metaphysis (red arrow).

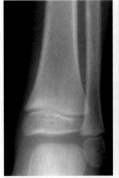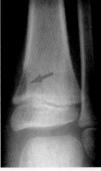

Fig. 12.17 Osteomyelitis of proximal femur. Bone scans aid in localizing the site of infection. The bone scan may be useful in determining the site for surgical drainage.

Evaluation

The child's medical history is important in the assessment of any previous injury or medical problem in the course of the current illness. The duration of symptoms in septic arthritis is of prognostic significance. Infections that are present for more than 3 days may cause residual joint damage, especially in the newborn. It is important to inquire about previous antibiotic treatment.

Physical Examination

Perform a screening examination first. Does the child appear ill (Fig. 12.13)? The presence of systemic signs distinguishes septic arthritis from toxic synovitis. Is spontaneous movement present? The most reliable sign of septic arthritis of the hip in the newborn is a reduction of spontaneous movement of the limb. The reduction of movement from infection is described as *pseudoparalysis*. Swelling, erythema, and increased temperature are signs of inflammation, often due to infection. Note the position of the limb. Most infected limbs are positioned with the joints in slight flexion to reduce the intraarticular pressure. The hip is usually positioned in slight flexion, lateral rotation, and abduction (Fig. 12.14).

Note the extent of soft tissue swelling and joint effusions. Try to localize the area of tenderness about the knee, ankle, wrist, or elbow to determine whether the primary problem is in the joint or the adjacent metaphysis. This is helpful in differentiating septic arthritis from osteomyelitis.

Move the joint through a gentle range of motion to assess guarding or limitation of the arc of motion. Medial rotation is limited by inflammation about the hip.

Imaging

Conventional radiographs may show soft tissue swelling (Fig. 12.15) and obliteration of the soft tissue planes, but little else during the early course of an infection. A reduction of bone density of about 30% is necessary before radiographic changes are present. This usually requires 10–14 days (Fig. 12.16).

Bone scans are useful in evaluating infection in the early stages of the illness. Technesium scans in septic arthritis are usually "warm." Scans in osteomyelitis are usually warm or hot but may be cold early in the disease. In the early phase of the disease, uptake may be reduced and a cold segment of bone may indicate the presence of a severe infection. In early osteomyelitis the phasic scan may be useful. The early phase includes vascular perfusion that parallels the physical findings of swelling and inflammation. In the second or osseous phase, uptake is greater over the site of involvement. Bone scans are not necessary if radiographic changes are already present. Often the bone scan is helpful in localizing the site of involvement (Fig. 12.17). Order a "pinhole colluminated" scan for increased resolution. The bone scan is unaffected by bone or joint aspiration.

Ultrasound evaluation for hip joint effusions (Fig. 12.18) may be helpful if the ultrasonologist is experienced. A negative study should not delay a diagnostic aspiration if the clinical signs suggest the possibility of an infected joint. Ultrasound is also useful in localizing abscess formations around long bones, and its use is underutilized.

MRI studies of infection may be useful in localizing an abscess (Fig. 12.19). MRI studies of discitis may be alarming and can lead to overtreatment. Use newer imaging techniques only as adjuncts to conventional well-understood techniques.

CT studies are sometimes useful in evaluating deep infections such as those about the pelvis. CT and MRI studies may be helpful in localizing abscess and planning the surgical approach for drainage.

Laboratory Studies

The erythrocyte sedimentation rate (ESR), C reactive protein (CRP), and cultures are the most valuable laboratory tests. Serial measures are useful in following the course of infection. Often the WBC is normal.

ESR is still valuable. Following the onset of infection the ESR slowly rises to peak at 3–5 days and remains elevated for about 3 weeks if treatment is successful (Fig. 12.20).

CRP peaks in 2 days and follows most closely the clinical course of the infection. If treatment is successful, the values return to normal in about a week.

Cultures are essential and usually include blood, joint fluid, wound and biopsy samples. Blood cultures are positive in 30–50% of patients. Be aware that negative cultures are common in both osteomyelitis and septic arthritis.

Differentiation from Neoplasm

The differentiation of infection from neoplasm is sometimes difficult. Infections are more common, especially in the younger subjects, and often show signs of inflammation. Subacute osteomyelitis may be confused with osteoid osteoma, osteosarcoma, chondroblastoma, Ewing sarcoma, fibrosarcoma, or eosinophilic granuloma. If necessary, establish the diagnosis with biopsy, curattage, and cultures. If the lesion is well demarcated, making a malignant tumor less likely, consider prescribing a course of oral antibiotics. If the lesion is due to an infection, the treatment is both diagnostic and therapeutic.

Eosinophilic granuloma may show inflammatory features.

Ewing sarcoma differentiation may pose a major problem. MRI and bone scans may be helpful (Fig. 12.21). Sometimes biopsy and cultures are necessary.

References

2000 Overview and new developments in childhood musculoskeletal infections. Morrissy, RT. AAOS symposium, Orlando, Fl.

1997 Subacute osteomyelitis presenting as a bone tumour. A review of 21 cases. Cottias P, et al. Int Orthop 21:243

1995 Usefulness of magnetic resonance imaging for the diagnosis of acute musculoskeletal infections in children. Mazur JM, et al. JPO 15:144

1994 Ultrasonic features of acute osteomyelitis in children. Mah ET, et al. JBJS 76B:969

1994 Isotope bone scanning for acute osteomyelitis and septic arthritis in children. Tuson CE, Hoffman EB, Mann MD. JBJS 76B:306

1994 The usefulness of C-reactive protein levels in the identification of concurrent septic arthritis in children who have acute hematogenous osteomyelitis. A comparison with the usefulness of the erythrocyte sedimentation rate and the white blood-cell count. Unkila-Kallio L, Kallio MJ, Peltola H. JBJS 76A:848

1993 Ultrasound in diagnosis and management of acute haematogenous osteomyelitis in children. Howard CB, et al. JBJS 75B:79

1993 Diagnostic aspects of subacute osteomyelitis in children and adolescents. Clinical and radiographic resemblance to primary malignant tumors. Saetersdal AB, et al. Nor Laegeforen 113:3240

1984 Fever, C-reactive protein, and erythrocyte sedimentation rate in monitoring recovery from septic arthritis: a preliminary study. Peltola H, Vahvanen V, Aalto K. JPO 4:170

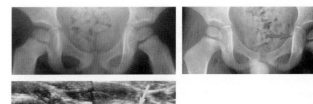
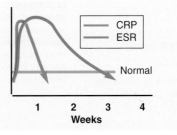

Fig. 12.18 Imaging in septic arthritis. This child developed hip pain and guarding. The initial radiograph (top left) was negative. The family refused aspiration. When seen the next day, the radiograph showed widening of the joint space (red arrow) and the ultrasound showed a joint effusion (yellow arrow).

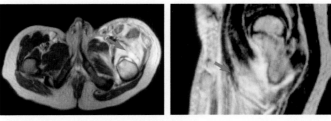

Fig. 12.19 MRI showing a thigh abscess. This study shows the massive upper thigh abscess (arrows) secondary to femoral osteomyelitis.

Fig. 12.20 CRP and ESR changes with time. Following a musculoskeletal infection, the CRP declines more rapidly than the ESR. Based on Unkila-Kallio (1993).

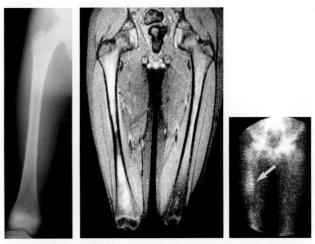

Fig. 12.21 Differentiating diaphyseal osteomyelitis from Ewing sarcoma. In this child with osteomyelitis, note that the conventional radiograph was negative (left). This differentiation was aided by the MRI study, which showed little soft tissue involvement (arrow). The bone scan (yellow arrow) showed that only the femur was involved.

Agent	Dose
Oxacillin	150–200 mg/kg/day
Nafcillin	150–200 mg/kg/day
Dicloxacillin	75–100 mg/kg/day
Cephalexin	100–150 mg/kg/day
Cefazolin	100–150 mg/kg/day
Cefotaxime	100–150 mg/kg/day
Cefuroxime	150–200 mg/kg/day
Gentamicin	5–7.5 mg/kg/day
Clindamycin	30–40 mg/kg/day

Fig. 12.22 Daily dosage of antibiotic treatment. These are some broad generalizations for infants over 1 month and for children.

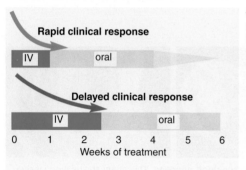

Fig. 12.23 Duration of IV antibiotic treatment. Base duration of parenteral antibiotics on clinical response.

Disease	Comment
Septic arthritis	7 days IV, 3–4 weeks total
Osteomyelitis	7 days IV, 4–6 weeks total or until ESR normal
Cellulitis	10–14 days
Surgical prophylaxis	Single dose prior to incision

Fig. 12.24 Duration of antibiotic treatment. These are some broad generalizations, which serve as an average duration of treatment.

Management Principles

Management of infections in children is guided by a number of principles that often differ from those that apply to adults.

Greater Healing Potential

The potential for healing infection is remarkable in children. For example, discitis usually resolves with time with or without treatment. Bone damaged by osteomyelitis heals. Infection of bone may be contained and localized to only a residual abscess or resolve completely without treatment. Chronic osteomyelitis can nearly always be cured in the child. Operative wound infections are uncommon in children.

Antibiotics

The selection of the antibiotic agent is complex. Consider the disease, organism, and special features of the child. These features include the age, concurrent illness, and the family situation. The route of administration and duration of treatment are other factors to consider. Initial therapy should be intravenous or, if access is difficult, intramuscular. Certain antibiotics are most commonly used for musculoskeletal infections (Figs. 12.22 and 12.25).

Oral antibiotic therapy is justified if the infection is minor, the agent is well absorbed, and the family is reliable. In most serious infections, treatment may begin with parenteral antibiotics and switch to oral agents when the disease is under control. Before switching to the oral route of administration, be certain that adequate blood levels are documented following oral administration and that the family is reliable.

Duration of antibiotic treatment is controversial. Several factors should be considered in determining the duration. Consider the severity and potential for disability that the infection poses, the rapidity of response to treatment (Fig. 12.23), serial determinations of the ESR and CRP, and the results of published studies. There are, however, some generalizations that can be made (Fig. 12.24). These can be modified according to the situation. Joint suppuration in septic arthritis reduces the effectiveness of the antibiotic treatment.

Consultant

Jane Burns, e-mail: jburns@chmc.org

Condition	Organism	Agent
Sepsis		
Neonate	Group A and B strep, coliforms	Nafcillin + gentamicin
Infant	*H. flu*, pneumococcus, meningococcus	Ceftriaxone or cefotaxime
Septic Arthritis		
Neonate	Group B strep, staph, coliforms	Nafcillin + gentamicin
Infant	*H. flu*, staph A, group A and B strep,	Cefotaxime
Child	*Staph. aureus*	Nafcillin
Osteomyelitis		
Neonate	Group B strep, staph A, coliforms,	Nafcillin + gentamicin
Infant/Child	staph A	Nafcillin
Nail Puncture		
Through Shoes	Pseudomonas	Ceftazidime or Ticarcillin
Barefoot	*S. aureus*	Nafcillin
Discitis	*S. aureus*	Nafcillin
Open Fractures	*S. aureus*	Nafcillin
Operative Prophylaxis	*S. aureus*	Nafcillin

Fig. 12.25 Commonly used antibiotics for musculoskeletal infections.

Indication	Comment
Abscess	Open drainage
Hip Joint	Open drainage
Other Joints	Drain by aspiration
Osteomyelitis	Drain abscess open
Brodie Abscess	Drain open if necessary
Sequestrum	Excise

Fig. 12.26 Indications for drainage. These are the common indications for operative drainage.

Operative Drainage

Drainage may be accomplished by needle aspiration, arthroscopic decompression, or open procedures.

Indications Drainage is necessary whenever antibiotic penetration into the infected site is impaired (Fig. 12.26). This penetration is most often due to the presence of an abscess or an accumulation of pus within a joint (Fig. 12.27). Impaired penetration may also be due to a loss of vascularity as occurs in chromic osteomyelitis with sequestration or in soft tissue with poor vascularization due to thrombosis of vessels and acute inflammation. The presence of an abscess may be demonstrated by clinical examination, imaging such as ultrasound or MRI, needle aspiration, or suggested by a failure of clinical response to antibiotic treatment. This failure of response to antibiotics (Fig. 11.28) is the failure of reduction in fever, pain, local inflammatory signs, and CRP during the first 48–72 hours after instituting antibiotic treatment. Keep in mind that this failed response may also be due to an ineffective antibiotic agent or to an immunocompromised child.

Technique may be simply needle aspiration (Fig. 11.29) as is feasible for most joints, arthroscopic or open drainage. Open drainage of abscess due to acute infections requires simply draining the abscess through a small window in the cortex. If the abscess is near a growth plate, take care to avoid injuring the physis (Figs. 12.30 and 12.31). Monitor the position of the curette with fluoroscopy.

References

1996 Percutaneous drainage of septic hip arthritis in children. Griffet J, El Hayek T. Rev Chir Orthop Reparatrice Appar Mot 82:251

1996 Subacute hematogenous osteomyelitis: are biopsy and surgery always indicated? Hamdy RC, et al. JPO 16:220

1994 Acute pyogenic osteomyelitis in children. Dirschl DR. Orthop Rev 23:305

1991 Arthroscopic treatment of septic arthritic knees in children and adolescents. Ohl MD, Kean JR, Steensen RN. Orthop Rev 20:894

1990 Acute septic arthritis in infancy and childhood. Shaw BA, Kasser JR. CO 257:212

1985 Percutaneous aspiration, drainage, and biopsies in children. Towbin RB, Strife JL. Radiology 157 :81

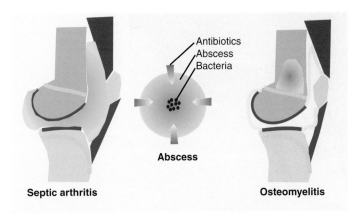

Septic arthritis — Antibiotics, Abscess, Bacteria — **Abscess** — **Osteomyelitis**

Fig. 12.27 Abscess protects bacteria from antibiotics. The abscess prevents antibiotic penetration, protecting bacteria.

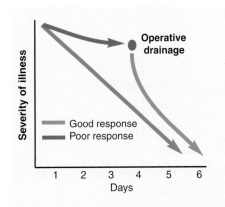

Fig.11.28 Indication for operative drainage. The failure of response to antibiotic treatment is often an indication for drainage.

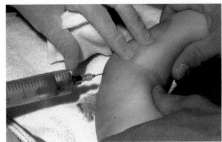

Fig. 11.29 Needle aspiration. This drainage is usually adequate for most joints with septic arthritis.

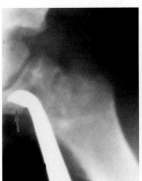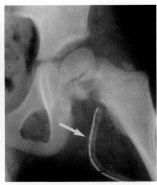

Fig.12.30 Drainage in difficult locations. Monitor position of curette with fluoroscopy and avoid the physis (red arrow). Usually a drain is placed (yellow arrow).

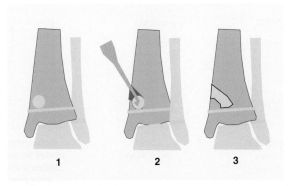

Fig. 12.31 Surgical drainage of acute or subacute osteomyelitis. The infection is drained locally with care taken to avoid injury to the growth plate. Bone fill is in the defect with time.

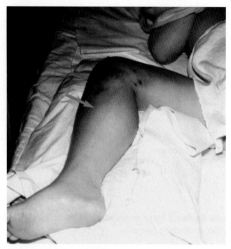

Fig. 12.32 Osteomyelitis. This boy has osteomyelitis of the upper tibia with an associated soft tissue abscess (arrow).

Osteomyelitis

Osteomyelitis is an infection of bone (Fig. 12.32). The infection may be acute, subacute, or chronic. The infection may involve any bone (Fig. 12.33). Osteomyelitis in the preantibiotic era often caused death or severe disability. Currently, osteomyelitis remains a relatively common problem but with a much better prognosis.

Natural History

The natural history of osteomyelitis depends upon the virulence of the organism, the resistence of the host, and the age of onset (Fig. 12.34). Virulent organisms may cause death of the child due to overwhelming sepsis or if localized progress to chronic osteomyelitis. Chronic osteomyelitis develops through stages, which include bone and soft tissue abscesses causing sequestrum formation (Fig. 12.35), intermittent drainage, and a lifelong disability. Chronic drainage may lead to development of squamous cell carcinoma of the sinus tracts during adult life.

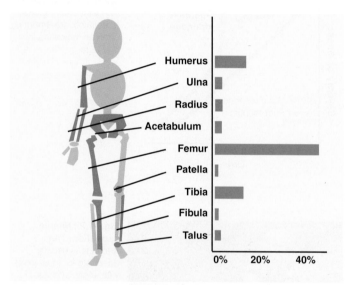

Fig. 12.33 Distribution of osteomyelitis. From a series of 66 patients reported by Perlman (2000).

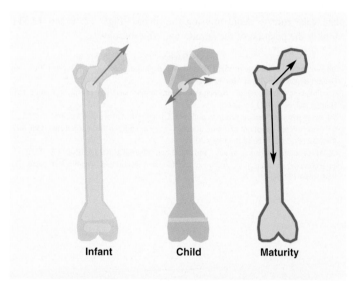

Fig. 12.34 Spread of osteomyelitis by age. Bone structure affects the spread of osteomyelitis. In the infant the absence of an epiphyseal plate may allow spread into a joint (red arrow). In the child the path of least resistance is through the adjacent cortex to an extramedullary abscess (blue arrow). In the mature adolescent the thick cortex and absence of growth plates allows extension throughout the medullary cavity (black arrows).

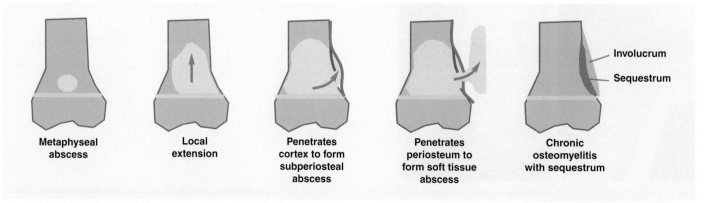

Fig. 12.35 Natural history of osteomyelitis. The infection starts in the metaphysis. Contained by the growth plate, the infection spreads through the metaphysis, then penetrates the cortex, creating a subperiosteal abscess. This may penetrate the periosteum to produce a soft tissue abscess. During healing, new bone (involucrum) forms around the devitalized cortical bone. This dead bone is called a "sequestrum."

Acute Osteomyelitis

Acute osteomyelitis produces local pain, swelling, warmth, erythema, tenderness, and systemic manifestations of fever and malaise. Laboratory findings usually include a leukocytosis and elevated CRP and ESR. The CRP and ESR elevations are the most consistent laboratory findings.

Image with conventional radiographs to provide a baseline and assess for soft tissue swelling. A bone scan may be useful in localizing the site of involvement. Ultrasound and MRI studies may be helpful in localizing any abscess. To isolate the organism, culture the blood and consider aspirating the site of infection. Aspiration is most successful if a subperiosteal abscess is present.

Management When planning management, estimate the stage of the disease (Fig. 12.35). Antibiotic treatment is usually successful without the need for drainage if the osteomyelitis is discovered early before suppuration has occurred. Start antibiotic treatment while awaiting the results of the cultures. The selection of agent is done empirically, taking into consideration the age of the patient and the presence of any special features. Antibiotics are first given parenterally to ensure effective blood levels. The clinical course is monitored. If the antibiotic is effective against the organism and no suppuration is present, clinical improvement will occur with reduction in local signs of inflammation and systemic manifestations. If such improvement fails to occur over a period of 24–48 hours, the most likely cause is the formation of an abscess. An abscess requires operative drainage (Fig. 12.36). See page 381.

Subacute Osteomyelitis

Subacute osteomyelitis is an infection with a duration longer than 2–3 weeks. Often this type of osteomyelitis is the residual of acute osteomyelitis that has been contained but not eradicated (Fig. 12.37). The child may show no or little systemic response but with local swelling, warmth, and tenderness. Sometimes the complaint is a limp.

Evaluation Radiographs will show the lesion. The appearance will be variable (Fig. 12.39) and may be confused with a primary bone tumor, especially when diaphyseal and showing periosteal elevation. The differentiation between infection and Ewing sarcoma or leukemia is usually not difficult.

Management Manage classic metaphyseal lesions by antibiotic treatment without drainage. Drain and culture if lesions are atypical, if concern exists about a neoplastic etiology, if the child is immologically impaired or the lesion or symptoms persist following antibiotic treatment (Fig. 12.38).

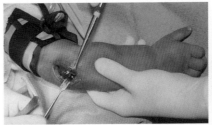
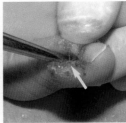

Fig. 12.36 Drainage of osteomyelitis. Drain by windowing the cortex and exploring adjacent bone with a curette (yellow arrow).

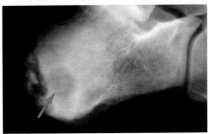
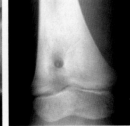

Fig. 12.37 Subacute osteomyelitis. Osteomyelitis is contained in a bone abscess (arrows).

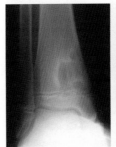
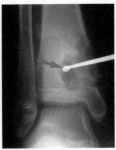
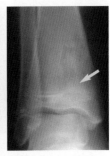

Fig. 12.38 Drainage of persistent subacute distal tibial osteomyelitis. Tenderness and inflammation and radiographic changes were indications for operative drainage. Avoid placing the curette across the physis (red arrow). Defect is healing 4 weeks later (yellow arrow).

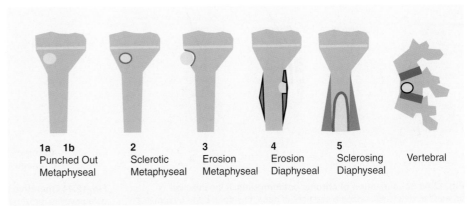

Fig. 12.39 Types of subacute osteomyelitis. Redrawn from Roberts (1982)

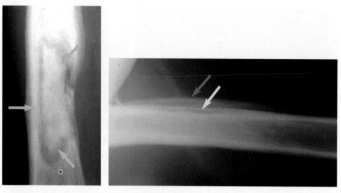

Fig. 12.40 Diaphyseal osteomyelitis. Note the classic appearance of a well-established sequestrum in the tibia (orange arrows). Uncommon pattern of osteomyelitis of the femoral diaphysis is present in an 8-year-old girl. New bone formation (red arrow) surrounds a linear sequestrum (yellow arrow). This sequestrum was removed surgically.

Chronic Osteomyelitis

Untreated acute osteomyelitis usually becomes chronic with the disease localized to a segment of bone. Long bones are most likely to develop chronic osteomyelitis as a segment of cortex may be devascularized to form a sequestrum (Fig. 12.40). Flat bones, such as those of the pelvis, are primarily cancellous with better blood supply and less likely to develop chronic disease. The patterns of chronic osteomyelitis are numerous (Figs. 12.41 and 12.42)

Management requires operative sequestrectomy and resection of infected tissue by saucerization to allow filling of the dead space with viable tissue (Fig. 12.43). See page 381. In very long-standing infections complex sinus tracts may develop. Assess the condition preoperatively with MRI, CT scans, and possibly by contrast injection of the sinus tract to determine its location, path, and depth of the sinus. Before resection, consider injecting dye into the sinus to stain the infected tissue (Fig. 12.44). Plan the operative approach that will allow excision of all infected tissue. Provide antibiotic coverage based on preoperative sinus cultures. If the periosteum is viable, new bone will fill in the surgically created bony defect.

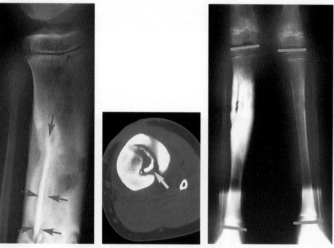
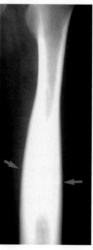

Fig. 12.41 Chronic osteomyelitis in a 12-year-old boy. The sequestrum is clearly shown on the lateral radiograph (red arrows) and CT scan (yellow arrow). Note the overgrowth and valgus deformity of the right tibia (green lines).

Fig. 12.42 Sclerosing osteomyelitis. The entire shaft of the femur was converted into an abscess cavity in this adolescent boy.

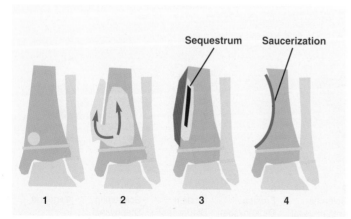

Fig. 12.43 Saucerization of chronic osteomyelitis. If the infection spreads and devascularizes a segment of bone, this dead bone becomes a sequestrum (black) under the involucrum (dark brown). Manage by *saucerization* to remove the sequestrum and infected tissue. The healthy overlying soft tissue fills in the saucer.

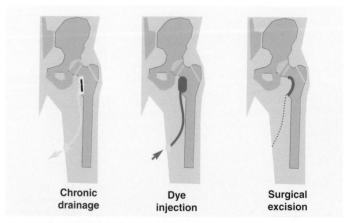

Fig. 12.44 Operative debridement. The site of drainage of chronic osteomyelitis (proximal medial femur) may be distant from the sequestrum (left). Define the sinus tract and infected tissue with a sinogram with methylene blue dye. Excise the sequestrum and all infected tissue (red).

Complications of Osteomyelitis

Systemic complications Untreated osteomyelitis may lead to systemic infections such as bronchopneumonia and septic pericarditis with life-threatening consequences.

Local complications are uncommon with current treatment. Complications due to deformity of bone can usually be reconstructed with a satisfactory outcome. This is in contrast to the complications of septic arthritis, which often damage joints with no satisfactory reconstruction usually possible.

Pathologic fracture is a serious complication of osteomyelitis (Fig. 12.45). Often the extent of the deossification is not appreciated and the child is discharged with the affected limb unprotected. Pathological fractures are slow to heal and may heal in a deformed position. The deossification resulting from osteomyelitis lags the activity of the infection by 2–3 weeks. The risk of pathological fracture should be anticipated and a protective cast applied before the deossification occurs.

Sequestrum formation is usually due to delay in diagnosis. Sequestrectomy is usually effective and curative for chronic disease.

Growth disturbance may be due to initial damage from the infection or operative drainage. Infections that destroy the growth plate or epiphysis may cause significant deformity (Figs. 12.46 and 12.47).

References

2000 The incidence of joint involvement with adjacent osteomyelitis in pediatric patients. Perlman MH, et al. JPO 20:40.

1996 Subacute hematogenous osteomyelitis: are biopsy and surgery always indicated? Hamdy RC, et al. JPO 16:220

1994 Humerus varus: a complication of neonatal, infantile, and childhood injury and infection. Ellefsen BK, et al. JPO 14:479

1991 The management of chronic osteomyelitis. Cole WG. CO 264:84

1991 Complications of suppurative arthritis and osteomyelitis in children. Porat S, et al. Int Orthop 15:205

1991 Influence of chronic osteomyelitis on skeletal growth: analysis at maturity of 26 cases affected during childhood. Tudisco C, et al. JPO 11:358

1990 Acute osteomyelitis in children: a review of 116 cases. Scott RJ, et al. JPO 5:649

1987 Acute hematogenous osteomyelitis in children. Vaughan PA, Newman NM, Rosman M. JPO 7:652

1983 Acute haematogenous osteomyelitis in infancy and childhood. Nade S. JBJS 65B:109

1982 Acute haematogenous osteomyelitis. O'Brien T, et al. JBJS 64B:450

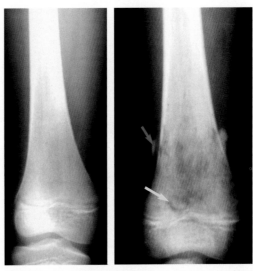

Fig. 12.45 Pathological fracture complicating osteomyelitis. This girl was treated only with antibiotics for a metaphyseal osteomyelitis. Her discharge radiographs showed no deossification. She returned 3 weeks later with a pathological fracture (red arrow) through the deossified metaphysis (yellow arrow).

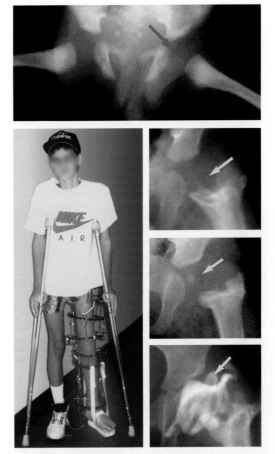

Fig. 12.47 Limb lengthening for residual of osteomyelitis. This boy developed osteomyelitis of the left upper femur in the neonatal period (red arrow). The growth plate was damaged, resulting in deformity of the femoral head (yellow arrows) and limb shortening of 8 cm. The shortening was corrected by an Ilizarov leg lengthening technique. The bone is divided and gradually distracted while being stabilized with the external fixator.

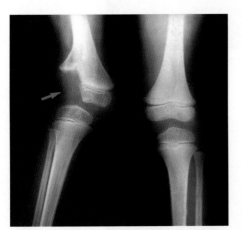

Fig. 12.46 Severe genu valgum due to infection. This child lost the lateral half of the distal femoral growth plate due to osteomyelitis in early infancy. The deformity is progressive and difficult to correct.

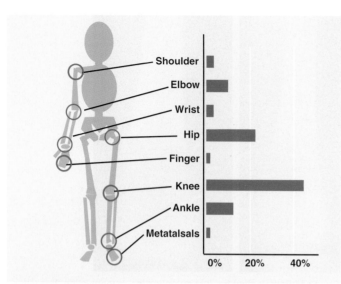

Fig. 12.48 Distribution of septic arthritis. From data of Jackson and Nelson (1982).

Organism	Comment
Staphylococcus	Most common
Hemophilus	Becoming rare
Streptococcus	
Meningococcus	Primary or secondary
Pneumococcus	Infant
E. Coli	Infant
Gonococcus	Adolescent
Lyme Disease	
Tuberculosis	Increasing frequency
Fungal Infections	Certain areas endemic
Viral Infections	Rare

Fig. 12.49 Organisms in septic arthritis. These organisms are listed in categories according to relative frequency.

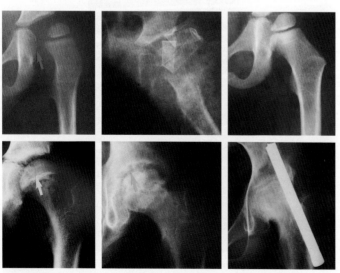

Fig. 12.50 Sequence of late treated septic arthritis. Treatment was delayed. Note the widening of the joint (red arrow). Open drainage was performed but avascular necrosis (yellow arrow) and joint destruction followed (orange arrow). The hip was eventually fused.

Septic Arthritis

Septic arthritis is a joint inflammation due to an infection usually involving synovial joints (Fig. 12.48). Many agents may cause septic arthritis (Fig. 12.49), but the vast majority are due to various strains of *Staphylococcus* and *Streptococcus* and *Kingella kingae* (see Fig. 12.10). Septic arthritis can cause severe deformity and disability, especially when involving the hip during the neonatal period. The joint is damaged by enzymes produced by the bacteria and leukocytes causing protoglycan loss and collagen degradation. Inflammation may cause secondary vascular damage from thrombosis or direct compression of vessels.

Natural History

Unlike osteomyelitis/ which may resolve without treatment, septic arthritis causes joint damage (Figs. 12.50 and 12.51). This makes septic arthritis a more serious disease than osteomyelitis.

Diagnosis

Clinical features are age related.

Neonate with septic arthritis may show few clinical signs. The most consistent finding is a loss of spontaneous movement of the extremity and posturing of the joint at rest. The hip is positioned in flexion, abduction, and some lateral rotation. Fever is often absent and the neonate may not appear ill.

Infant and child septic arthritis produces local and systemic signs of inflammation. The joint is swollen and tender, and the child resists movement. Hip infections result in severe limitation of rotation, a useful sign in separating septic arthritis from osteomyelitis. Radiographs early in the disease may be deceptive (Fig. 12.52). A negative study is not significant. Widening of the joint is significant. Ultasound studies may show joint effusions. Bone scans show slight to moderate increased uptake over the joint.

The most useful laboratory studies are the sedimentation rate and CRP. The ESR is usually elevated above 25 mm/hour. This test is not reliable for diagnosis in the neonate.

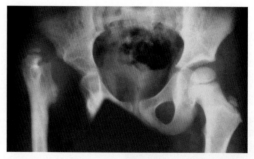

Fig. 12.51 Residual deformity of septic arthritis of the hip. Note the severe deformity or Choi type 4 (see Fig. 12.56).

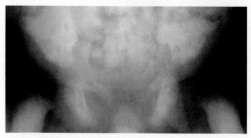

Fig. 12.52 False negative radiograph. The radiograph was read as negative, no treatment given, and the hip was destroyed by the septic arthritis.

The diagnosis of septic arthritis is established by joint aspiration (Fig. 12.53). See page 379. This evaluation should be performed early and not delayed to obtain a bone scan or other imaging studies. Joint fluid in septic arthritis is cloudy, with leukocyte counts above 50,000 and PMNs predominating. Perform a Gram stain and culture. Cultures will be negative in 20–30% of cases of septic arthritis and thus a negative study does not rule out a joint infection. Culture the blood before starting antibiotic treatment.

Differential diagnosis includes toxic synovitis, poststreptococcal reactive arthritis, and rheumatoid arthritis.

Management
Manage with antibiotics and drainage.

Antibiotic treatment Start with an agent that is statistically most likely to be effective (Fig. 12.54). Later, the antibiotics may be changed based on the culture reports. Parenteral treatment is continued for several days and the clinical course monitored. Failure to improve suggests that the antibiotic is ineffective or that the drainage is incomplete. The duration of parenteral antibiotics should be based on the rapidity of clinical response in reduction of fever, local inflammation, and C reactive protein response. Arbitrary rigid regimens prolong hospitalization and increase costs and patient discomfort without improving results. Most septic arthritis may be managed with parenteral antibiotics for 3 to 21 days followed by oral antibiotics for a total of about 4 weeks.

Joint drainage is necessary for all cases and should be done promptly. See page 380.

Serial needle aspiration is a traditional method of drainage. Aspirate initially and as necessary to keep the joint free of pus. Most joints should be drained several times. If response to needle aspiration is slow, consider open or arthroscopic drainage.

Open drainage is mandatory for the hip. Consider open drainage for other joints if the diagnosis is delayed or situation complicated.

Arthroscopic drainage is an option for large joints in children (Fig. 12.55). Place a drain.

Immobilization in septic arthritis is unnecessary. Avoid placing the child in traction as the child will naturally hold the limb in the position of greatest comfort, which is the position in which intraarticular pressure is least.

Residual Deformity

Knee Residual deformity is most likely if the infection occurs in infancy and treatment is delayed. Usually a valgus or varus deformity develops due to displacement or loss of the physis. The deformity is usually permanent and often progressive.

Hip Ischemic changes are common and varied. Absence or delayed ossification, loss then return of ossification, or most severe complete loss or collapse. In this more severe form, increasing deformity may be present. Deformity is varied depending upon the extent of articular and physeal cartilagenous damage (Fig. 12.56).

Consultant Jane Burns, e-mail: jburns@chmc.org

References
2000 A shortened course of parenteral antibiotic therapy in the management of acute septic arthritis of the hip. Kim HKW, Alman B, Cole WG. JPO 20:44.

1998 Late sequelae of neonatal septic arthritis of the shoulder. Bos CF, et al. JBJS 80B:645

1997 Avascular necrosis as a complication of septic arthritis of the hip in children. Vidigal EC, Vidigal EC, Fernandes JL. Int Orthop 21:389

1994 Sequelae from septic arthritis of the knee during the first two years of life. Strong M, et al. JPO 14:745

1990 Sequelae and reconstruction after septic arthritis of the hip in infants. Choi IH, et al. JBJS 72A:1150

1990 Acute septic arthritis in infancy and childhood. Shaw BA, Kasser JR. CO 257:212

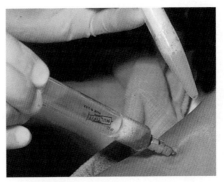

Fig. 12.53 Hip aspiration for diagnosis. Open drainage is required for septic arthritis of the hip.

Age	Organism	Antibiotic	Dose
Neonate	Group B streptococcus S. aureus E. coli	Cefotaxime	150 mg/kg/day
Infant	S. aureus Group A streptococcus Pneumococcus	Nafcillin	150-200 mg/kg/day
Child	S. aureus	Nafcillin	150–200 mg/kg/day

Fig. 12.54 Antibiotic management of septic arthritis by age group. The usual infecting organism and appropriate antibiotic are categorized by age group.

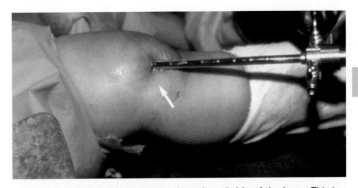

Fig. 12.55 Arthroscopic drainage of septic arthritis of the knee. This is an acceptable method of drainage.

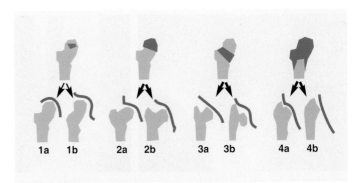

Fig. 12.56 Classification of sequelae from septic arthritis of the hip. This classification demonstrates that the initial necrosis (red) determines the severity of the final deformity. From Choi (1990).

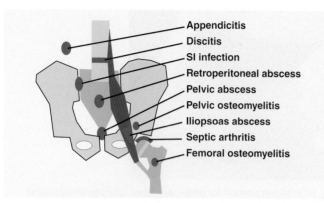

Fig.12.57 Sites of infections about the pelvis. Consider these possibilities in the differential diagnosis.

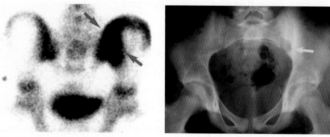

Fig. 12.58 Sacroiliac joint infection. Initial radiographs were negative but a bone scan demonstrated involvement of SI joint (red arrow). Radiographs 1 month later demonstrated a bone abscess (yellow arrow).

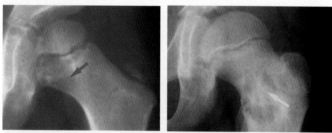

Fig.12.59 Osteomyelitis proximal femur. These lesions may be lytic (red arrow) or, when chronic, become more sclerotic (yellow arrow).

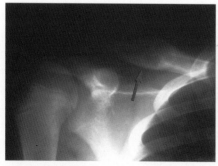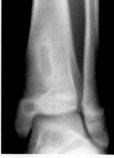

Fig. 12.60 Unusual forms of osteomyelitis. Chronic osteomyelitis of the clavicle produces bony overgrowth with a cystic appearance often confused with a neoplasm (red arrow). Rarely, lesions occur in the epiphysis (yellow arrow).

Pelvic Infections

The combination of hip or flank pain, limp, and fever suggests an infection about the pelvis (Fig. 12.57). As these infections are deep in location, localization by physical examination is more difficult than for infections of the extremities. Each infection has some unique characteristics that aid in diagnosis.

Evaluation

Physical examination may localize the infection. Tenderness and pain in the back or abdomen suggests discitis or an abdominal problem. Limitation of hip rotation suggest septic arthritis of the hip. Tenderness over the SI joints or proximal femur may help localize the process to those sites. Performing a rectal examination may help localize the problem.

Imaging is usually necessary. The bone scan is most helpful in localizing the infection (Fig. 12.58). CT scans may show soft tissue swelling. Ultrasound evaluation may demonstrate inflammatory changes in muscles.

Laboratory Growth of *Staphylococcus aureus* from a pelvic abscess indicates that the process is musculoskeletal in origin. Growth of fecal flora suggests an intraabdominal cause that warrants further study.

Differential Diagnosis

Septic arthritis of the hip requires most urgent management. Pain on passive rotation of the leg suggests this diagnosis. Confirm by aspiration. Urgent open drainage is necessary.

Iliopsoas abscess causes pain and positioning of the hip in flexion. Extension is painful. Iliopsoas abscess can be readily diagnosed by ultrasonography or computed tomography and treated by percutaneous retroperitoneal drainage.

SI infection of the joint or adjacent bone are best demonstrated by bone scan (Fig. 12.58). Manage with antibiotic treatment. Drainage is usually not necessary.

Pelvic osteomyelitis may occur in varied sites. Localize with bone scan, demonstrate any abscess by US or CT scans. Treat with antibiotics. If unresponsive, consider aspiration with image guidance.

Femoral osteomyelitis is more serious with the potential for joint or growth damage (Fig. 12.59). Open drainage is often necessary.

Unusual Forms of Osteomyelitis

Osteomyelitis of the Clavicle

The clavicle responds to osteomyelitis with thickening and cystic changes that give the appearance of a neoplasm (Fig. 12.60, left). CT scans may demonstrate a bone abscess, which may be drained. Cultures may be negative. Consider chronic recurrent multifocal osteomyelitis in the differential. Treat bacterial infections with drain and antistaphlococcal antibiotics.

Epiphyseal Osteomyelitis

Primary hematogenous osteomyelitis rarely affects the epiphysis primarily (Fig. 12.60, right). The infection may spread through the growth plate from a metaphyseal origin. The physeal erosion allowing this transphyseal spread usually heals without the formation of a physeal bridge. The exception is in meningococcemia and severe infections with delayed treatment.

Salmonella Osteomyelitis

Salmonella and staphlococcal auerus osteomyelitis occur in children with sickle cell disease (Fig. 12.61). The infection is characterized by polyostotic distribution, extensive diaphyseal involvement, massive involucrum, and frequent complications due to compromised immune status and poor circulation of blood in bone. Manage by decompression and parenteral antibiotics.

Soft Tissue Infections

Chicken Pox (Varicella)

Group A streptococcal infections may cause cellulitis, abscesses, septic arthritis, or extensive necrotizing fascitis.

Toxic Shock Syndrome (TSS)

TSS is due to a toxin elaborated by different types of *S. aureus* and streptococcus. TSS has been reported about 2 weeks following orthopedic procedures and under casts in children. About half are nonmenstrual. The characteristic features include high fever, vomiting, diarrhea, rash, hypotension, pharyngitis, headache, and myalgia. Management is directed toward controlling the effects of the toxemia.

Polymyositis

Muscle abscesses are infrequent as skeletal muscle is resistant to bacterial infections. A bacteremia seeds muscle abscess (Fig. 12.62). In some cases some underlying condition reduces resistance. Untreated, the generalized inflammation becomes focal with abscess formation in 2–3 weeks. The child becomes progressively more ill with the potential of death. *Tropical polymyositis* often occurs in anemic and malnourished children.

Initial stage The child presents with poorly localized aching pain and fever. The most common sites are the hip and thigh. Clinical and laboratory signs of infection are present. Radiographs show soft tissue swelling, bone scan shows increased uptake (12.63), and the MRI is most specific and diagnostic. Treat with parenteral antistaphlococcal antibiotics.

Suppurative stage The child shows more systemic signs and focal tenderness. The MRI demonstrates a muscle abscess. Confirm the diagnosis and determine the organism by aspiration of the abscess. In some this is adequate. Most require operative drainage.

Lyme Disease

Lyme arthritis in children may mimic other pediatric arthritides. The natural history of untreated Lyme disease in children may include acute infection followed by attacks of arthritis and then by keratitis, subtle joint pain, or chronic encephalopathy. Treat with amoxicillin, doxycycline, and ceftriaxone. With treatment complete, resolution is expected within 2–12 weeks and prognosis is excellent.

Puncture Wounds

Foot infections are often due to puncture wounds. The classic example is the nail puncture wound of the foot. When these occur through shoes, the infecting organism is *Pseudomonas*. Puncture wounds in other situations are usually due to staphylococcus. Retention of foreign material such as wood may be best imaged by ultrasound (Fig. 12.64). Removal of foreign bodies is often more difficult than expected. See page 378.

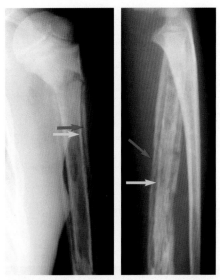

Fig. 12.61 Salmonella osteomyelitis in sickle cell disease. This osteomyelitis elicits an extensive subperiosteal new bone formation (red arrows) that completely surrounds the original diaphysis (yellow arrows).

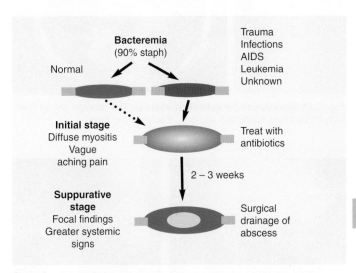

Fig. 12.62 Natural history of polymyositis. The natural history of this infection includes cellulitic and suppurative stages.

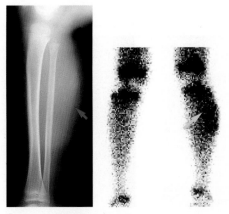

Fig.12.63 Polymyositis. Note the soft tissue swelling (red arrow) and increased muscle uptake (yellow arrow) on bone scan.

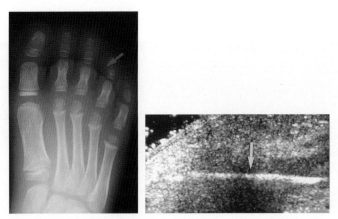

Fig. 12.64 Foreign body infections. The foot is swollen (red arrow) but without bony change. The ultrasound shows the wood fragment (yellow arrow).

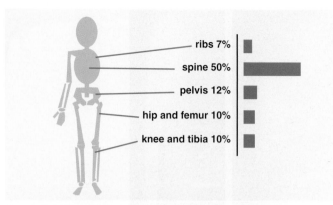

Fig. 12.65 Distribution of musculoskeletal tuberculosis.

ribs 7%
spine 50%
pelvis 12%
hip and femur 10%
knee and tibia 10%

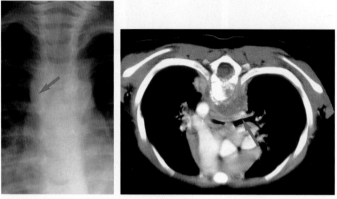

Fig. 12.66 Tuberculous paravertebral abscess. The abscess can be seen both on the chest radiograph and the CT scan (red arrows).

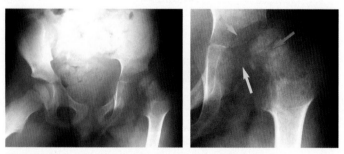

Fig. 12.67 Tuberculous hip infection. Note the infection involves the proximal femur (red arrow), joint (yellow arrow), and acetabulum (orange arrow).

Tuberculosis

More new cases of tuberculosis are being seen throughout the world. This is due to increasing number with suppressed immune systems, drug resistant strains of *Mycobacterium*, an aging population, and more exposed health care workers. Musculoskeletal tuberculosis most often involves the spine (Fig. 12.65).

Spinal Tuberculosis

In children the infection usually involves only bone (Fig. 12.66) leaving the disc and cartilagenous endplates intact. This improves prognosis and allows spontaneous correction of the kyphosis with growth. Medical management is the primary treatment. Treat all patients with at least three drugs for a prolonged period.

Operative management is controversial. Undisputed indications include a significant neurological deficit, a neurological deficit or kyphosis progressing despite adequate medical management, or compromised pulmonary function from the abscess.

Tuberculous Osteomyelitis

In young children this may be associated with BCG vaccination. The children are usually afebrile and show local swelling and discomfort, which may alter function. Mild leukocytosis and increased ESR are common. The CRP is usually normal. Radiographs show metaphyseal lesions with soft tissue swelling. Manage with operative drainage and long-term antituberculosis chemotherapy for about 1 year.

Tuberculous Arthritis

In contrast to pyogenic arthritis, tuberculosis causes a slow, progressive joint disintegration (Fig. 12.67). Management usually requires medical management, joint debridemen, and stabilization such as by arthrodesis.

Consultant Hugh Watts, e-mail: hwatts@ucla.edu

Meningococcal Infections

Purpura Fulminans

Meniongococcemia causes disseminated intravascular coagulation. This results in extensive soft tissue damage with compartment syndromes and skin necrosis most evident in the extremities (Figs. 12.68).

Meningococcal Multifocal Osteomyelitis

This infection is unique as it often affects the growth plate causing physeal fusions and severe deformities (Figs. 12.69 and 12.70).

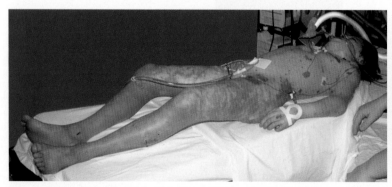
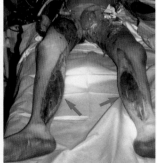

Fig. 12.68 Necrotizing fasciitis. This 12-year-old boy developed meningococcemia and four-extremity involvement. Despite fasciotomies (arrows), the limbs became gangrenous. The disease was fatal.

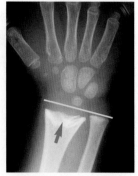

Fig. 12.69 Physeal arrest from meningococcemia. Note the sclerosis and shortening of the radius.

Chronic Recurrent Multifocal Osteomyelitis

Chronic recurrent multifocal osteomyelitis (CRMO) is a rare form of osteomyelitis of unknown etiology characterized by symmetrical bone lesions (Fig. 12.71). It is occasionally associated with palmoplantar pustulosis. The lesions were most often located at the metaphyseal region of tubular bones and the clavicle, but also at the spine, ischiopubic bone, and the sacroiliac joint. Progressive sclerosis and hyperostosis occurred mostly in the clavicle and occasionally in the tibia, femur, metatarsal, and ischiopubic bone, similar to those sclerosing bacterial osteomyelitis. Less common is unilateral involvement (Fig. 12.72) CRMO is often recurrent, but resolves slowly over an extended period. Cultures are negative and antibiotic treatment ineffective. Treat with nonsteroidal antiinflammatory drugs.

Chapter consultant Kit Song, e-mail: ksong@chrmc.org

References

1999 Pyomyositis in children and adolescents: report of 12 cases and review of the literature. Spiegel DA, et al. JPO 19:143

1999 Tuberculous osteomyelitis in young children. Wang MNH, et al. JPO 19:151

1998 Chronic recurrent osteomyelitis with clavicular involvement in children: diagnostic value of different imaging techniques and therapy with non-steroidal anti-inflammatory drugs. Girschick HJ, et al. Eur J Pediatr 157:28

1998 The conservative management of acute pyogenic iliopsoas abscess in children. Tong CW, et al. JBJS 80B:83

1997 Acute staphylococcal osteomyelitis of the clavicle. Lowden CM, Walsh SJ. JPO 17:467

1996 Orthopedic manifestations of invasive group A streptococcal infections complicating primary varicella. Mills WJ, Mosca VS, Nizet V. JPO 16:522.

1996 Tuberculosis of bones and joints (current concepts review). Watts HG, Lifeso RM. JBJS 78A:288

1995 Toxic shock syndrome as a complication of orthopedic surgery. Grimes J, Carpenter C, Reinker K. JPO 15:666

1995 Invasion of the growth plate by bone tumors and osteomyelitis in childhood. Jager HJ, et al. Radiologe 35:409

1995 Acute hematogenous osteomyelitis of the epiphysis. Longjohn DB, Zionts LE, Stott NS. CO 316:227

1994 Pediatric Lyme arthritis: clinical spectrum and outcome. Rose CD, et al. JPO 14:238

1993 Osteomyelitis in sickle cell disease. Piehl FC, Davis RJ, Prugh SI. JPO 13:225

1991 Osteomyelitis in patients who have sickle-cell disease. Diagnosis and management. Epps CH Jr, et al. JBJS 73A:1281

1989 Chondro-osseous growth abnormalities after meningococcemia. A clinical and histopathological study. Grogan DP, et al. JBJS 71A:920

1988 Chronic recurrent multifocal osteomyelitis: a follow-up study. Jurik AG, et al. JPO 8:49

1984 Foci of chronic circumscribed osteomyelitis (Brodie's abscess) that traverse the epiphyseal plate. Bogoch E, Thompson G, Salter RB. JPO 2:162

1983 Osteomyelitis of the pelvis in children. Highland TR, La Mont RL. JBJS 65A:230

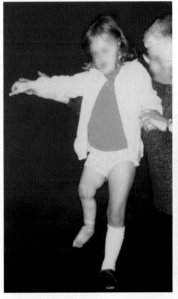
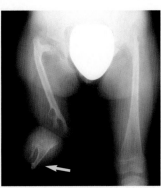

Fig.12.70 Meningococcemia with growth plate injury. This child developed meningitis and meningococcemia. Mengiococcal osteomyelitis damaged the growth plate causing severe residual shortening of the right leg. A below the knee amputation was performed to make prosthetic fitting possible (yellow arrow).

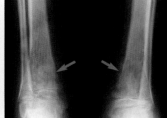
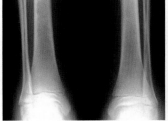

Fig. 12.71 Chronic recurrent multifocal osteomyelitis. This atypical form of osteomyelitis produces symmetrical bone lesions (red arrows).

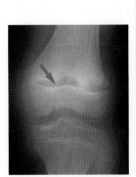
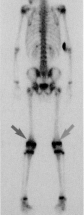
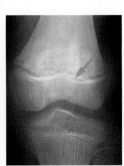

Fig. 12.72 Unilateral chronic recurrent multifocal osteomyelitis. Note the unilateral right distal femoral metaphysis involvement (red arrows). The left femur (green arrows) is not affected.

Alderson M, Speers D, Emslie K, et al. Acute haematogenous osteomyelitis and septic arthritis—a single disease: an hypothesis based upon the presence of transphyseal blood vessels. J Bone Joint Surg 1986;68B:268-274

Andrew TA, Porter K. Primary subacute epiphyseal osteomyelitis: a report of three cases. J Pediatr Orthop 1985;5:155-157.

Behr JT, et al. Herpetic infections in the fingers of infants. J Bone Joint Surg 1987;69A:137-139.

Betz RR, Cooperman DR, Wopperer JM, et al. Late sequelae of septic arthritis of the hip in infancy and childhood. J Pediatr Orthop 1990;10:365-372.

Biyani A, Sharma JC. Continuous suction and intermittent irrigation for septic coxitis. Acta Orthop Scand 1988;59:664.

Borman TR, Johnson RA, Sherman FC. Gallium scintigraphy for diagnosis of septic arthritis and osteomyelitis in children. J Pediatr Orthop 1986;6:317-325.

Cristofaro RL, Appel MH, Gelb RI, et al. Musculoskeletal manifestations of Lyme disease in children. J Pediatr Orthop 1987;7:527-530.

Danielsson LG, Gupta RP. Four cases of purulent arthritis of the shoulder secondary to hematogenous osteomyelitis. Acta Orthop Scand 1989;60:591.

Daoud A, Saighi-Bouaouina A. Treatment of sequestra, pseudarthroses, and defects in the long bones of children who have chronic hematogenous osteomyelitis. J Bone Joint Surg 1989;71A:1448-1468.

Farley T, Conway J, Shulman ST. Hematogenous pelvic osteomyelitis in children. Am J Dis Child 1985;139:946.

Fink CW, Nelson JD. Septic arthritis and rheumatism in children. Clin Rheum Dis 1986;12:423-435.

Gamble JG, Rinsky LA. Chronic recurrent multifocal osteomyelitis: a distinct clinical entity. J Pediatr Orthop 1986;6:579-584.

Green NE. Musculoskeletal infections in children: Part VI. Disseminated gonococcal infections and gonococcal arthritis. In Evarts CM (ed): AAOS Instruct Course Lect 1983;32:48-50.

Green NE, Edwards K. Bone and joint infections in children. Orthop Clin North Am 1989;18:555-576.

Grogan DP, Love SM, Ogden JA, et al. Chondro-osseous growth abnormalities after meningococcemia. A clinical and histopathological study. J Bone Joint Surg 1989;71A:920.

Gustilo RB, Gruninger RP, Tsukayama DT (eds). Orthopedic Infection: Diagnosis and Treatment. Philadelphia, WP Saunders, 1989.

Hamdan J, Asha M, Mallouh A, et al. Technetium bone scintigraphy in the diagnosis of osteomyelitis in children. Pediatr Infect Dis J 1987;6:529.

Hansen ES, Hjortdal VE, Noer I, et al. Three phase [Tc99m] diphosphonate scintimetry in septic and non-septic arthritis of the immature knee: an experimental investigation in dogs. J Orthop Res 1989;7:543.

Herndon WA, Alexieva BT, Schwindt ML, et al. Nuclear imaging for musculoskeletal infections in children. J Pediatr Orthop 1985;5:343-347.

Hoffman EB, de Beer, J de V, Keys G, et al. Diaphyseal primary subacute osteomyelitis in children. J Pediatr Orthop 1990;10:250-254.

Jackson MA, Nelson JD. Etiology and medical management of acute suppurative bone and joint infections in pediatric patients. J Pediatr Orthop 1982;2:313-323.

Jacobs RF, McCarthy RE, Elser JM. Pseudomonas osteochondritis complicating puncture wounds of the foot in children: a 10-year evaluation. J Infect Dis 1989;160:657-661.

Johanson PH. Pseudomonas infections in the foot following puncture wounds. JAMA 1968;204:262-264.

Kumar K, Saxena MBL. Multifocal osteoarticular tuberculosis. Int Orthop 1988;12:135.

Lewis JS, et al. Acute osteomyelitis in children: combined Tc-99m and Ga-67 imaging. Radiology 1986;158:795.

Medical Research Council Working Party on Tuberculosis of the Spine. A 10-year assessment of a controlled trial comparing debridement and anterior spinal fusion in the management of tuberculosis of the spine in patients on standard chemotherapy in Hong Kong: eighth report. J Bone Joint Surg 1982;64B:393-398.

Morrissy RT, Haynes DW. Acute hematogenous osteomyelitis: a model with trauma as an etiology. J Pediatr Orthop 1989;9:447-456.

Nade S. Acute septic arthritis in infancy and childhood. J Bone Joint Surg 1983;65B:234-241.

Norden CW, Budinsky A. Treatment of experimental chronic osteomyelitis due to staphylococcus aureus with ampicillin/sulbactam. J Infect Dis 1990;161:52.

Paterson MP, Hoffman EB, Roux P. Severe disseminated staphylococcal disease associated with osteitis and septic arthritis. J Bone Joint Surg 1990;72B:94-97.

Pelkonen P, Ryoppy S, Jaaskelainen J, et al. Chronic osteomyelitislike disease with negative bacterial cultures. Am J Dis Child 1988;142:1167.

Perry J, Burke S, Haddad RJ. Psoas abscess mimicking a septic hip. Diagnosis by computed tomography. J Bone Joint Surg 1985;67A:1281.

Rasool MN, Govender S. The skeletal manifestations of congenital syphilis. A review of 197 cases. J Bone Joint Surg 1979;79B:752-755.

Roberts JM, Drummond DS, Breed AL, et al. Subacute hematogenous osteomyelitis in children: a retrospective study. J Pediatr Orthop 1982;2:249-254.

Rud B, Halken S, Damholt V. Hematogenous osteomyelitis in children. Acta Orthop Scand 1986;57:440-443.

Scoles PV, Aronoff SC. Antimicrobial therapy of childhood skeletal infections. J Bone Joint Surg 1984;66A:1487-1492.

Scott RJ, Christofersen MR, Robertson WW Jr, et al. Acute osteomyelitis in children: a review of 116 cases. J Pediatr Orthop 1990;10:649-652.

Sorenson TS, Hedeboe J, Christensen RR. Primary epiphyseal osteomyelitis in children. Report of three cases and review of the literature. J Bone Joint Surg 1988;70B:818.

Staheli LT, Nelp WB, Marty, R. Strontium 87m scanning. early diagnosis of bone and joint infections in children. JAMA 1972, 221:1159.

Sueoka BL, et al. Infantile infectious sacroiliitis. Pediatr Radiol 1985;15:403.

Sundberg SB, Savage JP, Foster BK. Technetium phosphate bone scan in the diagnosis of septic arthritis in childhood. J Pediatr Orthop 1989;9:579-585.

Syrogiannopoulos GA, McCracken GH Jr, Nelson JD. Osteoarticular infections in children with sickle cell disease. Pediatrics 1986;78:1090-1096.

Van Howe RS, Starshak RJ, Chusid MJ. Chronic, recurrent multifocal osteomyelitis. Clin Ped 1989;28:54.

Whalen JL, Fitzgerald RH, Morrissy RT. A histological study of acute hematogenous osteomyelitis following physeal injuries in rabbits. J Bone Joint Surg 1988;70A:1383.

Wingstrand H, Egund N, Lidgren L, et al. Sonography in septic arthritis of the hip in the child: report of four cases. J Pediatr Orthop 1987;7:206-209.

Wopperer JM, White JJ, Gillespie R, et al. Long-term follow-up of infantile hip sepsis. J Pediatr Orthop 1988;8:322-325.

Chapter 13—Tumors

About 2000–3000 new cases of malignancies of the musculoskeletal system are diagnosed each year in United States. The number of benign neoplasms is estimated to be about ten times this number.

Evaluation

Evaluate tumors by taking the patient's history, performing a careful physical examination, and obtaining necessary laboratory and imaging studies. Usually the diagnosis of a tumor is made by the presence of pain, a mass, or a pathologic fracture, it may be as an incidental finding (Fig. 13.1).

History

Tumors usually present as a mass, produce pain, or cause disability. How long a mass has been present is often difficult to determine from a history. Frequently, a large lesion such as a slow-growing osteochondroma is not noticed until shortly before the consultation. The family incorrectly concludes that the tumor had grown quickly.

Pain is a more reliable indicator of the time of onset of a tumor. Inquire about the onset, progression, severity, and character of the pain. Night pain is characteristic of both malignant tumors and some benign lesions such as osteoid osteoma. Malignant lesions produce pain that progressively increases over a period of weeks. Night pain in the adolescent is especially worrisome and should be evaluated first with a conventional radiograph. An abrupt onset of pain is usually due to a pathologic fracture. Such fractures most commonly occur through bone cysts.

Age of the patient is helpful. Bone lesions in children under age 5 years are likely to be due to an infection or eosinophilic granuloma. Giant cell tumors and osteoblastomas occur in the late teen period.

Race is notable, as blacks seldom develop Ewing sarcoma.

Examination

A screening examination should be performed first. Some lesions, such as osteochondroma, are usually multiple. Look for asymmetry, deformity, or swelling. Palpate for masses. If a mass is present, measure its size, assess for tenderness, and note any associated inflammation. Malignant tumors are typically firm, often tender, and may produce signs of inflammation.

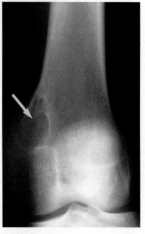
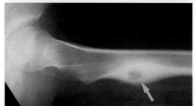
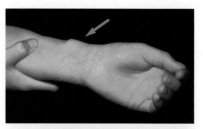
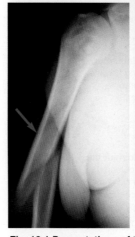

Fig. 13.1 Presentations of tumors in children. The common modes of presentation are with a mass, as in osteochondroma (green arrow); with pain, as in ostoid osteoma (orange arrow); with a pathologic fracture, as in osteosarcoma (red arrow); or as an incidental finding, such as this small nonossifying fibroma (yellow arrow).

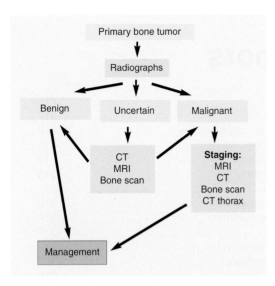

Fig. 13.2 Flowchart for imaging primary bone tumors.

Imaging

Order imaging studies with a plan in mind (Fig. 13.2). Start with good-quality radiographs. Conventional radiographs remain the basic tool for diagnosis. Consider several features in assessment.

Location Lesions tend to occur in typical locations both with respect to the bone involved (Fig. 13.3) and the position in the bone (Fig. 13.4).

Effect of lesion Note the lesion's effect on the surrounding tissue (Fig. 13.6).

Effect of lesion on bone Sharply punched out lesions are typical of eosinophilic granuloma. Osteolytic lesions are typical of most tumors; few are osteogenic on radiographs.

Effect on normal adjacent bone is useful in determining the invasiveness of the lesion. An irregular, moth-eaten appearance suggests a malignant lesion or an infection. A lesion that expands the adjacent cortex is usually benign and typical for aneurysmal bone cysts.

Diagnostic features suggest the aggressiveness of the lesion. Sclerotic margination suggests that the lesion is long-standing and benign. Periosteal reaction suggests a malignant, traumatic, or infectious etiology.

Special imaging Consider special types of conventional radiographs such as for soft tissue or bone detail (Fig. 13.5).

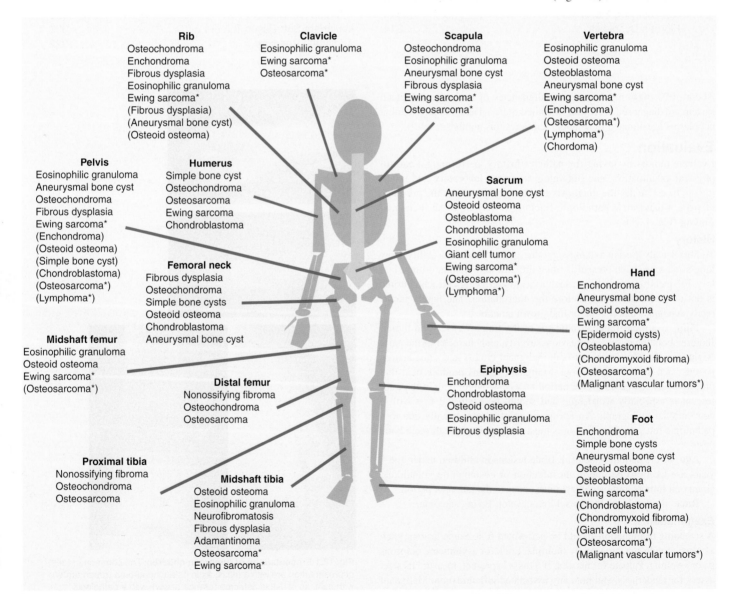

Fig. 13.3 Tumor types per site. Less common tumors at each site are in parentheses. Asterisks (*) indicate malignant tumors. Based on Adler and Kozlowski (1993).

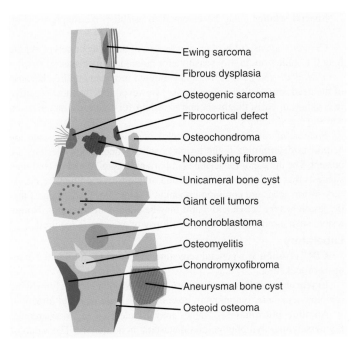

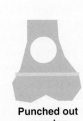

Ewing sarcoma
Fibrous dysplasia
Osteogenic sarcoma
Fibrocortical defect
Osteochondroma
Nonossifying fibroma
Unicameral bone cyst
Giant cell tumors
Chondroblastoma
Osteomyelitis
Chondromyxofibroma
Aneurysmal bone cyst
Osteoid osteoma

Fig. 13.4 Typical locations for various tumors.

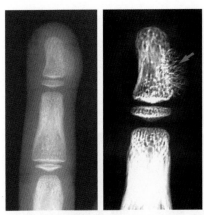

Fig. 13.5 High-resolution radiographs. Compared to conventional radiography (left), note the increased bony detail shown by the high-resolution radiograph (red arrow).

Effect of lesion on bone

Punched out margins
Eosinophilic granuloma

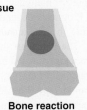
Destructive
Blurred margins
Malignant tumor
Infection

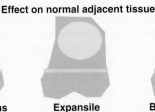
Aggressive
Crosses physis
Malignant tumor
Infection

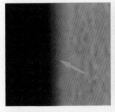
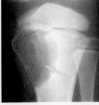
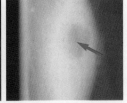

Effect of lesion on bone. Bone destruction from eosinophilic granuloma in an infant (green), destructive lesion in osteogenic sarcoma (yellow), and aggressive osteogenic sarcoma that readily crosses the physis (red).

Effect on normal adjacent tissue

Sclerotic margins benign
Nonossifying fibroma

Expansile benign
Aneurysmal bone cyst

Bone reaction varied
Osteogenic sarcoma
Eosinophilic granuloma
Infection

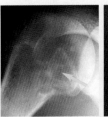
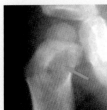

Effect of lesion on normal adjacent tissue. Note the sclerotic margins in the nonossifying fibroma (green), expanded cortex in an aneurysmal bone cyst (yellow), and marked periosteal reaction in an eosinophilic granuloma (red).

Diagnostic features of lesion

Ground glass
Diaphyseal fibrous dysplasia

Speckled
Cartilage tumor

Osteoblastic
Varied tumor
Infection

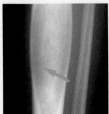
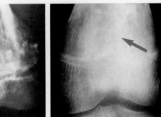

Diagnostic features. Note the ground glass appearance of fibrous dysplasia (green), speckled calcification in a cartilage tumor (yellow), and osteoblastic features of an osteoblastic osteogenic sarcoma (red).

Fig. 13.6 Diagnostic features by conventional radiography. Note the effect of the lesions on bone (top), the effect on normal adjacent tissues (middle), and special diagnostic features (bottom).

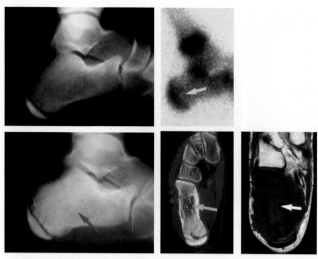

Fig. 13.7 Evaluation by imaging. This child had foot pain and a negative radiograph (upper left). A month later, the patient was seen again with increasing night pain. At that time, a bone scan showed increased uptake (yellow arrow), the radiograph showed increased density of the calcaneus (red arrow), a CT scan showed erosion of the calcaneus (orange arrow), and MRI showed extensive marrow involvement (white arrow). Ewing sarcoma was suspected by these findings.

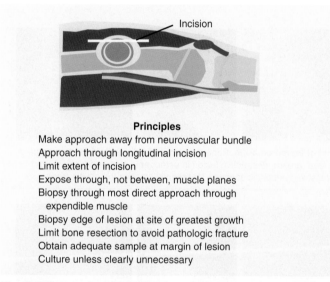

Incision

Principles
Make approach away from neurovascular bundle
Approach through longitudinal incision
Limit extent of incision
Expose through, not between, muscle planes
Biopsy through most direct approach through
    expendible muscle
Biopsy edge of lesion at site of greatest growth
Limit bone resection to avoid pathologic fracture
Obtain adequate sample at margin of lesion
Culture unless clearly unnecessary

Fig. 13.8 Biopsy principles. Follow these basic principles during biopsy procedures.

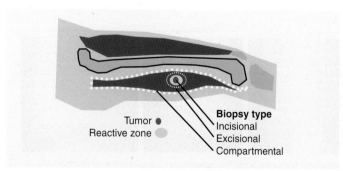

Tumor ●
Reactive zone ●

Biopsy type
Incisional
Excisional
Compartmental

Fig. 13.9 Biopsy types. These include incision, excision, and compartmental resection, depending upon the objective of the biopsy.

Special studies may be essential to establish the diagnosis (Fig. 13.7).

CT scans are useful in assessing lesions of the spine or pelvis. Whole lung CT studies are highly sensitive for pulmonary metastases.

MRI is the most expensive and is limited in young children because of the need for sedation or anesthesia. However, it is the most sensitive in making an early diagnosis and excellent for tissue characterization and staging of tumors.

Bone scans are the next most useful diagnostic tool. These scans are helpful in determining if the lesion is solitary and if other lesions are present. The uptake of the lesion is important to note. A cool or cold scan suggests that the lesion is inactive, and only observation may be necessary. Warm scans are common in benign lesions. Hot scans suggest that the lesion is very active and that it may be either a malignant or benign lesion, such as an osteoid osteoma. Biopsy or excision is required.

Laboratory
CBC is useful as a general screening battery and helpful in the diagnosis of leukemia.

Erythrocyte sedimentation rate (ESR) is often elevated in Ewing sarcoma, leukemia, lymphomas, eosinophilic granuloma, and infection.

Alkaline phosphatase values may be elevated in osteosarcoma, Ewing sarcoma, lymphoma, and metastatic bone tumors. The value of the study is limited because of the natural elevation of this value during growth, especially in the adolescent.

Biopsy
The biopsy is a critical step in management (Fig. 13.8) and should be performed thoughtfully by an experienced surgeon. In most cases, an open biopsy is appropriate. Needle biopsy is indicated for lesions located at inaccessible sites and for special circumstances. The biopsy should provide an adequate sample of involved tissue, and the tissue should be cultured unless the lesion is clearly neoplastic. The biopsy procedure should not compromise subsequent reconstructive procedures.

Biopsies can be incisional, excisional, or compartmental in type (Fig. 13.9). Excisional biopsy is appropriate for benign lesions such as osteoid osteoma (Fig. 13.10) or for other lesions when the diagnosis is known before the procedure and the lesion can be totally resected.

Staging
Staging of malignant tumors provides a means of establishing a prognosis. Prognosis depends on the grade of the lesion (potential for metastases), the extent and size of the lesion, and the response to chemotherapy. The extent of the lesion is categorized by whether the lesion is extracompartmental or intracompartmental (Fig. 13.11) and whether any distant metastases are present. A knowledge of the response to chemotherapy (Fig. 13.13) helps the surgeon to determine the appropriateness of limb salvage procedures and how wide the surgical margins must be to avoid local recurrence following resection.

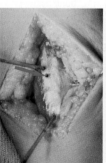
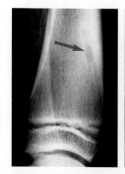
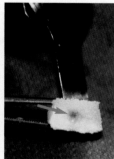

Fig. 13.10 Excisional biopsy of osteoid osteoma. The original lesion (red and blue arrows) is excised in a block of bone. This block is divided in the operating room to make certain the entire lesion is removed. The nidus of the tumor is clearly seen (green arrow).

Differential Diagnosis

Differentiating from Myositis Ossificans

Differentiating bone tumors from myositis ossificans (MO) is sometimes difficult. MO lesions have reactive bone that is most active on the margins. MRI studies are rarely necessary, but will show an inflammatory lesion with a tumor core (Fig. 13.12).

Differentiating Neoplasms, Infection, and Trauma

Sometimes a child presents with pain (Fig. 13.14) and tenderness over a long bone (usually the tibia or femur). The radiographs may be negative or show only slight periosteal elevation. The differential diagnosis often includes osteomyelitis, a stress fracture, or Ewing sarcoma (Fig. 13.15). This differentiation is usually established without a biopsy. The evaluation usually requires a careful physical examination, radiographs, a bone scan, and a determination of the ESR.

References

2000 Initial symptoms and clinical features of osteosarcoma and Ewing sarcoma. Widhe B, Widhe T. JBJS 82A:667.

1999 New developments in the staging and imaging of soft-tissue sarcomas. Cheng EY, Thompson RC. JBJS 81A:882

1996 Preface to pediatric orthopedic oncology. Heinrich SD, Scarborough MT, OCNA 27:421

1996 The staging of surgery of musculoskeletal neoplasms. Wolf RE, Enneking WF OCNA 27:473

1996 Evaluation of the child with a bone or soft-tissue neoplasm. Letson GD, Greenfield GB, Heinrich SD. OCNA 27:431

1993 Primary Bone Tumors and Tumorous Conditions in Children. Adler CP, Kazimierz Kozlowski K, Springer-Verlag, Berlin.

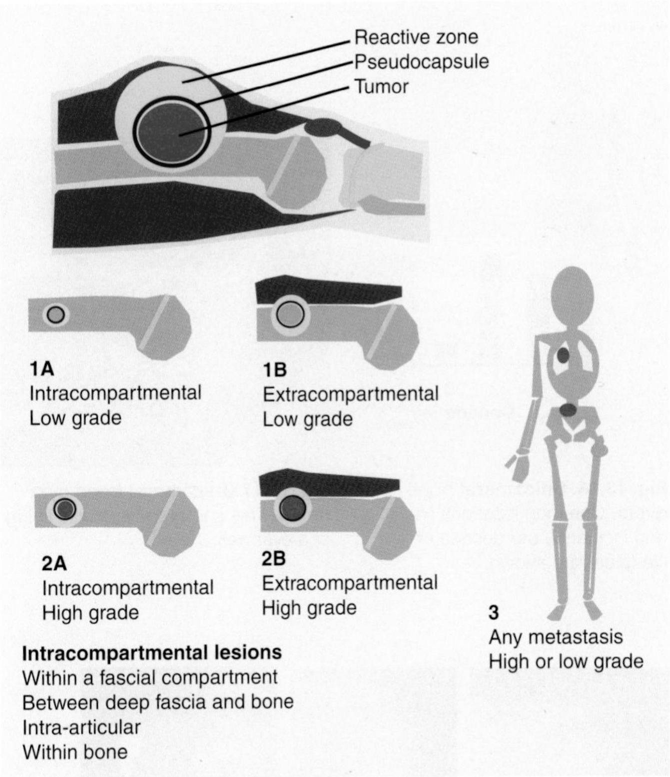

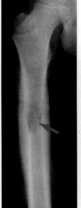

Reactive zone
Pseudocapsule
Tumor

1A Intracompartmental Low grade

1B Extracompartmental Low grade

2A Intracompartmental High grade

2B Extracompartmental High grade

3 Any metastasis High or low grade

Intracompartmental lesions
Within a fascial compartment
Between deep fascia and bone
Intra-articular
Within bone

Fig. 13.11 Staging of musculoskeletal tumors. Staging is determined by the grade and extent of the lesion. Based on Wolf and Enneking (1996).

Grade	Tumor response in osteosarcoma
1	Little or none
2	Extensive necrosis >10% viable tumor
3	Extensive necrosis <10% viable tumor
4	Complete necrosis

Fig. 13.13 Response to chemotherapy. The response to chemotherapy is helpful in determining the prognosis and subsequent management.

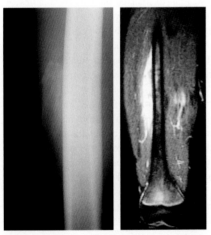

Fig. 13.12 Myositis ossificans. Note that the lesion appears to be extracortical in origin and that the inflammatory mass does not include the bone.

Category	Examination	Imaging or laboratory	Comment
Malignant tumor	Mass, diffuse tenderness and MRI findings	Hot bone scan	Pain progressive, often occurs at night
Osteomyelitis	Inflammatory signs Metaphyseal location	Elevated ESR Warm to hot bone scan Culture positive	Systemic illness Recent onset
Stress fracture	Localized tenderness Typical locations	Normal ESR, no mass	Overuse history Pain reduces with rest

Fig. 13.14 Differentiating tumor, infection, and traumatic lesions. Features of the lesion allow classification into diagnostic categories without the need for a biopsy.

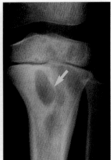

Fig. 13.15 Bone infections. Sometimes unusual bone infections may be difficult to differentiate from tumors, as a diaphyseal lesion (red arrow) or osteomyelitis that extends across the physis (yellow arrow).

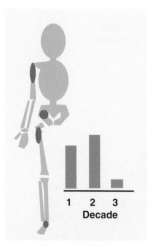

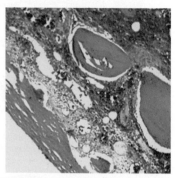

Fig. 13.16. Unicameral bone cysts. Common locations (red) and incidence per decade of life (blue) are shown.

Fig. 13.17 Unicameral bone cyst lining. This shows the synovial lining of a cyst wall.

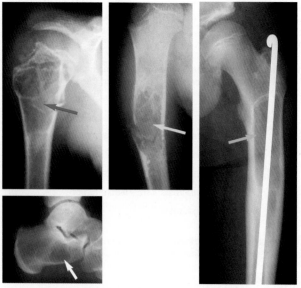

Fig. 13.18 Unicameral bone cysts. Note the typical active (red arrow) and inactive (yellow arrow) cysts with fractures. Flexible intramedullary rod fixation of an upper femoral cyst (orange arrow) is shown. A calcaneal cyst is an additional common site (white arrow).

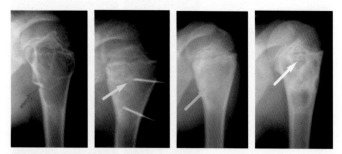

Fig. 13.19 Unicameral bone cyst. This is the classic location of this type of bone cyst. This 12-year-old boy developed pain in the right upper arm; a radiograph showed the typical cyst with a pathologic fracture (red arrow). The lesion was treated by steroid injection (yellow arrow) with satisfactory healing (orange arrow). A year later, the cyst has recurred (white arrow), but not to a degree that required additional treatment.

Unicameral Bone Cysts

Unicameral (UBC), solitary, or simple bone cysts are common lesions of unknown cause that generally occur in the upper humerus or femur (Fig. 13.16). Theories of etiology include a defect in enchondral bone formation or altered hemodynamics with venous obstruction causing increased interosseous pressure and cyst formation. The cysts are filled with yellow fluid and lined with fibrous tissue (Fig. 13.17).

Diagnosis

These cysts are most often first diagnosed when complicated by a pathologic fracture (Fig. 13.18). Their radiographic appearance is usually characteristic. The lesions are usually metaphyseal, expand the bone, have well-defined margins, evoke little reaction, and appear cystic with irregular septa. Sometimes a fragment of cortical bone (called *fallen leaf sign*) can be seen in the bottom of the cavity.

Active cysts abut the growth plate and occur in children less than 10 to 12 years of age. They are more likely to recur after treatment.

Inactive cysts are separated from the plate by normal bone and usually occur in adolescents over age 12 years.

Fractures are usually the presenting complaint. Sometimes the fracture line is difficult to separate.

Management

Management is complicated by recurrence. The usual natural history of these cysts is to become asymptomatic following skeletal maturation. The objective of treatment is to minimize the disability when cysts are likely to fracture. These lesions are not precancerous.

Humeral cysts Place the child in a sling to allow the fracture to heal and reestablish stability. Seldom does the effect of the trauma result in permanent healing of the cyst. Plan to manage the cyst by a series of injections (Fig. 13.19) with steroid, bone marrow, or bone matrix. Some doctors recommend breaking up the adhesion by forceful injections or perforating the septa with a trochar. Recurrence can be managed by repeated injections or curettage and grafting with autogenous or bank bone. Opinions differ regarding how aggressively recurrence is managed. See page 409.

Femoral cysts are much more difficult to manage. Plan to curette and graft the cyst and stabilize the fracture with flexible intramedullary fixation. Complications include malunion with coxa vara and avascular necrosis with displaced neck fractures. This fixation is permanent and may prevent additional fractures even if some recurrent cyst formation occurs. An alternative approach is injection followed by spica cast protection for 6 weeks.

Calcaneal cysts are best managed by curettage and bone grafting.

Complications

Recurrence and growth arrest of the upper humeral physis are most common. Growth arrest is usually due to the lesion, not the surgery. Recurrence is common and requires long-term thoughtful management.

References

2000 Unicameral bone cysts. Wilkins RM. JAAOS 8:217.

1998 Simple bone cysts treated with aspiration and a single bone marrow injection. A preliminary report. Delloye C, et al. Int Orthop 22:134

1998 Growth arrest resulting from unicameral bone cyst. Stanton RP, Abdel-Mota'al MM. JPO 18:198

1997 Incomplete healing of simple bone cysts after steroid injections. Hashemi-Nejad A, Cole WG. JBJS 79B:727

1996 Unicameral and aneurysmal bone cysts. Capanna R, Campanacci DA, Manfrini M. Orthop Clin North Am 27:605

1996 Contribution to the vascular origin of the unicameral bone cyst. Gebhart M, Blaimont P. Acta Orthop Belg 62:137

1994 Unicameral bone cyst of the calcaneus in children. Moreau G, Letts M. JPO 14:101

Aneurysmal Bone Cysts

An aneurysmal bone cyst (ABC) is considered to be a pseudotumor possibly secondary to subperiosteal or interosseous hemorrhage or a transitional lesion secondary to some primary bone tumor.

Diagnosis

The diagnosis can usually be established by a combination of the location of the lesion, the age of the patient (Fig. 13.20), and the appearance on conventional radiographs (Fig. 13.21). ABCs are eccentric, expansile, cystic lesions. They often present with defined patterns (Fig. 13.23). Sometimes the lesions are less eccentric and difficult to differentiate from simple bone cysts (Fig. 13.24).

Activity of the lesion The activity level can also be assessed by the appearance of the lesion's margins.

Inactive cysts have intact, well-defined margins.

Active cysts have incomplete margins but the lesion is well defined.

Aggressive cysts show little reactive bone formation and poorly defined margins.

Other imaging is often necessary, especially in aggressive cysts. Fluid levels are common and can be seen on CT scans and MRI studies (Fig. 13.22).

Management

Manage ABCs on the basis of the patient's age, the site, and the size of the lesion.

Age ABCs in early childhood are very likely to recur. Plan for this probability in discussing the procedure with the family.

Spine About 10–30% of these lesions are in the spine. Study with CT and MRI preoperatively. The possible need for a combined approach, complete excision, and stabilization, as well as the risk of recurrence, complicates management.

Long bones Options include complete excision or saucerization leaving a cortical segment intact, or curettage with cryotherapy or with a mechanical burr. Consider prophylactic intramedullary rodding to prevent refracture.

Pelvis Manage most lesions by curettage and bone grafting. Some recommend selective embolization. Be prepared for extensive blood loss.

References
1999 Aneurysmal bone cyst of the extremities. Gibbs CP, et al. JBJS 81A:1671
1998 Aneurysmal bone cysts: percutaneous embolization with an alcoholic solution of zein- -series of 18 cases. Guibaud L, et al. Radiology 208:369
1997 Embolization in the treatment of aneurysmal bone cysts. Green JA, Bellemore MC, Marsden FW. JPO 17:440
1997 Cementation of primary aneurysmal bone cysts. Ozaki T, et al. CO 337:240
1996 Unicameral and aneurysmal bone cysts. Capanna R, Campanacci DA, Manfrini M. Orthop Clin North Am 27:605
1994 Aneurysmal bone cysts in young children. Freiberg AA, et al. JPO 14:86
1985 Anerysmal cysts of long bones. Capanna R, et al. Ital J Orthop Traumatol 11:421.

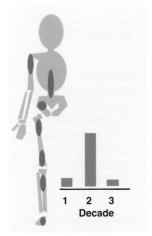

Fig. 13.20 Aneurysmal bone cysts. Shown here are the common locations (red) and incidence per decade of growth (blue).

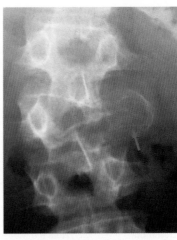

Fig. 13.21 Aneurysmal bone cyst of the vertebral column.

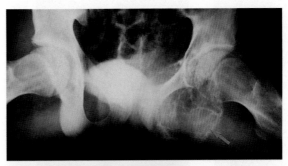

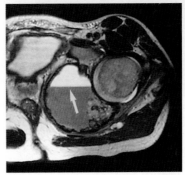

Fig. 13.22 Aneurysmal bone cyst of the pelvis. Note the extensive lesion (red arrow) and fluid level (yellow arrow) on the MRI.

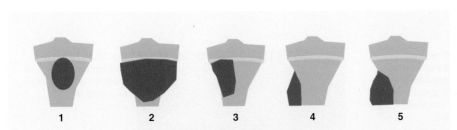

Fig. 13.23 Classification of aneurysmal bone cysts. Types 1–5 are various common patterns of lesions of long bones. Based on Capanna et al. (1985).

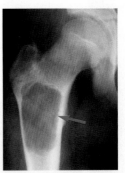

Fig. 13.24. Aneurysmal bone cyst of the upper femur.

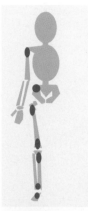

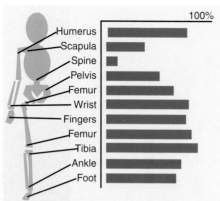

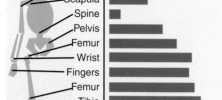

Humerus
Scapula
Spine
Pelvis
Femur
Wrist
Fingers
Femur
Tibia
Ankle
Foot

100%

Fig. 13.25 Common locations of solitary osteochondromatas.

Fig. 13.26 Multiple familial osteochondromatas. Note the widespread involvement. Based on data by Jesus-Garcia (1996).

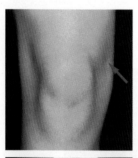

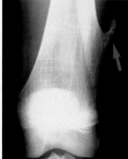

Fig. 13.27 Typical location for symptomatic lesions. Lesions about the knee are frequently irritated and painful (red arrows).

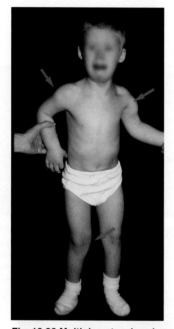

Fig. 13.28 Multiple osteochondroma. This child has multiple lesions (arrows).

Benign Cartilagenous Tumors

Osteochondroma

Osteochondromas (osteocartilagenous exostoses) include solitary (Fig. 13.25) and multiple lesions (Fig. 13.26). The multiple form is inherited but thought to be due to a loss or mutation of two tumor suppressor genes. Lesions sometimes develop after chemotherapy and radiation therapy. Most tumors develop by enchondral ossification under a cartilage cap.

Diagnosis Osteochondromas are usually first noted as masses that are painful when injured during play (Fig. 13.27). These lesions are usually pedunculated but may be sessile. They may grow to a large size. Osteochondromas are so characteristic in appearance that the diagnosis is made by conventional radiographs.

Solitary Osteochondromatas These lesions are most common in the metaphyses of long bones. They occur sporadically and present as a mass, often about the knee. Presentations in the spine may be associated with neurologic dysfunction.

Multiple Osteochondromatas The common multiple form (Fig. 13.28) is inherited in an autosomal dominant pattern and is more common in boys. Multiple lesions about the wrist and ankle often cause progressive deformity (Fig. 13.29). Others may cause valgus deformities about the knee.

Management depends on the location and size of the tumor.

Painful mass is the most common indication for removal (Fig. 13.30). Often several lesions are removed in one operative setting. Complications of excision include peroneal neuropraxia, arterial lacerations, compartment syndromes, and pathologic fracture.

Valgus knee can be managed by medial femoral or tibial hemistapling in late childhood.

Limb length inequality may require correction by an epiphysiodesis.

Ankle and wrist deformities result from growth retardation of the distal ulna or fibula. Management of these deformities is complex and controversial.

Prognosis Very rarely malignant transformation to chondrosarcoma occurs during adult life. Because the transformation is very rare, prophylactic removal is not appropriate.

References

2000 Clinical and radiographic analysis of osteochondromas and growth disturbance in hereditary multiple exostoses. Porter DE, et al. JPO 20:246

1999 Clinical correlation to genetic variations of hereditary multiple exostosis. Carroll KL, et al. JPO 19:785

1998 Clonal karyotypic abnormalities of the hereditary multiple exostoses chromosomal loci 8q24.1 (EXT1) and 11p11-12 (EXT2) in patients with sporadic and hereditary osteochondromas. Bridge J, et al. Cancer 82:1657

1997 Management of forearm deformity in multiple hereditary osteochondromatosis. Arms DM, et al. JPO 17:450

1997 Surgical risk for elective excision of benign exostoses. Wirganowicz P, Watts H. JPO 17:455

1996 The natural history of hereditary multiple exostoses. Schmale GA, Conrad EW, Raskind WH. JBJS 76A:986.

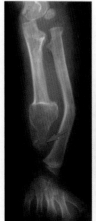

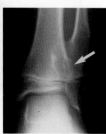

Fig. 13.29 Common deformities that cause disturbed growth. These are common about the wrist (red arrow) and ankle (yellow arrow).

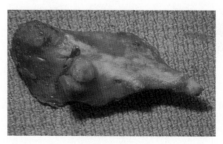

Fig. 13.30 Removed osteochondroma. This resected lesion is large and irregular.

Enchondroma

These cartilage tumors within bone are common in the phalanges and long bones and increase in frequency during childhood (Fig. 13.31). These lesions may expand bone and produce the classic characteristic of cartilage tumors: speckled calcification within the lesion (Fig. 13.32).

Types There are several different types of enchondromas.

Solitary lesions occur most commonly in the hands and feet. Removal and grafting is indicated if the lesions cause disability.

Ollier disease is a generalized disorder with cartilagenous enchondromas as one feature. These children often have limb shortening and varus deformities (Fig. 13.32). About one-fourth develop chondrosarcoma in adult life.

Maffucci syndrome is a rare disorder with subcutaneous hemangiomatas and multiple enchondromatas. Malignant transformation is usual in adult life (see Chapter 15).

Chondroblastoma

These uncommon tumors occur in the epiphysis of long bones often during adolescence (Figs. 13.33 and 13.34) and cause an inflammatory reaction. They can be confused with infection or arthritis. They are aggressive and prone to recur. Treat by thorough curettage and possibly cryotherapy or phenolization and bone grafting. Avoid operative injury to the growth plate or articular cartilage. Expect a recurrence of about 20%.

Chondromyxoid Fibroma

This is a rare primary bone tumor that occurs most commonly about the knee during the second decade. The radiographic appearance is often characteristic with an eccentric position, a sclerotic rim with lobulated margins, and prominent septa. Manage with local resection and grafting.

Dysplasia Epiphysialis Hemimelica

Dysplasia epiphysialis hemimelica (Trevor disease) is a rare cartilagenous tumor that arises from the growth plate or articular cartilage (Fig. 13.35). The most common sites of involvement are the distal tibia and the distal femur. Lesions often involve one side of the epihysis and may show multilevel involvement in the same limb. The diagnosis is often difficult early on, as the lesion is primarily cartilagenous and poorly imaged with conventional radiographs. MRI is helpful in showing the extent of the tumor and separating the lesion from the normal epiphysis or joint cartilage. Excise extraarticular lesions. Remove intraarticular lesions and correct secondary deformity with an osteotomy as necessary. Recurrence of the tumor is common, and multiple resections throughout childhood may be necessary.

References

1999 Chondroblastoma: MR characteristics with pathologic correlation. Jee W, et al. J Comput Assist Tomogr 23:721

1998 Chondroblastoma during the growing age. Schuppers H, et al. JPO-b 7:293

1998 Epiphyseal-metaphyseal enchondromatosis. A new clinical entity. Gabos PG, Bowen JR. JBJS 80A:782

1998 Ollier's disease: varus angulation at the lower femur and its management. Chew DK, Menelaus MB, Richardson MD. JPO 18:202

1998 Dysplasia epiphysialis hemimelica: clinical features and management. Kuo RS, et al. JPO 18:543

1996 MRI characteristics of chondroblastoma. Oxtoby J, Davies A. Clin Radiol 51:22

1992 Dysplasia epiphysialis hemimelica: diagnosis and treatment. Keret D, et al. JPO 12:365

1991 Chondromyxoid fibroma: radiographic appearance in 38 cases and in a review of the literature. Wilson AJ, Kyriakos M, Ackerman LV. Radiology 179:513

1988 The Maffucci syndrome. Ben-Itzhak I, et al. JPO 8:345

1987 The malignant potential of enchondromatosis. Schwartz HS, et al. JBJS 69A:269

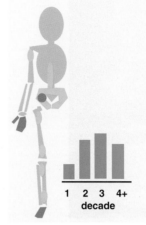

Fig. 13.31 Enchondromatas. Common (red) and less common (orange) locations are shown. Age pattern of involvement is shown in blue.

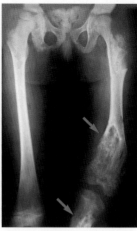

Fig. 13.32 Ollier disease. Note the extensive lesions of the distal femur and tibia (red arrows) with shortening and varus deformity.

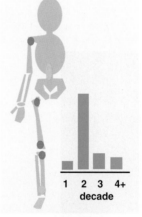

Fig. 13.33 Chondroblastoma. Common (red) and less common (orange) locations are shown. Age pattern of involvement is shown in blue. Based on Schuppers (1998).

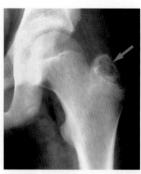

Fig. 13.34 Chondroblastoma. This is a greater trochanter lesion (arrow).

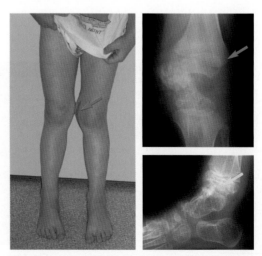

Fig. 13.35 Dysplasia epiphysialis hemimelica. Note the swelling of the knee (red arrows) and ankle involvement (yellow arrow).

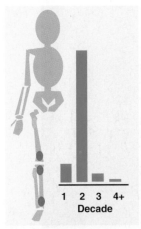

Fig. 13.36 Nonossifying fibroma. Common (red) and less common (orange) locations are shown. Age pattern of involvement is shown in blue.

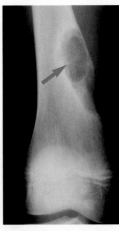

Fig. 13.37 Nonossifying fibroma of the distal femur.

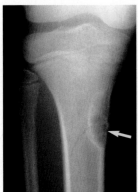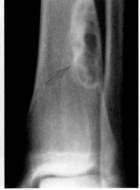

Fig. 13.38 Typical nonossifying fibroma.

Fibrous Tumors

Fibrocortical Defects

Fibrocortical defects (or *fibrous metaphyseal defects*) are fibrous lesions of bone that occur in normal children, produce no symptoms, resolve spontaneously, and are found incidentally. They occur at insertion of a tendon or ligament near the epiphyseal growth plate, which may be related to the etiology. They have a characteristic appearance that is eccentric and metaphyseal, with scalloped sclerotic margins. These lesions often cause concern that sometimes leads to inappropriate treatment. Fortunately, the lesions have a characteristic radiographic appearance that is usually diagnostic. They are small in size, cortical in location, and well-delineated by sclerotic margins. They usually resolve spontaneously over a period of 1 to 2 years.

Nonossifying Fibroma

A larger version of the fibrocortical defect is called a *nonossifying fibroma*. These lesions are present in classic locations and are usually diagnosed during adolescence (Fig. 13.36). They are metaphyseal, eccentric with scalloped sclerotic margins (Figs. 13.37 and 13.38), and may fracture when large or if present in certain locations. Manage most by cast immobilization. Resolution of the lesion occurs with time. Rarely, curettage and bone grafting are indicated if the lesion is unusually large or if a fracture through the lesion occurs with minimal trauma.

Fibrous Dysplasia

Fibrous dysplasia includes a spectrum of disorders characterized by a common bony lesion. The neoplastic fibrosis replaces and weakens bone, causing fractures and often a progressive deformity. Ribs and the proximal femur are common sites, and the lesions are most common in adolescents (Fig. 13.39).

Fibrous dysplasia can be monostotic or polystotic. The polystotic form is more severe and is more likely to cause deformity. This deformity is often most pronounced in the femur where a "shepherd's crook" deformity is sometimes seen (Fig. 13.40) and may show extensive involvement of the femoral diaphysis. Rarely, fibrous dysplasia is associated with café au lait skin lesions and precocious puberty, as described with Albright syndrome.

Management of fibrous dysplasia is surgical. Weakened bone can be strengthened by flexible intramedullary rods. Leave these rods in place indefinitely to prevent fractures and progressive deformity (Fig. 13.40).

References

1998 Fibrous dysplasia of the proximal part of the femur. Long-term results of curettage and bone-grafting and mechanical realignment. Guille JT, Kumar SJ, MacEwen GD. JBJS 80A:648
1997 Pathologic fractures through nonossifying fibromas: is prophylactic treatment warranted? Easley ME, Kneisl JS. JPO 17:808
1990 Fibrous metaphyseal defect. Ritschl P, et al. Int Orthop 14:205

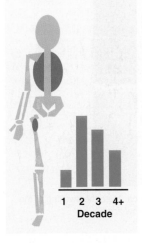

Fig. 13.39 Fibrous dysplasia. Common (red) and less common (orange) locations are shown. Age pattern of involvement is shown in blue.

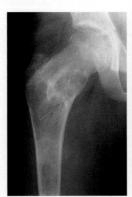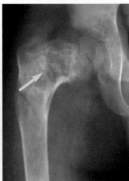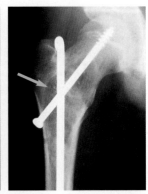

Fig. 13.40 Fibrous dysplasia of proximal femur. These patients show a femur at risk for deformity (red arrow), varus deformity (yellow arrow), and intramedullary fixation to prevent deformity (orange arrow).

Osseous Tumors

Osteoid Osteoma

This benign, bone-producing, highly vascular tumor induces an intense bony reaction and a characteristic pain pattern. These tumors occur most commonly in long bones during the second decade (Fig. 13.41)

Diagnosis The pain occurs at night, is well-localized, and is often relieved by aspirin. Spine lesions occur in the posterior elements of the spine and often cause secondary scoliosis. Lesions are tender and, if close to a joint, cause joint inflammation that may be confused with primary arthritis. Lesions may cause hemideossfication due to chronic pain and a limp (Fig. 13.42). The radiographic appearance is often characteristic for well-established lesions. A radiolucent nidus is surrounded by reactive bone (Fig. 13.43). The bone scan is diagnostic, with intense localized uptake at the nidus.

Management New options for management supplement the traditional approach of open excision.

Antiinflammatory Eventually, lesions resolve over many years. This option is rarely acceptable to families.

Percutaneous ablation using CT is accomplished by removal, alcohol injection, thermocoagulation, or interstitial laser photocoagulation.

Open excision is a standard practice.

Osteoblastoma

This benign bone-producing tumor is similar to the osteoid osteoma but larger. These lesions occur in the spine and long bones most frequently during the second decade (Fig. 13.44). One-third of these lesions occur in the spine (Fig. 13.45), causing back pain and often scoliosis. They are sometimes difficult to differentiate from osteosarcoma. Spinal lesions are most difficult to manage because of the adjacent vertebral artery in a cervical spine lesion. Manage by complete resection. Expect a recurrence rate of about 10–20%.

References

2000 Percutaneous CT guided resection of osteoid osteoma of the tibial plafond. Donley BG, et al. Foot Ankle Int 21:596

2000 Osteoid osteoma of the spine treated with percutaneous computed tomography-guided thermocoagulation. Cove JA, et al. Spine 25:1283

1999 Spinal osteoblastoma: CT and MR imaging with pathological correlation. Shaikh M, Saifuddin A, Pringle J, Natali C, Sherazi Z. Skeletal Radiol 28:33

1999 Osteoid osteoma. Direct visual identification and intralesional excision of the nidus with minimal removal of bone. Campanacci M, Ruggieri P, Gasbarrini A, Ferraro A, Campanacci L. JBJS 81B:814

1999 Intra-articular benign osteoblastoma of the acetabulum: a case report. Arauz S, Morcuende J, Weinstein S. JPO-b 8:136

1998 Osteoid osteoma and osteoblastoma of the spine. Factors associated with the presence of scoliosis. Saifuddin A, White J, Sherazi Z, Shaikh M, Natali C, Ransford A. Spine 23:47

1998 Evidence of the subperiosteal origin of osteoid osteomas in tubular bones: analysis by CT and MR imaging. Kayser F, Resnick D, Haghighi P, Pereira ER, Greenway G, Schweitzer M, Kindynis P. Am J Roentgenol 170:609

1997 Interstitial laser photocoagulation of osteoid osteomas with use of CT guidance. Gangi A, Dietemann J, Gasser B, Mortazavi R, Brunner P, Mourou M, Dosch J, Durckel J, Marescaux J, Roy C. Radiology 203:843

1996 Osteoid osteoma: comparative utility of high-resolution planar and pinhole magnification scintigraphy. Roach P, Connolly L, Zurakowski D, Treves S. Pediatr Radiol 26:222

1996 Evaluation of suspected osteoid osteoma. McGrath B, Bush C, Nelson T, Scarborough M. CO 247

1996 Clinicopathologic features and treatment of osteoid osteoma and osteoblastoma in children and adolescents. Frassica F, Waltrip R, Sponseller P, Ma L, McCarthy EJ. Orthop Clin North Am 27:559

1994 Percutaneous resection of osteoid osteoma under CT guidance in eight children. Baunin C, Puget C, Assoun J, Railhac J, Cahuzac J, Clement J, Sales GJ. Pediatr Radiol 24:1

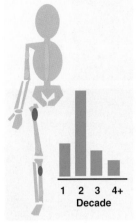

Fig. 13.41 Osteoid osteoma. Common (red) and less common (orange) locations are shown. Age pattern of involvement is shown in blue.

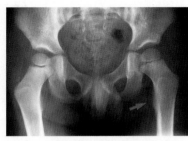

Fig. 13.42 Osteoid osteoma. Note the hemideossification of the left pelvis and femur. This is due to pain and limp over a period of months from a proximal femoral lesion.

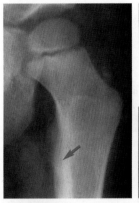

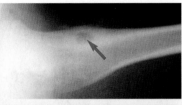

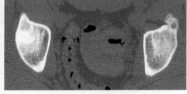

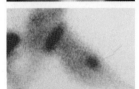

Fig. 13.43 Osteoid osteoma of the proximal femur. Lesions are common in this location. Note the typical nidus (red arrow) surrounded by reactive bone. Lesions are very "hot" on bone scan (yellow arrow).

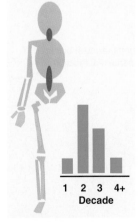

Fig. 13.44 Osteo-blastomas. Common (red) and less common (orange) locations are shown. Age pattern of involvement is shown in blue.

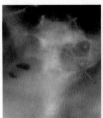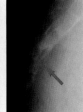

Fig. 13.45 Osteoblastoma of the sacrum.

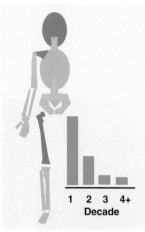

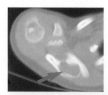
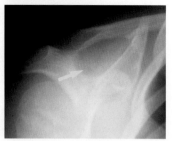

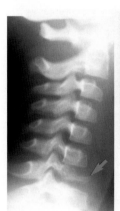

Fig. 13.46 Eosinophilic granuloma. Common (red) and less common (orange) locations are shown. Age pattern of involvement is shown in blue.

Fig. 13.47 Eosinophilic granuloma of the scapula. This lesion is shown by CT scan (red arrow) and conventional radiograph (yellow arrow).

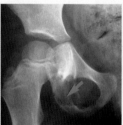
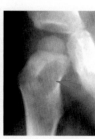

Fig. 13.48 Eosinophilic granuloma in varied locations.

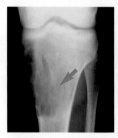
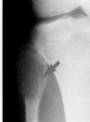

Fig. 13.49 Giant cell tumor of bone. These lesions (arrows) occurred shortly after the end of growth. Note the lack of periosteal reaction.

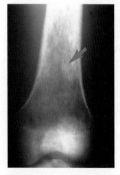

Fig. 13.50 Hemangioma of bone. These lesions (arrow) are often difficult to differentiate from malignant lesions.

Miscellaneous Bone Tumors

Eosinophilic Granuloma

Eosinophilic granuloma is the localized form of Langerhans' cell histiocytosis or histiocytosis X.

Diagnosis The peak age of onset is between 1 and 3 years of age (Fig. 13.46). Lesions are painful and are most often confused with osteomyelitis or sometimes Ewing sarcoma. Lesions often appear "punched out" on conventional radiographs (Figs. 13.47 and 13.48), but sometimes elicit periosteal reactions, suggesting a sarcoma. The child may have a low-grade fever and elevated ESR and CRP, making the differentiation from an infection difficult. Consider ordering skull films to aid in assessing a generalized disorder. Sometimes the diagnosis must be established by biopsy.

Management The natural history is of spontaneous resolution over a period of many months. Management options include simple observation, immobilization to improve comfort and reduce the risk of pathologic fracture, injection with steroid, limited curettage, or radiation treatment.

Spine lesions cause collapse (*vertebra plana*) and sometimes neurologic involvement. Manage by observation or brace immobilization. Rarely, curettage is necessary to hasten resolution.

Lower limb long-bone lesions, if large enough, may pose a risk of pathologic fracture. Curettage and cast protection may be appropriate.

Giant Cell Tumors

Giant cell tumors (GCT) are aggressive tumors that fall between the usual classification of benign and malignant lesions. They occasionally occur in adolescents. Lesions are usually metaphyseal or epiphyseal, eccentric, expansive, and show little sclerosis or periosteal reaction (Fig. 13.49). These tumors are locally invasive and often recur. Manage by curettage and grafting. Provide careful follow-up because recurrence is common.

Neurofibroma

Neurofibromatosis causes widespread pathology, including scoliosis, pseudoarthrosis of long bones, thoracic lordoscoliosis, protrusio acetabuli, and abnormal bone growth (see details in Chapter 15).

Osseous Hemangioma

This is often present in the vertebrae or skull but may appear in the extremities. Lesions are diffuse and suggest a malignant tumor (Fig. 13.50). Wide resection is necessary and recurrence is common.

References

1999 Medical management of eosinophilic granuloma of the cervical spine. Levy EI, et al. Pediatr Neurosurg 31:159

1999 Giant cell tumor of the foot phalanges in children: a case report. Alvarez RA, Valverde GJ, Garcia AM. JPO 8B:132

1998 Eosinophilic granuloma of bone: results of treatment with curettage, cryosurgery, and bone grafting. Schreuder H, et al. JPO 7B:253

1997 Eosinophilic granuloma of the spine. Floman Y, et al. JPO 6B:260

1997 Cast and brace treatment of eosinophilic granuloma of the spine: long-term follow-up. Mammano S, Candiotto S, Balsano M. JPO 17:821

1996 Giant cell tumor of bone. Yip K, Leung P, Kumta S. CO 323:60

1992 Unusual orthopedic manifestations of neurofibromatosis. Joseph KN, Bowen JR, MacEwen GD. CO 278:17

1991 Lower limb bone hemangiomas in children: report of two cases. Melchior B, et al. JPO 11:482

1986 Osseous manifestations of neurofibromatosis in childhood. Crawford AH Jr, Bagamery N. JPO 6:72

Benign Soft Tissue Tumors

Hemangioma

Hemangiomas are common during childhood. They may be part of a systemic condition (Fig. 13.51) or an isolated lesion (Fig. 13.52).

Diagnosis The clinical features depend on the location and size of the lesions. Subcutaneous lesions are usually locally tender. Intramuscular lesions cause pain and fullness, and very large or multiple lesions may cause overgrowth or bony deformity.

Imaging Punctate calcification in lesion is diagnostic. CT and MRI are most useful for diagnosis and preoperative planning.

Management Many patients are diagnosed clinically and treated symptomatically. Large and very painful lesions may require resection. Resection is often difficult, as the lesions are poorly defined and may be extensive. Recurrence is common.

Synovial Hemangioma

Hemangioma of the knee is a cause of pain and recurrent hemarthroses in the pediatric age group (Fig. 13.53). The diagnosis may be delayed and the condition misdiagnosed as an internal derangement of the knee. Historically, long delays in diagnosis have occurred. Conventional radiographs show soft tissue swelling. MRI is usually diagnostic. Diffuse lesions are difficult to excise arthroscopically, and open wide excision is often required. Recurrence is common.

Plantar Fibroma

Fibromas may occur in infants with a lump on the anteromedial portion of the heel pad. Most remain small and asymptomatic, some disappear, and rarely do they persist and require excision.

In the child, plantar fibroma usually occurs as nodular thickening of the plantar fascia (Fig. 13.55). Observe to determine the potential for enlargement. Resect enlarging lesions. Be aware that mitotic figures are common in the specimen. Recurrence is frequent; overtreatment is common. Sometimes differentiating from fibrosarcoma or desmoid tumors is difficult.

Other Tumors

A variety of other tumors occur in childhood, including lipomas (Fig. 13.54), lymphangiomas, and benign fibrous tumors.

References

2000 Vertebral hemangioma mimicking a metastatic bone lesion in well-differentiated thyroid carcinoma. Laguna R, et al. Clin Nucl Med 25:611

1997 Plantar fibromatosis of the heel in children: a report of 14 cases. Godette GA, O'Sullivan M, Menelaus MB. JPO 17:16

1997 Synovial hemangioma of the knee. Price NJ, Cundy PJ. JPO 17:74

1994 Skeletal-extraskeletal angiomatosis. A clinicopathological study of fourteen patients and nosologic considerations. Devaney K, Vinh TN, Sweet DE. JBJS 76A:878

1994 Soft tissue hemangiomas: MR manifestations in 23 patients. Suh JS, Hwang G, Hahn SB. Skeletal Radiol 23:621

1993 Vascular abnormalities of the extremities: clinical findings and management. Rogalski R, Hensinger R, Loder R. JPO 13:9

1990 YAG laser resection of complicated hemangiomas of the hand and upper extremity. Apfelberg DB, et al. J Hand Surg 15A:765

1988 Dupuytren's disease of the foot in children: a report of three cases. Rao GS, Luthra PK. Br J Plast Surg 41:313

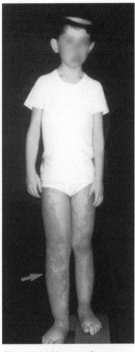

Fig. 13.51 Hemangioma. This boy has Klippel-Weber-Trenaunay syndrome with extensive hemangioma and limb hypertrophy (red arrow).

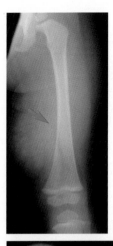
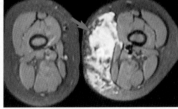

Fig. 13.52 Extensive thigh hemangioma. This large lesion involves much of the medial thigh muscles (red arrows).

Fig. 13.53 Synovial hemangioma. This child had a swollen knee with frequent bloody effusions. Repeated resections over a period of many years were required.

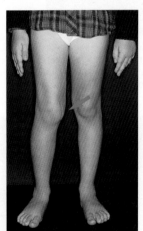

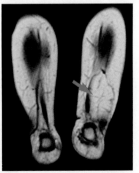

Fig. 13.54 Lipoma. Note the large lipoma (arrow) of the distal leg in a 16-month-old infant.

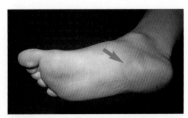

Fig. 13.55 Plantar fibromatosis. Note the plantar thickening with overlying thickening of the skin.

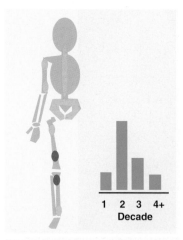

Fig. 13.56 Osteosarcoma. Common (red) and less common (orange) locations are shown. The age of onset in decades is shown in blue.

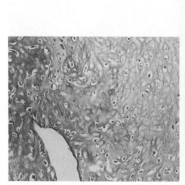
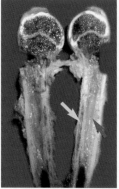

Fig. 13.57 Pathology of osteosarcoma. This photomicrograph (left) shows tumor cell and primitive bone matrix formation. The gross specimen of the proximal humerus from an adolescent shows the intramedullary tumor (red arrow) and periosteal new bone formation (yellow arrow).

Malignant Bone Tumors

Osteosarcoma

Osteogenic sarcoma is the most common malignant tumor of bone. Primary osteosarcoma occurs in children.

Diagnosis It commonly occurs during the second decade of life and often occurs about the knee (Fig. 13.56). Aching, nocturnal pain is often the initial complaint. Tenderness is often present, and a mass is sometimes palpable. Sometimes the patient presents with a pathologic fracture. Radiographs may identify either an osteolytic or osteogenic lesion of metaphyseal bone (Fig. 13.58). Bone scans are helpful in identifying other affected sites. CT and MRI are helpful in assessing the osseous and soft tissue components of the lesion and in staging the tumor (Fig. 13.59). The histology (Fig. 13.57) shows tumor cells with primitive bone matrix formation.

Management Chemotherapy followed by surgical eradication of the tumor is necessary. Manage the tumor by amputation or local resection. Limb salvage can be done by replacing the resected bone with an allograft or metallic implant. Rotationplasty includes lesion resection and rotational reconstruction, substituting the ankle for the knee. Limb salvage during growth results in significant limb shortening. This can be managed by procedures designed to spare the growth plate, expandable prosthetic implants, or contralateral epiphysiodesis. At present, the overall 5-year survival rate is about 75% following aggressive chemotherapy and resection.

Variants Osteosarcoma has several types.

Parosteal osteosarcoma These well-differentiated lesions develop on the surface of the bone, such as the posterior femoral metaphysis, with little or no medullary involvement. Manage by wide local resection.

Periosteal osteosarcoma develops on long tubular bones, especially the tibia and femur. In contrast to parosteal osteosarcoma, periosteal osteosarcoma is less differentiated, resulting in a poorer prognosis.

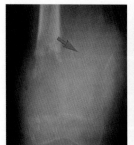
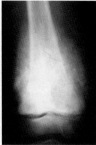
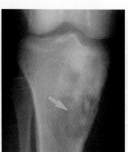
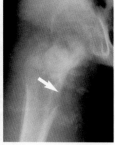

Fig. 13.58 Varied radiographic appearance of osteosarcoma. Lesions may be destructive (red arrow), osteogenic (yellow arrow), cause a motheaten appearance (orange arrow), or show combined osteoblastic and lytic features (white arrow).

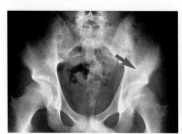
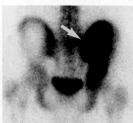
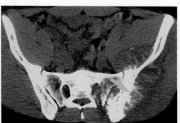
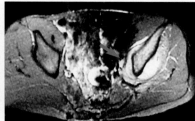

Fig. 13.59 Osteogenic sarcoma of the pelvis. Note that the lesion is not readily identified on conventional radiographs (red arrow), but it is well imaged by bone scan (yellow arrow), CT (orange arrow), and MRI (blue arrow).

Ewing Sarcoma

Ewing sarcoma is the second most common childhood malignant bone tumor. The tumor is most common in the second decade and occurs most commonly in the pelvis, femur, and tibia (Fig. 13.60). This is a very malignant round cell tumor (Fig. 13.61).

Diagnosis These tumors cause pain and often present with a large soft tissue mass. The lesion is usually diaphyseal (Fig. 13.63) and osteolytic or permeative in character. Bone scans and MRI are useful (Fig. 13.62). Because the tumor may cause fever, leukocytosis, anemia, and an elevated sedimentation rate, it can be confused with osteomyelitis. Confirm the diagnosis by biopsy.

Management Treatment by chemotherapy and resection has increased the 5-year survival rate into the 70% range. This malignancy differs from osteogenic sarcoma by a greater likelihood of metastasizing to bone and a lower suvival rate.

References

2000 Initial symptoms and clinical features in osteosarcoma and Ewing sarcoma. Widhe B, Widhe T. JBJS 82A:667

1998 Ewing sarcoma masquerading as osteomyelitis. Durbin M, et al. CO 176

1996 The surgical treatment and outcome of pathological fractures in localised osteosarcoma. Abudu A, et al. JBJS 78B:694

1996 Osteosarcoma and its variants. Vander Griend, RA. OCNA 27:575

1996 Ewing's sarcoma. Vlasak R, Sim FH. OCNA 27:591

1995 The management of limb-length discrepancies in children after treatment of osteosarcoma and Ewing's sarcoma. Gonzalez-Herranz P, et al. JPO 15:561

1995 Extendable tumour endoprostheses for the leg in children. Schiller C, et al. JBJS 77B:608

1994 Limb salvage for malignant bone tumors in young children. Cara JA, Canadell J. JPO 14:112

1994 Parosteal osteosarcoma. A clinicopathological study. Okada K, et al. JBJS 76A:366

1993 Physeal and epiphyseal extent of primary malignant bone tumors in childhood. Correlation of preoperative MRI and the pathologic examination. Panuel M, et al. Pediatr Radiol 23:421

1987 Periosteal osteosarcoma. Ritts GD, et al. CO 219:299

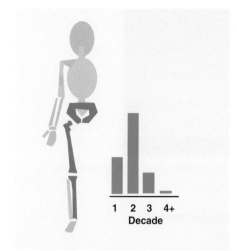

Fig. 13.60 Ewing sarcoma. Common (red) and less common (orange) locations are shown. The age of onset in decades is shown in blue.

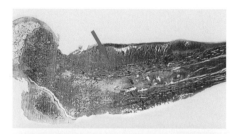

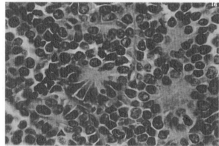

Fig. 13.61 Pathology of Ewing sarcoma. Note the cortical destruction and extracortical extension in the proximal femur. This photomicrograph shows small round cell tumor cells.

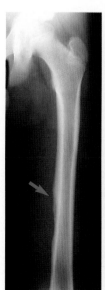
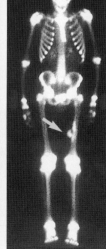
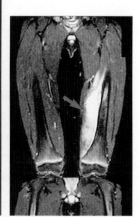

Fig. 13.62 Ewing sarcoma. Note the diaphyseal location (red arrow), the positive bone scan (yellow arrow), and extensive soft tissue involvement (blue arrow).

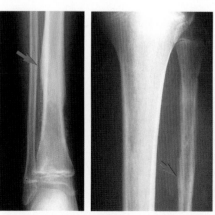

Fig. 13.63 Typical radiographic features of Ewing sarcoma. Note the diaphyseal location with periosteal reaction.

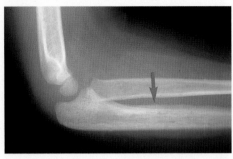

Fig. 13.64 Leukemia. Note the periosteal bone of the proximal ulna (arrow).

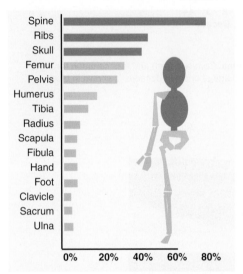

Fig. 13.65 Site and frequency of skeletal metastasis. From data of Leeson et al. (1985).

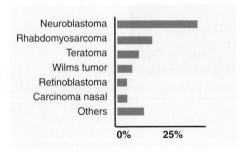

Fig. 13.66 Tumors producing skeletal metastasis. From data of Leeson et al. (1985).

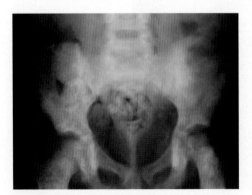

Fig. 13.67 Metastatic neuroblastoma. Note the extensive metatases in the pelvis and proximal femora.

Leukemia

About 20% of children with leukemia present with bone pain and may first be seen by an orthopedist or rheumatologist. Common findings include bone pain, joint pain and swelling, antalgic gait, mild lymphadenopathy and hepatosplenomegaly, and a moderate fever. Radiographic findings include diffuse osteopenia, metaphyseal bands, periosteal new bone formation (Fig. 13.64), sclerosis, and a combination of sclerosis and lytic features. Usual laboratory findings include an elevated ESR, thrombocytopenia, anemia, decreased neutrophils, increased lymphocytes, and blast cells on the peripheral blood smear. Confirm the diagnosis with a bone marrow biopsy.

Metastatic Bone Tumors

Metastatic tumors to bone are most likely to involve the axial skeleton (Fig. 13.65). The most common primary tumors are neuroblastoma followed by rhabdomyosarcoma (Fig. 13.66). Vertebrae metastases are most common in the lumbar spine, while thoracic and cervical involvement are less common. The primary site of tumors with spinal involvement are neuroblastoma and astrocytoma. Complications of spinal metastasis include paralysis, pathologic fractures, and kyphoscoliosis. Assess children with neuroblastoma for bony metastatic disease by CT, MRI, scintigraphy, or bone marrow biopsy. Extensive bony involvement is a relatively late finding (Fig. 13.67).

References

1999 Imaging of abdominal neuroblastoma in children. Hugosson CR, et al. Acta Radiol 40:534

1998 The limping child: a manifestation of acute leukemia. Tuten H, Gabos P, Kumar S, Harter G. JPO 18:625

1998 Acute lymphoblastic leukemia with severe skeletal involvement: a subset of childhood leukemia with a good prognosis. Muller H, Horwitz A, Kuhl J. Pediatr Hematol Oncol 15:121

1997 The management of spinal metastasis in children. Sinha A, Seki J, Moreau G, Ventureyra E, Letts R. Can J Surg 40:218

1997 Occult trauma mimicking metastases on bone scans in pediatric oncology patients. Lowry PA, Carstens MC. Pediatr Radiol 27:114

1994 The prognostic significance of the skeletal manifestations of acute lymphoblastic leukemia of childhood. Heinrich S, Gallagher D, Warrior R, Phelan K, George V, MacEwen G. JPO 14:105

1993 Metastatic vertebral disease in children. Freiberg AA, Graziano GP, Loder RT, Hensinger RN. JPO 13:148

1989 Comparison of radiolabeled monoclonal antibody and magnetic resonance imaging in the detection of metastatic neuroblastoma in bone marrow: preliminary results. Fletcher BD, Miraldi FD, Cheung NK. Pediatr Radiol 20:72

1985 Metastatic skeletal disease in the pediatric population. Leeson MC, Makley JT, Carter JR. JPO 5:261

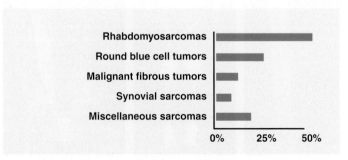

Fig. 13.68 Soft tissue sarcomas. From data of Conrad et al. (1996).

Malignant Soft Tissue Tumors

These tumors account for about 7% of malignant tumors of childhood. About half are rhabdomyosarcomas. These soft tissue malignancies are divided into five general categories (Fig. 13.68).

Rhabdomyosarcoma

This is a sarcoma of the skeletal muscle. It is the most common pediatric soft tissue sarcoma. Extremity tumors account for 20% and carry a poorer prognosis.

Lesions are firm, nontender, and within the muscle compartment. Tumors occur in childhood, and metastasize to lymph nodes and later to bone (Fig. 13.69). Manage by total excision and chemotherapy. Expect the 5-year survival in the 65–75% range.

Round Blue Cell Tumors

These tumors include primitive neuroectodermal tumors, soft tissue Ewing sarcoma, and Askin tumors. Askin tumors are round-cell tumors involving the central axis and chest wall.

Malignant Fibrous Tumors

Desmoid tumors, or fibromatosis, are sometimes considered to be benign. However, because of their tendency to recur, they are sometimes considered as low-grade fibrosarcomas. Most occur in the extremities, creating a soft tissue mass and sometimes erosion or deformity of the adjacent bone (Fig. 13.70). The natural history of fibromatosis is variable; lesions often recur and undergo spontaneous remission. Fibromatosis seldom metastasize or cause death.

Manage by total resection when possible. If surgical margins cannot be achieved without sacrificing the limb or its function, excisional resection is an acceptable alternative. The role of adjuvant chemotherapy or radiation is controversial.

Synovial Sarcoma

These tumors occur most commonly in adolescents (Fig. 13.71) and adults. Most occur in the lower extremities. Primary metastases are usually to regional lymph nodes or the lungs. Manage by chemotherapy, nonmultilating resection, and radiation. Expect 70–80% survival.

Miscellaneous Sarcomas

Peripheral nerve sheath sarcomas Malignant degeneration occurs in 5–10% of patients with neurofibromatosis (NF1). Enlarging lesions in these patients should be documented by MRI and excised or biopsied.

Other sarcomas These include a variety of tumors (Fig. 13.72): leiomyosarcoma, liposarcoma, angiosarcoma, and many others.

Chapter Consultants

Ernest Conrad, e-mail: chappiec@u.washington.edu
George Rab, e-mail: george.rab@ucdmc.ucdavis.edu

References

1999 Aggressive fibromatosis from infancy to adolescence. Spiegel DA. JPO 19:766
1998 Neuropathic arthropathy of the knee associated with an intra-articular neurofibroma in a child. Lokiec F, et al. JBJS 80B:468
1996 Pediatric soft-tissue sarcomas. Conrad EU, Bradford L, Chansky HA. OCNA 27:655
1995 Pediatric desmoid tumor: retrospective analysis of 63 cases. Faulkner LB, et al. J Clin Oncol 13:11.
1994 Synovial sarcoma in children and adolescents: the St Jude Children's Research Hospital experience. Pappo AS, et al. J Clin Oncol 12:2360

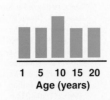
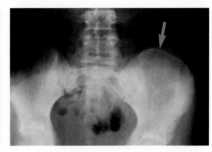

Fig. 13.69 Rhabdomyosarcoma age distribution. These tumors are common in infancy and early childhood. They can extend to bone (arrow).

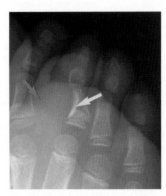

Fig. 13.70 Desmoid. Note the large soft tissue mass (red arrow) and deformation of the second proximal phalanx (yellow arrow).

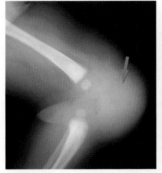
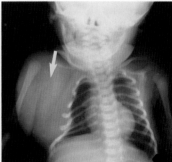

Fig. 13.72 Soft tissue malignancies in infants. This liposarcoma (red arrow) and fibrosarcoma (yellow arrow) have become massive lesions.

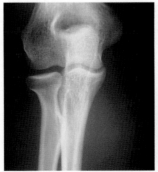
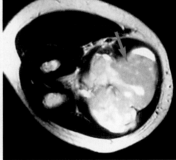

Fig. 13.71 Synovial sarcoma. This lesion in a 16-year-old boy involving the elbow joint is poorly seen on conventional radiographs but readily imaged by MRI (red arrow).

Alman BA, DeBari A, Krajbich JI. Massive allografts in the treatment of osteosarcoma and Ewing sarcoma in children and adolescents. J Bone Joint Surg 1995;77A:54-64.

Aprin H, Riseborough EJ, Hall JE. Chondrosarcoma in children and adolescents. Clin Orthop 1982;166:226-232.

Arata MA, Peterson HA, Dahlin DC. Pathological fractures through non-ossifying fibromas: Review of the Mayo Clinic experience. J Bone Joint Surg 1981;63A:980-988.

Bacci G, Toni A, Avella M. Long-term results in 144 localized Ewing's sarcoma patients treated with combined therapy. Cancer 1989;63:1477-1486.

Bechler JR, Robertson WW Jr, Meadows AT. Osteosarcoma as a second malignant neoplasm in children. J Bone Joint Surg 1992;74A:1079-1083.

Black B, Dooley J, Pyper A. Multiple hereditary exostoses: An epidemiologic study of an isolated community in Manitoba. Clin Orthop 1993;287:212-217.

Bohndorf J, Reiser M, Lochner B. Magnetic resonance imaging of primary tumours and tumour-like lesions of bone. Skeletal Radiol 1986;15:511-517.

Boyko OB, et al. MR Imaging of osteogenic and Ewing's sarcoma. AJR 1987;148:317.

Camissa FP Jr, Glasser DB, Otis JC. The Van Nes tibial rotationplasty: A functionally viable reconstruction procedure in children who have a tumor of the distal end of the femur. J Bone Joint Surg 1990;72A:1541-1547.

Campanacci M, Capanna R, Picci P. Unicameral and aneurysmal bone cyst. Clin Orthop 1986;204:25-36.

Campbell AN, Chan HS, et al. Malignant tumours in neonate. Arch Dis Child 1987;62:19-23.

Capanna R, Springfield DS, Ruggieri P. Direct cortisone injection in eosinophilic granuloma of bone: A preliminary report on 11 patients. J Pediatr Orthop 1985;5:339-342.

Cara JA, Canadell J. Limb salvage for malignant bone tumors in young children. J Pediatr Orthop 1994;14:112-118.

Catani F, Capanna R, Benedetti MG. Gait analysis in patients after Van Nes rotationplasty. Clin Orthop 1993;296:270-277.

Cole WG. Treatment of aneurysmal bone cysts in childhood. J Pediatr Orthop 1986;6:326-329.

Dabezies EJ, D'Ambrosia RD, Chuinard RG, et al. Aneurysmal bone cyst after fracture: A report of three cases. J Bone Joint Surg 1982;64A:617-21.

Donaldson SS: Rhabdomyosarcoma: Contemporary status and future directions. Arch Surg 1989;124:1015-1020.

Dubousset J, Missenard G, Kalifa C. Management of osteogenic sarcoma in children and adolescents. Clin Orthop 1991;270:52.

Eckhardt JJ, Safran MR, Eilber FR. Expandable endoprosthetic reconstruction of the skeletally immature after malignant bone resection. Clin Orthop 1993;297:188-202.

Enneking WF. A system of staging musculoskeletal neoplasms. In: Bassett FH III (ed): AAOS Instruct Course Lect 1988;37:3-10.

Enneking WF, Spanier SS, Goodman MA. A system for surgical staging of musculoskeletal sarcoma. Clin Orthop 1980;153:106-120.

Gebhardt MC, Ready JE, Mankin JH. Tumors about the knee in children. Clin Orthop 1990;255: 86-110.

Ghelman B. Radiology of bone tumors. Orthop Clin North Am 1989;20:287-312.

Gherlinzoni F, Rock M, Picci P. Chondroidmyxoid fibroma: The experience at the Istituto Ortopedico Rizzoli. J Bone Joint Surg 1983;65A:198-204.

Gille P, Nachin P, Aubert D, et al. Intraoperative radioactive localization of osteoid osteomas: Four case reports. J Pediatr Orthop 1986;6:596-599.

Gitelis S, Schajowicz F. Osteoid sarcoma and osteoblastoma. Orthop Clin North Am 1989;20: 313-325.

Glasser DB, Duane K, Lane JM. The effect of chemotherapy on growth in the skeletally immature individual. Clin Orthop 1991;262:93-100.

Goldwein JW. Effects of radiation therapy on skeletal growth in childhood. Clin Orthop 1991;262:101-107.

Greis PE, Hankin FM. Eosinophilic granuloma: The management of solitary lesions of bone. Clin Orthop 1990;257:204-211.

Hall TR, Kangarloo H. Magnetic resonance imaging of the musculoskeletal system in children. Clin Orthop 1989;244:119-30.

Healey JH, Ghelman B. Osteoid osteoma and osteoblastoma: Current concepts and recent advances. Clin Orthop 1986;204:76-85.

Huvos AG, Marcove RC. Chondroblastoma of bone: A critical review. Clin Orthop 1973;95: 300-312.

Jaffe N. Advances in the management of malignant bone tumors in children and adolescents. Pediatr Clin North Am 1985;32:801.

Jaffe N, Smith D, Jaffe MR, et al. Intraarterial cisplatin in the management of stage IIB osteosarcoma in the pediatric and adolescent age group. Clin Orthop 1991;270:15.

Jenkins NH, Freedman LS, McKibbin B. Spontaneous regression of a desmoid tumor. J Bone Joint Surg 1986;68B:780.

Kahn LB, Wood FW, Ackerman LV. Fracture callus associated with benign and malignant bone lesions and mimicking osteosarcoma. Am J Clin Pathol 1969;52:14-24.

Keeney GL, Unni KK, Beabout JW. Adamantinoma of long bones: A clinicopathologic study of 85 cases. Cancer 1989;64:730-737.

Keim HA, Reina EG. Osteoid-osteoma as a cause of scoliosis. J Bone Joint Surg 1975;57A:159-63.

Kirwan EO, Hutton PA, Pozo JL, et al. Osteoid osteoma and benign osteoblastoma of the spine: Clinical presentation and treatment. J Bone Joint Surg 1984;66B:21-6.

Kroon HM, Schurmans J. Osteoblastoma: Clinical and radiological findings in 98 new cases. Radiology 1990;175:783-790.

Kumar SF, Harcke HT, MacEwen GD, et al. Osteoid osteoma of the proximal femur: New techniques in diagnosis and treatment. J Pediatr Orthop 1984;4:669-72.

Lange TA. The evaluation of a soft-tissue mass in the extremities. In: Barr JS Jr (ed): AAOS Instruct Course Lect 1989;38:391-8.

Lewis MM, Sissons HA, Norman A, et al. Benign and malignant cartilage tumors. In: Griffin PP (ed): AAOS Instruct Course Lect 1987;23:87-114.

Makley JT. Preoperative staging techniques for soft-tissue neoplasms. In Barr JS Jr (ed): AAOS Instruct Course Lect 1989;38:399-405.

Makley JT, Joyce MJ. Unicameral bone cyst (simple bone cyst). Orthop Clin North Am 1989;20:407-415.

Makley JT. Carter JR. Eosinophilic granuloma of bone. Clin Orthop 1986;204:37-44.

Mankin HJ, Lange TA, Spanier SS. The hazards of biopsy in patients with malignant primary bone and soft-tissue tumors. J Bone Joint Surg 1982;64A:1121-1127.

Masada K, Tsuyuguchi Y, Kawai, H, et al. Operations for forearm deformity caused by multiple osteochondromas. J Bone Joint Surg 1989;71B:24.

Meyers PA. Malignant bone tumor in children: Ewing's sarcoma. Hematol Oncol Clin North Am 1987;1:667-73.

Mickelson MR, Bonfiglio M. Eosinophilic granuloma and its variations. Orthop Clin North Am 1977;8:933-945.

Milgram JW. The origins of osteochondromas and endochondromas: A histopathologic study. Clin Orthop 1983;174:264-284.

Moser RP Jr, Sweet DE, Haseman DB, et al. Multiple skeletal fibroxanthomas: Radiologic-pathologic correlation of 72 cases. Skeletal Radiol 1987;16:353-9.

Neff JR, Nonmetastatic Ewing sarcoma of bone: The role of surgical therapy. Clin Orthop 1986;204:111.

Oppenheim WL, Galleno H. Operative treatment versus steroid injection in the management of unicameral bone cysts. J Pediatr Orthop 1984;4:1-7.

Picci P, Manfrini M, Zucchi V. Giant-cell tumor of bone in skeletally immature patients. J Bone Joint Surg 1983;65A:486-490.

Pritchard DJ. Bone tumors: Part I. Small cell tumors of bone. In: Murrary JA (ed): AAOS Instruct Course Lect 1989;33:26-39.

Rogalsky RJ, Black GB, Reed MH. Orthopaedic manifestations of leukemia in children. J Bone Joint Surg 1986;68A:494.

Rosenborg M, Mortensson W, Hirsch G, et al. Technique. Considerations in the corticosteroid treatment of bone cysts. J Pediatr Orthop 1989;9:240-243.

Scaglietti O, Marchetti PG, Bartolozzi P. Final results obtained in the treatment of bone cysts and methylprednisolone acetate (Depo-Medrol) and a discussion of results achieved in other bone. Clinic Orthop 1982; 165:33-42.

Schubiner JM, Simon MA. Primary bone tumors in children. Orthop Clin North Am 1989;18:577.

Schwartz HS, Zimmerman NB, Simon MA. The malignant potential of enchondromatosis. J Bone Joint Surg 1987;69A:269-274.

Seimon LP. Eosinophil granuloma of the spine. J Pediatr Orthop 1981;1:371-6.

Shindell R, Huurman WW, Lippiello L, et al. Prostaglandin levels in unicameral bone cysts treated by intralesional steroid injection. J Pediatr Orthop 1989;9:516-9.

Sim FH, Wold LE, Swee RG. Bone tumors: Part II. Fibrous tumor of bone. In: Murray JA (ed): AAOS Instruct Course Lect 1984;33:40-59.

Simon MA, Aschliman MA, Thomas N. Limb-salvage treatment versus amputation for osteosarcoma of the distal end of the femur. J Bone Joint Surg 1986;68A:1331-1337.

Simon MA, Biermann JS. Biopsy of bone and soft-tissue lesions. J Bone Joint Surg 1993;75A: 616-621.

Simon MA. Limb salvage treatment versus amputation for osteosarcoma of the distal end of the tibia. J Bone Joint Surg 1986;678A:1331.

Simon MA, Finn HA. Diagnostic strategy for bone and soft-tissue tumors. J Bone Joint Surg 1993;75:622-631.

Simon MA. Biopsy of musculoskeletal tumors. J Bone Joint Surg 1982; 64A:1253-1257.

Simon MA. Causes of increased survival of patients with osteosarcoma: Current controversies. J Bone Joint Surg 1984;66A:306-310.

Snearly W.N., Peterson HA. Management of ankle deformities in multiple hereditary osteochondromata. J Pediatr Orthop 1989;9:427-32.

Springfield DS, Capanna R, Gherlinzoni F. Chondroblastoma: A review of seventy cases. J Bone Joint Surg 1985;67A:748-755.

Stephenson RB, London MD, Hankin FM, et al. Fibrous dysplasia. An analysis of options for treatment. J Bone Joint Surg 1987;69A:400-409.

Suit H, Mankin HJ, Wood WC, et al. Treatment of the patient with stage MO soft tissue sarcoma. J Clin Oncol 1988;6:854-862.

Tonai M, Campbell CJ, Ahn GH, et al. Osteoblastoma: Classification and report of 16 patients. Clin Orthop 1982;167:222-235.

Chapter 14 – Neuromuscular Disorders

Neuromuscular disorders (Fig. 14.1) are the most common cause of chronic disability in children. Because motor dysfunction is often an early manifestation of these diseases the orthopedist may be the first to see the child. The child with in-toeing may have mild spastic hemiparesis or the boy whose walking deteriorates in early childhood may have muscular dystrophy.

Statistics

Prevalence of cerebral palsy far exceeds other disorders (Fig. 14.2) with an estimated 750,000 affected individuals in United States alone. Poliomyelitis is still a problem in developing countries (Fig. 14.3).

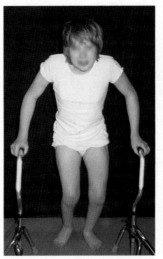
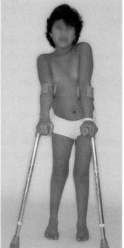

Fig. 14.1 Neuromuscular disorders. Children with neuromuscular disorders such as cerebral palsy (left) and myelodysplasia (right) are common.

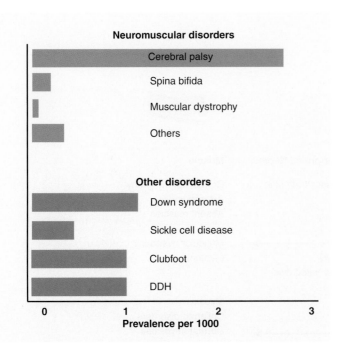

Fig. 14.2 Prevalence of neuromuscular disorders in North America. This graph shows the relative frequency of each disorder and a comparison with other conditions causing disability in children.

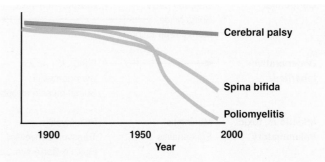

Fig. 14.3 Incidence of neuromuscular disorders with time in North America. Dramatic declines in incidence of poliomyelitis and spina bifida are shown.

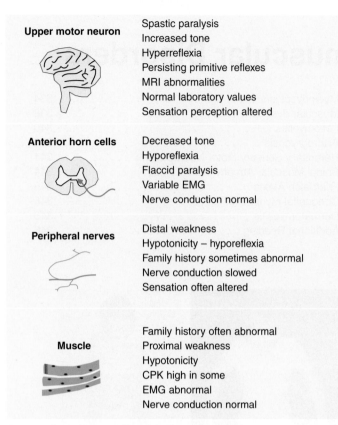

Upper motor neuron	Spastic paralysis Increased tone Hyperreflexia Persisting primitive reflexes MRI abnormalities Normal laboratory values Sensation perception altered
Anterior horn cells	Decreased tone Hyporeflexia Flaccid paralysis Variable EMG Nerve conduction normal
Peripheral nerves	Distal weakness Hypotonicity – hyporeflexia Family history sometimes abnormal Nerve conduction slowed Sensation often altered
Muscle	Family history often abnormal Proximal weakness Hypotonicity CPK high in some EMG abnormal Nerve conduction normal

Fig. 14.4 Physical and laboratory features by level. Each level of pathology has unique features that are useful in assessment.

Evaluation

An accurate diagnosis is essential for effective management. Classify the condition first by anatomical level and then match the clinical and laboratory findings with the various diagnostic possibilities to establish the diagnosis (Figs. 14.4 and 14.5).

Family History

A family history is often positive in peripheral neuropathies and muscular dystrophy.

Medical History

The time of onset is helpful. Mothers of children with neurological problems often note something unusual about the pregnancy or early infancy. The mother may note less than expected or late fetal movement during pregnancy. The pregnancy may be abnormal, delivery prolonged, birth weight low. The Apgar score may be low. Feeding problems, respiratory difficulties, and delay in acquiring motor skills are common during infancy. Mothers often sense that *something is wrong* during pregnancy or during early infancy. The mother's intuition is surprisingly accurate.

Acquisition of Motor Skills

Infants with neurological impairment usually show a variety of abnormal findings including abnormal reactions, retention of primitive reflexes, and delays in acquiring motor skills. The most useful and consistent finding is a delay in motor development. The normal infant shows head control by about 3 months, sitting by 6 months, standing with support by 12 months, and walking independently by about 14 months (Fig. 14.6). Although considerable individual variability exists, gross delay in developing these skills is worrisome.

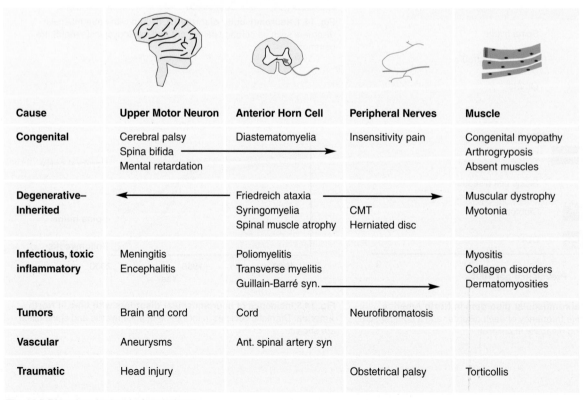

Cause	Upper Motor Neuron	Anterior Horn Cell	Peripheral Nerves	Muscle
Congenital	Cerebral palsy Spina bifida ⟶ Mental retardation	Diastematomyelia	Insensitivity pain	Congenital myopathy Arthrogryposis Absent muscles
Degenerative–Inherited	⟵	Friedreich ataxia ⟶ Syringomyelia Spinal muscle atrophy	CMT Herniated disc	Muscular dystrophy Myotonia
Infectious, toxic inflammatory	Meningitis Encephalitis	Poliomyelitis Transverse myelitis Guillain-Barré syn. ⟶		Myositis Collagen disorders Dermatomyosities
Tumors	Brain and cord	Cord	Neurofibromatosis	
Vascular	Aneurysms	Ant. spinal artery syn		
Traumatic	Head injury		Obstetrical palsy	Torticollis

Fig. 14.5 Disorders by level of pathology.

Physical Examination

Give special attention to the neurological examination of infants suspected of have a neuromuscular problem. Perform a screening examination. See page 20. Observe the child running. Gait disturbances that are minimal during walking become pronounced when the child runs.

Assess strength Does the infant show signs of weakness? If possible watch the child walk up and down stairs. Observe the child arising from a position on the floor. The Gower maneuver is a classic test for weakness seen in muscular dystrophy (Fig. 14.7). In the older child assess strength of specific muscle groups. For example, assess foot eversion strength if Charcot Marie Tooth disease is suspected. Grade muscle strength by standard criteria. See page 23.

Assess tone Tone is often altered in these children.

Hypotonus Infants with reduced tone are often described as *floppy infants*. There are many causes of hypotonia (Fig. 14.8). Head control is poor, motor development ia delayed, feeding and respiratory problems are frequent. Often infants with cerebral palsy show hypotonity in early infancy and spasticity later.

Hypertonus Increased tone may be due to spasticity or rigidity. Spasticity is most common and characterized by hyperreflexia, increased resting tone, an exaggerated response to suddenly applied stretch, and tone that increases when the child is stressed or upright positioned.

Sensation

Sensory abnormalities are classic in myelodysplasia and in the sensory neuropathies. Less appreciated are the sensory alterations that occur in cerebral palsy where the pathways are intact but appreciation and integration of the sensory input is impaired.

Deformity

Deformity may be dynamic, fixed, or a combination.

Dynamic deformities causes abnormal position or function without structural muscle shortening. For example, scissoring or a crossing of the legs may occur before fixed adduction contractures develop. An equinus position may precede the development of fixed triceps contractures. Assess the severity of dynamic deformity by noting the posture of the child while held in the upright position. The upright position increases tone that accentuates dynamic deformity.

Fixed contractures are due to shortening of the muscle-tendon complex. This shortening occurs over a period of months following the onset of dynamic contractures due to spasticity as seen in cerebral palsy. Shortening occurs more slowly, over a period of years, from chronic positioning of children with flaccid paralysis. An example is the development of hip flexion contractures in children with myelodysplasia who sit all day. Finally contractures of the capsular or ligaments about joints develop most slowly over a period of several years.

Combined contractures Most contractures have elements of both dynamic and fixed types. The proportion of fixed to dynamic congtracture gradually increases with time.

Progression Fixed contractures eventually cause joint deformity. The articular surfaces of the joint first become deformed. Later joint subluxation and sometimes dislocation develop. Scoliosis, hip subluxation or dislocation, or flattening of the femoral condyles from lack of normal motion are examples of the late effect on joints of fixed contractures.

Pelvic obliquity Assess pelvic obliquity with the child positioned over the edge of the examination table (Fig. 14.9). Assess the effect of rotating the pelvis in each direction to determine whether the deformity causing the obliquity has its origin is in the spine (suprapelvic), in the pelvis (pelvic) or from hip deformity (infrapelvic). Sometimes deformities are combined and complex.

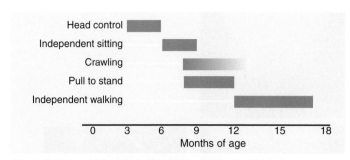

Fig. 14.6. Normal range of motor development. Motor milestones are reached on an average (green) and then 95% at end of bar (red).

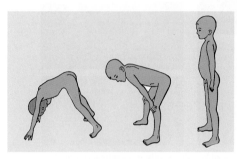

Fig. 14.7 Gower sign. Note the characteristic maneuver to stand from a position on the floor.

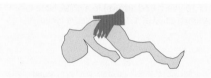

Fig. 14.8 Floppy infant. Note the lack of head control.

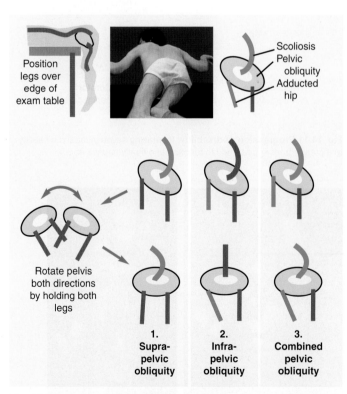

Fig. 14.9 Assessing cause of pelvic obliquity. Position the child with the legs over the end of the examining table. Rotate the legs as a unit from one side to the other. 1. Suprapelvic obliquity is present if the spine remains deformed and the pelvic–thigh position becomes neutral. 2. Infrapelvic obliquity is present if the spine straightens but the thigh remains adducted. 3. Combined deformity is present if deformities of the spine and adduction of the thigh persist when the pelvis is rotated in either direction.

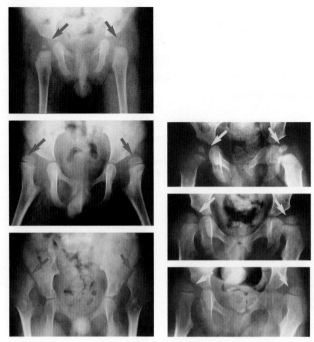

Fig. 14.10 Natural history of hip deformity in cerebral palsy. With adduction contractures, hips gradually dislocate with time. Note the sequence from ages 1, 4, and 10 years (red arrows) in a child. Note less symmetrical progression in another child at 1, 2, and 3 years (yellow arrows).

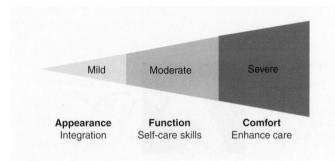

Fig. 14.11 Progression of disability. Increasing severity causes disability to increase from appearance to function and finally causes pain.

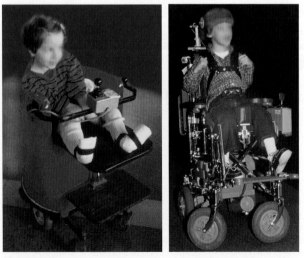

Fig. 14.12 Effective mobility. Various mobility / aids allow the child to be independent.

Management Principles

Management of neuromuscular problems is often complex. This complexity is due to the great variety of disorders, varied individual response to disease, and often the lack of effective treatment methods. Application of general principles of management often simplifies and improves management.

Natural History of Deformity

Neuromuscular disorders cause disability not only from weakness, altered sensation, and incoordination but also from acquired deformity. These acquired deformities develop in a definite sequence (Fig. 14.10). For example, the child with cerebral palsy is first hypotonic and then becomes spastic. This spasticity causes dynamic deformities that becomes a fixed contractures with time. These fixed contractures cause altered loading of joint cartilage, disturbed growth, and finally bony deformity. These acquired deformities limited function and mobility further increasing disability. Understanding this sequence of progressive deformity and disability is important in planning management.

Effectiveness of Orthopedic Treatment

Musculoskeletal procedures in neuromuscular disorders focus on the secondary problems of spasticity, contracture, and bony deformity. As our management can only alter the *affects* rather than the *cause* of the disease, treatment is not definitive.

Focus Management on Comfort, Function, and Appearance–Not Deformity

The objective of management is to improve comfort, function, and appearance, not to correct deformity. Individualize management based on the severity of the disability (Fig. 14.11). For example, in the severely disabled child the first priorities are to enhace comfort and to facilitate care. The objective is to correct only those deformities that interfere with these priorities.

Appreciate the Significance of Sensation and Perceptive Disabilities

Loss of sensation or perceptive impairments are often underrated in importance. The child with cerebral palsy is described as having *spastic paralysis*. Often the focus is on the *deformity* alone. Equally important but less obvious are sensory and perceptive disabilities. For example, the child with arthrogryposis who has more deformity but intact sensation functions at a higher level than a child with cerebral palsy with less deformity but impaired sensation. Recurrent ulcers of an insensate foot often cause more disability than the motor weakness for the child with myelodysplasia.

Establish Appropriate Priorities

Adults with disability rank communication and socialization above mobility in importance. Frequently the family's major concern is whether or not their child will walk. Help the family understand that the long-term objectives are independence and social integration. During each visit attempt to keep the focus on the essential needs of the child such as self-care capabilities and communication and away from trivial problems. For example, efforts to overcome minor variations in gait may waste energy and resources needed to help the child develop independence in self care, communication skills, and effective mobility.

Provide Effective Mobility

Establish effective, age-appropriate, independent mobility (Fig. 14.12). The 2-year-old child with normal mental development should have a means of mobility controlled and initiated by the child. This mobility is often a combination of methods, which may include rolling, crawling, and walking using splints, a walker, or a wheelchair–whatever works for the child. Mobility must be practical, effective, and energy efficient. Mobility is the goal; the method is much less important. Children with effective mobility develop intellectual and social abilities most rapidly. Provide a wheelchair early if necessary to enhance mobility. Children do not become *addicted* to wheelchairs.

Focus on Self-Care

During early and midchildhood, focus on self-care. Assess the child's self-care abilities – eating, dressing, and toileting. Order occupational therapy with specific objectives. Avoid simple stretching programs that waste time and accomplish little.

Focus on Assets

Often children with disability have talents that need to be identified. Time spent developing the child's assets may be more productive than attempting to overcome the child's disability.

Shift Priorities with Age

Focus on mobility early, self-care in early childhood, school, and socialization (Fig. 14.13) in midchildhood and early teens and on vocational training (Fig. 14.14) in late teen years. Make these age priorities.

Maintain Family Health

Avoid exhausting the family with nonessential or unproven treatments. Be aware that the strength of the marriage and the well-being of the siblings are important (Fig. 14.15) for the handicapped child. Recognize that all treatments have a price for the child and family. Ineffective treatments deprive the child of important play time and energy and waste the family's limited resources.

Treat the Whole Child

The objective is a child who meets its potential both emotionally and physically. Play is the occupation of the child. The child with a disability has need of play just as other children. Preserve time and energy for this experience. The individual is a child only once.

Avoid Management Fads

Attempt to steer the family away from interventions that are unproven or unrealistic. Such treatments sap the resources of the family and lead to eventual disappointment for the child. History of cerebral palsy management includes a vast number of treatments that were either harmful or ineffective. Extensive bracing, misguided operations, and exhaustive therapies are examples of treatments once in vogue but later abandoned. Often the outcome of treatment is studied and if the treatment is found ineffective, it is replaced by a new treatment, which is applied until it too is found unsatisfactory. Results are often poor because *cause* of the neurological problem cannot be corrected with current management techniques.

See Child Several Times before Deciding on Surgery

Delay major management decisions such as surgical procedures until the child is seen several times. This delay provides an opportunity to better understand the family and allows evaluation of the child in different situations. If after each assessment the surgeon's decision is the same, the odds for a successful outcome are improved.

Consider Regression

Motor regression following surgery is greatest following major procedures that require prolonged immobility in the older child. Be very cautious about performing procedures in late childhood or adolescence in marginal walkers as the child may never regain their preoperative walking ability.

Prevent Complications

Take active measures to prevent skin ulcers, pathological fractures, and motor regression.

Gait Lab Comparison with Normals

Be cautious about using laboratory data (Fig. 14.16) that campares data based on normal children as controls. The objective of management is not to create normal laboratory values but to enhance function.

Develop Appropriate Recreational Programs

Tailor recreational programs to the child. Often these children do better in individual rather than team sports. Special olympics and wheelchair basketball are examples of appropriate team sports.

Help Family Find Support Groups

Support groups provide information, perspective, and friendship, which can be invaluable for the family.

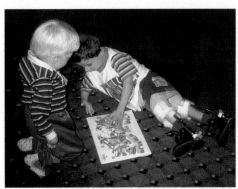

Fig. 14.13 Socialization skills. Integration and play with other children are essential childhood experiences and of special importance to those with disability.

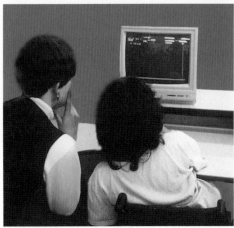

Fig. 14.14 Vocational planning. During the second decade the need for vocational training becomes a major priority.

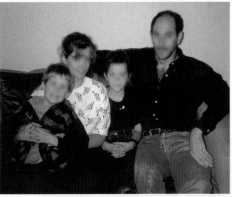

Fig. 14.15 Family health. A healthy family is especially important for a child with a disability.

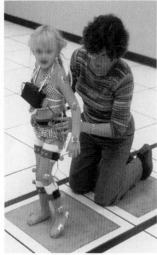

Fig. 14.16 Gait laboratory evaluation. Be aware that these evaluations should be viewed as only one part of a comprehensive assessment.

Causes of Cerebral Palsy

Prenatal
  Hypoplasia
  Genetic forms
  Infections
  Trauma
Prematurity
Paranatal problems
  Traumatic delivery
  Neonatal asphyxia
  Kernicterus
Infections
Trauma
  Head injury
  Near drowning
  Cardiovascular problems

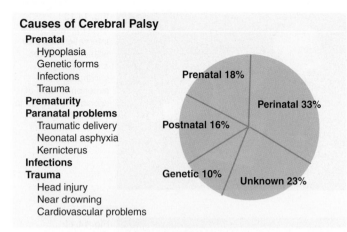

Fig. 14.17 Causes and timing of onset of cerebral palsy.

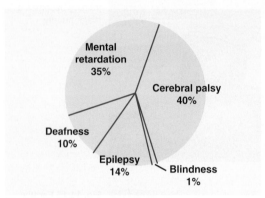

Fig. 14.18 CNS insult outcomes.

Cerebral Palsy

Cerebral palsy (CP), or static encephalopathy, is a nonprogressive central nervous system disorder that causes perceptual and neuromotor disability with an onset in infancy or early childhood. Most CNS insults are pre- or perinatal in origin (Fig. 14.17). CNS injury may cause a variety of clinical problems (Fig. 14.18).

Etiology

CP is an inclusive diagnosis with an extensive list of causes (Fig. 14.17). Common causes include trauma, infection, and toxins. Common associations include prematurity, low Apgar score, difficult delivery, and neonatal illnesses.

Pathology

Most infants with CP show pathologic changes in the brain that correlate poorly with the clinical features. Focal and generalized involvement of the cortex, basal ganglia, and brain stem result from ischemic damage, atrophy, agenesis, gliosis, and degenerative changes. MR imaging shows abnormalities, which include periventricular leukomalacia in preterm infants, a variety of abnormalities in term infants, and extrapyramidal cerebral palsy shows lesions in the putamen and thalamus.

Evaluation

Consider conditions that may be confused with cerebral palsy. Progressive diseases such as spinal cord or brain tumors are sometimes slow growing and can be confused with CP. Demyelinating, degenerative or familial (spastic paraplegia) disorders must be ruled out. If any question exists, refer to a neurologist to confirm the diagnosis.

Tone

Spasticity is increased tone with passive stretch. This response is greatest if the stretch is applied quickly. This is the common form of cerebral palsy (Fig. 14.19).

Rigidity is an increased resistance to passive stretch that is independent of the speed of application. Rigidity may be a uniform (lead pipe) or intermittent (cog wheel) type. This is uncommon in cerebral palsy.

Fig. 14.19 Spastic cerebral palsy. Note the adductor spasticity with the scissoring.

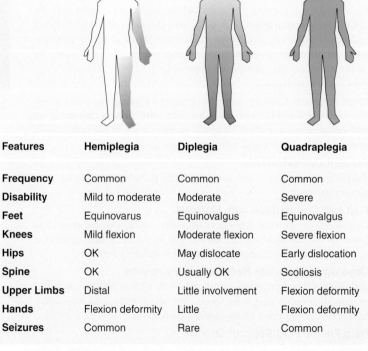

Features	Hemiplegia	Diplegia	Quadraplegia
Frequency	Common	Common	Common
Disability	Mild to moderate	Moderate	Severe
Feet	Equinovarus	Equinovalgus	Equinovalgus
Knees	Mild flexion	Moderate flexion	Severe flexion
Hips	OK	May dislocate	Early dislocation
Spine	OK	Usually OK	Scoliosis
Upper Limbs	Distal	Little involvement	Flexion deformity
Hands	Flexion deformity	Little	Flexion deformity
Seizures	Common	Rare	Common

Fig. 14.20 Classification of cerebral palsy based on distribution of involvement.

Athetosis is characterized by involuntary movement. The combination of athetosis and spasticity is referred to as *tension athetosis*.

Ataxia is a loss of muscular coordination and balance.

Dystonia is an intermittent distorted posturing.

Ballismus is an uncontrolled involuntary motion.

Distribution

Cerebral palsy is usually classified by distribution of involvement (Fig. 14.20) Be aware that on careful examination the so-called uninvolved extremity often shows subtle abnormalities. Slight upper limb involvement is seen in diplegia and opposite limb abnormalities in hemiplegia. Side-to-side asymmetry is also common in spastic quadraplegia and diplegia.

Monoplegia is uncommon and affects a single limb.

Hemiplegia is common and affects the limbs on one side. The upper limb are often more involved. Hemiparesis is the mild form.

Diplegia is common, and affects the lower limbs more than the upper limbs. This pattern is sometimes called *paraplegia*.

Triplegia is uncommon and involves three limbs.

Quadraplegia, or total body involvement, is common and most severe.

Deformity

Deformity changes during childhood as dynamic deformity becomes fixed with time (Fig. 14.21). Examine the child in both the supine and upright position. Dynamic deformity changes with positioning and stress. The physical examination increases stress, increasing tone and dynamic deformity. Separate dynamic deformity from fixed contracture. Assess fixed deformity by gentle and prolonged stretch with the patient as relaxed and comfortable as possible (Fig. 14.22). Record severity in degrees. Assess the torsional profile, pelvic obliquity. and spinal deformity.

Supine measurements are made first.

Ankle dorsiflexion Measure with the knee flexed and extended ankle neutral.

Knee extension Measure any loss of extension.

Popliteal angle Assess with hip flexed as a measure of hamstring contractures.

Hip abduction Assess using pelvis landmarks as bases of reference.

Prone measures

Rotational profile includes hip rotation, thigh-foot angle and shape of foot. See page 70.

Prone extension test for assessment of hip flexion deformity. See page 131. This test has been shown to be more reliable than the Thomas test in cerebral palsy.

Rectus femoris test is performed by slowly flexing the knee and noting how much elevation of the buttocks occurs due to secondary hip flexion.

Other Measures

The value of assessing reflexes, reactions, and patterns is helpful for the very experienced clinician in developmental medicine (Figs. 14.23 and 14.24). For most orthopedists, assessing motor development, head control, sitting, crawling, standing, and walking is most practical.

References

2000 Botulinum toxin type A improved ankle function in children with cerebral palsy and dynamic equinus foot deformity. Goldberg MJ. JBJS 82A:874

2000 Correlation of static to dynamic measures of lower extremity range of motion in cerebral palsy and control populations. McMulkin ML, et al. JPO 20:366

1997 Alterations in surgical decision making in patients with cerebral palsy based on three-dimensional gait analysis. De Luca PA, et al. JPO 17:608

1994 Gait laboratory analysis for preoperative decision making in spastic cerebral palsy: is it all it's cracked up to be? Watts HG. JPO 14:703

1994 The role of gait analysis in the treatment of cerebral palsy. Gage JR. JPO 14:701

1994 Clinical and MR correlates in children with extrapyramidal cerebral palsy. Menkes JH, Curran JA. Am J Neuroradiol 15:451

1992 Cerebral palsy: MR findings in 40 patients. Truwit CL, et al. Am J Neuroradiol 13:67

1985 Hip flexion contractures: a comparison of measurement methods. Bartlett MD, et al. Arch Phys Med Rehabil 66:620

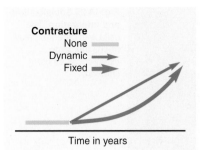

Fig. 14.21 Effect of time on contracture formation. In early infancy hypotonia is often present and no contracture develops (green). With the onset of spasticity, dynamic deformity (blue arrow) develops. With time, this dynamic contracture becomes fixed (red arrow).

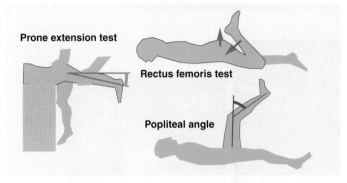

Fig. 14.22 Assess contractures. These are common tests to assess contractures in cerebral palsy.

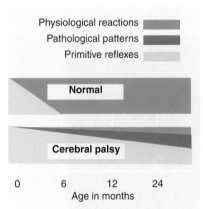

Fig. 14.23 Natural history of reactions, patterns, and reflexes. Note that primitive reflexes are replaced by normal reactions during normal development. In cerebral palsy, primitive reflexes and pathological patterns persist. These differences are useful for diagnosis determining severity of involvement.

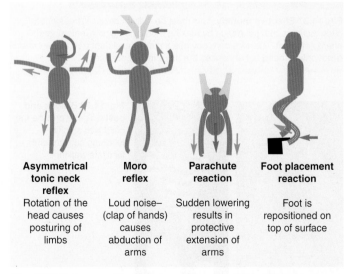

Fig. 14.24 Common reflexes and reactions. The test is initiated (red arrow) and the responses (green arrows) indicate a positive response.

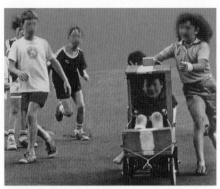

Fig. 14.25 Socialization and integration. The child with cerebral palsy needs the same experiences as other children.

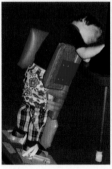
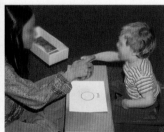

Fig. 14.26 Promoting upper extremity function. This may be done by positioning to free the hands and by occupational therapy to improve hand function.

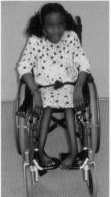
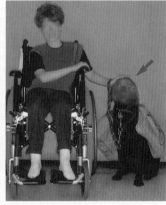

Fig. 14.27 Effective motility. This must be individualized. Wheelchairs often increase independence by making mobility safe, convenient, and energy efficient. This fortunate boy has a canine assistant (red arrow) who is not only a friend but ehnances the boy's independence.

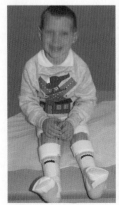
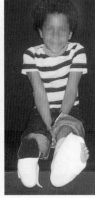

Fig. 14.28 Braces and casts. These provide the child with stability following surgery and facilitate walking.

Management Options in Cerebral Palsy

Management is challenging as the disease is complex, extensive, permanent, and varied. Manage with the perspective that the long-term success places priorities on communication, socialization (Fig. 14.25), independence, and, finally, mobility. Optimal management requires considered application of the best of many choices of interventions for the particular child. Avoid ineffective treatments as they are harmful to the child and draining on the family's energy and resources.

Therapy is valuable in assessment, providing family support, facilitating bonding, improving self-care skills, providing infant stimulation, promoting use of adaptive equipment, and facilitating family interaction with the child.

Neurodevelopmental therapy (NDT) has been shown to be equal to infant stimulation programs and is declining in use.

Inhibitory casting benefit is derived from immobilization in a functional position.

Adaptive equipment includes standing devices (Fig. 14.26) and aids for self-care. These devices are often very practical and effective in improving function.

Mobility aids include wheelchairs (Fig. 14.27), carts, and motorized devices, which allow the child greater independent mobility.

Cast correction is effective as a temporary means of overcoming recently acquired fixed contractures.

Night splinting is sometimes useful in managing the child following surgery to prevent early recurrence and provide comfort.

Botulinum toxin injections into the muscle belly provide 3–6 months of reduction in muscle tone. The high cost of the agent and short duration of effect limit its value of this treatment.

Intrathecal baclofen Continuous infusion reduces spasticity in the upper and lower extremities, and improves upper extremity function and activities of daily living. Complications from the intrathecal catheter occur in 20% of patients and infection in about 5%.

Rhizotomy Selective dorsal rhizotomy is effective in reducing spasticity, especially in spastic diplegia. Orthopedic procedures are still required in about 70% of patients but usually should be postponed for 1–2 years after rhizotomy.

Orthotics have very limited usefulness. The ankle-foot orthosis (AFO) is the only brace shown to be useful (Fig. 14.28). Whether the ankle is articulated or solid is controversial.

Musculoskeletal surgery is appropriate to improve function, reduce discomfort, or facilitate care. Deformity alone is not an indication for surgery. Recurrent deformity is common.

References

1998 Orthopedic procedures after rhizotomy. Carroll KL, Moore KR, Stevens PM. JPO 18:69

1998 Botulinum toxin A compared with stretching casts in the treatment of spastic equinus: a randomised prospective trial. Corry IS, et al. JPO 18:304

1997 A preliminary evaluation of ankle orthoses in the management of children with cerebral palsy. Hainsworth F, et al. Dev Med Child Neurol 39:243

1997 A comparison of intensive neurodevelopmental therapy plus casting and a regular occupational therapy program for children with cerebral palsy. Law M, et al. Dev Med Child Neurol 39:664

1996 Baclofen in the treatment of cerebral palsy. Albright AL. J Child Neurol 11:77

1996 Impact of orthoses on the rate of scoliosis progression in children with cerebral palsy. Miller A, Temple T, Miller F. JPO 16:332

1993 Management of cerebral palsy with botulinum-A toxin: preliminary investigation. Koman LA, et al. JPO 13:489

1988 The effects of physical therapy on cerebral palsy. A controlled trial in infants with spastic diplegia. Palmer FB, et al. N Engl J Med 318:803

Hemiplegia

The spectrum of severity is broad. Sometimes a child is seen for intoeing or clumsiness and found to have mild hemiplegia or hemiparesis. The family may not have been aware of any underlying neurologic problem.

Clinical Features Contractures are most severe distal in the limb. Typical deformities include equinus and varus or valgus feet, and flexed elbow, wrist, fingers, and adducted thumb (Fig. 14.30). Proximal joints have less consistent involvement. Scoliosis is uncommon. Limb shortening is mild and proportional to severity. Function is generally fair and proportional to severity. Walking is slightly delayed. The involved hand disability is proportional to overall severity (Fig. 14.31). Learning disability, seizures, and social problems are common. Sensory deficits are more significant than deformity in limiting hand function.

Management Tailor management based on the severity of the disability. Mainstream children when possible. As hand function requires sensation and fine motor function, disability in the upper limb is most severe.

Upper limb encourage use of hands early. Value of early stretching, splinting, casting are controversial. Base operative indications on level of discriminatory sensibility, intelligence, motivation, and overall function. Delay operative correction until at mid or late childhood (Fig. 14.32). Transfer muscle under voluntary control to improve finger, thumb, or wrist extension. Fuse joints for stability.

Lower limb Limb shortening insufficient to require epiphysiodesis. Patterns of involvement vary considerably (Fig. 14.33) and require that management be individualized. Triceps, posterior tibialis, and hamstring lengths often necessary at about 4–6 years of age.

Spastic Diplegia

Spastic diplegia (Figs. 14.34 abd 14.35) is the most common form of cerebral palsy. About twothirds are associated with prematurity. Spasticity usually develops during the second year. Motor development is delayed but gradually improves to about age 7 years (Fig. 14.36). Independent walking usually occurs if the infant achieves a motor level of about 12 months by the chronological age of 36 months.

Clinical features include typical deformities of the lower limbs. Mild upper limb involvement is detected by careful examination. Severity varies. Often involvement is asymmetrical. Perform standard examination. Assess for hip subluxation and cause of a crouch gait (Fig. 14.37, next page).

Management Consider providing walking aids, ankle-foot orthoses (AFOs), monitor the status of the hips for subluxation. This may require operative treatment. Operative procedures commonly indicated are adductor releases between 3–5 years, hamstring lengthening procedures between 6–10 years, and heel-cord lengthening after age 7. When possible correct equinus with gastrocnemius lengthening alone. Femoral rotational osteotomy may be helpful in correcting intoeing in the older child.

References

1999 Relation between clinical measures and fine manipulative control in children with hemiplegic cerebral palsy. Gordon AM, Duff SV. Dev Med Child Neurol 41:586

1998 Spastic hemiplegia of the upper extremity in children. Waters PM, Van Heest A. Hand Clin 14:119

1997 Developmental skills of children with spastic diplegia: functional and qualitative changes after selective dorsal rhizotomy. Buckon CE, et al. Arch Phys Med Rehabil 78:946

1997 Orthotic management of gait in spastic diplegia. Carlson WE, et al. Am J Phys Med Rehabil 76:219

1996 Gait patterns in children with hemiplegic spastic cerebral palsy. Hullin MG, Robb JE, Loudon IR. JPO 5B:247

1995 Selective posterior rhizotomy and soft-tissue procedures for the treatment of cerebral diplegia. Marty GR, Dias LS, Gaebler-Spira D. JBJS 77A:713

1991 Use of the Green transfer in treatment of patients with spastic cerebral palsy: 17-year experience. Beach WR, et al. JPO 11:731

1985 Analysis of tendon transfers in cerebral palsy. Mowery CA, Gelberman RH, Rhoades CE. JPO 5:69.

1966 Spastic paraplegia and diplegia. Beals RK, JBJS 48A:827

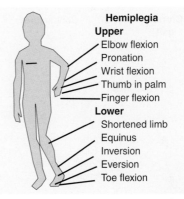

Hemiplegia
Upper
Elbow flexion
Pronation
Wrist flexion
Thumb in palm
Finger flexion
Lower
Shortened limb
Equinus
Inversion
Eversion
Toe flexion

Fig. 14.30 Deformities in hemiplegia. Note that the deformities are mostly distal in the limbs.

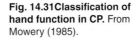

Hand function	
Excellent	Good use
Good	Helper hand
Fair	Helper hand no effective use
Poor	Paperweight function

Fig. 14.31 Classification of hand function in CP. From Mowery (1985).

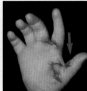

Fig. 14.32 Opertive correction of thumb-in-palm deformity. Note the improved correction following surgery (arrow).

Type	Clinical pattern	Underlying abnormality
1	Minimal, drop foot pattern	Anterior tibialis weakness
2	Flexed knee	Tight gastrocnemius
3	Flexed knee and hip	Tight gastro and hip flexors
4	Knee hyperextension	Tight soleus
5	Knee and ankle hyperextension	Abnormal fore–aft shear force

Fig. 14.33 Gait patterns in hemiplegia. From Hullin (1996).

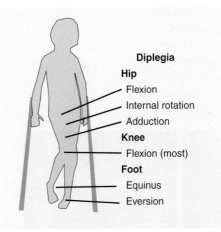

Diplegia
Hip
Flexion
Internal rotation
Adduction
Knee
Flexion (most)
Foot
Equinus
Eversion

Fig. 14.34 Common deformities in spastic diplegia.

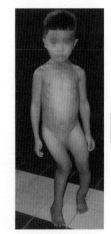

Fig. 14.35 Spastic diplegia.

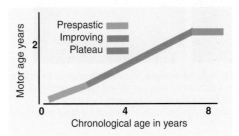

Prespastic
Improving
Plateau

Motor age years

2

0   4   8

Chronological age in years

Fig. 14.36 Motor development in diplegic children. Based on Beals (1966).

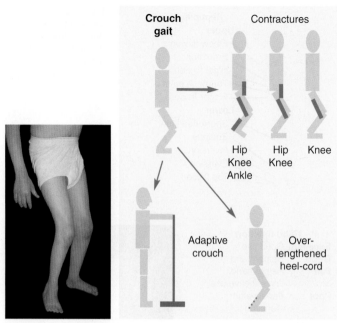

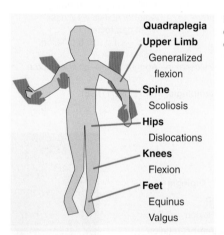

Fig. 14.37 Crouch gait. Determine the site(s) of contractures (red lines). Adaptive crouch position improves with support. An overlengthened heel-cord (dotted red line) causes a crouch without contractures.

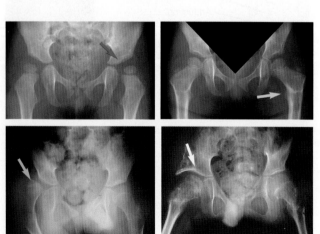

Fig. 14.38 Common deformities in quadraplegia.

Quadraplegia

Quadraplegia, or total body involvement, may be symmetrical or asymmetrical. Rarely, when asymmetrical with one limb minimally affected, the pattern is sometimes called *triplegia*.

Clinical features
Children with quadraplegia show greatest impairment in speech, mentation, nutrition, and self-care abilities, and are most demanding of caregivers. Deformities may be extensive (Fig. 14.38).

Management
Management is usually best provided in a center that provides multidiciplinary care. The goals are to maximize comfort, self-care, and independence. Functional walking is uncommon. Major orthopedic problems include multiple, severe extremity deformities, hip dislocations, and scoliosis.

Multiple Severe Contractures
Severe deformities may cause considerable disability and may require operative release. Postoperative management may be complicated by severe pain that increases spasticity that may cause recurrent deformity. Following release, immobilize for comfort and plan night splinting to prevent recurrence. The results of these release procedures is only fair.

Hip Subluxation–Dislocations
Natural history The hip is normal at birth. Dynamic adduction and flexion deformity develops during late infancy and converts to fixed contractures during early childhood. These contractures and increased tone cause progressive subluxation of the hip and erosion of the lateral acetabular margin. Dislocation often occurs during midchildhood. As the dislocation becomes fixed, femoral head deformation occurs, and if unilateral, infrapelvic obliquity develops. The relationship between hip dislocation and scoliosis is inconsistent. Hip dislocations cause pain, pelvic obliquity, and complicate care.

Management Attempt to interrupt the progression of the deformity by early adductor lengthening procedures. Perform procedures bilaterally for to enhance symmetry and to reduce the risk of recurrent deformity (Fig. 14.39). Management depends upon the severity of deformity (Fig. 14.40), and the child's age and functional level.

Scoliosis
Scoliosis is most common in severely affected children. Scoliosis usually develops independent of hip dislocations and may cause suprapelvic obliquity.

Progression Risk factors for progression include spinal curve of 40° before age 15 years, total body involvement, being bedridden, female gender, and thoracolumbar location. Progression after skeletal maturation is greatest if curves >50° with progression of about 1.5° per year.

Curve patterns fall into several categories (Fig. 14.41).

Disability is due to problems with sitting and care. Scoliosis is seldom a cause of decubiti or pulmonary compromise.

Orthotics and exercise treatments are not effective in altering the progression of the curve.

Operative correction maybe indicated for progressive severe curves to prevent progression and provide stability for sitting. Posterior fusion is adequate for curves below about 70°. Large curves require combined anterior-posterior releases, instrumentation, and fusion.

Fig. 14.39 Hip dislocation in quadraplegia. Subluxation was noted at age 3 years (red arrow). A varus osteotomy was performed (yellow arrow) at age 5 years. At age 8, right hip subluxation developed (orange arrow), which was managed by bilateral femoral osteotomies and a shelf procedure on the right (white arrow).

Athetosis

Athetosis has become uncommon because of improvements in obstretrical practices and neonatal care.

Clinical features

Athetosis causes dyskinesis with involuntary movement and labored volitional function (Fig. 14.42). Because of the excessive movement, contractures are uncommon except in combined forms, which include an element of spasticity. Scoliosis may develop. Intelligence is often normal.

Management

Traditional orthopedic procedures are usually not required. Provide effective mobility with an electric wheelchair, and adaptive equipment to facilitate self-care and independence. Speech and occupational therapy are most helpful. Teach computer skills and use of adaptive devices early.

Complications of Cerebral Palsy

Nutritional deficiencies

Nutritional problems should be resolved before severely affected patients undergo extensive releases or spinal surgery. Children with serum albumin <3.5 mg% and lymphocyte count of <1500 cells/cc are at risk for postoperative infections and for a prolonged hospitalization.

Postoperative Pain Syndrome

This distressing complication commonly occurs when children are mobilized following extensive operative procedures. Pain, irritability, increased tone, and recurrent deformity may occur. The pain may be due to stretch on the sciatic nerve following hamstring lengthening. Manage by gradual mobilization, pain relief, sedation, and patience.

Pressure Sores

Reduce the risk by applying extra cast padding, utilizing careful technique in cast application, relieving pressure over bony prominences, and periodically inspecting the skin.

Aspiration

Severely affected children in spica casts when positioned supine are at risk for aspiration. Prone or side-lying positioning may prevent this complication. In poorly nourished children, consider placing a nasogastric tube before surgery.

Consultants for Cerebral Palsy

Bill Oppenheim, e-mail: woppenhe@ucla.edu
Michael Sussman, e-mail: msussman@shrinenet.org

References

Hip dislocation

2000 Adductor tenotomies in children with quadriplegic cerebral palsy: longer term follow-up. Turker RJ, Lee R. JPO 20:370

1999 Resection arthroplasty of the hip for patients with cerebral palsy: an outcome study. Widmann RF, et al. J PO 19:805

1998 Natural history of scoliosis in spastic cerebral palsy. Saito N, et al. Lancet 351:1687

1993 Long-term follow-up of hip subluxation in cerebral palsy patients. Bagg MR, Farber J, Miller F. JPO 13:32

1991 Prevention of hip dislocation in cerebral palsy by early psoas and adductors tenotomies. Onimus M, et al. JPO 11:432

1989 Dislocation of the hip in cerebral palsy. Natural history and predictability. Cooke PH, Cole WG, Carey RP. JBJS 71B:441

Scoliosis

1996 Impact of orthoses on the rate of scoliosis progression in children with cerebral palsy Miller A, Temple T, Miller F. JPO 16:332

1993 The relationship between preoperative nutritional status and complications after an operation for scoliosis in patients who have cerebral palsy. Jevsevar DS, Karlin LI. JBJS 75A:880

1992 Untreated scoliosis in severe cerebral palsy. Kalen V, Conklin MM, Sherman FC. JPO 12:337

1988 Progression of scoliosis after skeletal maturity in institutionalized adults who have cerebral palsy. Thometz JG, Simon SR. JBJS 70A:1290

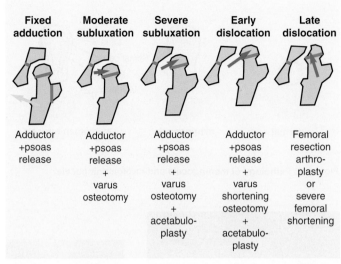

Fig. 14.40 Hip dysplasia and management. Hip deformity in cerebral palsy is usually progressive. With only adduction deformity (yellow arrow) soft tissue release is appropriate. Tailor the extent of bony correction to the severity of subluxation–dislocation and acetabular dysplasia (red arrows). Salvage long-standing dislocation with femoral head deformity (blue arrow) by a resection type of arthroplasty.

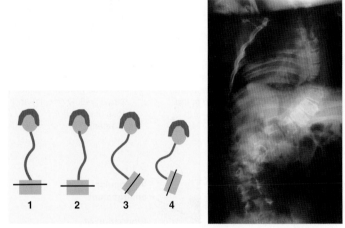

Fig. 14.41 Curve patterns in cerebral palsy. Based on Lonstein (1994).

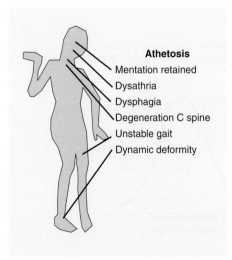

Fig. 14.42 Problems in athetosis.

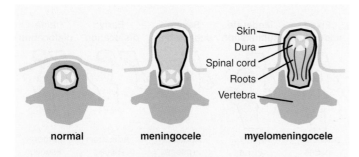

Skin
Dura
Spinal cord
Roots
Vertebra

normal   meningocele   myelomeningocele

Fig. 14.43 Pathology of meningocele and myelomeningocele.

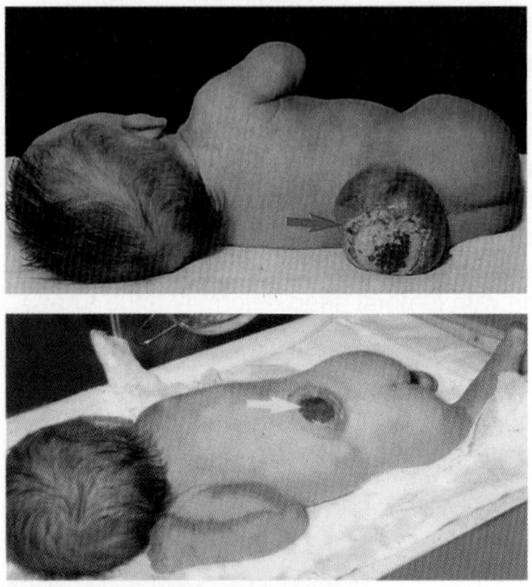

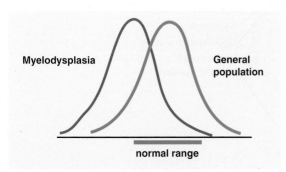

Fig. 14.44 Myelomeningocele. These lesions may be large. In the past (red arrow) large lesions were not repaired. Currently repairs are performed in the neonatal period (yellow arrow).

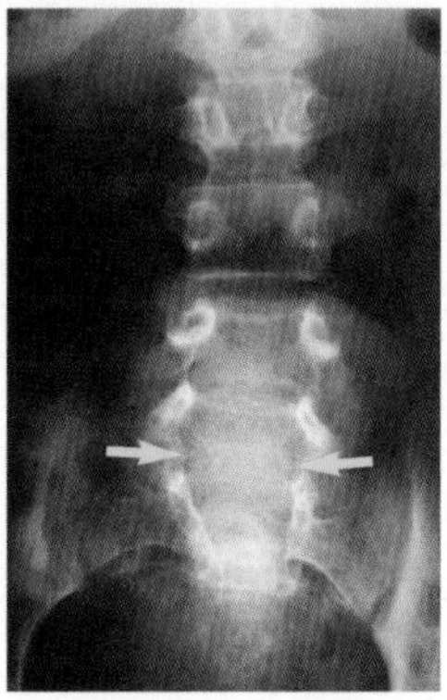

Fig. 14.45 Spina bifida. The vertebral defect includes widening of the canal (yellow arrows) and loss of posterior elements.

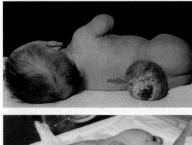

Ventricular enlargement

Elongation of cerebellum

Brain stem compression

Normal

Fig. 14.46 Chiari malformation. This deformity is common in myelodysplasia and includes several characteristic features as shown.

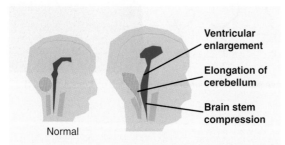

Myelodysplasia

General population

normal range

Fig. 14.47 Intelligence in myelodysplasia.

Myelodysplasia

Myelodysplasia is part of a spectrum of deformities (Fig. 14.43) resulting from failure of closure of the neural tube late in the first month following conception (Figs. 14.44 and 14.45).

Etiology

Factors include genetic, geography, and drugs (valproic acid and carbamazepine). The prevalence is reduced by periconceptional folic acid supplementation. The severity of paralysis is reduced by cesarean delivery before rupture of amniotic membranes and onset of labor.

Pathology

The spectrum of defects is broad with localized or extensive neurological defects.

Brain defects include hydrocephalus, and the varied Chiari malformations that may include herniation of the cerebellum into the upper cervical canal (Fig. 14.46). Mental retardation is most common in higher level lesions (Fig. 14.47).

Cord defect Lesions may be incomplete or complete, open or closed, and occur at different levels. An autonomous functioning cord below the primary lesion may result in segmental spasticity. Diastatomyelia, tethered cords, lipoma, and syringomyelia may be coexisting problems. The level of the defect usually determines the neurological level and pattern of musculoskeletal deformities (Fig. 14.48).

Multiple system involvement is common. Major problems include incontinence, urinary infections, and nutritional problems.

Bone and joint deformity are common associated problems. These include clubfeet, vertical talus, knee flexion or extension deformities, hip dislocations, and spinal kyphosis or scoliosis.

Secondary skeletal defects often develop with time and muscle imbalance. These include hip dislocations, progressive scoliosis, and lower limb deformities.

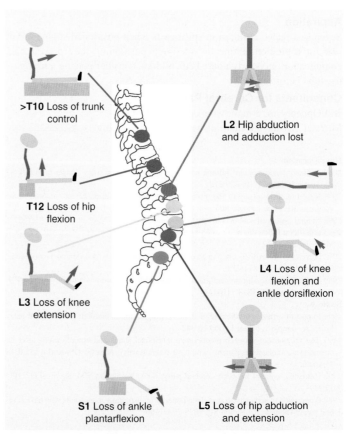

>T10 Loss of trunk control

L2 Hip abduction and adduction lost

T12 Loss of hip flexion

L4 Loss of knee flexion and ankle dorsiflexion

L3 Loss of knee extension

S1 Loss of ankle plantarflexion

L5 Loss of hip abduction and extension

Fig. 14.48 Weakness related to level of spinal defect. These tests are useful in determining the level of the defect. Function is lost distal to the defect. Tyical functional losses for each level are shown.

Walking

Walking ability is related to level ⟨
mental status, family compliance, ⟨
hip reduction status. Most sacral, m
patients walk (Fig. 14.57). Walking
and adolescence, when the body ⟨
mass. Provide walkers for gait trair
Walking must be energy efficient,
maintained. Combinations of ind
often provide a good long term solu

Problems

Pathologic fractures may fol
treatments, or operative procedure⟨
may be confused with osteomyeliti
fortable. Avoid long-term immobili
occur in the distal femur and upper

Cord tethering is suggested b⟨
mity or pain (Fig. 14.60). Untether
progression or eliminate the need f⟨

Skin breakdown includes sa⟨
14.61). These are common, seriou
disability. Reduce risk by correctin
pelvic obliquity.

Latex allergy occurs in about 5
history of latex allergy. Create a lat⟨
pital and at home. Before any op⟨
problem is accessed by an anesthes
ative prophylaxis.

Myelodysplasia Consultant Vincen

Refer

2000 Foot deformities in adolescents and you
  J PO-b 9:161
2000 Follow-up study after treatment of knee
  Snela S, Parsch K. JPO-b 9:154
1998 Incidence and type of hindfoot deform
  Frawley PA, Broughton NS, Menelaus MB.
1997 Surgical release of tethered spinal cord: ⟨
  Archibeck MJ, et al. JPO 17:773
1997 Surgical management of ankle valgus in
  olar screw. Davids JR, et al. JPO 17:3
1997 Chronic physeal fractures in myelodysp
  description, treatment, and outcome. Rodger
1997 Surgery of the spine in myelodysplasia.
  JB. CO 338:19
1995 Calcaneal lengthening for valgus deformi
  severe, symptomatic flatfoot and skewfoot. ⟨
1995 Epidemiology, etiologic factors, and pr
  Shurtleff DB, Lemire RJ. Neurosurg Clin N
1994 The high incidence of foot deformity in p
  NS, Graham G, Menelaus MB. JBJS 76B:5⟨
1994 Walking ability in spina bifida patients: a
  based on sitting balance and motor level. Sw
1993 Latex allergy in children with myelodysp
  E, et al. JPO 13:1
1993 Achilles tenodesis for calcaneus deform
  MA, Lynn MD, Demos HA. CO 292:239
1992 Neuropathic foot ulceration in patients w
  Burke SW. JPO 12:786
1991 Community ambulation by children with
  Charney EB, Melchionni JB, Smith DR. JPC

Clinical Features

Prenatal diagnosis is by alpha-fetoprotein determination and ultra-sound examination.

Initial assessment is best provided in a multidisciplinary facility with neurodevelopmental, neurosurgical, urologic, and orthopedic consultants available. Make certain management is whole-child oriented. Determine neurological level by neurological examination and muscle testing. Unilateral or incomplete lesions improve prognosis. Often the orthopedic concerns are the least of the child's problems.

Periodic evaluations are necessary throughout childhood (Fig. 14.49). During each visit, assess overall function, the spine and pelvis for symmetry, the skin for ulcers, and address specific problems identified by the parents.

Hip deformity

Hip deformity is related to the neurological level. In the past hip deformity was often over-treated (Fig. 14.50).

Flexion contractures increase with time and may require release.

Hip dislocations are most common in upper lumbar paralysis with muscle imbalance. Hip dislocation itself does not affect the ability to walk. Operative indications include painful dysplasia in the ambulatory patient and fixed pelvic obliquity, which makes sitting difficult or skin care unmanageable. Operative complications including recurrent deformity, stiffness, pathological fractures, and skin ulcers are common.

Spinal Deformity

Spinal deformity is most common in the more severely affected child. Progression is most likely when associated with cord tethering or hip contractures.

Kyphosis is usually congenital and may be severe (Figs. 14.51 and 14.52). Resection is indicated if the deformity prevents skin closure during neonatal repair of the defect or later if skin breakdown occurs over the apex of the deformity.

Scoliosis may cause suprapelvic obliquity increasing the risk of decubitus ulcer formation, sitting problems, and impaired hand function. Correct severe or progressive deformity and level the pelvis to distribute skin loading evenly under the pelvis. Manage with a focus on disability rather than deformity. Be aware that poor soft tissue coverage, contractures, impaired sensation, fragile bone, and deficient posterior elements complicate treatment. Pseudoarthrosis rates are decreased with combined anterior–posterior fusions and rigid segmental instrumentation.

Knee Deformity

Knee deformities may be congenital or develop during childhood.

Flexion deformity may make walking difficult or impossible. Correct significant disability with soft tissue releases, which often requires a posterior capsulotomy. Extension osteotomy may be necessary in the older child or adolescent.

Extension deformity may complicate sitting. Release persisting congenital contractures by early percutanous release.

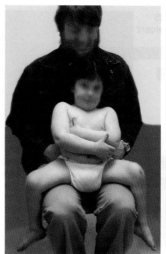
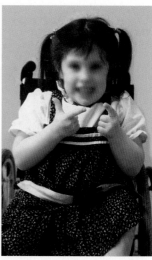

Fig. 14.49 Evaluation throughout childhood. Plan to see the child periodically throughout childhood. Become acquainted with the family.

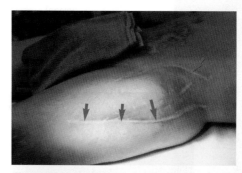

Fig. 14.50 Ineffective management. Hip reduction procedures are seldom helpful as recurrence is common, reoperations are frequent, complications are distressing, and functional improvement is minimal. This patient had several procedures (red arrows) with little or no improvement.

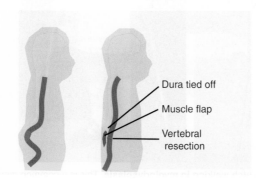

Dura tied off

Muscle flap

Vertebral resection

Fig. 14.51 Kyphosis repair. Repair usually requires bony and soft tissue procedures.

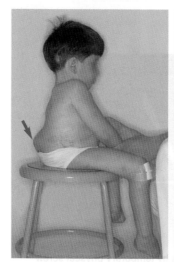
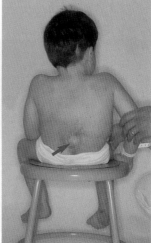

Fig. 14.52 Lumbar kyphosis. This prominence makes the overlying skin vulnerable to breakdown.

0

Upper level paralysis

Equinus

Calcaneus

Valgus

Varus

Vertical talus

Lower level paralysis

Equinus

Calcaneus

Valgus

Varus

Vertical talus

Fig. 14.53 Foot deformities in high-a
data of Broughton (1994) and Frawley

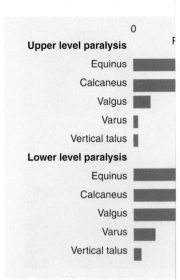

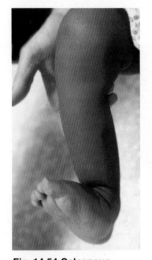

Fig. 14.54 Calcaneus deformity.

Fig.
com
Corr
nece
mob

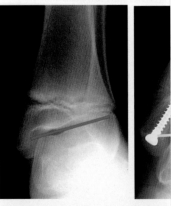

Fig. 14.56 Correction of ankle valgus placement. Correct ankle valgus (red l
screw to inhibit medial physeal growth.
deformity is corrected (yellow line).

Muscular Dystrophy

X-chromosomal

Duchenne muscular dystrophy

Becker muscular dystrophy

Emery–Dreifuss muscular dystrophy

Autosomal dominant

myotonic muscular dystrophy

fascioscapulohumeral dystrophy

Autosomal recessive

limb–girdle muscular dystrophy

congenital muscular dystrophy

Fig. 14.62 Types of muscular dystrophy.

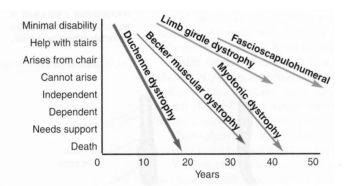

Fig. 14.63 Natural history of muscular dystrophies. The arrows show the average clinical course with level of disability and age.

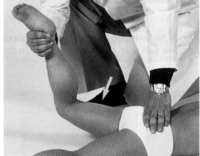

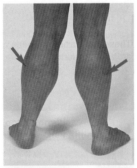

Fig. 14.64 Clinical features of Duchenne muscular dystrophy. Note the calf pseudohypertrophy (red arrows) and positive Ober test (yellow arrow). This positive Ober test demonstrates a tensor fascia contracture.

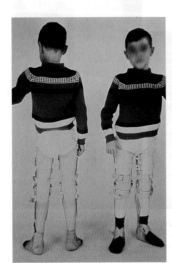

Fig. 14.65 Long-leg braces may prolong walking.

Muscular Dystrophy

Muscular dystrophies are a group of uncommon, genetically determined primary myopathies characterized by progressive muscle wasting (Fig. 14.62). The natural history is variable (Fig. 14.63).

Duchenne Muscular Dystrophy

Duchenne muscular dystrophy (DMD) is most common and caused by absence or impaired dystrophin. The dystrophin gene is located on the X chomosome. Dystrophin stabilizes the cell membrane and protein complexes within the muscle cell. A loss of this function causes the disease. Prenatal diagnosis can sometimes be made by special molecular studies or fetal muscle biopsy.

Clinical features include males with an onset in early childhood, a wide base gait, impaired running, positive Gowers sign, delayed motor development, intellectual slowness, calf pseudohypertrophy (Fig. 14.64), and often a positive family history. About onethird are new mutants.

Diagnosis Serum CPK is elevated 200–300 times normal values. Muscle biopsy shows variation in fiber size, loss of fibers, increased fat, and sometimes centralization of nuclei. EMG shows myopathic changes.

Natural history Most boys show progressive deterioration with flexion–abduction contractures of the hips, and flexion contractures of the knees and ankle with loss of walking about 10 years of age. Once walking ability is lost, scoliosis develops progressively. Cardiomyopathy and pulmonary compromise progress, and death usually occurs in late teens.

Lower limb management Use stretching exercises and night AFO splinting to delay contracture formation. Attempt to preserve walking by releasing contractures just before the ability to walk is lost. Release the Achilles tendon and consider an anterior transfer of the posterior tibialis tendon. Release knee flexion and hip flexion–abduction contractures if they limit function. Place in a long-leg brace made before surgery and mobilize on the first postoperative day (Fig. 14.65). This aggressive management may delay wheelchair dependence by 1–4 years.

Mobility Provide effective mobility. An electric wheelchair and a van for the family are useful. Make the home wheelchair accessible. Foot deformities should be corrected before the child becomes wheelchair dependent (Fig. 14.66).

Spine management Prepare the family in advance of the onset of scoliosis. Progressive scoliosis develops once the child becomes non-ambulatory (Fig. 14.67). Avoid bracing. Between about 11 and 13 years, when the curve approaches 20°, and before the vital capacity falls below 30%, perform a segmental instrumentation and fusion from T2 to L5 or the sacrum.

Family support This disease causes guilt in the mother, stress in the family, and depression in the child. Provide a support system and make available counseling as necessary.

Long-term ventilatory support Prolongation of survival is technically possible but creates many ethical issues.

Dystrophin replacement may be feasible in the future.

Becker Muscular Dystrophy

Becker muscular dystrophy (BMD) is a uncommon, mild, muscular dystrophy due to dystrophin abnormality with clinical findings similar to DMD but much less severe. Early features of BMD include leg cramps and gait problems during childhood. Scoliosis is rare. Survival into midadult life is usual. In some cases, the diagnosis is not established until adult life. Management problems are similar to DMD but required at an older age. Provide physical therapy, release of contractures, and effective mobility.

Emery-Dreifuss Muscular Dystrophy

This ia a rare sex-linked recessive muscular dystrophy with elbow, triceps, and posterocervical muscle contractures, slowly progressive muscle wasting, and cardiomyopathy. Weakness becomes apparent during the first decade, and more pronounced during adolescence. Differentiate this from BMD and DMD by only mildly elevated CPK levels and by dystrophin testing. Patients may require contracture releases, spinal stabilization and referal to a cardiologist for insertion of a cardiac pacemaker.

Autosomal Dominant Muscular Dystrophies

Myotonic dystrophies include a heterogeneous group of diseases characterized by myotonia. Myotonia is the inability of the muscle to relax after contracting. Severe forms are seen.

Myotonia congenita has an onset in infancy but becomes more evident during adolescence. Clinical features include generalized muscle hypertrophy, absence of skeletal deformities, and minimal long-term disability.

Congenital myotonic dystrophy shows variable expressions with potential for severe early involvement. Features include hypotonia, delayed development, feeding and respiratory difficulties, and mild mental retardation. Walking is delayed. Cataracts may develop in adolescence. Orthopedic problems include clubfeet, hip dislocations, and lower limb contractures (Fig. 14.68).

Myotonic dystrophy onset is during adult life. Clinical features include encephalopathy, facies myopathica, paresthesia, atrophy, myotonia, mental retardation, cataract, diabetes, and cardiac conduction defects.

Fascioscapulohumeral dystrophy (FSHD) is characterized by progressive weakness and atrophy of the facial, shoulder-girdle and upper arm muscles, and occasional later pelvic-girdle and lower limb involvement. Shoulder instability may be improved by scapulothoracic fusion (Fig. 14.69).

Autosomal Recessive Muscular Dystrophies

Congenital muscular dystrophy (CMD) includes a heterogeneous group of congenital disorders characterized by marked hypotonia, generalized muscle weakness, and frequently multiple contractures. Four categories of CMD include: (1) the classic form without severe impairment of intellectual development; (2) the Fukuyama type CMD with muscle and structural brain abnormalities; (3) the milder Finnish type, and (4) severe Walker-Warburg syndrome (CMD IV).

Limb–girdle muscular dystrophy is similar to FSHD but without involvement of the fascial muscles. Problems are similar to DMD and BMD except scoliosis is mild. Longevity is limited to middle age.

Consultant Michael Sussman, e-mail: msussman@shrinenet.org

References

Duchenne

1999 Lower limb surgery in Duchenne muscular dystrophy. Forst J, Forst R. Neuromuscul Disord 9:176

1999 Management of neuromuscular scoliosis. McCarthy R. Orthop Clin North Am 30:435

1999 Fetal muscle biopsy as a diagnostic tool in Duchenne muscular dystrophy. Nevo Y, et al. Prenat Diagn 19:921

1996 Spinal fusion in Duchenne's muscular dystrophy. Brook PD, et al. JPO 16:324

1996 Evaluation of a program for long-term treatment of Duchenne muscular dystrophy. Experience at the University Hospitals of Cleveland. Vignos PJ, et al. JBJS 78A:1844

Becker

1999 Clinical characteristics of aged Becker muscular dystrophy patients with onset after 30 years. Yazaki M, et al. Eur Neurol 42:145

1998 Pilot study of myoblast transfer in the treatment of Becker muscular dystrophy. Neumeyer A, et al. Neurology 51:589

Other

1998 Myotonic dystrophy: molecular genetics and diagnosis. Gharehbaghi-Schnell E, et al. Wien Klin Wochenschr 110:7

1997 Emery-Dreifuss syndrome. Tsuchiya Y, Arahata K. Curr Opin Neurol 10:421

1996 Congenital muscular dystrophy: a review of the literature. Leyten Q, et al. Clin Neurol Neurosurg 98:267

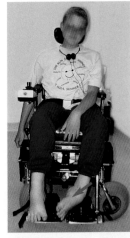
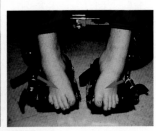

Fig. 14.66 Heel-cord contractures in DMD makes foot positioning difficult. These equinovarus deformities (red arrows) make positioning of the feet on the footrests difficult.

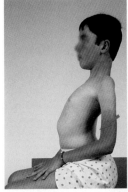
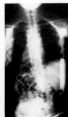
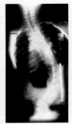
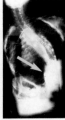

Fig. 14.67 Progressive scoliosis in DMD. Child has thoracolumbar lordosis (red arrow). Scoliosis becomes progressive once the patient becomes nonambulatory. Instrument and fused before curves become severe (yellow arrow).

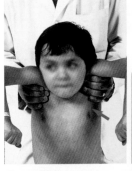

Fig. 14.68 Unusual forms of muscular disorders. Congenital muscular dystrophy (red arrow) and heel-cord contracture in congenital myotonia (yellow arrow).

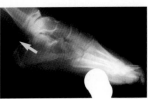
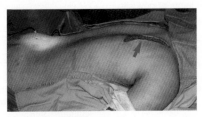

Fig. 14.69 Scapulothoracic fusion. Shoulder stabilization improves upper extremity function in FSHD.

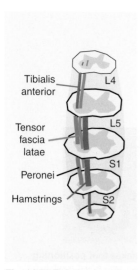

Fig. 14.70 Relative length of cell columns in spinal cord. Based on Sharrard (1955).

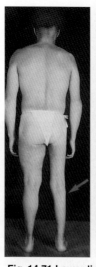

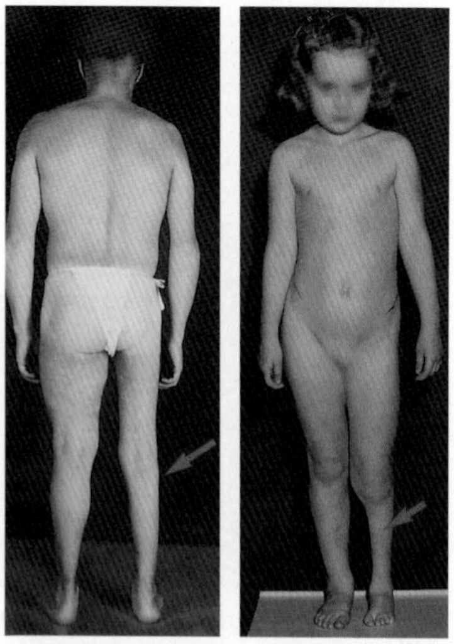

Fig. 14.71 Lower-limb atrophy due to poliomyelitis. This atrophy is associated with limb shortening (red arrows).

Poliomyelitis

Acute poliomyelitis is a viral infection that damages the anterior horn cells and brain stem motor nuclei, causing paralysis. From a human host, the disease is spread by the oropharyngeal route. Most develop only a mild gastroenteritis. About 1% develop paralysis.

Stages of Poliomyelitis

Acute stage After an incubation period of 1–3 weeks, a systemic flu-like illness develops. Rarely the infections spreads to the nervous system causing inflammatory changes with varying degrees of neuronal degeneration. Over a period of 1–2 weeks a progressively increasing paralysis develops without sensory involvement. Muscles with motor nuclei extending over several segments are most likely to be affected (Fig. 14.70). About twice as many muscles become weak as become totally paralyzed.

Convalescent stage This recovery phase extends over a period of about 2 years. Most recovery occurs during the first few months. Contractures start to develop during this period.

Chronic stage After about two years the disease becomes chronic. Muscle imbalance, contractures, and growth cause increasing deformities. Most severe deformities are seen in severely affected younger patients with many years of growth. Limb atrophy and shortening are characteristic deformities (Fig. 14.71).

Management Principles

Sensation and IQ are unaffected, improving prognosis as compared with children with cerebral palsy or myelodysplasia.

Prognosis is better for the young with minimal paralysis.

Contractures develop with time All soft tissue components–including muscle, tendon, joint capsules, fascia, and neurovascular structures–become contracted.

Gentle stretching and splinting An overcorrected position may improve or prevent progression of deformity (Fig. 14.72). Stretching must be performed carefully to avoid fractures of the fragile bone.

Operative correction is useful to correct deformity and provide stability. Sometimes function can be improved by tendon transfers.

Basic principles of tendon surgery are well established (Fig. 10.73).

Simple osteotomy fixation techniques are frequently utilized as these procedures are most commonly performed in developing countries with limited medical resources.

Bony procedures are best delayed until the end of growth to prevent recurrent deformity.

Bracing is often useful to provide stability and to facilitate walking.

Postpoliomyelitis syndrome (PPS) causes slowly progressive weakness, atrophy, muscle pain, and fasciculations that occur 15 or more years following the original disease. Management is usually conservative.

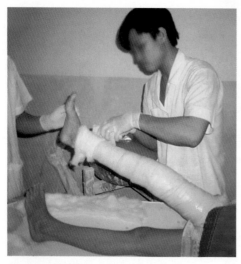

Fig. 14.72 Stretching casts for knee flexion deformity.

Principles of tendon transfers

Transfer only muscles of fair (3) or good (4) grade
Insure muscle excursion suitable
Loss of function from original site acceptable
Joint with adequate free passive motion
Transfer cannot overcome fixed deformity
Insure unrestricted motion of joints at new site
Preserve muscle neurovascular status
Transfer in straight line
Attach into bone preferable
Place transfer under proper tension

Fig. 14.73 Principles of tendon transfers. Based on Mayer (1956).

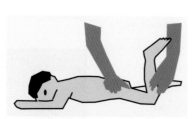

Fig. 14.74 Assessing hip abduction contracture in poliomyelitis. From Gautam 1998.

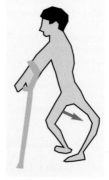

Fig. 14.75 Hyperextension knee deformity in polioyelitis.

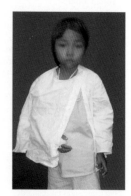

Fig. 14.76 Muscle transfers may improve hand function.

Orthopedic Management

Assessment requires a careful evaluation, which includes grading strength of muscle groups, determining the range of active and passive motion, assessing contracturs (Fig. 14.74), determine limb length differences, and documentation of deformity (Fig. 14.75). Function may be improved by tendon transfers. This requires a preoperative assessment of specific muscles to determine which have adequate strength to function effectively in a rerouted position.

Upper limb The objective is to place the hand in a position for optimum function and for stability to facilitate transfers and crutch walking. Children with little hand function may still use crutches and have prehension between the arm and the chest. These important adaptive functions should be preserved.

Shoulder stability is more important than mobility.

Elbow and hand require mobility for optimal function. Establish motion and correct deformity before performing tendon transfers (Fig. 14.76).

Spine Scoliosis (Fig. 14.77) occurs in about a third of children with paralysis. Curve patterns are usually either a double-major or long paralytic types. Pelvic obliquity is common (Fig. 14.78). Bracing may slow progression for 20°–40°curves. For curves 40°–60° a posterior segmental instrumentation and fusion is often indicated. Curves >60° may require anterior and posterior instrumentation and fusion.

Crawling is a form of mobility commonly used by children without medical care. With good medical care, about 60% of these children can become community and 30% household ambulators (Fig. 14.79).

Lower limb requires most attention as paralysis is more common and corrective procedures most effective. The objective is to provide stability and symmetry for walking with or without a brace. The foot should be plantigrade, the knee extended, and the hip stable. Symmetry requires an absence of significant pelvic obliquity and leg length inequality.

Common procedures in poliomyelitis include shoulder fusions (Fig. 14.80); tensor fascia releases; correction of knee flexion contractures, rotational osteotomies (Fig. 14.81), correction of calcaneus (Fig. 14.82), and cavus deformites; and limb length equalization procedures.

Topic consultant Hugh Watts, e-mail: hwatts@ucla.edu

References

2000 Appliances and surgery for poliomyelitis in developing countries. Huckstep RL. Instr Course Lect AAOS 49:593

1999 Prediction of walking possibility in crawling children in poliomyelitis. Arora S, Tandon H. JPO 19:715

1999 Triple arthrodesis: twenty-five and forty-four-year average follow-up of the same patients. Saltzman C, et al. JBJS 81A:1391

1998 A new test for estimating iliotibial band contracture. Gautam V, Anand S. JBJS 80B:474

1998 A simple method of shoulder arthrodesis. Mohammed N. JBJS 80B:620

1997 Late functional deterioration following paralytic poliomyelitis. Kidd D, et al. QJM 90:189

1997 Leg lengthening by the Ilizarov technique for patients with sequelae of poliomyelitis. Huang S. Formos. J Med Assoc 96:258

1997 Fixed pelvic obliquity after poliomyelitis: classification and management. Lee D, et al. JBJS 79B:190

1995 Review of Elmslie's triple arthrodesis for post-polio pes calcaneovalgus deformity. Faraj A. J Foot Ankle Surg 34:319

1994 Fibular shortening in poliomyelitis. Sharma O, Sharma N, Patond K. Indian J Pediatr 61:71

1991 Residual poliomyelitis of lower limb-pattern and deformities. Sharma J, et al. Indian J Pediatr 58:233

1990 Rotation osteotomy of the tibia after poliomyelitis. A review of 51 patients. Asirvatham R, Watts H, Rooney R. JBJS 72B:409

1989 Modified posterior soft tissue release for management of severe knee flexion contracture. Bhan S, Rath S. Orthopedics 12:703

1989 Calcaneal osteotomy and tendon sling for the management of calcaneus deformity. Pandey A, Pandey S, Prasad V. JBJS 71A:1192

1988 Transfer of half the calcaneal tendon to the dorsum of the foot for paralytic equinus deformity. Fernandez-Palazzi F, Medina J, Marcano N. Int Orthop 12:57

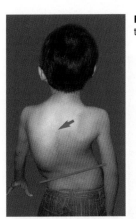

Fig. 14.77 Scoliosis from poliomyelitis. Note the scoliosis and pelvic obliquity.

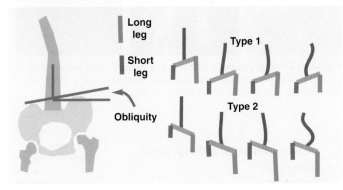

Fig. 14.78 Pelvic obliquity in poliomyelitis. Note that a variety of curve patterns occur with pelvic obliquity and limb shortening. Based on Lee (1997).

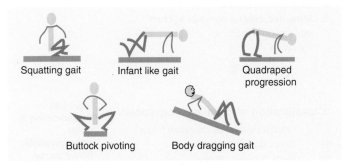

Fig. 14.79 Patterns of crawling in poliomyelitis. Based on Arora (1999).

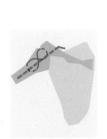

Fig. 14.80 Shoulder fusion. Using fig. 8 wiring and K wire fixation. From Mohammed (1998).

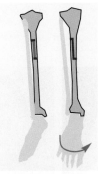

Fig. 14.81 Tibial rotational osteotomy. Removal of an anterior bone wedge (red) produces rotation. From Asirvatham (1990).

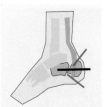

Fig. 14.82 Calcaneal osteotomy and tendon sling for calcaneus deformity. Osteotomy is fixed with a K wire. From Pandy, (1989).

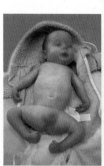
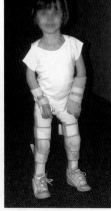
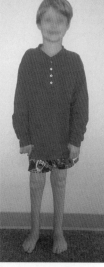

Fig. 14.83 Arthrogryposis in different age groups. The natural history is favorable. Multiple contractures at birth (left), treatments early childhood (middle), and a successful outcome in most patients (right).

Arthrogryposis

Arthrogryposis multiplex congenita includes a heterogenous group of disorders characterized by multiple congenital joint contractures. The disorder occurs in about 1/3000 births. Decreased fetal movement due to fetal or maternal abnormalities cause the deformities. The causes of fetal akinesis include disorders of nerves, muscles, or connective tissues, maternal disease, intrauterine constraint, or vascular compromise. The earlier and longer this loss of movement, the more severe the deformities. The most common deformities include clubfeet and hip dislocations. Most deformities are nonprogressive (Fig. 14.83).

Evaluation

More than 100 disorders are included in the differential diagnosis of multiple congenital contractures (Fig. 14.84). This differentiation may be complex and in some instances the exact diagnosis cannot be established. Deformities may be classified based on whether they primarily affect the limbs, include systemic involvement, or a clear neurological etiology. Certain types are most likely to be seen by the orthopedist.

Amyoplasia is the classic form of arthrogryposis making up about a third of the cases. The common features include clubfeet, flexed or extended knees, dislocated hips, internally rotated and abducted shoulders, flexed or extended elbows, pronated forearms, and flexed wrists and fingers. The trunk is less commonly affected. Muscles are hypoplastic or absent, joints are fibrotic and stiff. Joints show a loss of creases and dimpling. IQ is normal, sensation is intact, potential for walking is good, and most become independent and productive in adult life.

Distal arthrogryposis includes 6 subtypes (Fig. 14.85), often inherited and primarily involves the hands and feet. Fingers are flexed, medially deviated, and overlapping, and fist is clenched. Clubfeet or vertical tali are common.

Contractual arachnodactyly or Beal syndrome is an autosomal-dominant disorder with long extremities, joint contractures, and ear crumpling.

Pterygium syndromes include a group of varied disorders with characteristic features (Figs. 14.86 and 14.87).

Freeman–Sheldon syndrome or whistling face syndrome is a familial disorder with a characteristic *puckered appearance* to the face and multiple joint contractures.

Diastrophic dysplasia is a syndrome that includes short stature, multiple contractures, clubfeet, proximally placed thumbs, and progressive kyphoscoliosis.

Management

Management principles may be applied to most of the patients.

Accurate diagnosis is necessary to advise the family about the risk of recurrence.

Family counseling Deal with family guilt, which is usually present and unless resolved will interfere with management. Provide information regarding local or national arthrogryposis support groups. For parents of infants with amyoplasia, provide information regarding the favorable natural history with progressive reductions in deformity and the potential for an independent and productive life.

Classification of arthrogryposis

I **Mainly limbs**
Amyoplasia
Distal arthrogryposis type I

II **Limbs and other body areas**
Freeman–Sheldon syndrome
Diastrophic dysplasia

III **Limbs and central nervous system**
Fetal alcohol syndrome
Trisomy 21

Fig. 14.84 Classification of arthrogryposis – major categories and examples. From Hall (1997).

Classification of distal arthrogryposis

I	Overlapping, ulnar deviation fingers
IIa	Short stature, cleft palate
IIb	Hard muscles, ptosis
IIc	Cleft lip and palate
IId	Scoliosis
IIe	Trismus

Fig. 14.85 Classification of distal arthrogryposis. Based on Hall (1997).

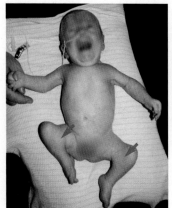
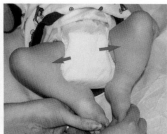

Fig. 14.86 Popliteal ptergium. Note the severe knee flexion deformities (arrows).

Multiple pterygium syndromes

Popliteal pterygium
Antecubital pterygium
Multiple pterygium – autosomal recessive
Multiple pterygium – autosomal dominant
Lethal multiple pterygium
Lethal popliteal pterygium
Pterygium and malignant hyperthermia

Fig. 14.87 Classification of multiple pterygium syndrome. Based on Hall (1997).

Physical therapy should be started early to reduce contractures and facilitate bonding. Encourage the family to provide the treatment. This is most convenient and economical for the family, and the parent-child interaction is emotionally therapeutic. Stretching should be gentle and atraumatic.

Bracing facilitates function by providing joint stabilization for standing and walking. Lightweight nonarticulated plastic AFO or KFO are most useful. Allow bracefree periods during the day for the child to crawl. Splinting at night is often essential to prevent recurrence of deformity once corrected by surgery.

Adaptive equipment such as walkers, electric wheelchairs, and devices to facilitate self-care are very valuable.

Operative correction is usually necessary to correct clubfeet, knee contractures, or hip dislocations. Minimizing the duration of immobilization during infancy and childhood by combining procedures, minimal duration of postoperative immobilization, and avoiding repeated procedures. Delay operative correction of upper-extremity deformities until early childhood when disability is clear. Surgery is necessary only to enhance function not correct deformity per se.

Clubfeet
Manage by early stretching, casting, percutaneous releases, repeated casting (Fig. 14.88). Correct residual deformity by extensive posteromedial release or talectomy. Provide night splinting for several years following correction to prevent recurrence. If recurrence does occur, correct with serial casting and reinstitute night splinting. Provide stretching exercises during the day. Avoid repeated procedures. Try to delay reoperation for rigid recurrent deformity until the end of growth.

Knee Flexion-Extension Deformity
Manage by early stretching to correct less fixed deformity. Correct fixed deformity by hamstring lengthening, capsulectomy, and femoral shortening if necessary (Fig. 14.89). Correct hyperextension deformity by quadriceps lengthening to center arc of motion to about 15° of flexion.

Hip Dislocation
Reduce dislocations in infancy (Fig. 14.90) by a medial approach open reduction and shorten postoperative immobilization to about 5 weeks. See page 407. Combine with other procedures when possible. Avoid repeated or extensive procedures that may cause stiffness. Establish symmetry and maintain mobility.

Upper limbs
Provide early manipulation to improve motion and retain with night splints. Teach use of adaptive devices to facilitate self-care. In early childhood, perform procedures to correct deformity that interferes with function. Because of good hand sensibility, function is often surprisingly good (Fig. 14.91).

Topic consultant: Lynn Staheli, e-mail: staheli @u.washington.edu

References

1999 Prenatal diagnosis of distal arthrogryposis type 1. Dudkiewicz I, Achiron R, Ganel A. Skeletal Radiol 28:233

1997 Arthrogrypotic joint contracture at the knee and the foot: correction with a circular frame. Brunner R, Hefti F. Tgetgel J. JPO 6B:192

1997 Arthrogryposis multiplex congenita: etiology, genetics, classification, diagnostic approach, and general aspects. Hall J. JPO 6B:159

1997 Management of clubfoot deformity in amyoplasia. Niki H, Staheli L, Mosca V. JPO 17:803

1997 Management of knee deformity in classical arthrogryposis multiplex congenita (amyoplasia congenita). Murray C, Fixsen J. JPO 6B:186

1997 Principles of treatment of the upper extremity in arthrogryposis multiplex congenita type I. Axt M, Niethard F, Doderlein L, Weber M. JPO 6B:179

1996 Medial-approach open reduction of hip dislocation in amyoplasia-type arthrogryposis. Szoke G, Staheli L, Jaffe K, Hall J. JPO 16:127

1985 The etiology of arthrogryposis (multiple congenital contracture). Swinyard C, Bleck E. CO 15

1985 Passive motion therapy for infants with arthrogryposis. Palmer P, MacEwen G, Bowen J, Mathews P. CO 54

1985 Spinal deformities in patients with arthrogryposis. A review of 16 patients. Daher Y, Lonstein J, Winter R, Moe J. Spine 10:60

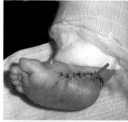
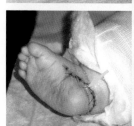
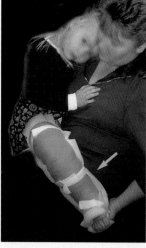

Fig. 14.88 Clubfoot correction. Correction often requires postoperative serial casting. Note improvement at 2 weeks (red arrow) and 4 weeks (yellow arrow). Night splinting is essential to prevent recurrence (orange arrow).

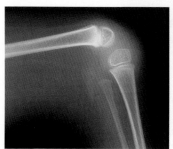
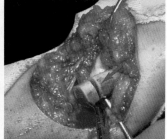

Fig. 14.89 Correction of knee flexion contracture. Correct severe contracture with femoral shortening (red arrow) and plate fixation.

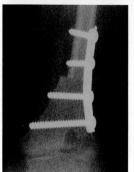

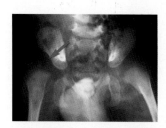
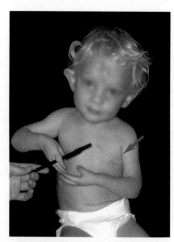

Fig. 14.90 Hip dislocations (arrow) should be reduced in early infancy.

Fig. 14.91 Upper extremity function is surprisingly good. This is due to normal sensation and excellent adaptive mechanisms.

Hereditary Sensory Motor Neuropathies (HSMNs I–VI)

Type I	Charcot–Marie–Tooth (CMT) disease
Type II	Axonal neuropathy
Type III	Hypertrophic interstitial neuropathy (Dejerine–Sottas disease)
Type IV	Refsum disease
Type V	Hereditary sensory neuropathy with spastic paraplegia
Type VI	Hereditary sensory neuropathy with optic atrophy

Fig. 14.92 Classification of hereditary sensory motor neuropathies.

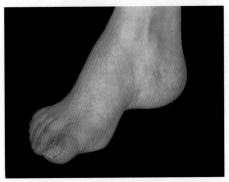

Fig. 14.93 Foot deformity in CMT disease.

Spinal Muscular Atrophy Classification

Traditional classification

Type I	Werdnig–Hoffman disease acute	onset <6 mo.
Type II	Werdnig–Hoffman disease chronic	onset 6–24 mo.
Type III	Kugelberg–Welander disease	onset >24 mo.

Current classification

Type I	Severe – unable to sit, usually dies in infancy
Type II	Moderate – diagnosis in infancy, unable to walk, dies mid–adult life
Type III	Mild – diagnosis after age 2, marginal walkers, independent adults

Fig. 14.94 Classification of spinal muscular atrophy. Two different classifications are in use. The traditional classification is based on age of onset. The current and more commonly used classification is based on severity with prognostic implications.

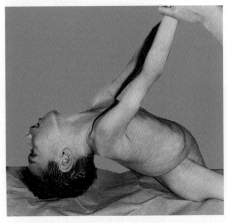

Fig. 14.94 Spinal muscular atrophy. Disability in severe form is profound with severe muscle weakness and disability. Note the lack of head control.

Miscellaneous Disorders

Hereditary Sensory Motor Neuropathies

This is a group of conditions that involve the sensory nerves, are often familial, and sometimes so mild in the parents that they may not be aware that their problem is a genetic disorder. The disability starts in childhood with gait disturbances; later, scoliosis and hand dysfuntion develop. Nerve condition is delayed. These disorders are progressive and recurrence often follows operative correction. This disease is commonly classified into six groups (Fig. 14.92). The first three are of most orthopedic significance.

Charcot-Marie-Tooth Disease (CMT) develops during childhood, is autosomal dominant (30% new mutations), often seen first for pes cavus. Check for loss of vibratory sense and foot eversion weakness. Examine parents as sometimes they show signs of the disease without being aware of the diagnosis.

Foot Bilateral pes cavovarus is the most common foot deformity (Fig. 14.93). The specific components include hindfoot varus, anterior or forefoot cavus, and, often, claw toes. The deformity is caused by the tibialis posterior overpowering peroneus brevis coupled with peroneus longus overpowering of the tibialis anterior. Manage pes cavus as outlined on page 111.

Spine Scoliosis, kyphoscoliosis, or kyphosis develops in about half by the end of growth.

Hand disability is increasing likely with advancing age. Disability results from decreased conduction velocity of the nerves, lack of opposition, weak pinch, and clawing of the fingers. Tendon transfers may be helpful in improving function.

Axon Neuropathy Like CMT disease but milder.

Hypertrophic Interstitial Neuropathy This condition may be associated with clubfeet. Weakness and sensory loss are progressive. Thickening of the peripheral nerves may be felt.

Spinal Muscular Atrophy

Spinal musclar atrophy (SMA) includes a heterogenous group of disorders that are rare, autosomal recessive, with anterior horn cell degeneration, causing muscle weakness and atrophy. Sensation and mentation are unaffected. SMA was traditionally classified by the age of onset but currently is being classified based on severity (Fig. 14.94).

SMA type I Infants are severely affected at birth, profound hypotonia, fragile, may have pathologic fractures. Maintain range of motion. Aggressive orthopedic care not appropriate.

SMA type II Children with this intermediate form live many decades with considerable disability. Prolongation of survival is possible with ventilatory assistance despite severe respiratory and bulbar muscle dysfunction. Common orthopedic problems include hip dislocations and spinal deformity.

Hip subluxation or dislocation may occur due to muscle imbalance, hypotonia, pelvic obliquity, and poor muscle tone. Attempt to maintain free mobile symmetrical motion. Avoid operative procedures as disability is minimal and recurrence is common.

Scoliosis occurs in nearly all of these patients. It occurs during the first decade and progresses at a rate related to the severity of the weakness. Bracing or modifications of seating may be helpful in supporting an upright posture. It is doubtful that bracing significantly affects progression. Posterior segmental fusion is indicated for curves approaching 40° and when forced vital capacity is still above 40%.

SMA type III Attempt to maintain walking as long as possible. Rarely hip dysplasia progresses making correction by femoral and pelvic osteotomy necessary. Progression of scoliosis is less severe than for type II but may require fusion. Be aware that long fusions may adversely affect walking.

Friedreich Ataxia

Friedreich ataxia (FRDA) is an autosomal recessive, progressive, spinocerebellar degeneration with a trinucleotide repeat defect found in chromosome 9.

Clinical features Friedreich ataxia is the most common cause of recessive ataxias. Neurological examination shows ataxia, dysarthria, areflexia, pyramidal signs, and sensory deficits. Cardiomyopathy and diabetes mellitus are common. Scoliosis and pes cavus are primary orthopedic problems. Walking becomes progressively more difficult and ceases to be functional by about 20 years of age. The disease progresses causing cardiopulmonary failure and usually death in mid-adult life.

Management Individualize management. Scoliosis is progressive (Fig. 14.95). Brace curves in the 25°–35° range if the bracing does not interfere with walking. Larger curves may require segmental instrumentation and fusion. Cavus foot deformities may be improved by plantar–medial release followed by tendon transfers and osteotomies. Provide effective mobility with electric wheelchairs.

Congenital Myopathies

These heterogenous disorders cause hypotonicity and muscle weakness in infants and children (Fig. 14.96). These disorders are non or slowly progressive. The diagnosis is established by histochemical analysis and electron microscopy of muscle biopsy specimens. Currently the classic list (Fig. 14.97) has been expanded to more than 40 disorders.

Dermatomyositis

Juvenile dermatomyositis is a multisystem disease causing inflammation affecting primarily the skin and muscle producing symmetrical weakness, and typical skin rashes that affect the face and hands. Confirm the diagnosis by an elevated CPK and muscle biopsy. Treatment often requires steroids or methotrexate.

Chapter Consultant Michael Sussman, e-mail: msussman@shrinenet.org

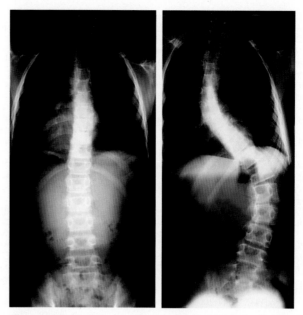

Fig. 14.95 Progressive scoliosis in Friedreich ataxia. Curves at age 9 and 14 years.

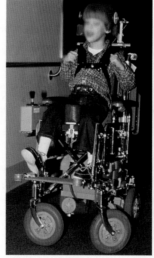
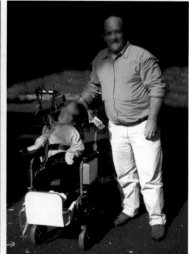

Fig. 14.96 Mobility aids in children with profound muscle weakness. Electric wheelchairs provide effective mobility and increased independence.

References

Charcot-Marie-Tooth disease

1996 Treatment of equinocavovarus deformity in adults with the use of a hinged distraction apparatus. Oganesyan O, Istomina I, Kuzmin V. JBJS 78A:546

1995 Treatment of the upper limb in Charcot-Marie-Tooth disease. Wood V, Huene D, Nguyen J. J Hand Surg 20B:511

1994 Spinal deformity in Charcot-Marie-Tooth disease. Walker J, et al. Spine 19:1044

1993 Foot and ankle manifestations of Charcot-Marie-Tooth disease. Holmes J, Hansen SJ. Foot Ankle 14:476

1993 The diagnosis and orthopaedic treatment of childhood spinal muscular atrophy, peripheral neuropathy, Friedreich ataxia, and arthrogryposis. Shapiro F, Specht L. JBJS 75A:1699

Spinal muscular atrophy

1995 Natural history in proximal spinal muscular atrophy. Clinical analysis of 445 patients and suggestions for a modification of existing classifications. Zerres K, Rudnik-Schoneborn S. Arch Neurol 52:518

1990 Surgical treatment of scoliosis in a spinal muscular atrophy population. Phillips DP, et al. Spine 15:942

Friedreich ataxia.

1999 Friedreich ataxia: recent developments and prospects for treatment. Legros B, Manto M. Rev Med Brux 20:73

1995 Natural history of muscle weakness in Friedreich ataxia and its relation to loss of ambulation. Beauchamp M, et al. CO 270

Congenital myopathy

1996 Congenital myopathies. Goebel H. Semin Pediatr Neurol 3:152

Juvenile dermatomyositis

1991 Juvenile dermatomyositis. Ansell BM. Rheum Dis Clin North Am 17:931

Congenital Myopathies

Central core disease
Nemaline myopathy
Myotubular myopathy
Congenital fiber–type disproportion
Metabolic myopathies

Fig. 14.97 Classic classification of congenital myopathies.

Albright AL, Barron WB, Fasick MP, et al. Continuous intrathecal baclofen infusion for spasticity of cerebral origin. JAMA 1993;270:2475-2477.

Alman BA, Craig CL, Zimbler S. Subtalar arthrodesis for stabilization of valgus hindfoot in patients with cerebral palsy. J Pediatr Orthop 1993;13:634-641.

Aronson DD, Zak PJ, Lee CL, et al. Posterior transfer of the adductors in children who have cerebral palsy: A long-term study. J Bone Joint Surg 1991;73A:59-65.

Bagg MR, Farber J, Miller F. Long-term follow-up of hip subluxation in cerebral palsy patients. J Pediatr Orthop 1993;13:32-36.

Barnes MJ, Herring JA. Combined split anterior tibial-tendon transfer and intramuscular lengthening of the posterior tibial tendon: Results in patients who have a varus deformity of the foot due to spastic cerebral palsy. J Bone Joint Surg 1991;73A:734-738.

Beach WR, Strecker WB, Coe J, et al. Use of the Green transfer in treatment of patients with spastic cerebral palsy: 17-year experience. J Pediatr Orthop 1991;11:731-736.

Beaty JH, Canale ST. Orthopaedic aspects of myelomeningocele. J Bone Joint Surg 1990;72A:626-630.

Bleck EE. Management of the lower extremities in children who have cerebral palsy. J Bone Joint Surg 1990;72A-140-144.

Boytim MJ, Davidson RS, Charney E, et al. Neonatal fractures in myelomeningocele patients. J Pediatr Orthop 1991;11:28-30.

Brinker MR, Rosenfeld SR, Feiwell E, et al. Myelomeningocele at the sacral level: Long-term outcomes in adults. J Bone Joint Surg 1994;76A:1293-1300.

Broughton NS, Graham G, Menelaus MB. The high incidence of foot deformity in patients with high-level spina bifida. J Bone Joint Surg 1994;76B:548-550.

Broughton NS, Menelaus MB, Cole WG, et al. The natural history of hip deformity in myelomeningocele. J Bone Joint Surg 1993;75B:760-763.

Brunner R, Baumann JU. Clinical benefit of reconstruction of dislocated or subluxated hip joints in patients with spastic cerebral palsy. J Pediatr Orthop 1994;14:290-294.

Buly RL, Huo M, Root L, et al. Total hip arthroplasty in cerebral palsy: Long-term follow-up results. Clin Orthop 1993;296:148-153.

Campos da Paz A, Burnett SM, Braga LW. Walking prognosis in cerebral palsy: A 22-year retrospective analysis. Dev Med Child Neurol 1994;36:130-134.

Carstens C, Paul K, Niethard FU, et al. Effect of scoliosis surgery on pulmonary function in patients with myelomeningocele. J Pediatr Orthop 1991;11:459-464.

Charney EB, Melchionni JB, Smith DR. Community ambulation by children with myelomeningocele and high-level paralysis. J Pediatr Orthop 1991;11:579-582.

Cuxart A, Iborra J, Melendez M, et al. Physeal injuries in myelomeningocele patients. Paraplegia 1992;30:791-794.

Damron TA, Breed AL, Cook T. Diminished knee flexion after hamstring surgery in cerebral palsy patients: Prevalence and severity. J Pediatr Orthop 1993;13:188-191.

Erken EH, Bischof FM. Iliopsoas transfer in cerebral palsy: The long-term outcome. J Pediatr Orthop 1994;14:295-298.

Fraser RK, Hoffman EB, Sparks LT, et al. The unstable hip and mid-lumbar myelomeningocele. J Bone Joint Surg 1992;74B:143-146.

Fraser RK, Menelaus MB. The management of tibial torsion in patients with spina bifida. J Bone Joint Surg 1993;75B:495-497.

Gage JR, DeLuca PA, Renshaw TS. Gait analysis: Principles and applications. Emphasis on its use in cerebral palsy. J Bone Joint Surg 1995;77A:1607-1623.

Gallien R, Morin F, Marquis F. Subtalar arthrodesis in children. J Pediatr Orthop 1989;9:59-63.

Georgiadis GM, Aronson DD. Posterior transfer of the anterior tibial tendon in children who have myelomeningocele. J Bone Joint Surg 1990;72A:392-398.

Harris MB, Banta JV. Cost of skin care in the myelomeningocele population. J Pediatr Orthop 1990;10:355-361.

Herndon WA, Bolano L, Sullivan JA. Hip stabilization in severely involved cerebral palsy patients. J Pediatr Orthop 1992;12:68-73.

Hoffer MM. The use of the pathokinesiology laboratory to select muscles for tendon transfers in the cerebral palsy hand. Clin Orthop 1993;288:135-138.

Hoffer MM, Barakat G, Koffman M. 10-year follow-up of split anterior tibial tendon transfer in cerebral palsied patients with spastic equinovarus deformity. J Pediatr Orthop 1985;5:432-434.

Hoffer MM, Lehman M, Mitani M. Long-term follow-up on tendon transfers to the extensors of the wrist and fingers in patients with cerebral palsy. J Hand Surg 1986;11A:836-840.

Hoffer MM, Stein GA, Koffman M. Femoral varus-derotation osteotomy in spastic cerebral palsy. J Bone Joint Surg 1985;67A:1229-1235.

Hoffer MM, Zeitzew S. Wrist fusion in cerebral palsy. J Hand Surg 1988;13A:667-670.

Hullin MG, Robb JE, Loudon IR. Ankle-foot orthosis function in low-level myelomeningocele. J Pediatr Orthop 1992;12:518-521.

Koman LA, Mooney JF III, Goodman A. Management of valgus hindfoot deformity in pediatric cerebral palsy patients by medial displacement osteotomy. J Pediatr Orthop 1993;13;180-183.

Koman LA, Mooney JF III, Smith BP, et al. Management of spasticity in cerebral palsy with botulinum-A toxin: Report of a preliminary, randomized, double-blind trial. J Pediatr Orthop 1994;14:299-303.

Lintner SA, Lindseth RE. Kyphotic deformity in patients who have a myelomeningocele: Operative treatment and long-term follow-up. J Bone Joint Surg 1994;76A:1301-1307.

Lock TR, Aronson DD. Fractures in patients who have myelomeningocele. J Bone Joint Surg 1989;71A:1153-1157.

Manske PR. Cerebral palsy of the upper extremity. Hand Clin 1990;6:597-709.

Maynard MJ, Weiner LS, Burke SW. Neuropathic foot ulceration in patients with myelodysplasia. J Pediatr Orthop 1992;12:786-788.

Mazur J, Menelaus MB, Dickens DR, et al. Efficacy of surgical management for scoliosis in myelomeningocele: Correction of deformity and alteration of functional status. J Pediatr Orthop 1986;6:568-575.

Mazur JM, Menelaus MB. Neurologic status of spina bifida patients and the orthopedic surgeon. Clin Orthop 1991;264:54-64.

McDonald CM, Jaffe KM, Mosca VS, et al. Ambulatory outcome of children with myelomeningocele: Effect of lower-extremity muscle strength. Dev Med Child Neurol 1991;33:482-490.

McHale KA, Bagg M, Nason SS. Treatment of the chronically dislocated hip in adolescents with cerebral palsy with femoral head resection and subtrochanteric valgus osteotomy. J Pediatr Orthop 1990;10:504-509.

McMaster MJ. The long-term results of kyphectomy and spinal stabilization in children with myelomeningocele. Spine 1988;13:417-424.

Mintz LJ, Sarwark JF, Dias LS, et al. The natural history of congenital kyphosis in myelomeningocele: A review of 51 children. Spine 1991;16:S348-S350.

Mubarak SJ, Valencia FG, Wenger DR. One-stage correction of the spastic dislocated hip: Use of pericapsular acetabuloplasty to improve coverage. J Bone Joint Surg 1992;74A:1347-1357.

Muller EB, Nordwall A. Brace treatment of scoliosis in children with myelomeningocele. Spine 1994;19:151-155.

Muller EB, Nordwall A, Oden A. Progression of scoliosis in children with myelomeningocele. Spine 1994;19:147-150.

Nene AV, Evans GA, Patrick JH. Simultaneous multiple operations for spastic diplegia: Outcome and functional assessment of walking in 18 patients. J Bone Joint Surg 1993;75B:488-494.

Payne LZ, DeLuca PA. Heterotopic ossification after rhizotomy and femoral osteotomy. J Pediatr Orthop 1993;13:733-738.

Phillips DL, Field RE, Broughton NS, et al. Reciprocating orthoses for children with myelomeningocele: A comparison of two types. J Bone Joint Surg 1995;77B:110-113.

Phillips DP, Lindseth RE. Ambulation after transfer of adductors, external oblique, and tensor fascia lata in myelomeningocele. J Pediatr Orthop 1992;12:712-717.

Pope DF, Bueff HU, DeLuca PA. Pelvic osteotomies for subluxation of the hip in cerebral palsy. J Pediatr Orthop 1994;14:724-730.

Renshaw TS, Green NE, Griffin PP. Cerebral palsy: Orthopaedic management. J Bone Joint Surg 1995;77A:1590-1606.

Root L, Goss GR, Mendes J. The treatment of the painful hip in cerebral palsy by total hip replacement or hip arthrodesis. J Bone Joint Surg 1986;68A:590-598.

Root L, Miller SR, Kirz P. Posterior tibial-tendon transfer in patients with cerebral palsy. J Bone Joint Surg 1987;69A:1133-1139.

Rose SA, DeLuca PA, Davis RB III, et al. Kinematic and kinetic evaluation of the ankle after lengthening of the gastrocnemius fascia in children with cerebral palsy. J Pediatr Orthop 1993;13:727-732.

Saji MJ, Upadhyay SS, Hsu LC, et al. Split tibialis posterior transfer for equinovarus deformity in cerebral palsy: Long-term results of a new surgical procedure. J Bone Joint Surg 1993;75B:498-501.

Samuelsson L, Eklof O. Scoliosis in myelomeningocele. Acta Orthop Scand 1988;59:122-127.

Schweitzer ME, Balsam D, Weiss R. Spina bifida occulta: Incidence in parents of offspring with spina bifida cystica. Spine 1993;18:785-786.

Segal LS, Thomas SE, Mazur JM, et al. Calcaneal gait in spastic diplegia after heel-cord lengthening: A study with gait analysis. J Pediatr Orthop 1989;9:697-701.

Stark A, Saraste H. Anterior fusion insufficient for scoliosis in myelomeningocele: Eight children 2-6 years after the Zielke operation. Acta Orthop Scand 1993;64:22-24.

Steinbok P, Irvine B, Cochrane DD, et al. Long-term outcome and complications of children born with meningomyelocele. Child Nerv Syst 1992;8:92-96.

Strecker WB, Emanuel JP, Dailey L. Comparison of pronator tenotomy and pronator rerouting in children with spastic cerebral palsy. J Hand Surg 1988;13A:540-543.

Sutherland DH, Davids JR. Common gait abnormalities of the knee in cerebral palsy. Clin Orthop 1993;288:139-147.

Sutherland DH, Santi M, Abel MF. Treatment of stiff-knee gait in cerebral palsy: A comparison by gait analysis of distal rectus femoris transfer versus proximal rectus release. J Pediatr Orthop 1990;10:433-441.

Swank M, Dias LS. Walking ability in spina bifida patients: A model for predicting future ambulatory status based on sitting balance and motor level. J Pediatr Orthop 1994;14:715-718.

Tenuta J, Shelton YA, Miller F. Long-term follow-up of triple arthrodesis in patients with cerebral palsy. J Pediatr Orthop 1993;13:713-716.

Thometz J, Simon S, Rosenthal R. The effect on gait of lengthening of the medial hamstrings in cerebral palsy. J Bone Joint Surg 1989;71A:345-353.

Thometz JG, Tachdjian M. Long-term follow-up of the flexor carpi ulnaris transfer in spastic hemiplegic children. J Pediatr Orthop 1988;8:407-412.

Tsoi LL, Buck BD, Nason SS, et al. Dislocation of the hip in myelomeningocele. J Bone Joint Surg 1996;78A:664-673.

Williams JJ, Graham GP, Dunne KB, et al. Late knee problems in myelomeningocele. J Pediatr Orthop 1993;13:701-703.

Wright JG, Menelaus MB, Broughton NS, et al. Lower extremity alignment in children with spina bifida. J Pediatr Orthop 1992;12:232-234.

Wright JG, Menelaus MB, Broughton NS, et al. Natural history of knee contractures in myelomeningocele. J Pediatr Orthop 1991;11:725-730.

Chapter 15 – Syndromes

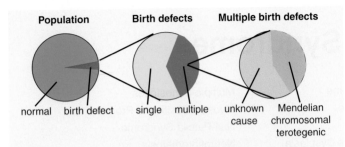

Fig. 15.1 Congenital defects in the population. Determining the site of abnormality is useful in differentiating syndromes. Based on Aase (1990).

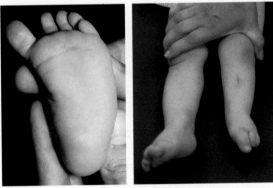

Fig. 15.2 Minor and major skeletal defects. Metatarsus adductus (left) is minor, fibular hemimelia (right) is a major defect.

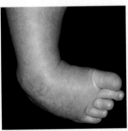

Clubfoot

Myelodysplasia
Amyoplasia
Distal arthrogryposis
Diastrophic dwarfism
Larsen syndrome
Trisomy 9, 9p, 20p syndromes
Camptomelic dysplasia
Caudal regression syndrome
Escobar syndrome
Freeman-Sheldon syndrome

Fig. 15.3 Clubfoot associations. These are some of the syndromes associated with this deformity.

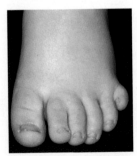

Polydactyly

Chondroectodermal dysplasia
Oto–Palato–Digital syndrome
Carpenter syndrome
Grebe syndrome
Trisomy 13 syndrome
Rubinstein–Taybe syndrome
Chondrodysplasia punctata
Bloom syndrome

Fig. 15.4 Polydactyly associations. These are some of the syndromes associated with polydacytly.

Introduction

In this chapter syndromes and other conditions are listed in alphabetical order to simplify finding a particular problem. Conditions may be generalized or focal. Conditions are cross referenced and discussed under the most commonly used name. The title *syndromes* is used for lack of a more inclusive term.

Generalized problems of the musculoskeletal system encompass thousands of disorders. As the human genome is developed, the number of possible DNA disorders continues to increase. Each of the traditional category of disorders is expanding with new subtypes.

Most orthopedic problems occur as single defects in an otherwise normal child. The diagnosis is usually not difficult and the challenge is providing successful treatment. In generalized disorders, diagnosis is often more difficult and the most important and critical first step in management. The first part of this chapter includes an approach to establishing the cause.

Prevalence

About 3% of the population have a birth defect (Fig. 15.1). Most defects are single, with the majority being minor (Fig. 15.2). Defects such as clubfeet or DDH are readily recognized.

In those with multiple defects, many are inherited by a Mendelian mechanism and are due to a chromosomal abnormality or to a terotegen. In some, the defects are not apparent at birth but develop during infancy or childhood. In about half, the diagnosis is never determined.

Orthopedic Involvement

The orthopedist becomes involved in management in several situations.

Musculoskeletal deformity such as a clubfoot in amyoplasia (Fig. 15.3), syndactylism as in Apert syndrome, bowlegs in achondroplasia, polydactyly in chondroectodermal dysplasia (Fig. 15.4), or scoliosis in Marfan syndrome appear as the major problems. The underlying diagnosis may be made before the orthopedic consultation. In some situations, an underlying disorder is not known and the orthopedist becomes responsible to establish the diagnosis or at least suspect that some underlying problem exists. The orthopedist may elect to pursue the diagnosis with physical, imaging (Fig. 15.5), and laboratory studies.

Delayed motor development may prompt an orthopedic consultation. Usually the question centers around delays in walking. Walking later than about 17 months is worrisome.

Specialist's opinion is sought by the primary care physician if the most obvious finding is a musculoskeletal deformity. The orthopedist is expected to give an opinion about diagnostic possibilities and decide whether the infant should be seen by a dysmorphologist or geneticist.

Skeletal Survey

Lateral skull
Lateral thoracolumbar spine
AP one arm to midhumerus
AP pelvis
AP one leg to midfemur

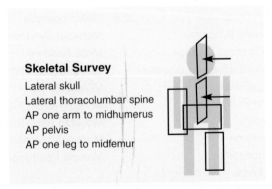

Fig. 15.5 Suggested radiographic studies to evaluate children with possible skeletal dysplasia.

Suspicious Features

Certain features suggest that the deformity or condition is not an isolated problem. These features can be identified by performing a screening examination (Chapter 2).

Atypical appearance is subjective but important (Fig. 15.6). Infants with Apert or Down syndrome have a typical facies. In others, the appearance *just doesn't look right.*

Altered stature as assessed by plotting the patient's length–height on standardized growth charts. Be aware that body proportions normally change with growth (Fig. 15.7).

Short stature below the 3rd percentile is a common finding in most generalized disorders. Compare the length or height of the patient with growth charts. Often the mother knows the percentile for height and weight as given by the primary care physician.

Tall stature is much less common and seen in only a few disorders, such as Marfan syndrome.

Disproportionate stature may be due to relative shortening of the trunk or limbs. Limb shortening is known as micromelia. Note which limb segment is most involved (Fig. 15.8): the proximal, in rhizomicromelia, the middle in mesomicromelia, or the distal in acromicromelia. Describe the site of shortening (Fig. 15.9).

Asymmetry of growth or size may result in hemihypertrophy or hemiatrophy. One limb or portion of the limb may be larger or smaller than normal.

Multiple defects increase the likelihood of an underlying problem.

Delayed maturation of motor, intellectual, speech or level of ossification as shown by radiographs is a suspicious feature.

Atypical response to treatment is a delayed but important sign of some underlying problem. The failure of a tibial fracture to heal may be a manifestation of neurofibromatosis; a scoliosis to respond to brace management, of Marfan syndrome; DDH to redislocate, to an underlying collagen disorder.

Other musculoskeletal problems such as fractures, finding of bone sclerosis, or epiphyseal abnormalities may prompt visit to the doctor.

References
1998 *Pediatric Orthopedic Secrets.* Page 385 Aase JM. Hanley & Belfus. Philadelphia.

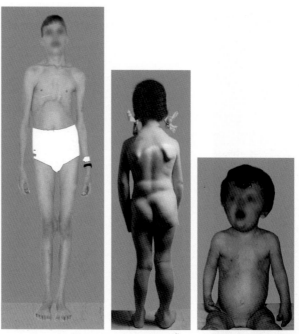

Fig. 15.6 Marfan syndrome, lipidosis, and Apert syndrome.

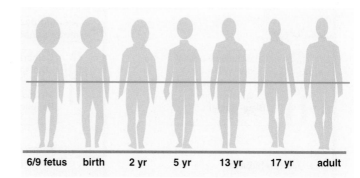

Fig. 15.7 Changes in body proportions with growth. At maturity, the position of the center of gravity (green line) is the level of the sacrum. From work of Palmer (1944).

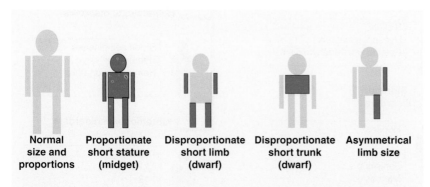

Fig. 15.8 Body proportions. Determining the site of abnormality is useful in differentiating syndromes.

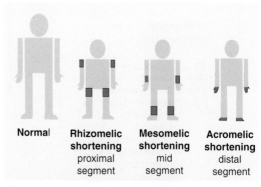

Fig. 15.9 Terminology for site of shortening. Proximal shortening involves the femora and humeri; midlimb shortening, the tibia and forearms; and distal shortening, the hands and feet.

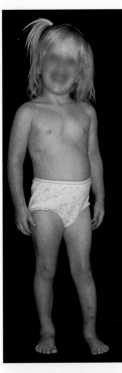

Fig. 15.10 The clinical appearance of this child with neurofibromatosis is diagnostic.

Evaluation

An early, accurate diagnosis is important to establish prognosis, to formulate an appropriate management plan, and to allow genetic counseling for the family. This differential is difficult because of the thousands of different disorders, the variety of expressions, and the changes that occur with growth.

Diagnostic Approaches

Generalized disorders are differentiated in several ways.

Clinical pattern recognition The best guess is made from the clinical features (Fig. 15.10) and then verified by imaging or laboratory studies. This approach requires considerable experience but is most efficient.

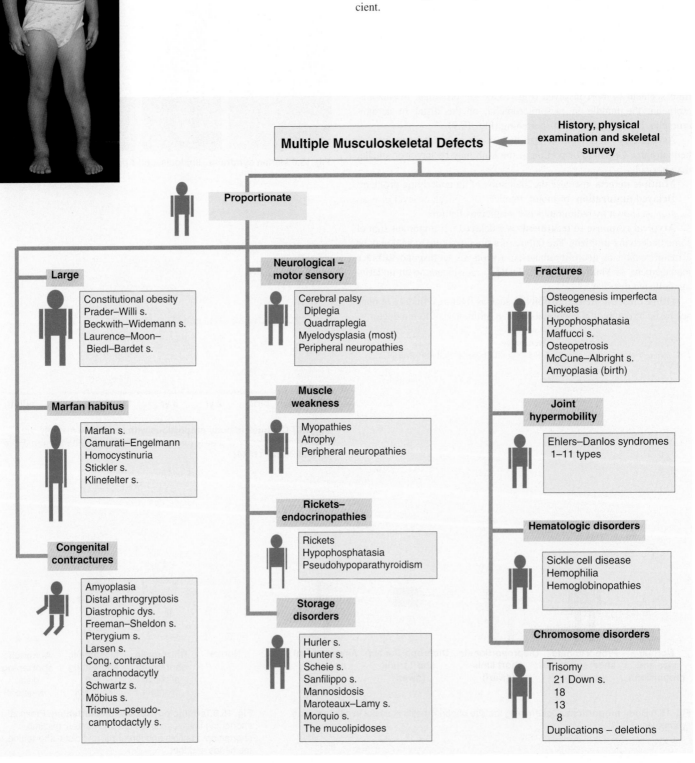

Multiple Musculoskeletal Defects ← History, physical examination and skeletal survey

Proportionate

Large
Constitutional obesity
Prader–Willi s.
Beckwith–Wiedemann s.
Laurence–Moon–
Biedl–Bardet s.

Marfan habitus
Marfan s.
Camurati–Engelmann
Homocystinuria
Stickler s.
Klinefelter s.

Congenital contractures
Amyoplasia
Distal arthrogryptosis
Diastrophic dys.
Freeman–Sheldon s.
Pterygium s.
Larsen s.
Cong. contractural
arachnodactyly
Schwartz s.
Möbius s.
Trismus–pseudo-
camptodactyly s.

Neurological – motor sensory
Cerebral palsy
Diplegia
Quadrraplegia
Myelodysplasia (most)
Peripheral neuropathies

Muscle weakness
Myopathies
Atrophy
Peripheral neuropathies

Rickets– endocrinopathies
Rickets
Hypophosphatasia
Pseudohypoparathyroidism

Storage disorders
Hurler s.
Hunter s.
Scheie s.
Sanfilippo s.
Mannosidosis
Maroteaux–Lamy s.
Morquio s.
The mucolipidoses

Fractures
Osteogenesis imperfecta
Rickets
Hypophosphatasia
Maffucci s.
Osteopetrosis
McCune–Albright s.
Amyoplasia (birth)

Joint hypermobility
Ehlers–Danlos syndromes
1–11 types

Hematologic disorders
Sickle cell disease
Hemophilia
Hemoglobinopathies

Chromosome disorders
Trisomy
21 Down s.
18
13
8
Duplications – deletions

Grouping then detailing Use an atlas or text and attempt to match the features of the patient and those in the atlas or written description. This requires that the condition be placed into categories to narrow the search (Figs. 15.11 and 15.12).

Flowchart This approach uses a stepwise progression to establish a diagnosis (Fig. 15.13). While it may have limitations, a flowchart provides a general framework into which most major categories of generalized disorders can be placed. This flowchart is based on major clinical features that can be recognized by an orthopedist. Other flowcharts are based on radiographic features, etiology, or nonmusculoskeletal features.

Chapter consultant
Mohammad Diab, e-mail: diab@chmc.org

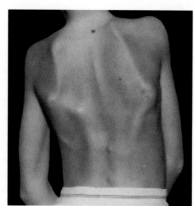

Fig. 15.11 Myositis ossificans progressiva. The presence of subcutaneous bone narrows the search to include only a few conditions.

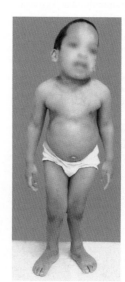

Fig. 15.12 Morquio syndrome. This proportional shortening and the unique radiographic features usually make possible establishing the diagnosis.

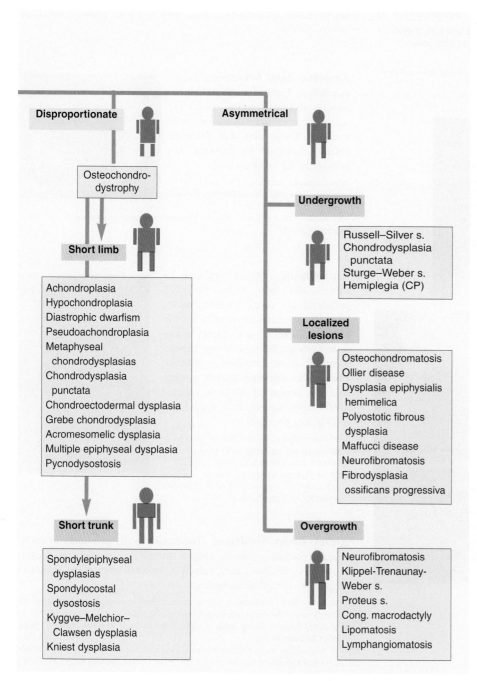

Disproportionate

Osteochondrodystrophy

Short limb

Achondroplasia
Hypochondroplasia
Diastrophic dwarfism
Pseudoachondroplasia
Metaphyseal chondrodysplasias
Chondrodysplasia punctata
Chondroectodermal dysplasia
Grebe chondrodysplasia
Acromesomelic dysplasia
Multiple epiphyseal dysplasia
Pycnodysostosis

Short trunk

Spondyloepiphyseal dysplasias
Spondylocostal dysostosis
Kyggve–Melchior–Clawsen dysplasia
Kniest dysplasia

Asymmetrical

Undergrowth

Russell–Silver s.
Chondrodysplasia punctata
Sturge–Weber s.
Hemiplegia (CP)

Localized lesions

Osteochondromatosis
Ollier disease
Dysplasia epiphysialis hemimelica
Polyostotic fibrous dysplasia
Maffucci disease
Neurofibromatosis
Fibrodysplasia ossificans progressiva

Overgrowth

Neurofibromatosis
Klippel-Trenaunay-Weber s.
Proteus s.
Cong. macrodactyly
Lipomatosis
Lymphangiomatosis

Fig. 15.13 Flowchart. This simple categorization by obvious features may aid in establishing the diagnosis or category of problem.

Conditions in Alphabetical Order

Aase–Smith Syndrome Characterized by multiple joint contractures, thin fingers with absent knuckles, cleft palate, cardiac anomalies and hydrocephalus (from Dandy-Walker anomaly).

1968 Dysmorphogenesis of joints, brain and palate: a new dominantly inherited syndrome. Aase JM, Smith DW. J. Pediat. 73:606

Achondroplasia (ACH) Most common nonlethal skeletal dysplasia. Fibroblast growth factor receptor 3 mutation. Autosomal dominant with >80% spontaneous mutation. Disordered endochondral with spared membranous ossification produces large head with narrow foramen magnum, "champagne pelvis" with constricted triradiate cartilage, long clavicles with broad shoulders, long fibulæ with varus ankles and knees, short pedicles with spinal stenosis. Rhizomicromelia, midface hypoplasia, trident hand, thoracolumbar kyphosis, joint contractures (including at the hips exaggerating lumbar lordosis), "chevron" metaphyses.

Figures below: Note the short proximal limb segments with preservation of trunk length [1], narrow lumbar canal [2], square iliac and horizontal acetabulae [3], and bowlegs with elongated fibula [4].

1996 Molecular genetic basis of the human chondrodysplasias. Horton WA. Endocrinol Metab Clin N Am 25:683
1976 Orthopædic complications of dwarfism. Kopits SE. CO 114:153

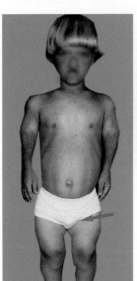
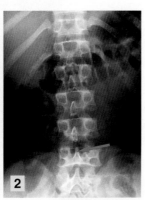
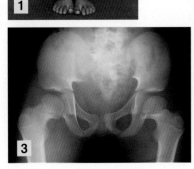
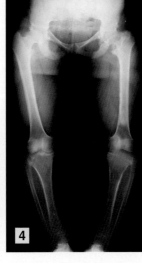

Acrodysostosis Autosomal dominant with incomplete penetrance. Facies, including nasal hypoplasia and prognathism. Mental retardation. Short tubular bones of hands and feet. Stippled and cone-shaped epiphyses.

1991 Acrodysostosis in two generations: an autosomal dominant syndrome. Hernandez RM, Miranda A, Kofman-Alfaro S. Clin Genet 39:376

Albers–Schönberg syndrome See osteopetrosis.

Albright Syndrome (McCune-Albright Syndrome) Triad of polyostotic fibrous dysplasia, endocrine abnormalities including precocious puberty and café au lait spots. Mutation in the GNAS1 gene. See page 314.

1986 Fibrous dysplasia of bone and the Weil-Albright syndrome. A study of thirteen cases with special reference to the orthopaedic treatment. Dohler JR, Hughes SP. Int Orthop 10:53
1986 McCune-Albright syndrome. Long-term follow-up. Lee PA, Van Dop C, Migeon CJ. JAMA 256:2980

Amniotic Band Syndrome Non-mendelian. Herniation of members through ruptured amnion results in constriction, vascular occlusion, and necrosis. Body wall and visceral defects explained by pressure on embryo during first four weeks.

1994 Congenital constriction band syndrome: a seventy-year experience. Foulkes GD, K Rienker. JPO 14:242
1992 Amniotic band sequence: Streeter's hypothesis reexamined. Bamforth JS. Am J Med Genet 44: 280-287

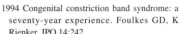
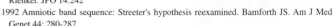

Amyoplasia Muscle replaced by fibrous and fatty tissue. So-called peripheral or "classic" arthrogryposis. Multiple congenital contractures, including medial rotation of shoulders, extension of elbows, flexion of wrists, hip dislocation, knee extension, clubfoot. Limited to musculoskeletal system. Sporadic, normal IQ. All limbs affected in 60%, lower limbs in 25%, upper limbs in 15%. See page 342.

1996 Amyoplasia, the most common type of arthrogryposis: the potential for good outcome. Sells JM, Jaffe KM, Hall JG. Pediatrics 97:225
1983 Amyoplasia: a common, sporadic condition with congenital contractures. Hall JB, Reed SD, Dricoll EP. Am J Med Genet 15:571

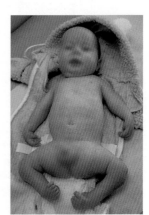

Antley–Bixler Syndrome Trapezoidocephaly secondary to lambdoid and coronal synostosis, midface hypoplasia, radiohumeral synostosis, joint contractures, camptodactyly, femoral bowing and fractures, urogenital and cardiac anomalies.

1996 Antley-Bixler syndrome: a disorder characterized by congenital synostosis of the elbow joint and the cranial suture. Kitoh H, et al. JPO 16:243
1994 Antley-Bixler syndrome: report of a patient and review of literature. Hassell S, Butler MG. Clin Genet 46:372
1975 Trapezoidocephaly, midface hypoplasia and cartilage abnormalities with multiple synostoses and skeletal fractures. Antley RM, Bixler D. Birth Def Orig Art Ser XI (2):397

Apert Syndrome Also called acrocephalosyndactyly. Mutation of fibroblast growth factor receptor 2. Variable mental retardation. Syndactyly produces "mitten" hand and "sock" foot. Synostosis produces pointed head. Cervical vertebral synostosis. Cleft palate, midface hypoplasia. Syndactyly release and craniectomy.

Figures below: Typical features include acrocephaly [1], osseous syndactyly [2], and syndactyly of both hands and feet [3].

*1906 De l'acrocephalosyndactyly. Apert E. Bull Soc Med Hôp Paris 23:1310
1996 Classification of hand anomalies in Apert's syndrome. al-Qattan MM, al-Husain MA. J Hand Surg Br. 21:266

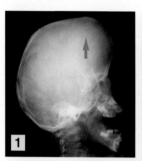
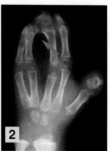

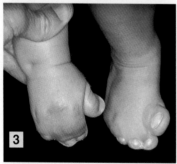

Arthrogryposis Also called arthrogryposis multiplex congenita. Heterogenous group of disorders of which the common feature is multiple congenital joint contractures. Occurs in 1/3000 births. Fetal akinesia at critical time in development causes abnormalities of nerves, muscles, or connective tissues. Akinesia due to maternal disease, intrauterine constraint, or vascular compromise. About half are subclassified as amyoplasia–the classic form. Condition detailed on page 342.

1923 Arthrogryposis multiplex congenita. Stern, WG. JAMA, 81:1507.

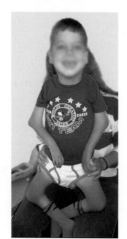

Beals I Syndrome Also called auriculo–osteodysplasia. Autosomal dominant, both sexes, short stature, auricular anomalies, radiocapitular dysplasia, and hip dysplasia.

*1967 Auriculo–osteodysplasia, a syndrome of multiple osseous dysplasia, ear anomaly, and short stature. Beals RK. JBJS 49A:1541

Beals II Syndrome Also known as congenital contractural arachnodactyly. True Marfan syndrome, without visceral involvement. Both sexes, multiple contractures, long and slender bones, osteopenia, kyphoscoliosis, "crumpled" ears.

*1971 Delineation of another heritable disorder of connective tissue. Beals RK, Hecht F. JBJS 53A:987

Beckwith–Wiedemann Syndrome Chromosome 11p15.5 mutation. Umbilical anomalies, macroglossia, hypertrophy of limbs and viscera, increased risk of tumors (particularly abdominal). Polycythemia, hypoglycemia, history of hydramnios and prematurity.

*1964 Hyperplastic fetus visceromegaly with macroglassia, omphalocele, cytomegaly or adrenal fetal cortex, postnatal somatic gigantism and other abnormalities: Newly recognized syndrome. Beckwith, et al. Proc Am Pediatr Soc, Seattle.

Blount Disease Uncommon, also called tibia vara or ostreochondrosis deformans tibiae. Deformity due to a focal growth disturbance of the medial portion of the proximal tibial epiphysis. See page 84.

*1937 Tibia vara, ostoechondrosis deformans tibiae. Blount WP. JBJS 19:1

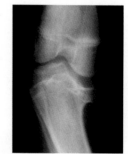

Brachydactyly Classified into groups A-E, each of which are subclassified. First syndrome in which Mendelian inheritance is described. Digital lengthenings may be indicated.

1903 Hereditary and sexual influence in meristic variation: a study of digital malformations in man. Farabee WC. Harvard Univ. Press 1903
*1951 On brachydactyly and symphalangism. Bell J. In Treasury of Human Inheritance, vol 5 pp 1–31, Cambridge University Press
1994 Digital lengthening in congenital hand deformities. Ogino T, Kato H, Ishii S, Usui MJ. Hand Surg Br 19 :120

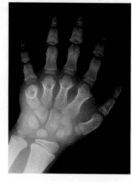

Brachyrachia "Short spine," with vertebral anomalies and kyphoscoliosis. Proximal femoral epiphyseal dysplasia leads to coxa vara. Resembles musculoskeletal manifestations of Morquio syndrome.

1933 Morquio's disease. Brown DO. Med. J. Aust. 1: 598-600, 1933
1995 "Brachyolmia: a report of two cases". Ikegawa S, et al. JPO 15:105

Bruck Syndrome Multiple joint contractures resemble arthrogryposis. Fractures, wormian bones resemble osteogenesis imperfecta. Normal sclerae and teeth. Pterygia, scoliosis, clubfoot. Abnormal type I collagen telopeptide crosslinking due to deficiency of lysyl hydroxylase.

* 1897 Über eine seltene Form von Erkrankung der Knochen und Gelenke. Bruck A. Dtsch Med Wsch. 23:152-155
1989 Osteogenesis imperfecta with congenital joint contractures (Bruck syndrome). Viljoen D, Versfeld G, Beighton P Clin Genet 36:122-126
1998 Bruck syndrome: a rare combination of bone fragility and multiple congenital joint contractures. Breslau-Siderius EJ, et al. JPOb 7:35

Caffey Disease Also called infantile cortical hyperostosis. Idiopathic, resolves spontaneously but may recur. Occurs in utero to 6 months. Acute inflammatory stage. Hyperostosis with diaphyseal periosteal deposition. Most often affects mandible and long bones.

Figures below: Note the typical extensive hyperostosis [1] and characteristic mandibular involvement [2].

* 1945 Infantile cortical hyperostosis, preliminary report on new syndrome. Caffey J, Silverman W. Am J Roentgen 54:1-16
1995 Familial aspects of Caffey's disease. Bernstein RM, Zaleske DJ. Am J Orthop 10: 777
1996 MR findings in a patient with Caffey's disease. Saatci I, Brown JJ, McAlister WH. Pediatr Radiol 26:68

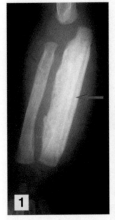
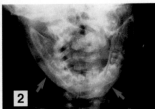

Camptomelic Dysplasia "Bent limbs" characterized by long bone bowing, especially of the tibiae with cutaneous dimple. Hypoplastic scapulae, scoliosis, clubfoot, hip dislocation. Cleft palate, micrognathia, flat face. Sex reversal. Chromosome 17 reversal with haploinsufficiency of SOX 9.

* 1971 Le syndrome campomelique. Maroteaux P et al. Presse Med. 22: 1157-1162
1994 Campomelic dysplasia and autosomal sex reversal caused by mutations in an SRY-related gene. Foster J, et al. Nature 372: 525-530
1997 The treatment of progressive kyphoscoliosis in camptomelic dysplasia. Thomas S, Winter RB, Lonstein JE. Spine 22:1330

Carpenter Syndrome Also called acrocephalopolysyndactyly II. Craniosynostosis produces a "pointed head." Deletion or release for preaxial polysyndactyly. Variable mental retardation, hypogonadism.

*1901 Carpenter, G: Two sisters showing malformation of the skull and other congenital abnormalities. Rep Soc Study Dis Child (London)1:110
1998 Islek I, et al. Carpenter syndrome: report of two siblings. Clin Dysmorphol 7:185

Caudal Regression Syndrome Sacral agenesis combined with variable lower extremity deformities, neurologic impairment, contractures of the lower extremities, hip dislocations, and spine instability.

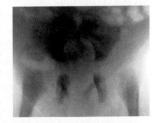

1991 Caudal regression: a review of seven cases, including the mermaid syndrome. Guidera KJ, et al. Pediatr Orthop 11:743

Charcot-Marie-Tooth One type of hereditary motor and sensory neuropathy. Autosomal dominant and recessive, as well as sex-linked forms. Autosomal dominant form results from mutation of myelin protein 0 gene on chromosome 1q22. Peroneal, tibialis anterior and intrinsic muscle weakness produce cavus, varus, and claw foot deformity. See page 344.

1886 Sur une forme particulière d'atrophie muscolaire progressive, sovent familiare débutant pas les pieds et les jambes et atteigant plus tard les mains. Charcot JM, Marie P. Rev Med 6:97
1886 The peroneal type of progressive muscular atrophy. Tooth HH, London, HK Lewis

Chondroectodermal dysplasia Also called Ellis–Van Creveld syndrome. Micromelia, postaxial polydactyly, genua valga, dysplasia of nails and teeth, cardiac anomalies. Largest pedigree in Amish.

1888 Ueber einen Fall von hereditaeren Polydaktylie mit Anomalien der Zaehne. Thomas. Dtsc Mschr Zaehnheilkd 6:407
1940 A syndrome characterized by ectodermal dysplasia, polydactyly, chondrodysplasia, and congenital morbus cordis: Report of three cases. Ellis RBW, Van Creveld S. Arch Dis Child 15:65
1994 Ellis-Van Creveld syndrome (chondroectodermal dysplasia). Avolio A Jr., Berman AT, Israelite CL. Orthopedics 17:735

Cleft hand–foot Ectrodactyly, monodactyly, "lobster-claw" deformity. Absence of central ray(s) represents malformation and not deformity. Autosomal dominant linked to chromosome 7q. Hand function good, repair foot deformity to allow shoeing.

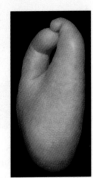

1990 Teratogenic relationship between polydactyly, syndactyly and cleft hand. Ogino T. J Hand Surg Br 15:201
1992 Cleft hand, syndactyly and hypoplastic thumb. Miura T, et al. J Hand Surg Br 17:365
1997 Cleft-foot closure: a simplified technique and review of the literature. Wood VE, Peppers TA, Shook J. JPO 17:501

Cleidocranial dysplasia Midline defects, including hypoplastic clavicles with hypermobile shoulders, bulging calvaria, coxa vara, symphysis pubica diastasis. Transcription factor CBFA1 mutation on chromosome 6p.

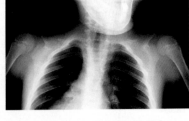

1968 The classic: on hereditary cleido-cranial dysostosis (transl.). Bick EM. CO 58:5

Conradi-Hünermann Syndrome Also called chondrodystrophia calcificans congenita and chondrodysplasia punctata. Autosomal or X-linked. Epiphyseal calcification produces shortened proximal long bones, joint contractures, scoliosis, cataracts, ichthyosis. X-linked form due to mutation in arylsulfatase E on Xp22.3.

1914 Vorzeitges Auftreten von Kochen und eigenartigen Verkalkungskernen bei Chondrodystrophia fötalis hypoplastica, Histologische und Röntgenuntersuchungen. Conradi E. J Kinderheilk 80:86
1931 Chondrodystrophia calcificans congenita als abortive form der chondrodystrophie. Hünermann C. Z Kinderheilkd 51:1
1974 Chondrodystrophia calcificans congenita: report of 2 cases. Vink TH, Duffy FP. JBJS 29A:509

Cornelia De Lange Syndrome Characteristic facies, including synophrys, crescentic or "carp" mouth, anteverted nares. Mental and growth retardation. Micromelia, ulnar dysgenesis, proximally placed thumb, clinodactyly of small finger, radial head dislocation.

Figures below: Elbow dysplasia with dislocation of radial head [1], shortened, wide phalanges both in the hand [2] and foot [3].

1933 Sur un type nouveau de dé–génération (typus Amstelodamensis). De Lange C. Arch Med Enfant 36:713 1982 Cornelia de Lange's syndrome. A review article (with emphasis on orthopedic significance). Joubin J, Pettrone CF, Pettrone FA. CO 171:180

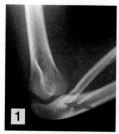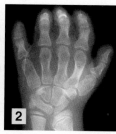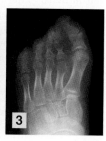

Craniodiaphyseal Dysplasia Both sexes, congenital, mental retardation. Craniofacial and diaphyseal hyperostosis produces leonine facies, midface obstruction with anorexia, widened ribs and clavicles.

1927 Leontiasis Ossea. Porto Alegre (Brazil) De Souza O. Faculdade de Med Rev Dos Cursos 13:47
1990 Craniodiaphyseal dysplasia. Brueton LA, Winter RM. J Med Genet 27:701

Craniometaphyseal Dysplasia Recessive or dominant. Craniofacial and metaphyseal hyperostosis produces leonine facies, facial nerve palsy, "Erlenmeyer flask" deformity in long bones. Mutation linked to chromosome 5p.

1954 Metaphyseal dysplasia, epiphyseal dysplasia, diaphyseal dysplasia, and related conditions. I. Familial metaphyseal dysplasia and craniometaphyseal dysplasia: their relation to leontiasis ossea and osteopetrosis: disorders of 'bone remodeling'. Jackson WPU, Albright F, et al. Arch Intern Med 94:871

De Barsy Syndrome Sporadic. Characteristic facies, multiple joint dislocations and subluxations, including of the hip, scoliosis, congenital vertical talus. Lax and translucent skin, cataracts, psychomotor delay.

1968 Dwarfism, oligophrenia and degeneration of the elastic tissue in skin and cornea. A new syndrome? De Barsy, AM, Moens E, Dierckx L, Helv. Paediat. Acta 23: 305-313
1994 Orthopaedic manifestations in De Barsy syndrome. Stanton RP; Rao N, Scott CI Jr. JPO 14:60

Diastrophic Dysplasia "Twisted" feet and spine. Clubfoot, thoracolumbar scoliosis, cervical hypoplasia with kyphosis and atlantoaxial instability, joint contractures, short first metacarpal producing "hitch-hiker thumb." Pinna calcification producing "cauliflower ear." cleft palate, micrognathia, respiratory obstruction. Hips show flattening and a double-hump deformation causing early osteoarthritis. Mutation linked to sulfate transporter on chromosome 5q.

1960 Le nanisme diastrophique. Lamy M, Maroteaux P. Presse Med 68:1977
1991 The spine in diastrophic dysplasia. Poussa M, et al. Spine 16:881
1992 Foot deformities in diastrophic dysplasia. An analysis of 102 patients. Ryoppy S, et al. JBJS 74B:441
1998 Development of the hip in diastrophic dysplasia. Vaara P, et al. JBJS 80B:315

Down Syndrome Common, trisomy 21, incidence related to maternal age, delayed physical, intellectual, and language development, typical facies, simian crease, square hands, short fingers, stubby feet, wide iliac wings, low acetabular index, flatfeet, unstable hips, patella, and C1–2. Cardiac and gastrointestinal disease, hearing loss, leukemia.

Figures below: A child with Down syndrome and recurrent hip dislocations shows flat iliae, low acetabular index, concentric hip reduction [1]. While under anesthesia, flexion and adduction causes the hip to dislocate [2]. In an adolescent with Down syndrome, hip dysplasia and pain, the AP pelvic radiograph shows a small femoral head and a dysplastic acetabulum, resulting in a reduction of load bearing area [3]. The CT reconstruction shows the dysplasia and subluxation [4].

1866 Observations on an ethnic classification of idiots. Down JLH. Clin Lect Rep London Hosp 3:259
1998 Should children with Down syndrome be screened for atlantoaxial instability? Pueschel SMS. Arch Pediatr Adolesc Med 152:123
1992 The hip joint in Down's syndrome. A study of its structure and associated disease. Shaw ED, Beals RK. CO 278:101
1995 Clubfoot deformity in Down's syndrome. Miller PR, Kuo KN, Lubicky JP. Orthopedics 18:449

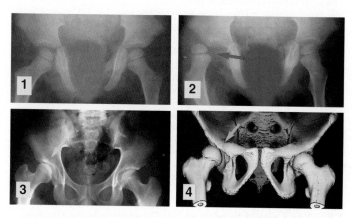

Dyggve–Melchior–Clausen Syndrome Resembles Morquio and Hurler syndromes. Mental retardation, microcephaly in autosomal form normal intelligence and mild microcephaly in X-linked form. Hip subluxation with waddling gait, odontoid hypoplasia with C1-2 instability, platyspondyly, camptodactyly, "lace border" iliac crests

1962 Morquio–Ulrich's disease; An inborn error or metabolism? Dyggve HV, Melchior JC, Clausen J. Arch Dis Child 37:525
1987 Case report 431: Dyggve-Melchior-Clausen syndrome (DMCS). Hall-Craggs MA, Chapman M. Skeletal Radiol 16:422
1998 Treatment of hip subluxation in Dyggve-Melchior-Clausen syndrome. Hosny GA, Fabry G. JPOB 7:32

Dysplasia Epiphysealis Hemimelica Rare developmental bone dysplasia, also called Trevor disease. Non-Mendelian, nonfamilial. Osteocartilaginous tumors arising from an epiphysis. Lesions cause pain, swelling, and deformity, often unilateral, starting during infancy or early childhood. Diagnosis often delayed as lesions are primarily cartilage and shown poorly by radiographs. Manage by excision and correct secondary bony deformity by osteotomy.

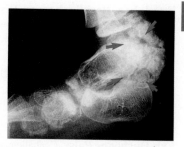

1994 Dysplasia epiphysealis hemimelica. Upper limb involvement with associated osteochondroma. Rao SB, Roy DR. CO 307:103
1998 Dysplasia epiphysealis hemimelica: clinical features and management. Kuo RS, et al. JPO 18:543

Ehlers–Danlos Syndrome Joint laxity causes hip, patellar, elbow, and shoulder dislocation, kyphoscoliosis, flat foot, recurrent deformity after operation. Cutis laxa with subcutaneous spherules, "lop ears," "cigarette-paper" skin. Soft tissue fragility causes

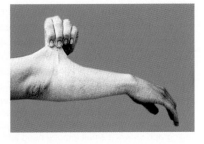

vascular aneurysm, bleeding, wound breakdown, thoracic and abdominal hernias, and visceral rupture.

Table below: Types of Ehlers–Danlos syndrome. Most are inherited by AD (autosomal dominant), some by AR (autosomal recessive) or X–linked modes.

1901 Curtis laxa, Neigung zu Haemorrhagien in der Haut lockering meherer Artikulationen. Ehlers E. Dermatol Z 8:173
1908 Un cas de cutis laxa avec tumeurs par contusion chroniquedes coudes et des genoux. Danlos H. Bull Soc Fr Dermat Syph 19:7
1994 Spinal deformity in Ehlers-Danlos syndrome. Five patients treated by spinal fusion. McMaster MJ. JBJS 76B:773

Type		Clinical features	Inheritance
1	classic	lax joints, fragile skin	AD
2	mild type	mild features of type 1	AD
3	benign	severe hypermobility	AD
4	ecchymotic type	collagen type III mutation	AD or AR
5	X–linked type	type 2 features	X–linked
6	ocular–scoliotic	ocular & skin frag. + scoliosis	AR
7	arthrochalasis	collagen type I mutation	AD or AR
8	peridonitis	laxity and peridonitis	AD
9	occipital horn s.	cutis laxa	X–linked
10	--	laxity, fragility, bruising skin	AR

Ellis–Van Creveld Syndrome see Chondroectodermal Dysplasia.

Engelmann-Camurati Disease Progressive inflammatory sclerosing diaphyseal hyperostosis produces painful fusiform limb swelling and anemia. Most often affects femora, tibiae, vertebral arch, skull base. Muscular hypoplasia and weakness lead to peculiar gait. "Malnourished" appearance. Linked to chromosome 19q.

1928 Ein Fall von Osteopathia hyperostotica multiple infantilis. Engelmann G. Fortschr Geb Röntgehstr 39:1101
1922 Di un raro caso di osteitis simmetrica ereditaria degli arti inferiori, Camurati M. Chir Orgi Mov 6:662
1981 Engelmann's disease and the effect of corticosteroids: a case report. Minford AMB, et al. JBJS 63B:597
1996 Engelmann's disease: a 45-year follow-up. Grey AC, et al. JBJS 78B:488

Engel–Von Recklinghausen Disease Rare, also called osteitis fibrosa generalisata, parathyroid osteitis, or renal osteodystrophy. Caused by chronic nephritis and hyperparathyroidism causing long bone bowing, spinal and chest deformity.

1910 Imtersicjimgem über Rachitis und Osteomalacie. von Recklinghausen F. Jena, G Fisher.

Epiphyseal Dysplasia See multiple epiphyseal dysplasia and spondyloepiphyseal dysplasia.

Erb-Duchenne Palsy Cephalic part of brachial plexus injury leading to paralyis of muscles supplied by C5-6. May follow traumatic delivery.

1855 De L'eléctrisation localiséeet de son application á la pathologie et á la therapeutique. Duchenne GB. Paris, Baillière
1877 Über eine eigenthümlichen localisation von lähmungen im plexus brachialis. Erb WH. Verhandl Natur-Med Versamml. Heidelberg 2:130
1996 Obstetric brachial plexus palsy. Lindell-Iwan HL, Partanen VS, Makkonen ML. JPO-b 5:210

Fabella syndrome Rare, congenital adolescent onset of intermittent posterolateral knee pain, localized tenderness over compressed fabella when compressed against femur.

1982 The "fabella syndrome": an update. Weiner DS, Macnab I. JPO 2:405

Fairbank Disease See multiple epiphyseal dysplasia.

Familial Dysautonomia Also called congenital insensitivity to pain, Riley-Day syndrome. Children lack normal pain avoidance, leading to self-inflicted injuries. Paroxysmal hypertension, hyperhidrosis, decreased lacrimation, cutaneous blotching, drooling, absence of fungiform papillae on tongue. Orthopedic problems include fracture, autoamputation, osteomyelitis, septic arthritis, neuropathic joints, scoliosis, and dislocation. Manage by patient/parent education to prevent complications. Treat fractures conservatively, fuse scoliosis.

1990 Orthopaedic manifestations in congenitally insensate patients. Guidera KJ, et al. JPO 10:514
1995 Scoliosis in familial dysautonomia. Operative treatment. Rubery PT, et al. JBJS 77A:1362

Fanconi Syndrome Myelophthisis with pancytopenia requires bone marrow transplant. Short stature, radial ray defects, including hypoplastic or absent thumb or radius require reconstruction. Urogenital and ocular anomalies, brown cutaneous pigmentation. Complimentation groups A-D: A linked to chromosome 20q, C to 9q.

1936 Die pseudoluetische, subakute hilifugale Bronchopneumonie des heruntergekommenen Kindes. Fanconi G. Schweiz Med Wochenschr 66:821
1993 The cellular basis of Fanconi syndrome. Baum M. Hosp Pract 28:137

Femoral–Facial Syndrome Upslanted paplebral fissures, thin upper lip, long philtrum, short nose, cleft palate, micrognathia. Short legs due to femoral hypoplasia or absence and bowing, preaxial polydactyly.

1986 Femoral hypoplasia-unusual facies syndrome: autopsy findings in an unusual case. De Palma L, Duray PH, Popeo VR. Pediatr Pathol 5:1

Fetal Alcohol Syndrome Common, (2/1000 children in USA), caused by teratogenic effect of alcohol, microcephaly, facial abnormalities such as hypoplastic maxilla, mild to moderate mental retardation, delayed bone age, digitial shortening and tapering, radioulnar synostosis, and coxa valga.

1899 A note on the influence of maternal inebriety on the offspring. Sullivan WC. J Ment Sci 45:489
1981 Bone fusion in the foetal alcohol syndrome. Jaffer Z, Nelson M, Beighton P. JBJS 63B:569

Fibular Dysgenesis Rare, congenital idiopathic elongation and bowing of the distal fibula (see radiograph right).

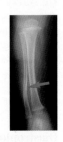

Focal Fibrocartilaginous Dysplasia Rare, idiopathic, onset in infancy, unilateral tibial bowing with fibrocartilaginous tissue in the defect.

1985 Tibia vara caused by focal fibrocartilaginous dysplasia: Three case reports. Bell SN, et al. JBJS 67B:780
1990 Three additional cases of fibrocartilaginous dysplasia causing tibia vara. Olney BW, Cole WG, Menelaus MB: JPO 10:405
1991 Focal fibrocartilaginous dysplasia consideration of a healing process. Kariya Y, et al. JPO 11:545

Freeman–Sheldon Syndrome Also called whistling face, windmill vane hand syndrome, craniocarpotarsal dystrophy. Small pursed mouth. Normal stature. Camptodactyly with ulnar deviation, windmill vane hand position, metacarpophalangeal joint contracture of fingers 2-5, adducted thumbs, clubfoot, hip dysplasia, scoliosis, steep anterior cranial fossa. Sometimes considered a form of arthrogryposis.

1938 Cranio-carpotarsal dystrophy: undescribed congenital malformation. Freeman EA, Sheldon JH. Arch Dis Child 13:277

Freiberg Infraction Idiopathic incomplete subchondral fracture of second or third metatarsal heads, leading to joint deformity.

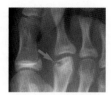

1920 Eine typische Erkrankung des 2 Metatarsophalangeal –gealaelenkes. Kohler A: MMW 67:1289
1926 The so–called infraction of the second metatarsal bone. Freiberg AH. JBJS 8:257

Friedreich Ataxia Triad of cerebellar ataxia, diminished deep tendon reflexes and preadolescent onset. Pes cavus, scoliosis. Cardiomyopathy, diabetes mellitus. Linked to chromosome 9. See Chapter 14.

1863 Über degenerative Atrophie der spinalen, Hinterstränge. Friedreich N. Arch Anat Physiol 26:391

Garré Syndrome Uncommon, infectious, also called sclerosing non-suppurative osteomyelitis or osteitis Garré. Night bone pain, swelling, tenderness, sclerosis of diaphysis. See Chapter 12.

1893 Ueber besondere Formen und Folgezunstände der akuten intektiösen Osteomyelitis. Garré C. Beitr Klin Chir 10:241

Gaucher Disease Autosomal recessive cerebroside lipidosis. Mutation in gene encoding glucocerbrosidase linked to chromosome 1q. Glucocerbrosidase-laden macrophages, known as Gaucher cells, accumulate in bone marrow, spleen, liver, and ocular limbus, leading to anemia, thrombocytopenia, hepatosplenomegaly, pingueculae. Three types of disease with different ages of onset. Orthopedic problems include osteolysis, bone crises, osteonecrosis of femoral head, pathologic fractures. Widening of the distal femoral metaphyses produces "Erlenmayer flask" deformity, shown on radiograph (arrows).

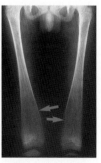

1882 De l'epithelioma primitif de la rate Gaucher P: (thesis) p 212. Paris
1987 Fractures in children who have Gaucher disease. Katz K, et al. JBJS 69A:1361
1995 Gaucher disease--the orthopaedic aspect. Report of seven cases. Tauber C, Tauber T. Arch Orthop Trauma Surg 114:179
1996 The natural history of osteonecrosis of the femoral head in children and adolescents who have Gaucher disease. Katz K, et al. JBJS 78A:14

Goldenhar Syndrome Also called oculoauriculovertebral dysplasia, hemifacial microsomia. Ear and eye anomalies, vertebral anomalies, and scoliosis. Normal IQ. Cosmetic facial surgery, fusion for scoliosis.

1861 Arrest of development of the left perpendicular ramus of the lower jaw, combined with malformation of the external ear. Canton E. Tr Path Soc London 12:237
1988 Orthopaedic manifestations of Goldenhar syndrome. Avon SW, Shively JL. JPO 8:683
1996 Abnormalities of the spine in Goldenhar's syndrome. Gibson JN, Sillence DO, Taylor TK. JPO 16:344

Guillain–Barré Syndrome Sporadic acute demyelinating polyneuropathy. Possible autoimmune or aberrant immune mechanism suggested by preceding upper respiratory or *C. jejuni* infection. Ascending flaccid paralysis, proximal muscles more affected. Involvement of respiratory muscles may necessitate ventilator support. Treat with pasmapheresis or immunoglobulin. Better prognosis in children.

1915 Le réflexe médico–plantaire: Étude de ses caracteres graphiques et de son temps perdu. Guillain G, Barré JA, Strohl A. Bull Soc Med Hop Paris 40:1459
1997 Clinical and epidemiologic features of Guillain-Barré syndrome. Hughes RA, Rees JH. J Infect Dis 176:S92

Hand–Foot Syndrome Rare, occurs in infants with sickle cell disease. Metacarpals, metatarsals, and phalanges infarcted during sickling crisis. Spontaneous recovery in 1–4 weeks, recurrence until 3 years old.

1941 Sickle cell anemia, with unusual bone changes. Danford EA, Marr R, Elsey EC. Am J Roentgen 45:223
1995 The hand-foot syndrome in sickle-cell haemoglobinopathy. Babhulkar SS, Pande K, Babhulkar S. JBJS 77B:310

Hand–Schüller–Christian Syndrome Rare, idiopathic, systemic histiocytosis with widespread symptoms including multiple osteolytic well-marginated bone lesions frequent in the ribs, femora, skull, and ribs.

1893 Polyuria and tuberculosis. Hand A Jr Arch Pediatr 10:673
1994 Treatment of Langerhans-cell histiocytosis in children. Experience at the Children's Hospital of Nancy. Sessa S, Sommelet D, Lascombes P, Prevot J. JBJS 76A:1513

Hemihypertrophy Uncommon, heterogenous group of overgrowth syndromes that involve nerves, blood and lymphatic vessels, endocrine and chromosomal abnormalities causing hypertrophy of muscle, bones, and viscera. Limb equalization procedures, abdominal tumor screening.

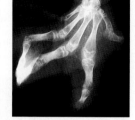

1822 Ueber die Seitliche Asymmetrie im tierischen Körper. Meckel JF. Anatomische physiologische Beobachtungen und Untersuchungen 147 Halle, Renger
1997 Hemihypertrophy. Concepts and controversies. Ballock RT, et al. JBJS 79A:1731

Hemophilia Uncommon, classic X-linked recessive inheritance, congenital deficiency of Factor VIII. Males with a few exceptions in homozygous females, onset from birth. Multiple bleeding sites including recurrent hemarthroses causing articular damage, progressive contractures. Manage by continuous prophylaxis to prevent need for synovectomies, hip arthroplasties, and radial head resections previously commonly necessary.

1803 An account of an hemorrhagic disposition existing in certain families. Otto JC. M Repository 6:1
1996 Orthopaedic surgery in hemophilia. 20 Years' experience in Sweden. Lofqvist T, Nilsson IM, Petersson C. CO 332:232
1997 Prophylactic transfusion for hypertrophic synovitis in children with hemophilia. Greene WB, McMillan CW, Warren MW. CO 232:19

Holt–Oram Syndrome Autosomal dominant caused by mutation in TBX5 gene on chromosome 12q. Congenital cardiac defects. Radial club hand and hypoplasia, radioulnar synostosis, thumb anomalies, anomalies of shoulder girdle.

1960 Familial heart disease with skeletal malformations. Holt M, Oram S. Br Heart J 22:236
1994 The clinical and genetic spectrum of the Holt-Oram syndrome (heart-hand syndrome) Basson CT, et al. N Engl J Med 330:885

Homocystinuria Autosomal recessive. Mutation in gene encoding cystathionine beta-synthase on chromosome 21q. Mental retardation, seizures, ectopia lentis, cardiac anomalies, pectus excavatum, thromboembolism, osteoporosis, "codfish" vertebrae, kyphoscoliosis, dolichostenomelia, limited joint mobility.

1984 Bone changes in homocystinuria in childhood. Tamburrini O, et al. Radiol Med 70:1293

Hunter Syndrome Also called mucopolysaccharidosis II, subtypes A and B. Mutation in gene encoding iduronate sulfatase on chromosome Xq. Short stature, cervical anomalies, thoracic kyphosis, joint contractures, mental retardation, hypertrichosis, cardiac disease, hepatosplenomegaly, abdominal hernias.

1917 A rare disease in two brothers. Hunter C. Proc R Soc Med 10:104
1995 Hunter's syndrome as a cause of childhood carpal tunnel syndrome: a report of three cases. Norman-Taylor F, Fixsen JA, Sharrard WJ. JPO-b 4:106
1997 Cervical decompression in mild mucopolysaccharidosis type II (Hunter syndrome). O'Brien DP, Cowie RA, Wraith JE. Childs Nerv Syst 13:87

Hurler Syndrome Also called mucopolysaccharidosis I, gargoylism. Autosomal recessive. Mutation in gene encoding alpha-L-iduronidase on chromosome 4p. Short stature, thoracolumbar kyphosis, coxa vara, joint contractures, brachydactyly, diaphyseal widening. Mental retardation, coarse facies, corneal opacities, respiratory insufficiency, cardiac disease, hepatosplenomegaly, abdominal hernias. Enzyme-replacement therapy or bone marrow transplantation improves life expectancy.

Figures below: Hurler syndrome showing lumbar kyphosis [1], broad and short bones [2], short stature [3] and enlarged pituitary fossa [4].

1919 Ueber einen Typ multipler Abartungen, vorwiegend am Skelettsystem. Hurler G. Z Kinderheilkd 24:220
1996 Hip dysplasia in Hurler's syndrome: orthopaedic management after bone marrow transplantation. Masterson EL, et al. JPO 16:731
1996 Spinal problems in mucopolysaccharidosis I (Hurler syndrome). Tandon V, et al. JBJS 78B:938

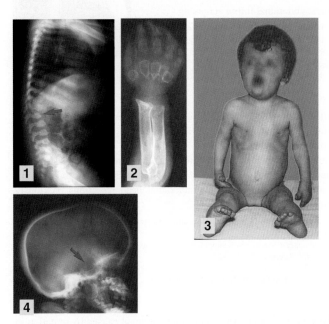

Hypochondroplasia Mutation in fibroblast growth factor receptor-3 on 4p, as in achondroplasia. Autosomal dominant, micromelia, macrocephaly, lumbar lordosis and stenosis, joint contractures, genua vara. Distinguished from achondroplasia by absence of trident hand and mild or absent midface hypoplasia.

1988 Hypochondroplasia. Review of 80 cases. Maroteaux P, Falzon P. Arch Fr Pediatr 45:105

Infantile Cortical Hyperostosis See Caffey disease.

Kienböck Disease Osteochondrosis of the lunate. See Chapter 9.

1910 Ueber traumatische Malazie des Mondbeins und ihre Folgezustaende: Entartungsformen und Kompressions-frakturen. Kienböck, R. Forschr Roentgen 16:77

Klein–Waardenburg Syndrome Abnormality of the PAX3 gene. Partial albinism, deaf mutism, blepharophimosis, flexion contractures, carpal synostosis, syndactyly, microcephaly, spasticity, winged scapulae.

1950 Albinism partial (leucisme) avec surdi–mutism, blepharophimosis et dysplasie myo–osteo–articulaire. Klein D. Helv Paediatr Acta 5:38

Klippel–Feil Syndrome Failure of vertebral segmentation in cervical with or without thoracic and lumbar spine, associated with hearing loss, cardiac and renal anomalies. See page 179.

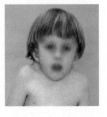

1912 Un cas d'absence des vertebres cervicales avec cage thoracique remontant jusqua la base du crane (cage thoracique cervicale). Klippel M, Feil A. Nouv Icon Salpetière 25:223

Klippel–Trenaunay–Weber Syndrome Cutaneous hemangiomas associated with hypertrophy of soft tissue and bone. Arteriovenous fistulae, lymphangiomas, and lymphaedema. Limb length equalization often necessary. See page 317.

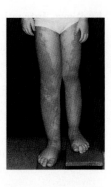

1900 Naevus variqueux osteohypertrophique. Klippel M, Trenaunay P. Arch Gen Med (Paris) 3:641
1993 Overgrowth management in Klippel-Trenaunay-Weber and Proteus syndromes. Guidera KJ, et al. JPO 13:459
1996 Wound healing in orthopaedic procedures for Klippel-Trenaunay syndrome. Gates PE, Drvaric DM, Kruger L. JPO 16:723

Kniest Dysplasia Mutation of COL2A1 gene. Macrocephaly, retinal detachment, hearing loss, cleft palate, occiptocervical instability, kyphoscoliosis [1 and 2], "swiss cheese" epiphyseal degeneration, joint contractures, coxa vara, abdominal herniae.

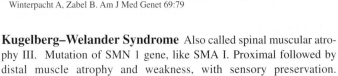

1952 Zur Abgrenzung der Dysostosis enchondrialis von der Chondrodystrophie. Kniest W. Z Kinderheilkd 70:633
1989 Occipitoatlantal instability in a child with Kniest syndrome. Merrill KD, Schmidt TL. JPO 9:338
1989 Kniest disease and total joint replacement for functional salvage. Sayli U, Brooker AF Jr. Adv Orthop Surg 13:85
1997 Kniest dysplasia: Dr. W. Kniest, his patient, the molecular defect. Spranger J, Winterpacht A, Zabel B. Am J Med Genet 69:79

Kugelberg–Welander Syndrome Also called spinal muscular atrophy III. Mutation of SMN 1 gene, like SMA I. Proximal followed by distal muscle atrophy and weakness, with sensory preservation. Diagnose by muscle biopsy and EMG. See page 344.

1956 Heredofamilial juvenile muscular atrophy simulating muscular dystrophy. Kugelberg E, Welander L. Arch Neurol Psychiatr 75:500

Larsen Syndrome Multiple congenital dislocations, including of knees, hips, and cervical spine. "Dish" facies, scoliosis, brachydactyly, clubfoot, accessory calcaneal and carpal ossification centers. Monitor spine, reduce dislocations, correct clubfoot.

1950 Multiple congenital dislocations associated with characteristic facial abnormality. Larsen LJ, Schottstaedt ER, Bost FC. J Pediatr 37:574
1994 Larsen's syndrome: review of the literature and analysis of thirty-eight cases. Laville JM, Lakermance P, Limouzy F. JPO 14:63

Lemierre Syndrome Rare, systemic anaerobic infection caused by *Fusobacterium necrophorum*. Causes acute oropharyngeal infection, septic thrombophlebitis of the internal jugular vein, sepsis, and multiple metastatic infections including septic arthritis and osteomyelitis.

1996 Fusobacterium osteomyelitis and pyarthrosis: a classic case of Lemierre's syndrome. J Stahlman GC, De Boer DK, Green NE. JPO 16:529

Lesch–Nyhan Syndrome X-linked, with deficiency in hypoxanthine-guanine phosphoribosyltransferase. Mental retardation, self-mutilation, choreoathetosis and spasticity, uric acid urinary stones, megaloblastic anemia, hip dislocation, scoliosis, fractures, autoamputations, infections.

1999 Orthopedic problems in Lesch–Nyhan syndrome. Sponseller, PD, et al. JPO 19:596

Letterer–Siwe Disease Familial, disseminated histiocytosis with severe presentation, including encephalopathy, hepatosplenomegaly, pulmonary infiltration and compromise, myelophthisis with pancytopenia, osteolysis.

1924 Aleukämische Retikulose. Letterer E. Frank Z Pathol 30:377.

Madelung Deformity Growth disturbance of the volar and ulnar distal radial physis producing forearm shortening, volar and ulnar subluxation of the hand with dorsal prominence of the distal ulna. Occurs in Leri-Weill dyschondrosteosis, characterized by short stature, mesomicromelia, joint contractures, ulnar and radial bowing. See page 195.

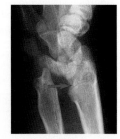

1878 Die spontane subluxation der hand nach vorne. Madelung OW. Verh Dent Ges Chir 7:259
1966 Dyschondrosteosis, the most common cause of Madelung's deformity. Herdman, RC, Langer LO Jr, Good RA. J Pediat 68:432
1998 Osteotomy of the radius and ulna for the Madelung deformity. Reis FB, et al. JBJS 80B:817

Marfan Syndrome Mutation of fibrillin-1 gene. Disproportionate tall stature, dolichocephaly and dolichostenomelia, which in the hands produces arachnodactyly. Craniofacial dysmorphism, ectopia lentis, retinal detachment, aortic and valvular anomalies, thoracic cage deformity, scoliosis, spondylolisthesis, ligamentous laxity, including patellar instability and pes planus, protrusio acetabuli, distensible skin.

Figures below: Marfan syndrome usual tall and slender stature [1], high, arched palate [2], and arachnodactyly [3–4].

1896 Un cas de déformacion congénitale des quatre membres, plus prononcée aux extrémités, caractérisée par l'allongement des os avec un certain degre d'amincissment. Marfan AB. Bull Soc Med Hôp Paris 13:220
1995 The thoracolumbar spine in Marfan syndrome. Sponseller PD, Hobbs W, Riley LH III, Pyeritz RE. J Bone Joint Surg 77A:867
1999 Changes in elastic fibers in musculoskeletal tissues of Marfan syndrome: a possible mechanism of joint laxity and skeletal overgrowth. Gigante A, Chillemi C, Greco F. JPO 19:283

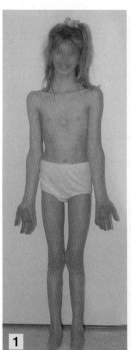
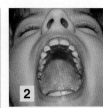
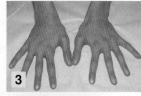
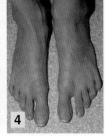

Maffucci Syndrome Cutaneous and mucous membrane hemangiomas associated with enchondromatosis (of Ollier). Risk of malignant transformation, skeletal (chondrosarcoma) and nonskeletal, is high, dictating periodic follow-up.

1881 Di un caso di encondroma ed angioma multiplo. Contribuzione alla genesi embrionale dei tumori. Maffucci A. Movimiento Medico–Chirurgico Nap 13:399
1988 The Maffucci syndrome. Ben-Itzhak I, et al. JPO 8:345

McCune–Albright Syndrome Mutation of GNAS 1 gene. Polyostotic fibrous dysplasia of long and craniofacial bones, café-au-lait spots with irregular or "coast of Maine" margins (as opposed to smooth or "coast of California" margins seen in neurofibromatosis), and precocious puberty resulting from autonomous cellular response. Deformity and pathological fractures produced by fibrous dysplasia require orthopedic intervention.

1936 Osteitis fibro–cystica: The case of a nine year old girl who also exhibits precocious puberty, multiple pigmentation of the skin and hyperthyroidism. McCune DJ. Am J Dis Child 52:743

Melnick–Needles Syndrome "Ribbon" ribs, short and bowed long bones with flared metaphyses, joint and cutaneous laxity, scoliosis, exophthalmos, glaucoma, hearing loss, micrognathia, calvarial sclerosis, cardiac and genitourinary anomalies.

1966 An undiagnosed bone dysplasia: A 2 family study of 4 generations and 3 generations. Melnick JC, Needles CF. Am J Roentgenol 97:39
1983 Melnick-Needles syndrome: osteodysplasty with kyphoscoliosis. Bartolozzi P, et al. JPO 3:387
1998 Melnick-Needles syndrome. Report of a case. Greco F, et al. Pediatr Med Chir 20:149

Melorheostosis Asymmetrical longitudinal flowing sclerosis in long bones, likened to wax dripping along a candlestick. Involvement of periarthritic tissues leads to painful and deforming contractures. Associated vascular anomalies of surrounding soft tissues.

Figures below: Melorheostosis. Note the linear irregular hyperostosis at these varied sites [1–3].

1997 Melorheostosis. Rozencwaig R, Wilson MR, McFarland GB Jr. Am J Orthop 26:83

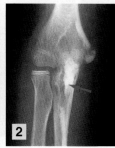
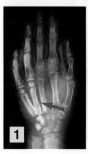
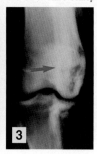

Mermaid Syndrome See Caudal Regression Syndrome.

Metachondromatosis Combines features of enchondromatsosis and hereditary multiple exostosis. Distinguished by lack of malignant potential and by direction of exostoses away from adjacent joints. May produce changes in the hip resembling Legg-Calvé-Perthes disease.

1985 Metachondromatosis: report of four cases. Bassett GS, Cowell HR. JBJS 67A:811

Metaphyseal Chondrodysplasias Metaphyseal involvement leads to joint contracture and bowing, including coxa vara and genu varum. Several types, including Schmidt, which results from mutation of COL10A1 gene, and Jansen, which results from mutation of parathyroid hormone receptor.

Table below: Types of metaphyseal chondrodysplasias. The major forms with mode of inheritance AD (autosomal dominant), AR (autosomal recessive), Sp (sporadic), clinical features and severity.

Figures below: Schmidt type (red arrows) metaphyseal chondrodysplasias. Note the coxa vara and metaphyseal defects [1–2]. McKusick type metaphyseal chondrodysplasias (yellow arrows). Note the metaphyseal changes and the cone-shaped epiphyses [3–5].

1963 Le formes partielles de la dysostose metaphysaire. Maroteaux P, Savart P, Lefebre J, et al. Presse Med 71:1523

Clinical features			
Schmidt	AD	short stature, coxa vara, genu varum	moderate
McKusick	AR	mod short stature, joint laxity, fine hair	moderate
Jansen	Sp	very short, severe bony deformity	severe
		Malabsorption and neutropenia form	
		Retinitis pigmentosa and bachydactyly	

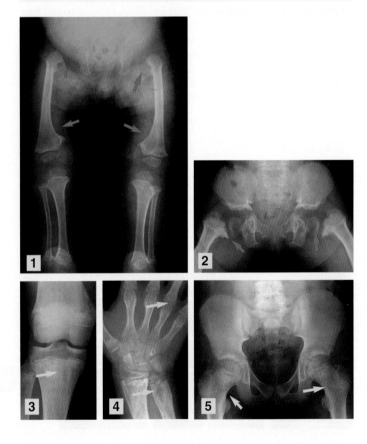

Möbius II Rare, chromosomal abnormalities, congenital facial diplegia, form of arthrogryposis, facial paralysis, tongue and palate atrophy, possible absence of pectoralis muscles, clubfoot, syndactyly.

1880 von Graefe A. Graefe–Saemisch Handbuch, 6:60 Leipzig, Engelmann
1996 Möbius syndrome: electrophysiologic studies in seven cases. Aradeh S, et al. Muscle Nerve 19:1148

Morquio-Brailsford Syndrome Type IV mucopolysaccharidosis, subtype A caused by N-acetylgalactosamine-6-sulfatase deficiency, while subtype B is caused by deficiency of β-galactosidase. Characterized by corneal opacity, hearing loss, aortic valve disease, odontoid hypoplasia with upper cervical instability, kyphoscoliosis, platyspondyly, joint derangement, including hip dysplasia. See Mucopolysaccharidosis.

Figures below: Morquio syndrome. Typical features including short stature [1], platyspondyly [2], and flared iliac wings [3].

1929 Sur une forme de dystrophie osseuse familiale. Morquio L. Bull Soc Pediatr Paris 27:145
1996 Occipito-atlanto-axial fusion in Morquio-Brailsford syndrome. A ten-year experience. Ransford AO, et al. JBJS 78B:307
1997 A review of Morquio syndrome. Mikles M, Stanton RP. Am J Orthop 26:533

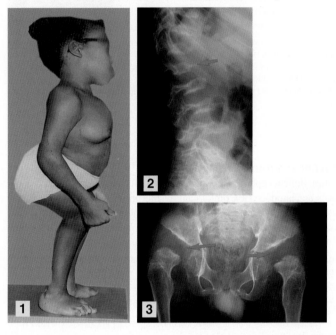

Moulded Baby Syndrome The moulded baby syndrome comprises: head moulding (plagiocephaly); pelvic obliquity with unilateral loss of hip abduction in flexion; and occasionally scoliosis, torticollis, and bat ears. The hips, however, are radiologically normal and do not require the treatment used in the management of congenital dislocation or dysplasia.

1984 The hip in the moulded baby syndrome. Good C, Walker G. JBJS 66B:491

Mucopolysaccharidosis Abnomality of degradation of, leading to intracellular accumulation and urinary excretion of, mucopolysaccharide. Several types are distinguished.

Table below: Mucopolysaccharidoses. The major features of the different diseases.

Clinical features	
I-H Hurler	Severe, involves CNS, viscera, skeleton, progressive
I-S Scheie	Joint contractures, IQ, stature and longevity normal
II Hunter	Males, similar to Hurler but less severe
III Sanfilippo	Like Scheie but with mental retardation
IV Morquio	Normal IQ, stort stature, joint laxity, cervical instability
VI Maroteaux –Lamy	Like Hurler syndrome but with normal IQ and flattening of femoral capital epiphysis
VII Sly	May be recognizable in neonatal period

Multiple Epiphyseal Dysplasia

(MED) Mutations in COL9A2 and cartilage oligomeric matrix protein (COMP) genes. Ribbing described mild form, Fairbanks the severe form. Moderate short stature, normal intelligence, delayed and irregular epiphyseal formation leading to premature osteoarthritis, brachydactyly, ovoid vertebrae. Multiple epiphyseal involvement distinguishes this from Legg-Calvé-Perthes disease.

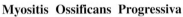

1935 Generalized disease of skeleton. Fairbank, HAT. Proc R Soc Med 28:1611

1937 Studien ueber hereditaere, multiple Epiphysenstoerungen. Ribbing S. Acta Radiol Suppl 34:1

1992 Early diagnosis of multiple epiphyseal dysplasia. Ingram RR. JPO 12:241

1998 Stature and severity in multiple epiphyseal dysplasia. Haga N, et al. JPO 18:394

Multiple Synostosis

Mutation of Noggin gene. Multiple synostoses, including of elbows, fingers, wrists, and feet, producing multiple tarsal coalitions. Brachydactyly, radial head dislocation, hypoplastic nails, hearing loss, pectus deformity.

1972 La maladie des synostoses multiples. Maroteaux P, Bouvet JP, Briard ML. Nouv Presse Med 1:3041

Myositis Ossificans Progressiva

Also called fibrodysplasia ossificans progressiva. Heterotopic ossification of striated muscle, in craniocaudal, axial to appendicular, and proximal to distal directions, producing pain and stiffness. Halluceal malformation, clinodactyly, reduction defects of all digits, cervical vertebral anomalies, hearing loss, baldness. No consistently effective treatment.

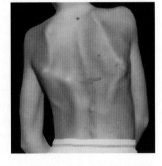

1982 Fibrodysplasia ossificans progressiva. The clinical features and natural history of 34 patients. Connor JM, Evans DA. JBJS 64B:76

1998 Fibrodysplasia (myositis) ossificans progressiva. Clinical lessons from a rare disease. Smith R. CO 346:7

Nail-Patella Syndrome

Mutation of the LIM-homeodomain protein LMX1B. Autosomal dominant. Nail malformation, absent or hypoplastic patellae, iliac horns, limited elbow motion with radial head dislocation. May be associated with nephropathy.

Figures below: Typical features of nail-patella syndrome include absence or hypoplasia of the patella and dysplastic nails [1–2].

1933 An hereditary arthrodysplasia associated with hereditary dystrophy of the nails. Turner JW. JAMA 100:882

1991 Nail patella syndrome: a review of 44 orthopedic patients. Guidera KJ, et al. JPO 11:73

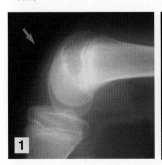

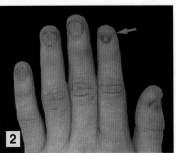

Neurofibromatosis (NF)

Type 1 caused by mutation of neurofibromin gene. Type 2 caused by mutation of schwannomin gene. Type 2 is characterized by fewer peripheral but more intracranial lesions, including acoustic neuromata. Simple neurofibromata, made up of Schwann cells and fibrous tissue, rarely produce deficit. Plexiform neurofibromas, which are highly vascular, lead to disfigurement and gigantism, which may require orthopedic intervention, such as limb equalization. Café-au-lait spots have smooth or "coast of California" borders (versus rough or "coast of Maine" borders in McCune-Albright syndrome). Scoliosis may be idiopathic or dystrophic. The former is treated as such. The latter is characterized by short and sharp angulation, osseous erosion by intraspinal lesions and dural ectasia, and spinal instability. Bracing plays no role, and early anterior together with posterior fusion is indicated because of the risk of pseudarthrosis. See page 181. Pseudarthrosis often involves the tibia, presenting as an anterolateral bow. This is treated by prophylactic bracing, and medullary fixation with osseous grafting after fracture. See page 127.

Table below: shows the features necessary to establish a diagnosis of neurofibromatosis. Two or more criteria are necessary for type 1.

Chart below: shows the features in neurofibromatosis. From Simone, et al. (1988) – orthopedic center data.

Figures below: Typical features of neurofibromatosis with anterior tibial bowing [1], pseudarthrosis tibiae [2], and soft tissue overgrowth and bony scalloping of the hand [3].

1986 Long-term follow-up of von Recklinghausen neurofibromatosis. Survival and malignant neoplasms. Sorensen SA, Mulvihill JJ, Nielsen A. N Engl J Med 314:1010

1994 Pathophysiology of spinal deformities in neurofibromatosis. An analysis of seventy-one patients who had curves associated with dystrophic changes. Funasaki H, et al. JBJS 76A:692

1995 Spinal tumors in patients with neurofibromatosis type 2: MR imaging study of frequency, multiplicity, and variety. Mautner VF, et al. AJR Am J Roentgenol 165:951

1997 Spine update. The management of scoliosis in neurofibromatosis. Kim HW, Weinstein SL. Spine 22:2770

Clinical features – 2 or more required for diagnosis

Café-au-lait spots	6 or more >5 mm.
Neurofibroma	2 or more or single plexiform neurofibroma
Freckling	in axillae or inguinal region
Optical glioma	
Lisch nodules	(iris hamartoma) 2 or more
Bone lesion	typical for NF1
Family history	First degree relative with NF1

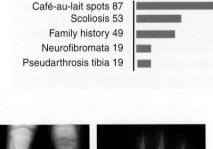

Café-au-lait spots 87
Scoliosis 53
Family history 49
Neurofibromata 19
Pseudarthrosis tibia 19

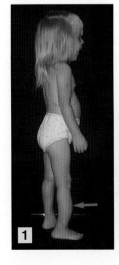

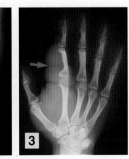

Niemann–Pick Disease Deficient activity of the enzyme that catalyzes cleavage of sphingomyelin to phosphorylcholine and ceramide. Accumulation of sphingomyelin in ganglia and reticuloendothelial cells leads to central nervous system disease, including mental retardation and seizures, and hepatosplenopathology, including ascites and recurrent infections. Five types are distinguished: classical infantile (type A), visceral (type B), subacute or juvenile (type C), Nova Scotia variant (type D), adult (type E).

1914 Ein Unbekanntes. Niemann A. Krankheitbild. Jahrb Kinderh NF 29:1

Nievergelt Syndrome Micromelia characterized by radioulnar synostosis, radial and ulnar capital subluxation, rhomboidal tibiae and fibulae, tarsal coalition and metatarsal synostosis, brachydactyly, camptodactyly.

1944 Positiver Vaterschafs nachweis auf Grund erblicher Missbildungen der Extremitäten. Nievergelt K. Arch Klaus Stift Vererbungforsch 19:157
1989 Longitudinal tibial epiphyseal bracket in Nievergelt syndrome. Burnstein MI, et al. Skeletal Radiol 18:121

Oculodentodigital Dysplasia Syndrome Includes smallest finger camptodactyly, syndactyly of ring and smallest fingers, aphalangia of the feet, spinal cord compression with spastic tetraparesis.

1998 The different appearance of the oculodentodigital dysplasia syndrome. Thomsen M, et al. JPO-b 7:23

Ollier Disease Multiple enchondromata in metaphyses of long bones, which are often asymmetric, deforming, and inhibit growth. Malignant transformation, to chondrosarcoma, observed in 10-30%. Hands and feet most often involved. Orthopedic intervention includes limb equalization and angular osteotomy.

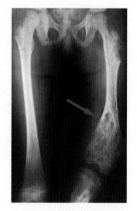

1899 De la dyschondroplasia. Bull Soc Chir (Lyon) 3:22
1982 Ollier's Disease. An assessment of angular deformity, shortening, and pathological fracture in twenty-one patients. Shapiro JBJS 64A:95
1987 Bone sarcomas associated with Ollier's disease. Liu J, et al. Cancer 59:1376
1998 Ollier's disease: varus angulation at the lower femur and its management. Chew DK, Menelaus MB, Richardson MD. JPO 18:202

Osteopetrosis Also called marble bone disease, Albers–Schönberg disease. Osteoclast dysfunction leads to defective bone resorption. Encroachment upon bone marrow results in pancytopenia and infection. Cranial nerve compression results in blindness and deafness. Extramedullary hematopoiesis results in hepatosplenomegaly. Abnormal bone turnover results in morbid fractures. Sclerosis hinders bone fixation. Autosomal recessive, or malignant, form presents in childhood. It is caused by mutation in the TCIRG1 subunit of the vacuolar proton pump. Treatment is bone marrow transplant. Adult form is autosomal dominant and more benign.

Figures, next column: Spine shows anterior notching [1], "bone in a bone" [2–3], and dense bone with fracture [4].

1904 Roentgenbilder einer seltenen Knochenerkrankung. Albers–Schönberg H. München Med Wochenschr 51:365
1995 Bilateral nonunited femoral neck fracture in a child with osteopetrosis. Steinwender G, Hosny GA, Koch S, Grill F. JPO-b 4 :213
1995 Long-term treatment of osteopetrosis with recombinant human interferon gamma. Key LL, et al. N Engl J Med 332:594
1997 Martin RP, Deane RH, Collett V. Spondylolysis in children who have osteopetrosis JBJS 79A:1685

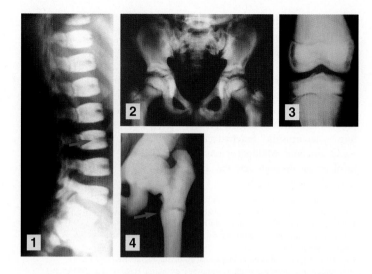

Osteogenesis Imperfecta Most common lethal osteochondrodysplasia. Caused by mutation of type I collagen gene. Location of mutation in the collagen molecule and type of mutation determine phenotype. Phenotype reflects distribution of type I collagen in bone, dentin, soft tissues such as sclerae, ligaments, and tendons, skin. Mild phenotype explained by haplo insufficiency, or reduced amount of normal collagen. Severe phenotypes explained by dominant negative mutation, that is abnormal collagen chains poison normal chains, thereby preventing formation of normal collagen. Four clinical types (see table), subtyped as A or B based upon absence or presence of dentinogenesis imperfecta. Multiple fractures produce shortening and deformity, including "saber" tibiae and "accordion" femora. Increased woven:lamellar bone and hypercellularity produce weak bone, which heals readily. Medullary fixation with solid or telescoping rods for fractures and in conjunction with osteotomies for deformed tubular bones. Minimize immobilization to decrease stress shielding of bone and joint stiffness. Ambulatory potential proportional directly to age of onset and inversely to deformity. Early fusion for scoliosis. No role for bracing. Spinal instrumentation hindered by bone fragility. No effective treatment for basilar invagination. Conductive (otosclerosis) and sensorineural hearing impairment. Bisphosphonates may delay onset and reduce number of fractures. Wormian bones, "codfish" vertebrae, malignant hyperthermia with anesthesia.

Table below: Shows type of osteogenesis imperfecta. Based on Sillence, et al. (1979).

Figures, next page: Radiographic features of osteogenesis imperfecta. Type 2 lethal form [1]; wormian bones [2]; OI type 4, 5 [3–4]; type 3 with IM rod fixation [5]; and lateral spine [6]. Note rod in femur.

1979 Genetic heterogeneity in osteogenesis imperfecta. Silence DO, Senn A, Danks DM. J Med Gen 16:101
1998 The Nicholas Andry Award–The molecular pathology of osteogenesis imperfecta. Cole WG. CO 343:235
1998 Osteogenesis imperfecta. Kocher MS, Shapiro F. J Am Acad Orthop Surg 6:225
2000 The Sofield-Miller operation in osteogenesis imperfecta. Li YH, Chow W, Leong JCY. JBJS 82B:11

Type	1	2	3	4
Inheritance	dominant	new mut.	recessive	dominant
Frequency	40%	10%	30%	20%
Severity	mild	lethal	progressive	deforming
Sclera	blue	blue	white	white
Ambulation	yes	-	rare	variable

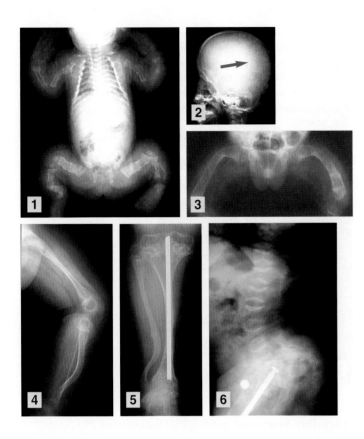

Panner Disease Osteochondritis dissecans of capitulum. See page 193.

1927 An affection of the capitellum humeri resembling Calve–Perthes disease of the hip. Panner HJ. Acta Radiol (Stockh) 8:617
1995 Panner's disease: X-ray, MR imaging findings and review of the literature. Stoane JM, et al. Comput Med Imaging Graph 19:473

Pfeiffer Syndrome Also called acrocephalosyndactyly, type V. Mutation of fibroblast growth factor receptor–1 and 2 gene. Polydactyly distinguishes this from Apert syndrome. Involvement of the hands and feet distinguishes it from Crouzon syndrome. Craniosynostosis with "tower" skull, syndactyly of hands and feet with broad thumbs and halluces, cervical vertebral anomalies, radiohumeral synostosis, hydrocephalus, and Chiari malformation.

1964 Dominante erbliche Akrocephalosyndactylie. Pfeiffer RA. Z Kinderheilkd 90:301
1996 Cervical spine in Pfeiffer's syndrome. Anderson PJ, et al. J Craniofac Surg 7:275

Poland Syndrome Symbrachydactyly associated with ipsilateral aplasia of the sternal head of the pectoralis major muscle. Cosmetic more than functional problem. Absence of other shoulder muscles may limit reconstructive surgery and necessitates preoperative MRI. Vascular insult *in utero*, termed sublavian artery supply disruption sequence, has been proposed as etiology. One bilateral case has been reported.

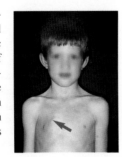

1841 Deficiency of the pectoral muscles. Poland A. Guy Hosp Rep 6:191
1982 Anatomical findings in the hands of patients with Poland's syndrome. Senrui H, Egawa T, Horiki A. JBJS 64A:1079
1986 Subclavian artery supply disruption sequence: hypothesis of a vascular etiology for Poland, Klippel-Feil, and Moebius anomalies. Bouwes Bavinck JN, Weaver DD, Am J Med Genet 23:903

Popliteal Pterygium "Wing" in popliteal fossa producing flexion contracture and possible subluxation of tibia on femur. Popliteal pterygium may be part of larger "musculus calcaneoischiadicus." Simple syndactyly, bifid halluceal nail. Pterygia produce facial and genital distortion. Treat by release and progressive extension of knee using Ilizarov frame. Rate of recurrence is high.

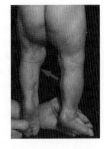

1869 Sur un vice conformation trés-rare de la lévre inférieure. Trélat V. J Med Chir Pract 40:442
1990 Popliteal pterygium syndrome: an orthopedic perspective. Oppenheim WL, et al. JPO 10:58

Prader–Willi Syndrome Caused by deletion of paternal copies of imprinted SNRPN and necdin genes. Poor fetal movement, mental retardation, neonatal failure to thrive followed by polyphagia and obesity, short stature, hypersalivation, hypoventilation, hypogonadism, cryptorchidism, kyphoscoliosis, small hands and feet, hypotonia, hyporeflexia.

1956 Ein Syndrom von Adipositas, Kleinwuchs, Kryptochidismus, und Oligophrenia nach myatonieartigem Zustand in Neugeborenenalter. Prader A, Labhart A, Willi H. Schbweitz Med Wochenschr 86:1260
1989 Scoliosis surgery in the Prader-Willi syndrome. Rees D, et al. JBJS 71B:685

Proteus Syndrome Diffuse, unilateral or local tissue hypertrophy leading to gigantism of trunk and/or limbs. Lymphatic and vascular tumors in skin and subcutaneous tissue. Orthopedic intervention consists of limb equalization and decompression and fusion for spinal stenosis and kyphoscoliosis.

1907 Zur Pathologie der dystrophischen Form des angeborenen partiellen Riesenwuchses. Wieland E. Jahrb Kinderheilk 65:519
1992 Proteus syndrome: musculoskeletal manifestations and management: a report of two cases. Demetriades D, et al. JPO 12:106

Pseudoachondroplasia Mutation of cartilage oligomeric matrix protein gene. Resembles achondroplasia with sparing of the face. Other distinguishing features include normal presentation at birth, odontoid hypoplasia producing instability, absence of lumbar spinal stenosis.

1984 Pseudoachondroplasia: biochemical and histochemical studies of cartilage. Pedrini-Mille A, Maynard JA, Pedrini VA. JBJS 66A:1408

Prune Belly Syndrome Viscera protrude through abdominal wall with absent muscles and lax, wrinkled skin. Urinary obstruction, cryptorchidism, imperforate anus, congenital heart defects, pectus deformity. Refractory hip dislocation, clubfoot, scoliosis, vertical talus, and congenital muscular torticollis.

Figures below: Note the typical appearance of the abdomen in prune belly syndrome [1] and the hip dislocation [2] that are common and difficult to manage because of tendency of recurrence.

1993 Orthopedic aspects of prune belly syndrome. Green NE, Lowery ER, Thomas R. JPO 13:496
1995 The orthopaedic manifestations of prune-belly (Eagle-Barrett) syndrome. Brinker MR, Palutsis RS, Sarwark JF. JBJS 77A:251

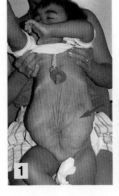

Pterygium Syndrome "Winging" in neck, across flexion creases in limbs, and between digits. Scoliosis, vertebral segmentation defects, camptodactyly, syndactyly, vertical talus, muscle hypoplasia, pectus deformity. Pterygia distort the genitalia. Cleft lip and palate, gastrointestinal and cardiac anomalies. Early pterygium release to limit disability. Neurovascular structures may limit extent of release. Early fusion for scoliosis, as no role for brace and correction is limited. Evaluate spine with MRI and kidneys with ultrasonogram preoperatively. Lethal and multiple forms are distinguished as autosomal recessive from popliteal form, which is autosomal dominant.

Table below: The major features of the pterygium syndrome.

Figures below: Note the webbing of the knee in the newborn [1] and multiple ptergyium [2] typical of these syndromes.

1988 Multiple pterygium syndrome. An overview. Ramer JC, Ladda RL, Demuth WW. Am J Dis Child 142:794

1992 Treatment of multiple pterygium syndrome. McCall RE, Budden AB. J Orthopedics 15:1417

Pterygium syndromes	
Multiple	Rare, recessive, short stature, CNS involvement, scoliosis, clubfeet, multiple pterygium
Popliteal	Rare, dominant, face, genitals and knee pterygium from pelvis to heel, early operative release
Lethal	Several forms

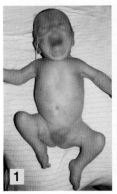 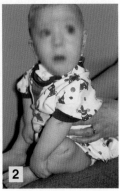

Pycnodysostosis Mutation of cathepsin K gene. Short stature, craniofacial dysmorphism with delayed closure of fontanels, bone hyperdensity or sclerosis, bone fragility leading to stress fractures, dysplastic clavicles, hip dislocation, spondylolisthesis, phalangeal acrosteolysis.

1992 Pycnodysostosis. Orthopedic aspects with a description of 14 new cases. Edelson JG, et al. CO 280:263

Pyle Syndrome See metaphyseal chondrodysplasia.

Reflex Sympathetic Dystrophy (RSD) Autonomic dysfunction results in disproportionate response to noxious stimulus, including dysesthesia, vasodilation or vasoconstriction, and edema in acute state, followed by atrophy, stiffness, and osteopenia in chronic state. See page 58.

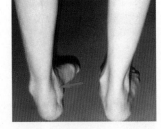

1990 Reflex sympathetic dystrophy in children. Dietz FR, Mathews KD, Montgomery WJ. CO 258:225

1992 Reflex sympathetic dystrophy in children. Clinical characteristics and follow-up of seventy patients. Wilder RT, et al. JBJS 74A:910

Rett Syndrome Mutation of methyl-CpG-binding protein-2 gene. Onset 6-18 months. X-linked dominant affecting girls. Progressive encephalopathy, seizures, autism, stereotypic hand movements, spasticity, hyperreflexia. Scoliosis not amenable to bracing and treated with fusion to pelvis. Short metacarpals and metatarsals, joint contractures.

Figures below: Rett syndrome. Note the severe scoliosis before [1] and after fusion [2].

1968 Ueber ein cerebral–atrophisches. Syndrom bei Hyperammonaemie. Rett A. Monatsschr Kinderheilkd 116:310

1989 Orthopedic aspects of Rett syndrome: a multicenter review. Loder RT, Lee CL, Richards BS. JPO 9:557

1994 Scoliosis in Rett syndrome. Huang TJ, Lubicky JP, Hammerberg KW. Orthop Rev 23:9

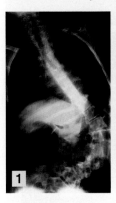 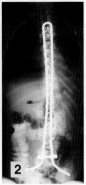

Riley–Day Syndrome See Familial Dysautonomia.

Rubinstein–Taybi Syndrome Mutation of the transcriptional coactivator CREB-binding protein gene. Broad thumbs and hallucis, facies, psychomotor retardation, vertebral anomalies and scoliosis, slipped capital femoral epiphysis, patellar hypoplasia and instability, cardiac and genitourinary anomalies, hirsutism.

1963 Broad thumbs and toes and facial abnormalities: A possible mental retardation syndrome. Rubinstein JH, Taybi H. Am J Dis Child 105:588

1987 Surgical treatment of the thumb in the Rubinstein-Taybi syndrome. Wood VE, Rubinstein JH. J Hand Surg Br 12:166

1998 Instability of the patellofemoral joint in Rubinstein-Taybi syndrome. Mehlman CT, Rubinstein JH, Roy DR. JPO 18:508

1999 Duplicated longitudinal bracketed epiphysis "kissing delta phalanx" in Rubinstein–Taybi syndrome. Wood VE, Rubinstein J. JPO 19:603

Sanfilippo Syndrome See mucopolysaccharidosis

SAPHO Syndrome Synovitis, acne, pustulosis, hyperostosis, and osteitis.

1999 The SAPHO syndrome in children: a rare cause of hyoperostosis and osteitis. Letts M, et al. JPO 19:297

Silver-Russell Syndrome Hemihypertrophy, body asymmetry, hand and foot anomalies, including brachydactyly, clinodactyly, syndactyly. Vertebral anomalies, scoliosis, slipped capital femoral epiphysis, hip dysplasia. Small triangular facies, variation in sexual development.

1953 Syndrome of congenital hemihypertrophy, shortness of stature, and elevated urinary gonadotropins. Silver KH, et al. Pediatrics 12:368

1954 A syndrome of "intra-uterine" dwarfism recognizable at birth with craniofacial dysostosis, disproportionately short arms and other anomalies. Russell A. Proc R Soc Med 47:1040

Small-Patella Syndrome Also called ischiopatellar dysplasia, coxopodopatellar syndrome. Patellar hypoplasia and instability, ischial hypoplasia, brachydactyly and widened web spaces in the feet.

1996 The 'small-patella' syndrome. Hereditary osteodysplasia of the knee, pelvis and foot. Dellestable F, et al. JBJS 78B:63

Spondyloepimetaphyseal Dysplasia Several types. Micromelia, delayed epiphyseal ossification, flared tubular bone metaphyses, joint laxity, kyphoscoliosis, clubfoot, cleft palate, retinal detachment.

1990 Spine deformity in spondyloepimetaphyseal dysplasia. Winter RB, Bloom BA. JPO 10:535

1995 Dominant mutations in the type II collagen gene, COL2A1, produce spondyloepimetaphyseal dysplasia, Strudwick type. Tiller GE, et al. Nature Genet 11:87

Spondyloepiphyseal Dysplasia (SED) Mutation of type II collagen gene. Heterogenous group. Delayed epiphyseal ossification, dens hypoplasia, and atlantoaxial instability. Kyphoscoliosis, platyspondyly, coxa vara, joint contractures, hypotonia, cleft palate, retinal detachment, sensorineural deafness.

Table below: This categorization is based on recommendations by Wynne–Davies (1985).

1966 Dysplasia spondyloepiphysaria congenita. Spranger JW, Wiedemann HR. Helv Paediat Acta 21:598

1985 Atlas of General Affections of the Skeleton. Wynne-Davies, R. Longman.

1990 Tandem duplication within a type II collagen gene (COL2A1) exon in an individual with spondyloepiphyseal dysplasia. Tiller GE, et al. Proc Nat Acad Sci 87:3889

Spondyloepiphyseal dysplasia	
Congenita	Severe, very short, short trunk, epiphyseal and meta-physeal changes, coxa vara, cleft palate, deafness
Tarda	X–linked, affects large proximal joints, late onset, not severe, only males
Tarda	Dominant and recessive, as with tarda X–linked
Tarda	Progressive arthopathy, recessive, clinically like JRA

Spondylometaphyseal Dysplasia Heterogenous group. Vertebral bodies extend beyond pedicles like an "open staircase." Flaring of tubular bone metaphyses resembles rickets. Platyspondyly, kyphoscoliosis, dens hypoplasia, coxa vara. Subclassified based upon delayed ossification of femoral neck and greater trochanter as severe, moderate or mild.

1967 La dysostose spondylo-metaphysaire. Kozlowski K, et al. Presse Med 75:2769

1991 The spondylometaphyseal dysplasias. A tentative classification. Maroteaux P, Spranger J. Pediatr Radiol 21:293

Stickler Syndrome Three types: I caused by type II collagen mutation, II and III caused by type XI collagen mutation. Also called hereditary arthro-opthalmopathy after osteoarthritis and ocular anomalies. Platyspondyly and kyphoscoliosis, Marfanoid features including arachnodactyly and protrusio acetabuli.

1990 Stickler syndrome. Bennett JT, McMurray SW. JPO 10:760

Streeter Dysplasia See Amniotic Band Syndrome.

Taybi Syndrome Also called otopalatodigital syndrome, type I: conductive deafness, cleft palate, broad distal phalanges of thumbs and toes with short nails. X-linked, small stature, mild mental deficiency, craniofacial dysmorphism, limited elbow extension, spina bifida, carpal synostosis, accessory ossification center at base of second metatarsal bone.

1962 Generalized skeletal dysplasia with multiple anomalies. Taybi H. Am J Roentgenol Rad Ther Nucl Med 88:450

Tarsal Tunnel Sndrome Rare, foot positioned in supination. Often use crutches, operative results good.

1982 The tarsal tunnel syndrome in children. Albrektsson B, Rydholm A, Rydholm U. JBJS 64B:215

Thrombocytopenia Absent Radius (TAR) Syndrome Thrombocytopenia, radial aplasia and clubhand, hip dislocation, knee subluxation and stiffness, cardiac anomalies. Distinguished from Fanconi syndrome by absence of panmyelopathy, leukemia, thumb anomalies, and pigmentary changes.

1956 Kongenitale hypoplastische Thrombopenie mit Radius-Aplasie, ein Syndrom multipler Abartungen. Gross H, et al. Neue Oest Z Kinderheilk 1:574

1999 Management of thrombocytopenia-absent radius (TAR) syndrome. McLaurin TM, et al. JPO 19:289

Trevor Disease See Dysplasia Epiphysealis Hemimelica.

Trichorhinophalangeal Dysplasia Mutation of zinc finger protein that is a putative transcription factor. Thin hair, piriform nose, conoid phalangeal epiphyses with brachydactyly.

1966 Das Tricho-rhino-phalangeal Syndrom. Giedion A. Helv Paediat Acta 21:475

1986 The trichorhinophalangeal dysplasia syndrome: report of eight kindreds, with emphasis on hip complications, late presentations, and premature osteoarthrosis. Beals RK, Bennett RM. JPO 6:133

1995 Hip pathology in the trichorhinophalangeal syndrome. Dunbar JD, Sussman MD, Aiona MD. JPO 15:381

Turner Syndrome Also called XO syndrome. Small stature female, gonadal dysgenesis with delayed sexual development, mental retardation, lymphaedema, webbed neck, broad chest with widely spaced nipples, elbow and knee anomalies, including cubitus valgus and patellofemoral instability, hip dysplasia, brachydactyly, renal and cardiac anomalies.

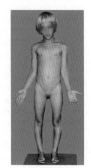

1938 A syndrome of infantilism, congenital webbed neck, and cubitus valgus. Turner HH. Endocrinology 23:566

1994 Recurrent dislocation of the patella in Turner's syndrome. Mizuta H, et al. JPO 14:74

1996 Leg lengthening in Turner dwarfism. Trivella GP, Brigadoi F, Aldegheri R. JBJS 78B:290

VACTERL Association Expanded acronym from VATER. **V**ertebral anomalies (hemivertebrae), **a**nal **a**tresia, **c**ardiac anomalies (septal defects), **t**racheo**e**sophageal fistula, **r**enal anomalies (urethral atresia, renal agenesis), **l**imb anomalies–radial aplasia, proximal origin of thumb, hexadactyly, humeral hypoplasia, hydrocephalus, scoliosis.

1972 The VATER association: vertebral defects, anal atresia, tracheoesophageal fistula with esophageal atresia, radial dysplasia. Quan, L, Smith, DW. Birth Defects Orig Art Ser VIII(2):75

1986 Orthopaedic aspects of the VATER association. Lawhon SM, MacEwen GD, Bunnell WP. JBJS 68:424

Van Neck Syndrome Painful swelling of normal ischiopubic synchondrosis. Usually a stress reaction, but may represent osteomyelitis. Incidental radiographic finding may be confused with neoplasm.

1988 The scintigraphic and radiographic appearance of the ischiopubic synchondroses in normal children and in osteomyelitis. Kloiber R, et al. J Pediatr Radiol 18:57

1995 Swollen ischiopubic synchondrosis: a dilemma for the radiologist. Kozlowski K, Hochberger O, Povysil B. Australas Radiol 39:224

Velocardiofacial Syndrome Also called Shprintzen syndrome. Cleft palate, cardiac anomalies, typical facies. Other features include intellectual impairment, hearing loss, short stature, hypotonia, scoliosis, clubfoot, Sprengel anomaly, joint laxity, arachnodactyly.

1978 A new syndrome involving cleft palate, cardiac anomalies, typical facies, and learning disabilities; velo-cardio-facial syndrome. Shprintzen RJ, et al. Cleft Palate J 15:56

1999 Musculoskeletal abnormalities in velocardiofacial syndrome. Pollard ME, et al. JPO 19:607

Whistling Face Syndrome See Freeman–Sheldon Syndrome.

Aase JM, *Diagnostic Dysmorphology* Plenum Medical Books NY, London.1990.

Ainsworth SR, Aulicino PL. A survey of patients with Ehlers-Danlos syndrome. Clin Orthop 1993;286:250-256.

Akbarnia BA, Gabriel KR, Beckman E, et al. Prevalence of scoliosis in neurofibromatosis. Spine 1992;17(Suppl 8):S244-S248.

Alter BP. Arm anomalies and bone marrow failure may go hand in hand. J Hand Surg 1992;17A:566-571.

Andrisano A, Soncini G, Calderoni PP, et al. Critical review of infantile fibrous dysplasia: Surgical treatment. J Pediatr Orthop 1991;11:478-481.

Baraitser M, Reardon W, Oley C, et al. Femoral hypoplasia unusual facies syndrome with preaxial polydactyly. Clin Dysmorphol 1994;3:40-45.

Beals RK, Rolfe B. VATER association: A unifying concept of multiple anomalies. J Bone Joint Surg 1989;71A:948-950.

Boers GH, Polder TW, Cruysberg JR, et al. Homocystinuria versus Marfan's syndrome: The therapeutic relevance of the differential diagnosis. Neth J Med 1984;27:206-212.

Bowen JR, Ortega AK, Ray S, et al. Spinal deformities in Larsen's syndrome. Clin Orthop 1985;197:159-163.

Brinker MR, Palutsis RS, Sarwark JF. The orthopaedic manifestations of prune-belly (Eagle-Barrett) syndrome. J Bone Joint Surg 1995;77A:251-257.

Brochstein JA, Shank B, Kernan NA, et al. Marrow transplantation for thrombocytopenia-absent radii syndrome. J Pediatr 1992;121:587-589.

Burke SW, French HG, Roberts JM, et al. Chronic atlanto-axial instability in Down syndrome. J Bone Joint Surg 1985;67A:1356-1360.

Calvert PT, Edgar MA, Webb PJ: Scoliosis in neurofibromatosis: The natural history with and without operation. J Bone Joint Surg 1989;71B:246-251.

Cetta G, Ramirez F, Tsipouras P (eds). Third international conference on osteogenesis imperfecta. Ann N Y Acad Sci 1988;543:1-185.

Chestnut R, James HE, Jones KL. The VATER association and spinal dysraphia. Pediatr Neurosurg 1992;18:144-148.

Cohen MM Jr. Further diagnostic thoughts about the Elephant Man. Am J Med Genet 1988;29:777-782.

Cole DE. Psychosocial aspects of osteogenesis imperfecta: An update. Am J Med Genet 1993;45:207-211.

Cole WG. Etiology and pathogenesis of heritable connective tissue diseases. J Pediatr Orthop 1993;13:392-403.

Craig JB, Govender S. Neurofibromatosis of the cervical spine: A report of eight cases. J Bone Joint Surg 1992;74B:575-578.

Crawford AH. Pitfalls of spinal deformities associated with neurofibromatosis in children. Clin Orthop 1989;245:29-42.

Crawford AH Jr, Bagamery N. Osseous manifestations of neurofibromatosis in childhood. J Pediatr Orthop 1986;6:72-88.

Dent JA, Patterson CR. Fractures in early childhood: Osteogenesis imperfecta or child abuse? J Pediatr Orthop 1991;11:184-186.

Dugdale TW, Renshaw TS. Instability of the patellofemoral joint in Down syndrome. J Bone Joint Surg 1986;68A:405-413.

Egelhoff JC, Bates DJ, Ross JS, et al. Spinal MR findings in neurofibromatosis types 1 and 2. Am J Neuroradiol 1992;13:1071-1077.

Ernhart CB, Sokol RJ, Martier S, et al. Alcohol teratogenicity in the human: A detailed assessment of specificity, critical period, and threshold. Am J Obstet Gynecol 1987;156:33-39.

Field RE, Buchanan JA, Copplemans MG, et al. Bone-marrow transplantation in Hurler's syndrome: Effect on skeletal development. J Bone Joint Surg 1994;76B:975-981.

Funasaki H, Winter RB, Lonstein JB, et al. Pathophysiology of spinal deformities in neurofibromatosis: An analysis of seventy-one patients who had curves associated with dystrophic changes. J Bone Joint Surg 1994;76A:692-700.

Gamble JG. Hip disease in Hutchinson-Gilford progeria syndrome. J Pediatr Orthop 1984;4:585-589.

Goldberg MJ. Spine instability and the Special Olympics. Clin Sports Med 1993;12:507-515.

Graham JM Jr, Hanson JW, Darby BL, et al. Independent dysmorphology evaluations at birth and 4 years of age for children exposed to varying amounts of alcohol in utero. Pediatrics 1988;81:772-778.

Green NE, Lowrey ER, Thomas R. Orthopaedic aspects of prune-belly syndrome. J Pediatr Orthop 1993;13:496-501.

Guidera KJ, Borrelli J Jr, Raney E, et al. Orthopaedic manifestations of Rett syndrome. J Pediatr Orthop 1991;11:204-208.

Guidera KJ, Satterwhite Y, Ogdan JA, et al. Nail patella syndrome: A review of 44 orthopaedic patients. J Pediatr Orthop 1991;11:737-742.

Gutmann DH, Collins FS. The neurofibromatosis type I gene and its protein product, neurofibromin. Neuron 1993;10:335-343.

Hall JG, Reed SD, Rosenbaum KN, et al. Limb pterygium syndromes: A review and report of eleven patients. Am J Med Genet 1982;12:377-409.

Hanscome DA, Winter RB, Lutter L, et al. Osteogenesis imperfecta: Radiographic classification, natural history, and treatment of spinal deformities. J Bone Joint Surg 1992;74A:598-616.

Hsu LCS, Lee PC, Leong JCY. Dystrophic spinal deformities in neurofibromatosis: Treatment by anterior and posterior fusion. J Bone Joint Surg 1984;66B:495-499.

Jaffer Z, Nelson M, Beighton P. Bone fusion in the foetal alcohol syndrome. J Bone Joint Surg 1981;63B:569-571.

Johnson JP, Carey JC, Gooch WM III, et al. Femoral hypoplasia-unusual facies syndrome in infants of diabetic mothers. J Pediatr 1983;102:866-872.

Jones KL, Robinson LK. An approach to the child with structural defects. J Pediatr Orthop 1983;3-238-244.

Joseph KN, Kane HA, Milner RS, et al. Orthopaedic aspects of the Marfan phenotype. Clin Orthop 1992;277:251-261.

Joubin J, Pettrone CF, Pettrone FA. Cornelia de Lange's syndrome: A review article (with emphasis on orthopedic significance). Clin Orthop 1982;171:180-185.

Laville MB, Lakermance P, Limouzy F. Larsen's syndrome: A review of the literature and analysis of thirty-eight cases. J Pediatr Orthop 1994;14:63-73.

Malkawi H, Tarawneh M. The whistling face syndrome, or craniocapotarsal dysplasia: Report of two cases in a father and son and review of the literature. J Pediatr Orthop 1982;3:364-369.

Mandell GA, Harcke HT, Scott CI, et al. Protusio acetabuli in neurofibromatosis: Nondysplastic and dysplastic forms. Neurosurgery 1992;30:552-556.

Marini JC. Osteogenesis imperfecta: Comprehensive management. Adv Pediatr 1988;35:391-426.

Marion RW, Wiznia AA, Hutcheon RG, et al. Fetal AIDS syndrome score: Correlation between severity of dysmorphism and age at diagnosis of immunodeficiency. Am J Dis Child 1987;141:429-431.

Mathoulin C, Gilbert A, Azze RG. Congenital pseudarthrosis of the forearm: Treatment of six cases with vascularized fibular graft and a review of the literature. Microsurgery 1993;14:252-259.

McGroy BJ, Amadio PC, Dobyns JH, et al. Anomalies of the fingers and toes associated with Klippel-Treaunay syndrome. J Bone Joint Surg 1991;73A:1537-1546.

Mitnick JS, Axelrod FB, Genieser NB, et al. Aseptic necrosis in familial dysautonomia. Radiology 1982;142:89-91.

Moen C. Orthopaedic aspects of progeria. J Bone Joint Surg 1982;64A:542-546.

Naidu S, Murphy M, Moser HW, et al. Rett syndrome: Natural history in 70 cases. Am J Med Genet 1986;1(Suppl):61-72.

Nicholls RD. Genomic imprinting an uniparental disomy in Angelman and Prader-Willi syndromes: A review. Am J Med Genet 1993;46:16-25.

Olive PM, Whitecloud TS III, Bennett JT. Lower cervical spondylosis and myelopathy in adults with Down's syndrome. Spine 1988;13:781-784.

Oppenheim WL, Larson KR, McNabb MB, et al. Popliteal pterygium syndrome: An orthopaedic perspective. J Pediatr Orthop 1990;10:58-64.

Ostrowski DM, Eilert RE, Waldstein G. Congenital pseudarthrosis of the ulna: A report of two cases and a review of the literature. J Pediatr Orthop 1985;5:463-467.

Pilarski RT, Pauli RM, Engber WD. Hand-reduction malformation: Genetic and syndromic analysis. J Pediatr Orthop 1985;5:274-280.

Pueschel SM, Moon AC, Scola FH. Computerized tomography in persons with Down syndrome and atlantoaxial instability. Spine 1992;17:735-737.

Pueschel SM, Scola FH. Atlantoaxial instability in individuals with Down syndrome: Epidemiologic, radiographic, and clinical studies. Pediatrics 1987;80;555-560.

Pueschel SM, Scola FH, Pezzullo JC. A longitudinal study of atlanto-dens relationships in asymptomatic individuals with Down syndrome. Pediatrics 1992;89:1194-1198.

Pyeritz RE, Fishman EK, Bernhardt BA, et al. Dural ectasia is a common feature of the Marfan syndrome. Am J Hum Genet 1988;43:726-732.

Rees D, Jones MW, Owen R, et al. Scoliosis surgery in Prader-Willi syndrome. J Bone Joint Surg 1989;71B:685-688.

Robin GC. Scoliosis in familial dysautonomia. Bull Hosp Jt Dis Orthop Inst 1984;44:16-26.

Sirois JL III, Drennan JC. Dystrophic spinal deformity in neurofibromatosis. J Pediatr Orthop 1990;10:522-526.

Skovby F. Homocystinuria: Clinical, biochemical and genetic aspects of cystathionine beta-synthase and its deficiency in man. Acta Pediatr Scand Suppl 1985;321:1-21.

Snodgrass SR. Cocaine babies: A result of multiple teratogenic influences. J Child Neurol 1994;9:227-233.

Soriano RM, Weisz I, Houghton GR. Scoliosis in the Prader-Willi syndrome. Spine 1988;13:2009-2011.

Spiegel PG, Pekman WM, Rich BH, et al. The orthopedic aspects of the fetal alcohol syndrome. Clin Orthop 1979;139:58-63.

Sponseller PD, Hobbs W, Riley LH III, et al. The thoracolumbar spine in Marfan syndrome. J Bone Joint Surg 1995;77A:867-876.

Stevenson GW, Hall SC, Palmieri J. Anesthetic considerations for patients with Larsen's syndrome. Anesthesiology 191;75:142-144.

Stricker S. Musculoskeletal manifestations of Proteus syndrome: Report of two cases with literature review. J Pediatr Orthop 1992;12:667-674.

Strong ML, Wong-Chung J. Prophylactic bypass grafting of the prepseudarthrotic tibia in neurofibromatosis. J Pediatr Orthop 1991;11:757-764.

Treble NJ, Jensen FO, Bankier A, et al. Development of the hip in multiple epiphyseal dysplasia: Natural history and susceptibility to premature osteoarthritis. J Bone Joint Surg 1990;72B:1061-1064.

Van Regemorter N, Dodion J, Druart C, et al. Congenital malformations in 10,000 consecutive births in a university hospital: Need for genetic counseling and prenatal diagnosis. J Pediatr 1984;104:386-390.

Vaughn RY, Selinger AD, Howell CG, et al. Proteus syndrome: Diagnosis and surgical management. J Pediatr Orthop 1993;28:5-10.

White KS, Ball WS, Prenger EC, et al. Evaluation of the craniocervical junction with Down syndrome: Correlation of measurements obtained with radiography and MR imaging. Radiology 1993;186:377-382.

Wilde PH, Upadhyay SS, Leong JC. Deterioration of operative correction in dystrophic spinal neurofibromatosis. Spine 1994;19:1264-1270.

Winter RB, Lonstein JE, Anderson M. Neurofibromatosis hyperkyphosis: A review of 33 patients with kyphosis of 80 degrees or greater. J Spinal Disord 1988;1:39-49.

Zimmerman EF. Substance abuse in pregnancy: Teratogenesis. Pediatr Ann 1991;20:541-547.

Chapter 16 Procedures

Introduction

The number of procedures in pediatric orthopedics is immense. Often procedures are combined or modified to best suit the unique problem of the child. In this section, common procedures are presented. In addition, the scope of options is sometimes presented to allow consideration of more than one method of correction. Because the orthopedist or resident is familiar with operative approaches and use of fixation devices, these details are omitted. General principles of surgical management are covered in Chapter 3. For more information, consult the references or question our consultants by e-mail.

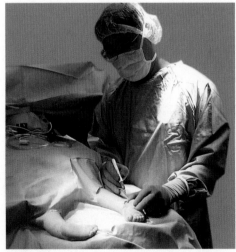

Operative procedures in pediatric orthopedics are numerous and varied.

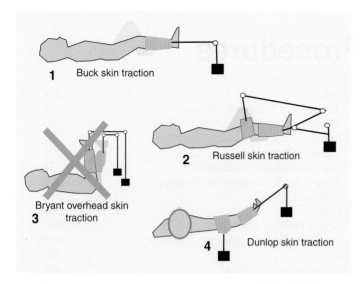

1. Buck skin traction
2. Russell skin traction
3. Bryant overhead skin traction
4. Dunlop skin traction

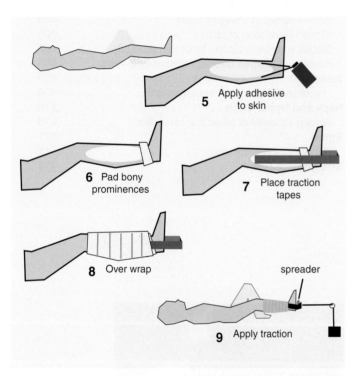

5. Apply adhesive to skin
6. Pad bony prominences
7. Place traction tapes
8. Over wrap
9. Apply traction

spreader

Skin Traction

Skin traction was one of the first management techniques in orthopedics. Currently skin traction is primarily used in managing trauma. The use has declined but still finds occasional application.

Indications for Skin Traction

Initial management Buck traction [1] provides temporary alignment while awaiting definitive treatment. Current indications include femur fractures prior to early spica cast application or operative fixation. Unstable slips may be managed by initial skin traction while awaiting internal fixation.

Definitive management Russell traction [2 & 10] is the traditional standard for management of young children with femoral shaft fractures. Bryant overhead traction [3] was used for managing femoral fractures in infants. Because of the risk of vascular compromise, this treatment has been abandoned. Dunlop traction [4] is sometimes used for managing supracondylar humeral fractures.

Fractures with operative contraindications Excessive swelling, fracture blisters, or infected skin wounds may contraindicate or at least delay internal fixation.

Temporary cervical taction Head halter traction may be used for the initial management of acute torticollis and rotatory subluxation.

Technique

Apply adhesive to the skin [5] as necessary.

Apply padding to the malleoli or bony prominences [6] before applying the traction tape.

Apply traction tapes of fabric backed foam to the skin [7]. Select a large size to reduce the load per unit area.

Overwrap to secure traction tapes [8]. Apply evenly with limited pressure. Avoid using the whole roll of material. Use only one or two layers of overwrap. Cut off and discard unused material.

Apply weight carefully, just enough to align the limb [9].

Insert spreader to avoid pressure over malleoli or wrist.

Place supports for the elevated limb. This may be a pillow under the knee or slings with separate support.

Complications to Avoid

Consider possible complications. These include blisters under the traction tapes or wrapping, or excessive compression causing excessive vessel or nerve compression. Careful application, avoiding excessive compression and traction, and good nursing care will minimize risks.

Monitoring

Skin condition Inspect the skin condition under the overwrap daily for the first few days.

Neurovascular status Inspect daily. Check dorsiflexion of the great toe to assess peroneal nerve function.

Consultant: Kaye Wilkins, e-mail: dkwilkins@aol.com

References

1998 Management of subtrochanteric fractures of the femur in children. Theologis TN, Cole WG. JPO 18:22

1996 Compartment syndrome as a complication of skin traction in children with femoral fractures. Janzing H, Broos P, Rommens P. J Trauma 41:156

1994 Comparison of inpatient and outpatient traction in developmental dislocation of the hip. Camp J, Herring JA, Dworezynski C. JPO 14:9

1993 Skeletal fixation: a review. Vangsness CT Jr, Hunt TJ. Bull Hosp Jt Dis 52:44

1987 Skeletal traction for fractures of the femoral shaft in children. A long-term study. Aronson DD, Singer RM, Higgins RF. JBJS 69A:1435

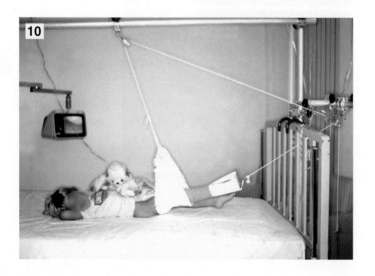

10

Skeletal Traction

Apply traction directly to bone. Modifications include single or multiple pins, use of eye-screws (upper tibia and proximal ulna), and pins combined with special frames (halo traction).

Indications for Skeletal Traction

Skeletal traction is usually selected over skin traction when greater weight or duration are required. The most common indication is 90°/90° traction for management of proximal or shaft fractures of the femur [1 & 12], olecranon pin traction for supracondylar fracture management [2 & 13], and spine traction through a halo-pin combination [3].

Technique

Traction bow or frame are selected. Bows may be simple to just support the pin or specially designed for small-diameter pins.

Pin selection Select a pin that fits the traction bow. Smooth pins are more easily inserted and removed but may slide in the bone. Smooth pins may be inserted with local anesthesia and removed in clinic. Threaded pins usually require more sedation or a general anesthetic to apply and remove.

Site for insertion Avoid growth plates. For femoral fractures, apply in the distal metaphysis, usually at the level of the superior margin of the patella.

Position of limb during insertion [4]. Avoid tenting of the skin or fascia by holding the limb in the position required for treatment.

Skin preparation Use 1% iodine or equivalent [5].

Anesthesia Inject local anesthetic agent into the skin fascia and periosteum at the sites of entry and exit of the pin [6].

Place the pins at right angles to the axis of traction [7 & 8].

Release skin if tented with a pointed scalpel. Some recommend an antibiotic ointment around the entry and exit of the pin through the skin.

Apply dressing to protect pin sites [9].

Apply traction bow Narrow the bow to reduce the potential for side to side movement on smooth pins [10].

Apply stops of felt or other material if necessary to avoid sliding on the smooth pin.

Apply weights to support the limb [11].

After Care

Inspect and clean pin sites daily. Should pins become inflamed or infected, first relieve any tenting of the skin or underlying fascia, culture wounds, and administer antibiotics as necessary.

Pin Removal

Cut the pin at the skin level on the exit side. Remove the pin with a drill. Place a protective dressing.

Break Adhesions

Divide adhesions between the dermis and underlying fascia with a pointed scalpel. This frees the skin and allows subcutaneous fat to fill the space between the skin and fascia, reducing the risk of a residual unsightly depressed scar.

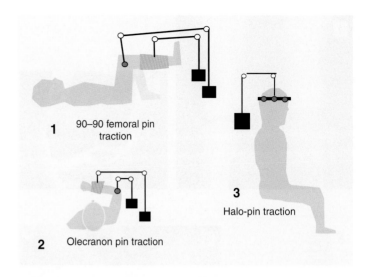

1 90–90 femoral pin traction

2 Olecranon pin traction

3 Halo-pin traction

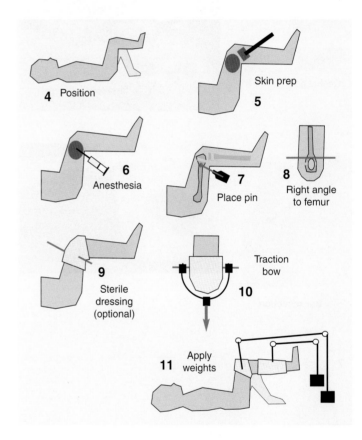

4 Position

5 Skin prep

6 Anesthesia

7 Place pin

8 Right angle to femur

9 Sterile dressing (optional)

10 Traction bow

11 Apply weights

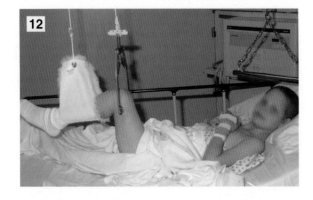

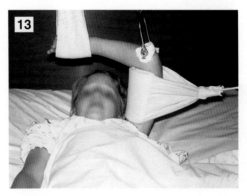

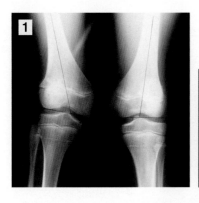

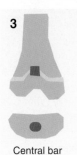

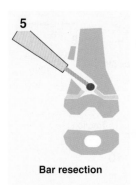

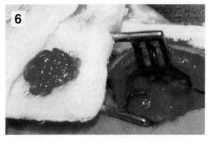

Central bar

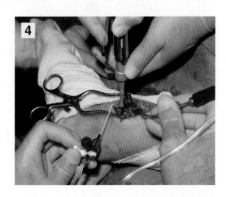

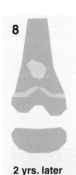

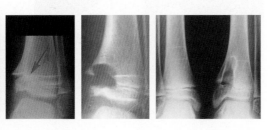

Bar resection

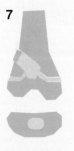

Fat in cavity

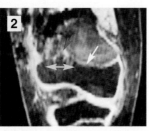

2 yrs. later

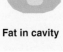

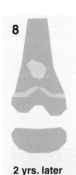

Partial Physeal Bar Resection

Indications

Resect bars that occupy less than 50% of the physis and have two years of growth remaining. Once resected, bone growth may be accelerated, normal, retarded, or absent. Outcomes are related to the location of the bar, its size, and the health of the adjacent growth plate. Following successful resection some correction of angulatory deformity may occur. This correction seldom exceeds 10°. For unacceptable deformity exceeding about 10°, consider a concurrent osteotomy. The osteotomy may not only correct the acquired deformity but may also facilitate excision of the bar.

Preoperative Planning

Assess the deformity clinically and image the bar. Clinical assessment includes determining the length inequality and angular deformity in all three planes. Document shortening by an orthodiagram. Determine the child's bone age. Document deformity with radiographs [1]. Comparative bilateral study on the same X-ray is useful. Assess the bar by CT or MR reconstructions [2]. On the MRI, the physis (white arrow) is abnormal on the lateral side (red arrow). A portion of the physis (yellow arrow segment) has been replaced by a bony bar. Estimate size and location of the the bar using frontal and sagittal reconstructions or use templates to make these determinations more accurately. Some computer software may make this calculation by generating a transverse plane image of the physis that provides this image. Make certain the exact location and size of the bar is known before resection [3]. Based on the location of the bar, plan the operative approach. Make available an air drill, abundant saline irritation, good lighting, fluoroscopy, and a dental mirror [4].

Technique

Drape the limb to allow free mobility and allow exposure to the site of bar resection and fat harvest. Mark the site of the physis with the image intensifier. Perform an osteotomy if indicated. Approach the bar through the osteotomy or a metaphyseal window [5]. Using the air drill, under image guidance, create a window about 1 cm in diameter and extend the window toward the bridge. Locate the normal physis adjacent to the bar. Use the suction tip with irrigation to clear away cancellous bone from the physis. Identify the bar by seeing normal cartilage on both sides of the lesion. Resect the bar. When normal physeal cartilage is seen all the way around the operative window, resection is complete. Harvest subcutaneous fat for interposition [6]. This may be possible from the operative site, behind the knee, or in the buttocks folds. Bone-wax cavity surfaces to reduce ooze. Place fat graft to fill cavity completely [7] to provide hemostasis and ensure complete interposition. Replace cortical graft. Close soft tissue over replaced cortical window. Close wound and apply a cast. Immobilize for 2–8 weeks depending upon extent of resection. Restrict activity until bone strength recovers. Following bar resection, a neophysis develops spanning the site of the previous bar, and growth resumes [8]. Follow with AP comparative radiographs.

Consultants

Ham Peterson, e-mail: peterson.hamlet@mayo.edu
Kaye Wilkins, e-mail: dkwilkins@aol.com

References

1996 MR imaging of physeal bars. Borsa JJ, Peterson HA, Ehman RL. Radiology 199:683
1996 Comparison of various interpositional materials in the prevention of transphyseal bone bridge formation. Martiana K, et al. CO 325:218
1992 Surgical technique of physeal bar resection. Birch JG. Instr Course Lect 41:445
1990 Physeal bar resections after growth arrest about the knee. Kasser JR. CO 255:68
1990 Partial physeal growth arrest: treatment by bridge resection and fat interposition. Williamson RV, Staheli LT. JPO 10:769
1984 Partial growth plate arrest and its treatment. Peterson HA. JPO 4:246
1975 An operation for partial closure of an epiphyseal plate in children and its experimental basis. Langenskiöld A. JBJS 57B:325

Ankle Fractures Reduction and Fixation

Undisplaceed Fractures

Manage undisplaced fractures in cast for 6 weeks. Apply a long-leg cast with the knee flexed about 30 degrees. Repeat radiographs in the cast at 1 and 2 weeks to confirm maintenance of reduction. After 3 weeks the cast may be converted to a short-leg walker cast. Continue the immobilization for a total of 6 weeks.

Metaphyseal and Salter–Harris 1 and 2 Fractures

These ankle fractures do not require anatomic reduction. The amount of acceptable displacement depends on the age of the child. Varus or valgus deformity in the older child should be corrected as remodeling may be incomplete. Internal fixation is sometimes necessary.

Displaced S–H 3 and 4 Fractures

Displaced fractures that exceed 2 mm of displacement require reduction. Assess degree of displacement with supplemental oblique or CT radiographs if degree of displacement is uncertain. Attempt a closed reduction under anesthesia. Reduce by reversing the direction of the injury. If reduction is not satisfactory, perform an open reduction. Establish the pattern of deformity before undertaking the procedure. Arrange intraoperative imaging. Make the approach based on the fracture pattern. Do not hesitate to make two incisions to aid visualization and fixation. Fix with metallic or absorbable pins or screws. Limited internal fixation is adequate as fixation is supplemented by a long-leg cast.

Medial malleolus fracture is a SH-3, SH-4, or rarely a SH-5 injury. Growth arrest and deformity are common sequelae. Consider placing a prophylactic fat graft to fill any residual defect that spans the growth plate. Fix with a horizontal screw [1] that remains within the epiphysis or with small smooth K wires [2] that may transverse the physis and can be removed in about 3 weeks.

Tillaux fracture is the SH-3 anterolateral epiphyseal fracture [3 and 4]. Expose the fracture through an anterolateral approach, reduce by internal rotation of the foot, and fix with a lag screw [5]. Usually the growth plate is closing, so growth disturbance is seldom a problem.

Triplane fractures are SH-4 injuries that include a variety of fracture patterns, which are often complex. Medial triplane fractures often include two [6] or three [7] fragments. Fracture patterns are varied and include many patterns [8] requiring tailoring approach and fixation based on the situation. Reduction can sometimes be difficult. Approach through two incisions if necessary. Fix with horizontal screws [9 & 10].

Consultant Kaye Wilkins, e-mail: dkwilkins@aol.com

References

1997 The triplane fracture: four years of follow-up of 21 cases and review of the literature. Karrholm J. JPO-b 6:91

1997 Intramalleolar triplane fractures of the distal tibial epiphysis. Shin AY, Moran ME, Wenger DR. JPO 17:352

1996 Distal tibial triplane fractures: long-term follow-up. Rapariz JM, et al. JPO 16:113

1995 Triplane fractures of the distal tibia. van Laarhoven CJ, Severijnen RS, van der Werken AG. J Foot Ankle Surg 34:556 discussion 594

1988 Triplane fracture of the distal tibial epiphysis. Long-term follow-up. Ertl JP, et al. JBJS 70A:967

1987 Distal tibial triplane fractures: diagnosis with CT. Feldman F, et al. Radiology 164:429

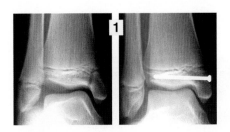

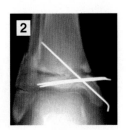

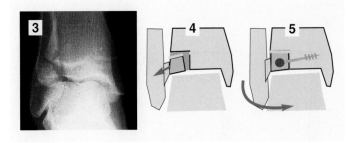

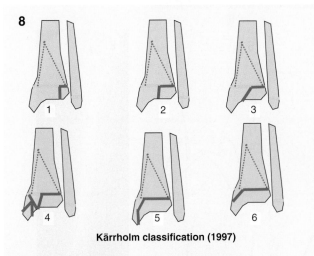

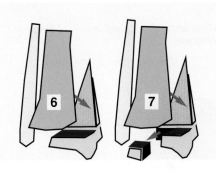

Kärrholm classification (1997)

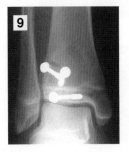

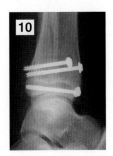

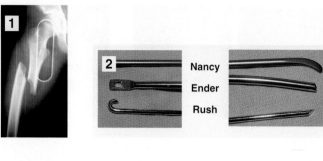

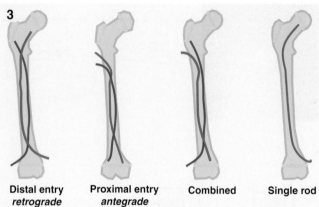

Distal entry
retrograde   Proximal entry
antegrade   Combined   Single rod

Drawings based on Metaizeau

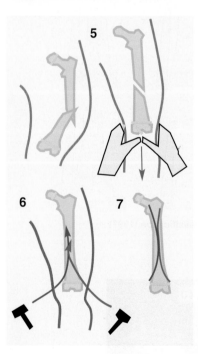

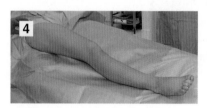

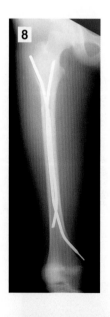

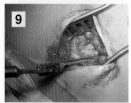

Flexible IM Fixation of Femoral Fractures

This is the best fixation for most fractures in ages 6 to the end of growth. Contraindications include comminution and unstable fracture patterns, or unacceptable anesthetic risk.

Technique

Preoperative planning Evaluate the fracture. Place leg in Buck traction to provide alignment and immobilization while awaiting operative stabilization [1]. Assess for other injuries, hip, knee, neurovascular status. Assess family situation and advise regarding management choices.

Select nails for fixation [2]. Basic choices include Nancy nails of titanium that are most flexible; Ender nails with fenestrated end for easy extraction; and Rush rods with beveled tip and hooked end. Make certain length and diameter are suitable for femur size. Generally two nails are placed. Consider placing a third nail in a large adolescent. Make available appropriate imaging.

Fixation strategy [3] Retrograde nailing is suitable for most fractures. Antegrade nailing is necessary for distal fractures. Single rod fixation may be adequate for the small child or may be supplemented with a single hip walking cast.

Procedure Postion and drape with limb freely moveable [4]. Apply traction to align the limb [5]. Select nails of appropriate diameter and length and prebend. Make small stab incisions at sites for nail entry. Make certain the sites avoid injury to the epiphyseal plate. Drill the cortical window at sites of rod entry. Place both rods [6] and alternately advance through medullary canal. Make certain rods extend far enough to provide adequate fixation. Adjust length so end of rods are outside the cortex to facilitate removal [7]. Ender nails may be fixed to the metaphysis with a screw to prevent migration. Nails may be left longer to make removal easier but may be prominent enough to become irritated in the months following fixation. Document fixation with an AP and lateral long radiographs [8]. Apply a single hip spica cast to supplement single nail fixation as necessary. Make certain the cast is well padded about the knee and ankle. Lightweight fiberglass single hip spica casts allow considerable mobility, usually permitting the child to return to school. If the cast is applied with the hip and knee flexed about 20 degrees, the cast may end at the ankle leaving the foot free for shoes.

Postoperative management Early discharge from the hospital is feasible. See in clinic in 1 week for initial assessment. See monthly until union is complete. Plan nail removal about 4–6 months. Allow return to sports about 1 month following hardware removal.

Rod removal Removal is simple if the end is left long. Special extractors facilitate nail removal [9].

Complications

Complications are uncommon following this procedure.

Discomfort from prominent rod end or from migration of the rod rarely is the most common problem. This irritation is usually not serious enough to require repositioning of the rod. Reducing the child's activities may be adequate to control the pain.

Loss of position may occur from shortening due to unrecognized comminution or an additional injury before union.

Consultant: Kaye Wilkins, e-mail: dkwilkins@aol.com

References

1996 Flexible intramedullary nail fixation of pediatric femoral fractures. Carey TP, Galpin RD. CO 332:110

1996 Flexible intramedullary nailing as fracture treatment in children. Huber RI, et al. JPO 16:602

1994 The operative stabilization of pediatric diaphyseal femur fractures with flexible intramedullary nails: a prospective analysis. Heinrich SD, et al. JPO 14:501

1988 Ostéosynthèse Chez l'enfant. Metaizeau JP. Sauramps Medical, Montpellier, France

Percutaneous Pinning of Supracondylar Fractures

Percutaneous pinning is the preferred method of managing displaced supracondylar fractures. The technique provides good fixation with the least number of complications. This procedure is indicated for displaced fractures without serious vascular compromise. See page 248.

Technique

Preoperative preparations Evaluate carefully before undertaking the procedure [1 & 2]. Have available 1 and 2 mm smooth pins, a power driver, an imaging device, and an assistant. Position thoughtfully. This is a matter of preference. The prone position allows gravity to help maintain the reduction while placing the pins [3].

Reduction Apply traction and hyperextension. First realign in frontal plane. The second step is to align in the sagittal plane. Confirm the reduction by AP and lateral imaging [4]. Maintain reduction by flexing the elbow. Perform a surgical skin prep and continue utilizing sterile technique.

Pin fixation Crossed pins, 2 or 3 lateral pins are acceptable fixation configurations. Using only lateral pins avoid risks of injury to the ulnar nerve, a complication of the procedure. Place a pin over the elbow and image to visualize best position for the pins. When elbow is very swollen, determine starting point with lateral imaging. Insert the lateral pin at about 45° to the axis of the humerus [5]. Be certain to penetrate the proximal fragment. Confirm position by AP and lateral imaging. Make decision regarding additional pins. If elbow is very swollen, consider placing two more lateral pins in diverging configuration to enhance stability. Usually a medial pin is placed with care to avoid the ulnar nerve [6]. If the elbow is very swollen, consider making a small incision to visualize the ulnar nerve to prevent nerve injury from the pin. Advance the pin under image control to engage proximal fragment [7]. Confirm pin placement with imaging in two planes [8]. Extend elbow gently to assess carrying angle. If angle seems abnormal, check accuracy of reduction. Once satisfied that reduction is accurate and fixation secure, bend over ends of pins outside skin and cut pins [9]. Assess vascular status of limb in different degrees of flexion. Dress and splint the arm in the degree of flexion that permits optimal circulation.

Postoperative Care

Place the splinted arm in a sling. Monitor circulation and avoid narcotics to avoid masking ischemia. Discharge home the next day. Advise the family to call if child has undue pain. Return to clinic in 1 week for AP and lateral radiographs in splint and 3 weeks for pin removal in clinic. Maintain sling for another week. Allow gradual return to activities and sports at 12 weeks. Follow monthly to assess motion. Allow reestablishment of range of motion to occur naturally. Physical therapy is unnecessary and may be harmful.

Complications

Reduce risk of **compartment syndrome** by careful monitoring, achieving an accurate reduction, and avoiding excessive flexion postfixation. Reduce risk of **cubitus varus** by accurate reduction, secure fixation. Reduce risk of **ulnar nerve injury** by careful pin placement.

Consultant Kaye Wilkins, e-mail: dkwilkins@aol.com

References

2000 Displaced supracondylar fractures of the humerus in children. Audit changes practice. O'Hara L, et al. JBJS 82B:204

1995 Closed reduction and percutaneous pinning for type III displaced supracondylar fractures of the humerus in children. Cheng J, Lam T, Shen W. J Orthop Trauma 9:511

1995 Clinical evaluation of crossed-pin versus lateral-pin fixation in displaced supracondylar humerus fractures. Topping R, Blanco J, Davis T. JPO 15:435

1994 Torsional strength of pin configurations used to fix supracondylar fractures of the humerus in children. Zionts L, McKellop H, Hathaway R. JBJS 76A:253

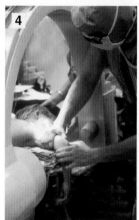

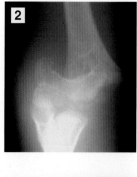

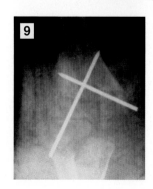

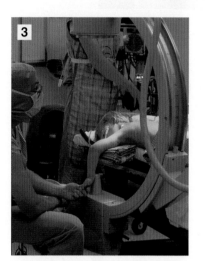

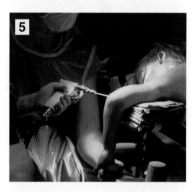

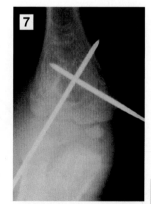

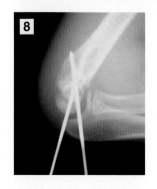

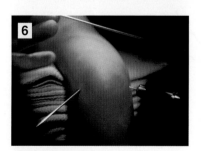

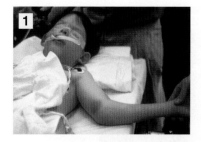

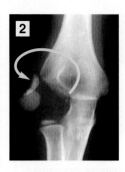
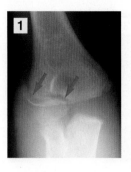

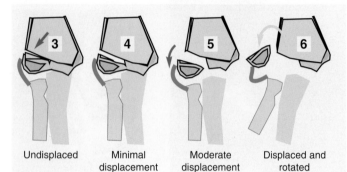

Undisplaced   Minimal   Moderate   Displaced and
displacement   displacement   rotated

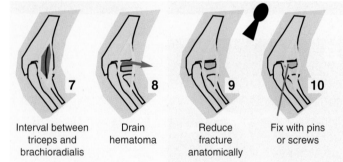

Interval between   Drain   Reduce   Fix with pins
triceps and   hematoma   fracture   or screws
brachioradialis   anatomically

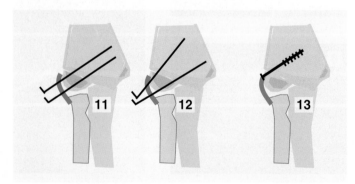

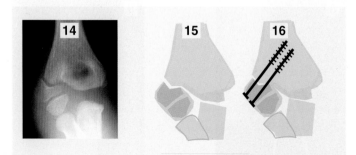

Lateral Condylar Fracture Reduction

Lateral condyle fractures are unique as they are intraarticular, involve the growth plate, and are prone to nonunion. Accept only minimal displacement of <2 mm. Reduce anatomically and fix securely.

Pathology

Fractures usually extend through metaphyseal bone and with varying degrees of displacement. Displacement may be minimal [1] or the fragment may be displaced and rotated [2].

Classification

Classification is based on the extent of displacement.

Undisplaced fractures show only a linear fracture line [3]. These fractures may be difficult to identify by conventional radiographs.

Minimal displacement fractures have 0–2 mm of displacement [4]. Such fractures do not require reduction but do require careful follow-up as they may be unstable and displace if the fracture line extends completely through cartilage and into the joint.

Moderate displacement fragment is separated but not rotated [5].

Severe displacement fragment is rotated and severely displaced [6].

Reduction

Use supine position, tourniquet, imaging, good lighting, and small retractors.

Approach Make a lateral longitudinal incision over the distal humerus [7] and develop the interval between the triceps and brachioradialis muscles. Drain the hematoma [8] and identify the fracture.

Reduction Avoid removing soft tissues from the fracture fragment to preserve its blood supply. Identify the margins of the fracture and visualize the direction of displacement. Reduce the fracture anatomically with aid of imaging [9]. The reduction is best visualized anteriorly and by aligning the metaphyseal margins.

Fixation Fix with pins or screws [10]. Usually two 1–2 mm smooth K wires either parallel [11] or diverging [12] provide adequate fixation. Leave the wires through the skin and bend the ends to prevent migration. If a metaphyseal fragment is large enough, screw fixation of this fragment to the humerus [13] as an acceptable alternative.

Postoperative management Remove the pins in clinic in 4–6 weeks. Maintain in a sling for 2 more weeks. Follow at 3, 6, and 12 months with a radiograph to assure union. Physical therapy is unnecessary.

Delayed or Nonunion

Most delayed or nonunions [14 and 15] require operative correction to avoid progressive displacement and atrophy of the fragment and cubitus valgus.

0–12 months Reduce and fix as with an acute injury. Often fixation with screws securing the metaphyseal fragment to the distal humerus provides firm fixation.

12+ months Remodeling often causes the fragment to no longer fit and reduction is not appropriate. Create union *in situ* by placing a screw across the metaphyseal fragment and humerus [16].

Consultant Kaye Wilkins, e-mail: dkwilkins@aol.com

References

1999 Assessment of stability in children's minimally displaced lateral humeral condyle fracture by magnetic resonance imaging. Kamegaya M, et al. JPO 19:570

1998 Nonoperative treatment for minimally and nondisplaced lateral humeral condyle fractures in children. Bast SC, MM Hoffer, S Aval. JPO 18:448

1995 Lateral condylar fractures of the humerus in children: fixation with partially threaded 4.0-mm AO cancellous screws. Sharma J, et al. J Trauma 39:1129

1991 Late surgical treatment of lateral condylar fractures in children. Roye DJ, et al. JPO 11:195

1989 Nonunion of slightly displaced fractures of the lateral humeral condyle in children: an update. Flynn J. JPO 9:691

1986 Lateral condylar fracture of the elbow. Herring J, Fitch R. JPO 6:724

Radial Neck Fracture Reduction and Fixation

Under fluroscopy, rotate the forearm while observing the fracture to show maximum displacement and tilt. If this displacement exceeds about 10% and the tilt 30°, reduction is necessary. Reduction of radial neck fractures can sometimes be successful by manipulation. Apply firm thumb pressure on the skin overlying the edge of the displaced fragment (arrow) while rotating the forearm [1]. If this is not successful, percutaneous reduction will be necessary. The simplest method involves levering the fragment back into place with a K wire. The more sophisticated method achieves reduction using an intramedullary pin.

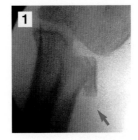
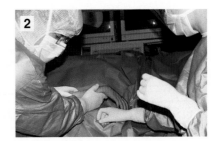

Technique – K Wire Leverage Method of Steele and Graham

Under general anesthesia, prep and drape the arm free [2]. Under fluoroscopic guidance, bring the fracture into profile. Place a 1.5–2 mm smooth K wire on a T handle chuck. Under fluoroscopy, position the entry point as far proximal as possible to avoid injury to the posterior interosseous nerve [3]. Advance the tip of the pin through the fracture site to the opposite cortex [4]. Move the K wire proximal to lever the head onto the radial neck [5]. Overcorrection is prevented by the capitellum. To improve apposition, move the radial head with the K wire [6]. Assess stability and motion by rotating the forearm [7]. Rotation of 60° should be possible in both directions. If the fracture is unstable, transfix with a single oblique percutaneous K wire left out through the skin [8]. Avoid transcapitellar fixation. Immobilize with the elbow flexed to a right angle in a posterior splint for 3 weeks. Remove the optional fixation and allow gradual return to full activity.

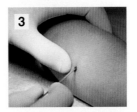
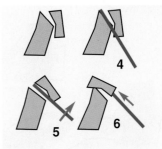
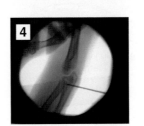

Technique – Closed Intramedullary Fixation of Metaizeau

Make a short lateral incision about 1–2 cm proximal to the distal radial growth plate while avoiding injury to the cutaneous branch of the radial nerve. Perforate the cortex with a drill and insert a curved K wire 1.2–2 mm (depending upon the child's age) with the terminal 3 mm bent more sharply [9]. The pin is hammered into the medullary canal and manipulated to enter the displaced radial head [10]. The pin is advanced moving the radial head against the capitellum [11]. The radial head is positioned against the capitellum with the periosteum (green) as a tether correcting the tilt of the articular surface [12]. Rotate the handle to medially displace the radial head to correct apposition and stabilize the reduction [13]. The pin may be cut off under the skin or left protruding to facilitate removal. A splint is applied for 2–3 weeks. The K wire is removed at 2 months.

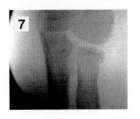
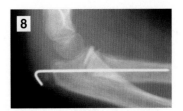

Complications

Avascular necrosis This complication is likely the result of the injury.

Malunion The risk of this complication is reduced by an accurate reduction.

Nonunion This is an uncommon complication.

Nerve injury Nerve injuries nearly always resolve with time.

Consultant Kaye Wilkins, e-mail: dkwilkins@aol.com

References

2000 Fractures of the proximal radial head and neck in children with emphasis on those that involve the articular cartilage. Leung AG, Peterson HA. J PO 20:7

1998 Displaced fractures of the radial neck in children: long-term results and prognosis of conservative treatment. Vocke AK, Von Laer L. JPOB 7:217

1998 Controversies regarding radial neck fractures in children. Radomisli TE, Rosen AL. CO 353:30

1997 Displaced radial neck fractures in children treated by closed intramedullary pinning (Metaizeau technique). Gonzalez-Herranz P, et al. JPO 17:325

1994 Percutaneous reduction of displaced radial neck fractures in children. Rodriguez Merchan EC. J Trauma 37:812

1993 Management of radial neck fractures in children: a retrospective analysis of one hundred patients. D'souza S, Vaishya R, Klenerman L. JPO 13:232

1993 Reduction and fixation of displaced radial neck fractures by closed intramedullary pinning. Metaizeau JP, et al. JPO 13:355

1992 Angulated radial neck fractures in children. A prospective study of percutaneous reduction. Steele JA, Graham HK. JBJS 74B:760

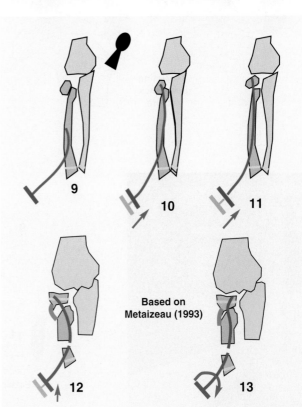

Based on Metaizeau (1993)

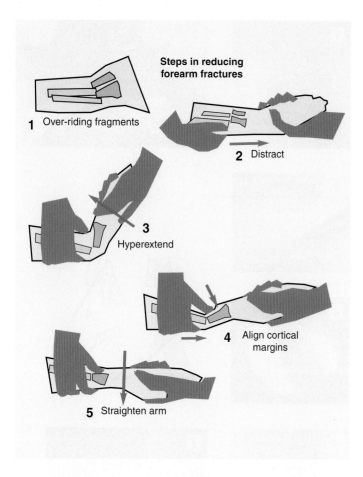

Steps in reducing forearm fractures

1 Over-riding fragments

2 Distract

3 Hyperextend

4 Align cortical margins

5 Straighten arm

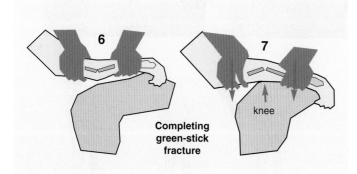

6

7 knee

Completing green-stick fracture

Closed Reduction of Forearm Fractures

Forearm fractures are the most common childhood fracture. Midshaft fractures require more accurate reduction as remodeling is much less than for distal forearm fractures.

Distal Forearm Fracture Reduction

Bayonette apposition may be accepted if angulation <20° and 2 years of growth remain. For fractures requiring reduction [1] follow several steps. Provide anesthesia for displaced fractures. Local, regional, or general anesthesias are acceptable options.

Distraction Apply firm traction [2] to overcome the shortening.

Hyperextend Extend the fracture to accentuate the deformity [3]. The distal fragment is brought into a position that allows reduction.

Align cortical margins With thumb pressure and traction, the cortical margins are approximated [4] to achieve appositional alignment.

Straighten arm This completes the reduction [5].

Midshaft Fractures

Midshaft fractures require an accurate reduction due to the greater distance between the fracture and the adjacent joint. Residual malalignment reduces forearm rotation.

Plastic deformation bowing may be straightened by manipulation.

Green-stick fractures may be completed [6 and 7] by or simply straightened based on the surgeon's preference.

Complete fractures may be reduced by the same general maneuver as for distal fractures.

Postion for Immobilization

Distal forearm fractures are placed in slight wrist flexion and supination for the common dorsal angulated fractures.

Midshaft fractures are immobilized in the position of rotation that occurs when traction is applied to the arm [8].

Proximal fractures are immobilized in supination.

Immobilization

Immobilize the arm in a long-arm cast or splint-cast combination. The splint-cast accommodates forearm volume changes that occur from the increase and decline of soft-tissue swelling. First apply padding [9], place anterior and posterior splints [10], overwrap the forearm with an elastic bandage [11], secure with a circumferential cast above [12], and then apply moulding [13] while the cast material hardens.

Post-Reduction Management

Obtain radiographs at 1 and 2 weeks to be certain the reduction is maintained. Cast immobilization is discontinued at 6 weeks for distal and 8 weeks for midshaft fractures. Be aware of the risk of refracture of midshaft fractures.

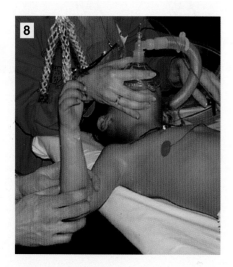

8

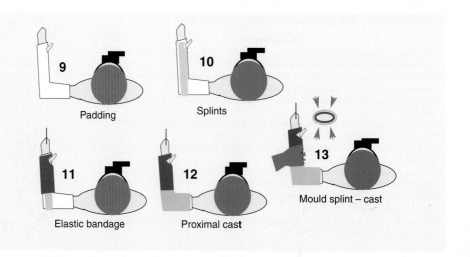

9 Padding

10 Splints

11 Elastic bandage

12 Proximal cast

13 Mould splint – cast

Flexible IM Fixation of Forearm Fractures

Manage most forearm fractures by closed reduction and casting. Those that require internal fixation are best fixed with flexible intramedullary pins or rods. This fixation was detailed by Metaizeau. Several recent studies confirm the effectiveness of this fixation.

Percutaneous K Wire-Fixation

This method was described by Yung et al. (1998).

Reduction Under anesthesia and on a radiolucent table, attempt closed reduction. If unsuccessful, perform an open reduction through a 2 cm incision directly over the fracture site. At least 50% apposition is required for fixation.

Fixation Perform percutaneously using 1.6 mm K wires guided by imaging. Entry points are radial styloid or olecranon [1]. For both-bone fractures reduce and fix the radius first. Drive the pins just short of the growth plates [2].

Immobilization Place a long-arm cast with the elbow flexed to 90° [3] and the forearm rotated based on fracture level and best alignment as determined by imaging. Remove the cast and wires in 4–6 weeks in clinic. Others recommend burying the pins and leaving them in place for 3–4 months to reduce the risk of refracture.

Titanium Nail Fixation

This technique is described by Richter et al. (1998).

Fixation Select nails about a third the diameter of the medullary canal. Nails are usually 2–3 mm. Make a small incision on the dorso-medial aspect of the proximal ulna [4]. Open the medullary canal with an awl distal to the epiphyseal plate. Bend an elastic titanium nail and insert it into the medullary canal. Make a small incision on the dorsora-dial side of the distal radius proximal to the epiphyseal plate and insert the second titanium nail. This nail should be bent so the convex side is radial to maintain the interosseous space. Position the nails under imaging to achieve optimal reduction and alignment [5]. Cut off the nails at skin level. A cast is usually not necessary.

After treatment Remove the nails at about 12 weeks under local anesthesia.

Single Bone Fixation

Single bone fixation maintains forearm alignment and is suitable for most children. Usually the ulna only is rodded. Supplement the IM fixation [6] with a long-arm cast [7]. See Flynn and Waters (1996).

Complications

Be aware of the complications that can occur [8] and take measures necessary to avoid these problems. See Cullen et al. (1998).

Consultant Kaye Wilkins, e-mail: dkwilkins@aol.com

References

2000 Intramedullary Steinmann pin fixation of forearm fractures in children. Long-term results. Pugh DM, Galpin RD, Carey TP. CO 39

1999 Intramedullary Kirschner wire fixation of open or unstable forearm fractures in children. Shoemaker SD, et al. JPO 19:329

1998 Complications of intramedullary fixation of pediatric forearm fractures. Cullen MC, et al. JPO 18:14

1998 Intramedullary fixation of unstable both-bone forearm fractures in children. Luhmann SJ, Gordon JE, Schoenecker PL. JPO 18:451

1998 Forearm and distal radius fractures in children. Noonan KJ, Price CT. J Am Acad Orthop Surg 6:146

1998 Elastic intramedullary nailing: a minimally invasive concept in the treatment of unstable forearm fractures in children. Richter D, et al. JPO 18:457

1998 Intramedullary nailing versus plate fixation for unstable forearm fractures in children. Van der Reis WL, et al. JPO 18:9

1998 Percutaneous intramedullary Kirschner wiring for displaced diaphyseal forearm fractures in children. Yung SH, et al. JBJS 80B:91

1996 Single-bone fixation of both-bone forearm fractures. Flynn JM, Waters PM. JPO 16:655

1988 Ostéosynthèse Chez l'enfant. Metaizeau JP. Sauramps Medical, Montpellier, France

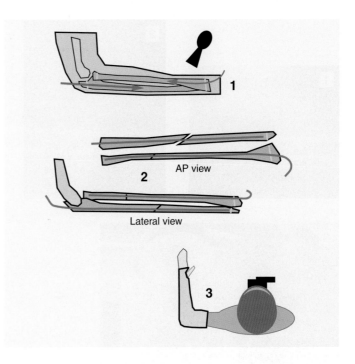

1

2   AP view

Lateral view

3

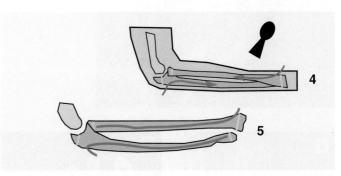

4

5

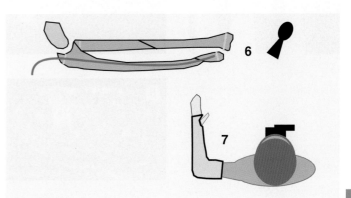

6

7

8   **Complications of IM fixation**

Hardware migration
Infection
Loss of reduction
Nerve injury
Loss of motion
Synostosis
Malreduction
Delayed union
Tendon entrapment
Refracture

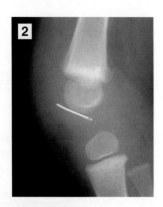

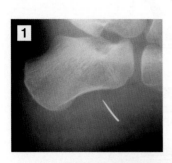

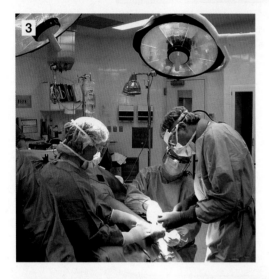

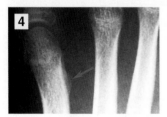

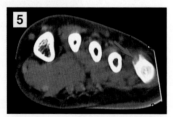

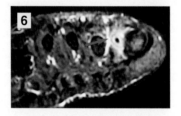

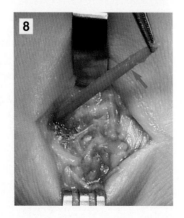

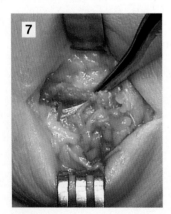

Foreign Body Removal

Retained foreign bodies are fairly common in children. Entry may occur from stepping on the object [1] or a fall [2]. Most foreign bodies can be identified and removed without difficulty. In others the bodies may remain for months or years causing intermittent symptoms before removal. Nonmetallic bodies are most difficult to identify. Often glass with a lead content is visible on standard radiographs. Sometimes no history of penetrating injury is given at all and the problem may be thought to be osteomyelitis or a soft tissue infection. Most foreign bodies should be removed.

Removal in the Emergency Room

If the object can be seen or felt it can usually be removed in the emergency room. Administer tetanus prophylaxis. Image and remove the object. Be aware that if the patient is anxious and any question exists about the ease of removal, remove the object in the operating room.

Removal of Deeply Imbedded Foreign Bodies

Plan removal with anesthesia, adequate assistance and good lighting [3]. Metallic objects can be easily imaged, and fluoroscopic guidance is helpful. Objects deeply imbedded in the foot are often more difficult to remove than initially imagined.

Nonmetallic objects may be identified by ultrasound. Intraoperative imaging may be very helpful. Long delays in removal may allow considerable foreign body reactions, which may be seen radiographically, on CT or MRI scans.

Clinical Example

This illustration is of 15-year-old girl who had chronic pain over the lateral aspect of the foot. She had several courses of antibiotics, each time followed by recurrence. An AP radiograph [4] and CT scan [5] demonstrated periosteal reaction of the 5th metatarsal. The MRI [6] showed a possible foreign body. Operative exposure of the site revealed a splinter of wood [7]. This was removed. It measured 6 cm in length [8].

Consultant Kaye Wilkins, e-mail: dkwilkins@aol.com

References

1998 Wooden foreign bodies in soft tissue: detection at US. Jacobson JA, et al. Radiology 206:45

1994 Late infections of the foot due to incomplete removal of foreign bodies: a report of two cases. Markiewitz AD, Karns DJ, Brooks PJ. Foot Ankle Int 15:52

1992 A retained wooden foreign body in the foot detected by ultrasonography. A case report. Kobs JK, Hansen AR, Keefe B. JBJS 74A:296

1992 Identification of non-metallic foreign bodies in soft tissue: Eikenella corrodens metatarsal osteomyelitis due to a retained toothpick. A case report. Siegel IM. JBJS 74A:1408

1990 Removal of foreign bodies from the foot, a technique using high elevation and local anaesthesia. Mardel SN. Arch Emerg Med 7:111

Joint Aspiration

Joint aspiration is useful for diagnosis and treatment. Treatment may include joint decompression in sepsis and steroid instillation for arthritis.

General Approach

Equipment includes culture tube, plain and anticoagulated sterile fluid collection containers.

Skin preparation is surgical with sterile drape [1].

Anesthetic If the joint is distended, quick placement of the needle into the joint may be least traumatic for the child. In most situations, inject local anesthesia through a #22 or #25 needle.

Aspiration Perform aspiration with a #18 or #20 needle [2 and 3]. Evacuate the joint completely [4].

Fluid evaluation Observe the viscosity, turbidity, and color. Consider for gram stain and cultures. Tests commonly ordered include a cell count and differential, sugar, protein, immunologic tests for arthritis.

Specific Joints

Shoulder Approach the shoulder from either an anterior or lateral approach just below the acromial process [5].

Elbow Aspirate the joint with a posterolateral approach between the radial head and capitellum [6].

Wrist Aspirate the joint from a dorsal radial approach [7].

Finger With the digit slightly flexed, approach on either the dorsal ulnar or radial sides.

Hip The hip is more difficult to aspirate due to the deep location. Imaging is helpful. The approach is influenced by the size of the child [8]. In infants and small chidren the medial approach is usually best. In most children and adolescents, make an anterolateral approach by directing the needle just proximal to the greater trochanter.

Knee A medial or lateral approach may be used [9]. Direct the needle just inferior to the proximal portion of the patella.

Ankle An anterolateral approach is appropriate [10].

Toes With the toe slightly flexed, aspirate from a dorsomedial or lateral approach.

References

1998 Joint aspiration. Kuo KN. Secrets of pediatric orthopedics 80, Hanley and Belfus, Philadelphia.

1995 Technical note: identifying and aspirating hip effusions. Berman L, et al. Br J Radiol 68:306

1993 Joint effusion in children with an irritable hip: US diagnosis and aspiration. Zawin JK, et al. Radiology 187:459

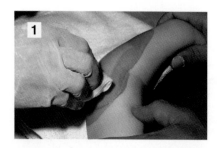

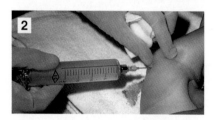

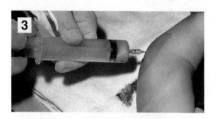

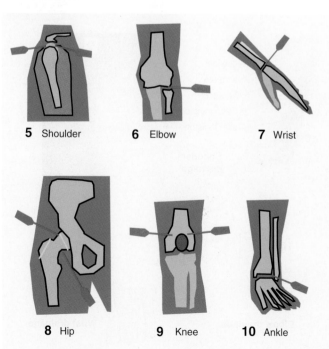

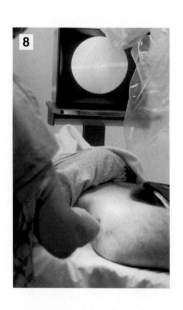

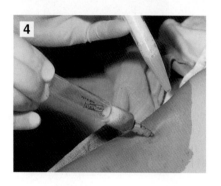

5 Shoulder   **6** Elbow   **7** Wrist

8 Hip   **9** Knee   **10** Ankle

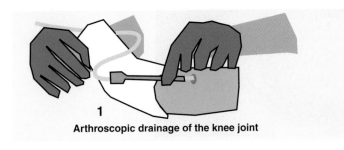

1
Arthroscopic drainage of the knee joint

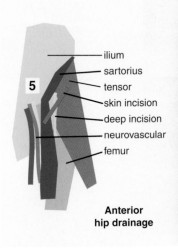

2 3

Ankle drainage

4

Knee drainage

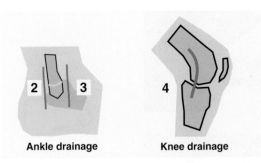

6

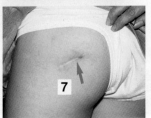

5
- ilium
- sartorius
- tensor
- skin incision
- deep incision
- neurovascular
- femur

Anterior hip drainage

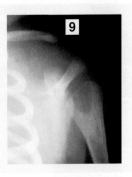

7

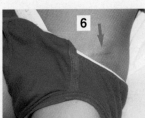

8
- clavicle
- scapula
- humerus
- deep incision
- skin incision

Shoulder drainage

9

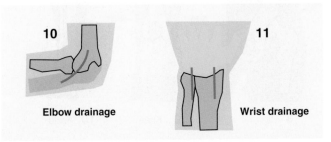

10

Elbow drainage

11

Wrist drainage

Drainage of Septic Joint

Drain septic joints as soon as the diagnosis is made to prevent cartilage damage. The drainage technique depends upon the joint, the duration of disease, and special considerations.

Technique

Needle drainage is suitable for most accessible joints early in the disease. Aspirate with a #18 gauge needle. Make the approach as described on page 379. Irrigation or antibiotic instillation is unnecessary. If joint content is too thick to aspirate, plan open or arthroscopic drainage.

Arthroscopic drainage is most suitable for the knee. Plan an anterolateral portal. Joint lavage may be necessary. Plan to introduce a drain through the scope at the end of the procedure to prevent reaccumulation of pus [1].

Open drainage is appropriate for nearly all cases of hip involvement and sometimes for the shoulder. Consider the need for drainage of the metaphysis in addition to the joint as both may be affected.

Metaphyseal drainage Consider the potential for coexisting osteomyelitis of the adjacent metaphysis. Concurrent infections are more common than often appreciated. To drain the metaphysis, wider exposure is required. Imaging is useful to identify the growth plate to avoid operative injury.

Specific Joints

Ankle Drainage Drain through a lateral approach either posterior [2] or anterior [3] to the fibula.

Knee drainage is through either a medial or lateral approach [4].

Hip drainage is best performed open as thorough drainage is necessary due to the vulnerability of the hip to residual deformity and the deep position, which makes repetitive arthrocentesis impractical. Anterior drainage is preferable [5] as the approach is less likely to damage the joint vascularity and the residual scar [6 and 7] is more acceptable. Make a 3 cm oblique incision 2 cm distal to the iliac crest. Develop the interval between the tensor and sartorius and lateral to the rectus femoris. Open the hip joint. Excise a small segment of capsule. Thoroughly drain the joint. Consider the need for metaphyseal drainage. Place a drain in the joint and secure its position with a single skin suture. Approximate skin. If the hip was subluxated or dislocated due to sepsis or metaphyseal osteomylitis present, immobilize in a spica cast positioned with the hip in abduction to reduce the joint and prevent pathological fracture of the upper femur.

Shoulder Drain through an anterior skin line axillary incision to minimize residual scaring [8]. Drain both the joint and the bursa for the biceps tendon. Place a small drain and secure it with a single skin suture to prevent premature displacement. Close the skin with a few subcutaneous sutures at the margins. Consider the possibility of concurrent osteomyelitis [9] that may need drainage. Avoid wide skin sutures, as permanent scars are unsightly. Place in a sling with the arm held to thorax with a dressing.

Elbow Drain through a direct lateral approach [10] between the triceps and biceps muscles. Open the joint capsule just anterior to the lateral collateral ligament.

Wrist Drain most by needle aspiration. Open drainage is performed on the dorsomedial or lateral aspect of the joint [11]. Avoid the superficial radial nerve on the lateral side.

Post Drainage Management

Antibiotics Start IV antibiotic treatment immediately after taking the joint fluid for culture. Gram stains are sometimes useful to identify the category of organism to help with selection of an antibiotic.

Drains Remove the drain only after significant drainage has ceased. Usually drains can be removed in 2–3 days.

Activities Allow active use as the child becomes comfortable. Physical therapy is usually unnecessary as joint motion recovers spontaneously.

Drainage of Osteomyelitis

Osteomyelitis presents in many forms. Abscesses may be extensive, involving bone and adjacent soft tissues, or localized. Localized bone abscesses are often subacute infections that are contained but not eradicated. Chronic infections are often associated with sequestration of dead bone, requiring removal.

Acute Osteomyelitis

Before surgery, attempt to localize the bone and soft tissues abscess by careful examination, ultrasound, or needle aspiration. Expose the cortex over the suspected site of the abscess. Look for sites of cortical erosion and spontaneous medullary abscess drainage by observation or probing with a curette. If the cortex is intact, explore by making drill holes [1]. Remove the drill and observe the drainage. If the drainage is purulent [2], window the cortex to provide better drainage [3]. If only blood drains [4], explore with additional drill holes until the site of abscess is found [5]. Window the cortex with a small osteotome [6]. Avoid penetrating the growth plate by imaging if necessary [7]. Avoid an excessively large window to reduce the risk of pathological fracture. Gently curette the medullary cavity to ensure complete drainage. Place a drain and perform a limited wound closure. Immobilize in a well-padded cast that extends above the knee for distal femur or upper tibia or below the knee [8] for ankle or foot procedures.

Subacute Osteomyelitis

Often these lesions are effectively managed by antibiotic treatment alone. Simple direct drainage is indicated if the diagnosis is uncertain or the lesion is refractory to antibiotic treatment alone, painful, or causes systemic signs. Make a simple direct approach and drain the bony abscess [9].

Chronic Osteomyelitis

Usually a sequestrum is present [10]. Sequestra may be subperiosteal, cortical, or medullary. Identify preoperatively with imaging. CT scans are usually indicated. Manage most by sequestrectomy [11] and saucerization [12]. Sometimes bone grafting is performed [13]; however, in most cases fill the space with adjacent muscle [14]. Consider the need for sending a specimen to pathology as sometimes tumors and infection are confused. If bone resection is significant, immobilize with a cast to prevent fracture. Continue antibiotic treatment until the ESR becomes normal.

Consultant Kit Song, e-mail: ksong@chmc.org

References

1995 Incorporation of diaphyseal sequestra in chronic haematogenous osteomyelitis. Jain AK, et al. Int Orthop 19:238

1993 Ultrasound localization of subperiosteal abscesses in children with late-acute osteomyelitis. Abernethy LJ, Lee YC, Cole WG. JPO 13:766

1993 Treatment of septic arthritis of the hip by arthroscopic lavage. Chung WK, Slater GJ, Bates EH. JPO 13:444

1991 Arthroscopic treatment of septic arthritic knees in children and adolescents. Ohl MD, Kean JR, Steensen RN. Orthop Rev 20:894

1990 Acute septic arthritis in infancy and childhood. Shaw BA, Kasser JR. CO 212

1990 Outcome after acute osteomyelitis in preterm infants. Williamson JB, Galasko CS, Robinson MJ. Arch Dis Child 65:1060

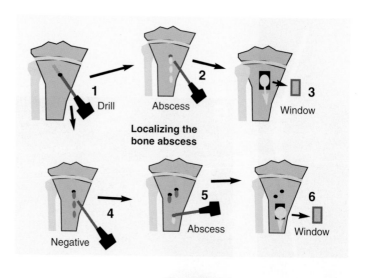

Localizing the bone abscess

1 Drill 2 Abscess 3 Window
4 Negative 5 Abscess 6 Window

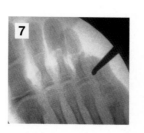
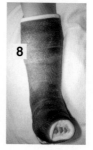
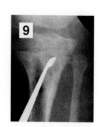

7 8 9

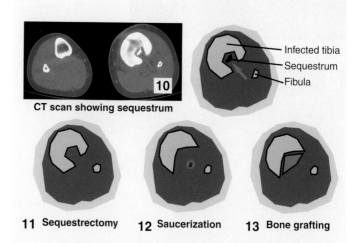

10 CT scan showing sequestrum

Infected tibia
Sequestrum
Fibula

11 Sequestrectomy **12** Saucerization **13** Bone grafting

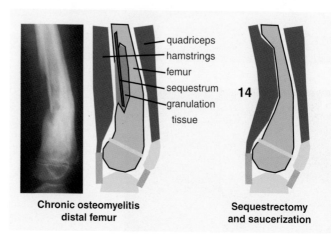

quadriceps
hamstrings
femur
sequestrum
granulation tissue

14

Chronic osteomyelitis distal femur

Sequestrectomy and saucerization

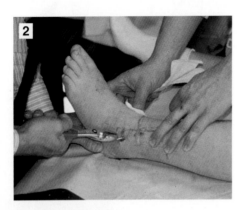

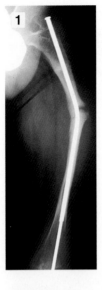

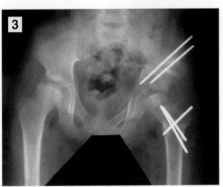

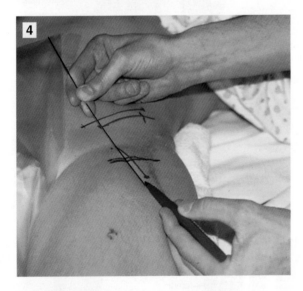

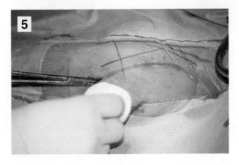

Hardware Removal

Removing hardware may be more difficult than expected—both in establishing appropriate indications and performing the procedure itself. Concern regarding the long-term effect of metal implants has made hardware removal in children more common than adults. This uncertainty must be weighed against the risks and costs of routine removal. Bioabsorbable fixation may solve these problems in the future.

Indications for Hardware Removal

The indications may be classified into categories:

Absolute indications include external pins, prominent fixation that causes skin irritation, infected devices, or hardware penetrating joints.

Usual indications include large fixation devices, those causing stress risers that may promote fractures, fixation considered likely to complicate operative procedures, concern that the fixation will become incased in bone and difficult to remove later.

Seldom justified are single screws, small implants, and spinal fixation devices.

Contraindicated are flexible rods in osteopenic bone, fibrous dysplasia, osteogenesis imperfecta [1].

Technique

Smooth pin removal Generally smooth pins can be removed in the clinic without sedation or anesthesia [2]. Obtain permission from the parent, have tools ready, tell the child what is to happen, place a visual barrier, and without delay remove the pin. Cover the field with a towel to hide the inevitable bleeding, and return in about 10 minutes once the drainage has stopped, to place a small dressing over the wound.

Deep threaded pin removal The decision regarding removal should be made at the original operation [3]. Pins to be left can be cut off at bone level. Those to be removed are left long to facilitate removal. Their length may be a source of discomfort before removal. Mark the position of the pins using fluoroscopy [4]. Make a small incision in line with the pins to insert a needle holder, grasp the end, and remove the pin [5].

Plates Plates may become overgrown with bone, making removal risks unacceptable. If a significant amount of bone is removed, the child may require a walking cast for a month to prevent a fracture.

Complications

Fracture Refracture or a pathological fracture may occur following removal. Avoid this complication by allowing adequate time for bone strength recovery prior to removal.

References

1999 Complication of blade plate removal. Becker CE, et al. JPO 19:188

1998 Late complication after single-rod instrumentation. Hatch RS, Sturm PF, Wellborn CC. Spine 23:1503

1998 Reasons for removal of rigid internal fixation devices in craniofacial surgery. Orringer JS, Barcelona V, Buchman SR. J Craniofac Surg 9:40

1997 The significance of positive cultures from orthopedic fixation devices in the absence of clinical infection. Moussa FW, et al. Am J Orthop 26:617

1996 Metallic or absorbable fracture fixation devices. A cost minimization analysis. Bostman OM. CO 329:233

1996 Routine implant removal after fracture surgery: a potentially reducible consumer of hospital resources in trauma units. Bostman O, Pihlajamaki H. J Trauma 41:846

1991 Electromagnetic metal localization for removal of retained hardware in children. Nugent PJ, et al. JPO 11:548

1991 Metal removal in a pediatric population: benign procedure or necessary evil? Schmalzried TP, et al. JPO 11:72

1988 Tissue reaction to implant corrosion in 38 internal fixation devices. Thomas KA, et al. Orthopedics 11:441

1985 Deep, late infections associated with internal fixation in children. Highland TR, La Mont RL. JPO 5:59

Spica Cast Application

Spica casts are the most difficult casts to apply. Some general points of application may be helpful to keep in mind during application.

Positioning

The infant or child should be supported in the correct position during the cast application. The hammock, spica boxes, or frames are used in different hospitals [1]. Some means of stabilizing the arms is helpful. A custom spica support can secure the arms [2].

Cast Application

For children with neuromuscular problems such as cerebral palsy or myelodysplasia, plan to supplement the usually padding with extra felt over bony prominences–sacrum, trochanters, patella, malleoli, and heels [3]. Once positioned, apply the liner that will be used to trim the cast [4]. Place the padding and folded towel for chest [5]. Some extra padding at the trim ends of the cast will be helpful. Trim the cast with the saw, turn back the liner and apply an additional layer of cast material to create a smooth padded edge [6]. Skin irritation is a common problem in infants [7]. Special liners may be useful but often the problem exists if the cast remains wet. Encourage the mother to avoid tucking in the diaper, change diapers frequently, and allow the cast to air dry without a diaper should irritation be present.

Spica Cast Types

Double spica casts are often necessary following procedures in cerebral palsy [8]. Sometimes the foot can be left out. This reduces the risk of pressure sores over the malleoli and heel. Incorporating a cross-bar in the cast adds strength with little extra weight [8]. Be sure to support the end of the cast on a pillow to unweight the heel. An abdominal window provides comfort [9]. For additional comfort, divide the cast at the upper margin of this window (red arrow) to relieve the sense of compression about the thorax. Be prepared for the toddler to stand in the spica cast [10]. A child in a single hip spica cast may be ambulatory [11]. Flex the knee about 20° to keep the cast from sliding down and add extra padding about the knee and lower edge of cast for comfort.

References

1995 The hammock suspension technique for hip spica cast application in children. Fraser KE. JPO 15:27

1995 The prevention of skin excoriation under children's hip spica casts using the Goretex pantaloon. Wolff CR, James P. JPO 15:386

1993 Upper extremity restraint during hip spica cast application. Buckley SL, et al. JPO 13:529

1993 One-piece stockinet for a spica cast. Farber JM, et al. Orthop Rev 22:640

1989 Transporting children in body casts. Bull MJ, et al. JPO 9:280

1981 Hip spica application for the treatment of congenital dislocation of the hip. Kumar SJ. JPO:97

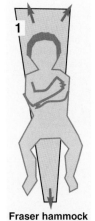

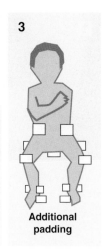

Fraser hammock

Buckley arm supports

Additional padding

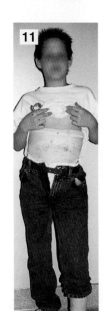

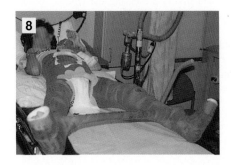

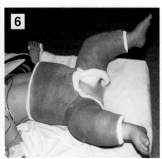

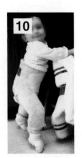

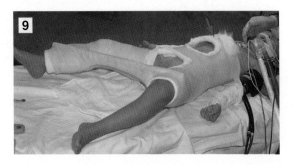

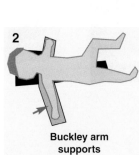

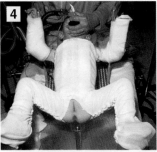

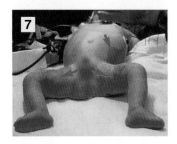

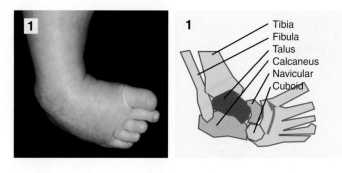

1

Tibia
Fibula
Talus
Calcaneus
Navicular
Cuboid

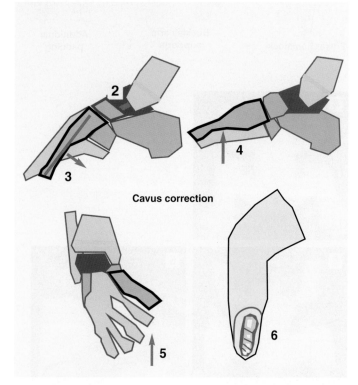

Cavus correction

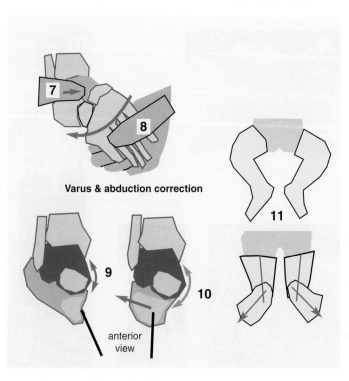

Varus & abduction correction

anterior view

Ponseti Clubfoot Management

The Ponseti approach to management of clubfeet has been refined over a period of 50 years, has been shown to produce good long-term results, and is becoming more widely used. Correction is achieved by manipulation and cast correction in a definite sequence. Correction is usually achieved in 5–6 weekly sessions (casts). An early percutaneous heel-cord tenotomy is commonly added to facilitate equinus correction and in many patients a lateral transfer of the anterior tibialis is performed in early childhood. The correction is best appreciated by using a skeletal model. This description is based on the publications and personal discussion with Dr. Ponseti.

Principles

Pathology The calcaneus, navicular, and cuboid are adducted and inverted in relation to the talus and held in adduction and inversion by contracted ligaments and tendons [1].

Severity The severe clubfoot is characterized by a very short distance between the medial malleolus and tubercle of the navicular [2].

Early treatment Treatment should be started as soon after birth as possible to take advantage of the favorable fibroelastic properties at that age.

Manipulation for a few minutes prior to cast application.

Casting follows initial gentle manipulation and held is continued for 5–7 days in a well molded long-leg plaster cast. Long-leg casts are necessary to control rotation. Most correction may be achieved in 4–6 weeks with weekly cast changes. Do not continue with more than 2–3 casts if correction is not being achieved.

Learning technique This technique is best learned under supervision of someone experienced with this technique. Faulty cast application may create deformities that are difficult to later correct.

Manipulation and Casting Sequence (Ponseti)

Correct cavus and adduction Supinate the forefoot [3 and 4]. This corrects the plantarflexion of the first ray [3 and 5]. The foot is immobilized in marked supination in the cast [6].

Correct supination and adduction With counterpressure by the thumb against the head of the talus [7], abduct the distal foot [8] in supination. Allow the calcaneus to abduct under the subtalar joint. By full abduction of the midfoot and forefoot, the tight medial tarsal ligament contractures are overcome [9 and 10]. This correction allows the calcaneus to abduct, extend, and evert under the talus [10], correcting the heel varus. Be aware that this correction occurs at the subtalar level, not in the ankle joint. During the process of rotating and sliding the calcaneus under the talus, progressively increase the thigh-foot angle in the casts until about 65° is achieved [11].

Equinus correction Before dorsiflexing the foot, make certain the foot is fully abducted and the medial contracted ligaments and tendons are stretched out in the casts [12]. Correct equinus by dorsiflexing the fully abducted foot. A percutaneous heel-cord tenotomy [13] is necessary in about 90% of cases.

Percutaneous tenotomy [13] may be performed in the outpatient clinic or in the operating room. Provide general anesthesia or inject a small amount of local anesthesia (0.1 cc to avoid obscuring the tendon) or apply EMLA cream (lidocaine 2.5% + prilocaine 2.5%) one hour before the procedure. Insert a small blade just medial to the heel-cord, feel the tendon with blade, and divide preserving the tendon sheath. Immobilize in a long-leg cast [14] for 3 weeks for the foot positioned in abduction and dorsiflexion. Mold sole of foot carefully to prevent rocker-bottom deformity. Extend the cast under toes to stretch long toe flexors. Leave dorsum of the cast uncovered to allow dorsiflexion of the toes and to observe circulation of the foot.

Post-Correction Management

Splinting The infant is managed in a foot abduction orthosis (Denis Browne splint) full-time for 3 months and at nighttime for 2–4 years [15]. The width of the bar should equal the width of the infants shoulders. Use stiff, open toed shoes on the bar. Place a plastizote pad to prevent the foot from slipping out of the shoes [15]. Set the foot in about 70°foot abduction (lateral rotation) on clubfoot side and about 45° on the normal side. The use of this splinting is an essential part of this management method.

Recurrence Recurrence can usually be corrected by a series of 2–3 long-leg casts, each worn for 2 weeks.

Tendon transfer If relapse occurs twice and the tibialis anterior tendon is strong and deforming, transfer the tendon to the 3rd cuneiform during early childhood [16]. Correct any recurrence fixed with a series of casts (needed for about 20% of feet). Avoid transfers before the cuneiform is ossified. Often a concurrent open heel lengthening should be combined with the the AT tendon transfer. This balances the foot, prevents recurrence, and is a relatively simple procedure.

Common Errors in Management

Pronation Avoid pronation of the foot that accentuates the cavus component. Although the whole foot is supinated, the forefoot is in relative pronation causing a cavus deformity.

Abduction of the foot Avoid abduction of the foot while the calcaneus is in varus to avoid posterior displacement of the lateral malleolus –an iatrogenic deformity.

Fixation on radiographs Good long-term results are related to mobility and strength, not radiographic appearance.

Relying on physical therapy alone without a period of cast immobilization allows relapse between therapy sessions, delaying correction.

Consultation

Ignacio Ponseti, e-mail: ignacio-ponseti@uiowa.edu
John Herzenberg, e-mail: jherzenberg@stapa.ummc.umaryland.edu

References

2000 Evaluation of Ponseti method for conservative management of idiopathic clubfoot. Herzenberg JE, Radler C, Bor N. Poster exhibit, POSNA 2000 Vancouver, BC, Canada

2000 Personal communication. Herzenberg J.

2000 Personal communication. Ponseti IV.

1997 Common errors in the treatment of congenital clubfoot. Ponseti IV. International Orthopedics 21:137

1996 Congenital clubfoot. Fundamentals of treatment. Ponseti, IV. Oxford University Press, Oxford, New York

1980 Long term results of treatment of congenital clubfoot. Laaveg SJ, Ponseti IV. JBJS 62A:23

1963 Congenital club foot: the results of treatment. Ponseti IV. JBJS 45A:261

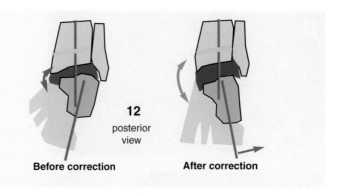

12 posterior view

Before correction · **After correction**

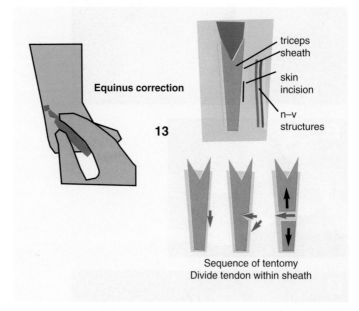

Equinus correction

triceps sheath

skin incision

n–v structures

13

Sequence of tentomy
Divide tendon within sheath

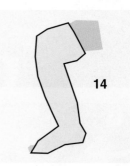

14

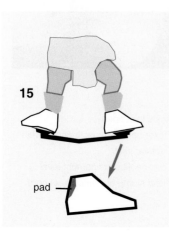

15

pad

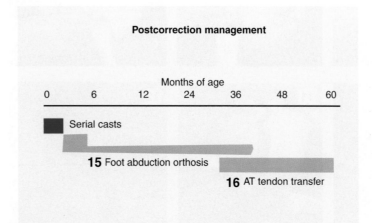

Postcorrection management

Months of age

0   6   12   24   36   48   60

Serial casts

15 Foot abduction orthosis

16 AT tendon transfer

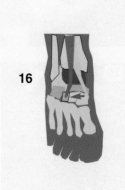

16

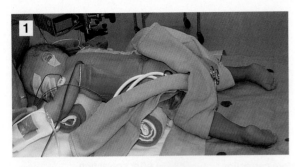

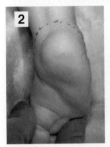

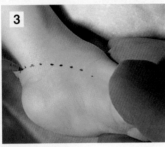

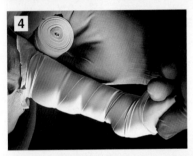

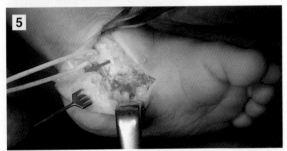

Posteromedial-Lateral Release

The posteromedial-lateral release is presented in detail because the procedure is complex with many important steps. See indications Chapter 5.

Preparation

The infant is intubated and catheterized. A caudal is optional. The infant is placed in the prone position, tourniquets applied, and the skin is prepared [1]. The level of the transverse incision is marked [2 and 3]. Make the incision about 1 cm above the heel crease. The limb is exsanguinated [4] and the tourniquet inflated to about 200 mm Hg.

Medial Exposure and Initial Release

Incision Make a transverse incision guided by the skin markings that extends from about the midfoot beyond the heel to the posterolateral aspect of the foot. Deepen the incision through the subcutaneous fat on the posteromedial aspect of the foot.

Mobilize the neurovascular bundle Expose the neurovascular (nv) bundle, mobilize the bundle, and place a tag [5] to allow retraction.

Release abductor origin Identify the abductor origin [6]. Develop the plane between the muscle origins and nerve [7]. Release the three origins of the abductor hallucis while protecting the medial and lateral plantar n–v bundle. Release the plantar fascia at the level of the lateral plantar n–v structures [8].

Open sheaths of toe flexors Dissect above the nerve and deep to expose and open the sheaths of the common and great toe flexors [9].

Posterior Release

In mild deformities, a posterior release may be performed as the only procedure.

Heel-cord lengthening Expose the tendon [10] and perform a "Z" lengthening of the tendon, releasing it medially from the calcaneus. To make certain the length of the "Z" is adequate for a substantial lengthening, retract the skin proximally [11] to expose the upper portion of the tendon.

Posterior capsulotomy Identify the flexor hallucis longus tendon. Trace the tendon distally to identify the capsule over the subtalar joint. Move the ankle joint to identify the joint level. Open the joint circumferentially while preserving the talocalcaneal interosseous ligaments [12].

Calcaneofibular ligament section Identify this ligament just medial to the peroneal tendon. Section of this ligament is essential for adequate correction.

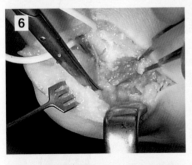

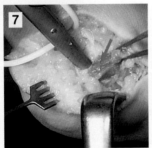

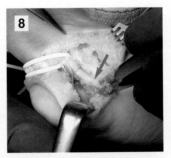

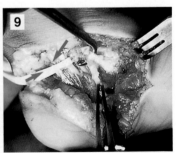

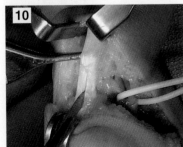

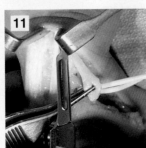

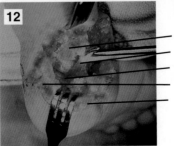

— Ankle joint open
— Flexor hallucis muscle and tendon
— Subtalar joint
— Calcaneofibular ligament level
— Distal stump of divided heel-cord

Deep Medial Release

Return to the medial side of the incision to perform the second phase of the medial release.

Posterior tibialis lengthening Identify the sheath of the posterior tibialis tendon. Open the sheath and lengthen the tendon with a long "Z" incision.

Open talonavicular joint Identify the level of the joint by moving the midfoot. Open the joint [13] and extend the capsulotomy above and below the joint to allow full exposure [14].

Division of Toe Flexor Tendons

With each toe extended to make the flexor tendon prominent, divide the toe flexors with a #11 blade through a midline 2–3 mm stab incision [15]. Division at this level preserves the tendon sheath, allowing rapid tendon regeneration without adhesion formation.

Imaging

Consider imaging the foot at this point to determine whether correction is adequate [16]. Dorsiflexion of the calcaneus to 20°–30° should be possible. The talus and calcaneus should no longer be parallel.

Optional Procedures

At this point, consider the necessity for a release of the plantar fascia and/or the calcaneocuboid joint. The need for these releases depends upon the adequacy of correction as judged by the visual and radiographic appearance of the foot. Perform these releases through the medial incision.

Stretch the Skin

Apply firm abduction of the foot to stretch the skin in preparation for the cast [17].

Skin Closure

Apply an elastic bandage [18] and release the tourniquet. After a few minutes, remove the bandage and cauterize any major bleeders. Close the skin in two layers. The primary closure is subcutaneous [19] and supplemented with a subcuticular dermal closure with absorbable sutures [20].

Cast Immobilization

Place sterile dressing and padding. The foot should show good correction [21]. With the foot held by the surgeon in a position of lateral rotation and about neutral dorsiflexion, a short-leg well-molded cast is applied [22]. Extend the cast above the knee [23]. The completed cast should show an externally rotated thigh–foot angle (arrows) and about neutral ankle dorsiflexion [24].

Postoperative Care

Change the cast in clinic in 2 weeks. Dorsiflex the ankle to about 10°–15° in the second cast. Apply the third cast at 6 weeks. Remove this third cast at 9 weeks. Follow with nighttime use of a Denis-Browne splint set with about 45° of external rotation. Continue nightsplinting until ages 2–3 years if possible. Allow normal shoes during the day following cast removal.

Consultant Mosca VM, e-mail: mosca@chmc.org

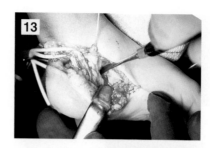

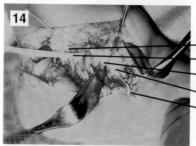

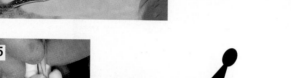
Neurovascular bundle — Tibialis posterior prox stump — Talus — Navicular — Tibialis posterior distal stump

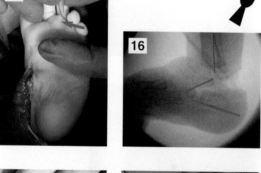

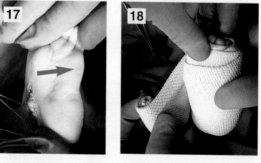

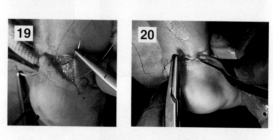

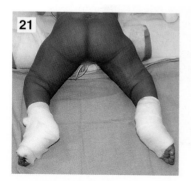

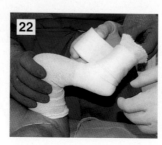

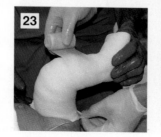

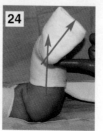

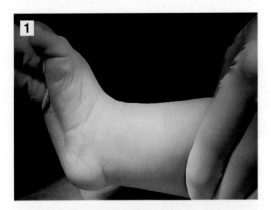

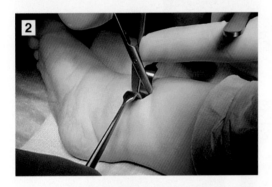

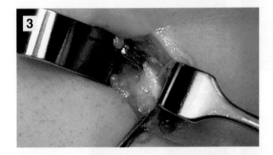

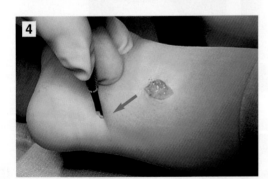

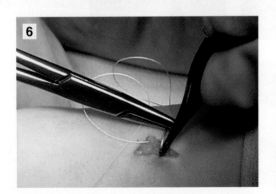

Limited Posteromedial Clubfoot Release

This procedure is an option for management of moderate and severe clubfeet for deformities that are too severe or late for Ponseti management. It is used in conjunction with pre- and postoperative casting. Consider this procedure for management of the clubfoot in arthrogryposis as this limited procedure may be combined with open reduction of the hips. Continue the serial cast correction of the feet by weekly cast changes of just the foot portion of the spica cast.

Technique (Mosca)

Prep and drape the leg free with the opposite pelvis elevated to facilitate access to the medial aspect of the foot and leg [1]. Perform the posterior tibialis tendinotomy through a 1.5 cm incision over the midportion of the distal medial leg [2]. Identify and divide the tendon within the distal body of the posterior tibial muscle [3]. Perform a percutaneous tendinotomy of the heel-cord. With dorsiflexion tension applied to the ankle, insert a scalpel just above the insertion and divide the tendon from anterior to posterior to avoid damage to the neurovascular bundle [4]. Perform a percutaneous lengthening of the flexor hallucis longus. While dorsiflexing the great toe, insert the scapel in the midline of the base of the great toe and divide the flexor tendon [5]. If the common toe flexors are also very tight, divide these tendons in a like fashion. Close the open tenotomy incision with a single subcuticular suture [6]. Apply a long-leg cast with the foot in a position of gentle correction [7].

Follow-up Care

After 2–3 weeks, resume weekly or biweekly serial cast correction. Once correction is achieved, confirm with radiographs, including a maximum dorsiflexion lateral study. This should show a tibial calcaneal angle of >15°. Maintain correction with a night splint fabricated from a bivalved fiberglass cast in the corrected position.

Consultant Mosca VM, e-mail: mosca@chmc.org

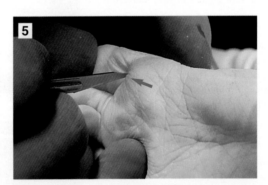

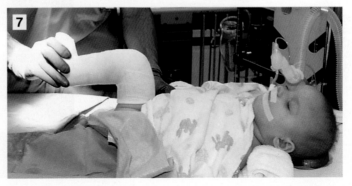

Triceps Lengthening Procedures

Lengthening of the triceps includes lengthening of the heel-cord or selective lengthening of the gastrocnemius fascia. Base the choice on the preoperative examination. Assess ankle dorsiflexion with the knee flexed and extended [1]. If the contracture involves only the gastrocnemius, dorsiflexion above a right angle will be possible with the knee flexed [2]. If the contracture includes the soleus alone or with the gastrocnemius, the limitation of dorsiflexion will remain regardless of the position of the knee [3].

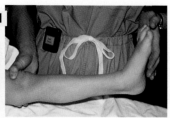

Technique for Gastrocnemius Recession

Prep and drape in the prone position [4]. Make a 3 cm midline longitudinal incision centered over the junction of the middle and distal thirds of the leg [5]. Identify the sural nerve and retract to the side. Incise the gastrocnemius fascia completely on both the medial and lateral aspects. The fascia may be incised at one or more levels. The ankle should then be dorsiflexed to >20° with the knee extended [6]. Close only the skin and apply a short-leg walking cast with the ankle in slight dorsiflexion. Remove the cast in about 4 weeks in the clinic.

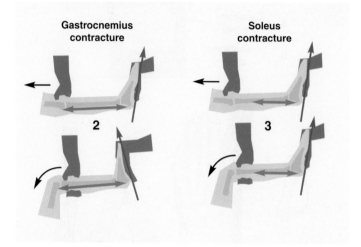

Gastrocnemius contracture

Soleus contracture

Techniques for Tendo Achilles Lengthening

There are numerous techniques for lengthening based on the training and preferences of the surgeon. Percutaneous techniques produce little scar and can be done quickly but provide less control of the amount of lengthening. Regardless of method, after lengthening, immobilize in a short-leg walking cast for about a month. Remove the cast in the clinic.

Open Tendo-Achilles Lengthening Make a longitudinal incision (yellow line) on the medial aspect of the distal leg just anterior to the tendon [7]. Expose the tendon and perform a step-cut lengthening. Make certain the long arm of the incision is long enough to allow the desired lengthening with enough overlap for suturing. Dorsiflex the ankle to about 10° and suture the tendon with interrupted sutures [8]. Close the subcutaneous tissue and dermis separately.

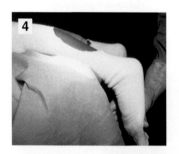

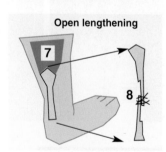

Technique for White Sliding Lengthening Make a 2 cm posteromedial distal incision [9] just above the tendon insertion (yellow line). Through this incision identify the tendon and divide about 60% of the medial fibers [10]. About 5 cm more proximal, make a second incision. With the tendon stretched by passive dorsiflexion of the ankle, divide about 60% of the posterolateral fibers until dorsiflexion of the ankle to about 10° is possible.

Technique of Percutaneous Lengthening With the child in the prone position, dorsiflex the ankle to tension the heel-cord [11]. Divide about 60–70% of the heel-cord at three levels through stab incision on alternate sides of the tendon [12]. The distalmost cut should be lateral to make it distant from the neurovascular bundle. Dorsiflex the ankle to achieve the desired amount of correction.

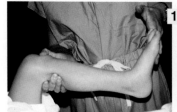

Open lengthening

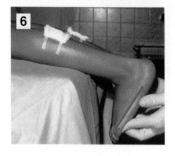

Complications

Overcorrection is most likely in the child with spastic diplegia. Avoid by patient selection and by avoiding excessive lengthening.

Recurrence may occur in children with cerebral palsy when the lengthenings are performed at a young age.

Scar irritation can be avoided by placing the incision to the side of the tendon. Avoid a midline scar over the tendon.

References

1998 Duration of immobilization after percutaneous sliding heel-cord lengthening. Blasier RD, White R. JPO 18:299

1989 Calcaneal gait in spastic diplegia after heel cord lengthening: a study with gait analysis. Segal LS, et al. JPO 9:697

1988 Lengthening of the calcaneal tendon in spastic hemiplegia by the White slide technique. A long-term review. Graham HK, Fixsen JA. JBJS 70B:472

1987 Outpatient percutaneous heel cord lengthening in children. Moreau MJ, Lake DM. JPO 7:253

White sliding lengthening

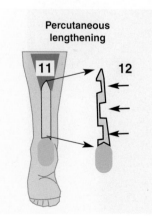

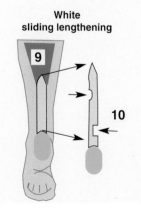

Percutaneous lengthening

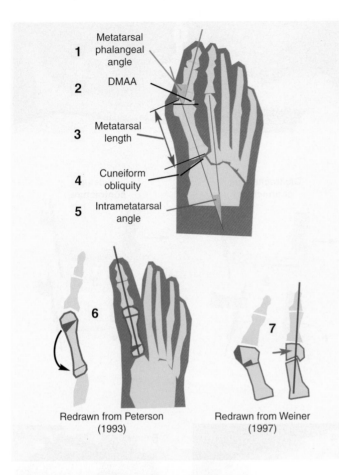

1 Metatarsal phalangeal angle

2 DMAA

3 Metatarsal length

4 Cuneiform obliquity

5 Intrametatarsal angle

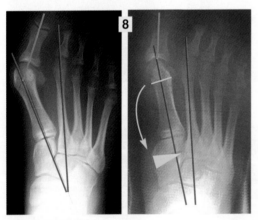

6

7

Redrawn from Peterson (1993)

Redrawn from Weiner (1997)

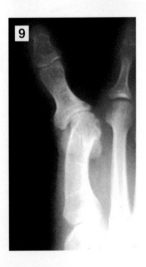

8

9

Bunion Correction

Bunion correction in the child is complicated by the effects of growth and varied pathology. When feasible, delay operative correction until the end of growth to reduce the risk of recurrence.

Indications

Correct bunions when symptoms are unacceptable and nonsurgical measures fail.

Preoperative Planning

Measure the metatarsal phalangeal angle [1]. This is normally 5°–15°. More severe deformities may indicate the need of a double-level osteotomy. Measure the distal metatarsal articular angle (DMAA). This is normally less 8° [2]. Note the congruity of the first metatarsal-phalangeal joint. If the joint is congruous with significant angular deformity, a distal osteotomy is indicated to preserve this congruity. Note the relative lengths of the first and second metatarsals [3]. Note the obliquity of the cuneiform-metatarsal joint [4]. Assess the intrametatarsal angle [5]. This is normally below 10°. Higher values describe metatarsus primus varus, typical of juvenile onset bunions. If the first metatarsal is short, plan opening wedge osteotomies to maintain or improve length. Base choice of procedure on the pathological anatomy. Plan full but not overcorrection; correct intrametatarsal and metatarsal phalangeal alignment while preserving normal metatarsal length relationships and congruity of the metatarsal phalangeal joint. Be careful to avoid sagittal plane deformity to cause uneven metatarsal loading.

Technique (Peterson and Newman)

This procedure is indicated for moderate or severe deformity with congruity of the metatarsal-phalangeal joint [6]. Expose the distal metatarsal and excise the bony prominence of the bunion. Remove a wedge of bone from the distal metaphysis. This wedge is usually about 20°. Correct any malrotation. Make a second medial incision to expose the proximal metatarsal metaphysis. Perform an osteotomy, leaving the lateral cortex intact. Wedge open the osteotomy and insert the graft taken from the first osteotomy site. Fix with a longitudinal 3/16 inch smooth K wire. Close the wounds and apply a compressive dressing. Before discharge, apply a short-leg non-weight-bearing cast. At 6 weeks ,remove the pin and apply a weight-bearing cast for 5–6 additional weeks.

Technique (Weiner et al.)

This is a modification of the Mitchell bunionectomy [7]. This procedure is indicated if the metatarsus primus varus is mild. The modification includes the use of smooth pin fixation and a trapezoidal step-off to preserve length.

Other Techniques

Other procedures include simple excision of the bunion prominence, opening wedge osteotomy of the cuneiform to correct excessive obliquity, and wedge osteotomies of the base of the proximal phalanx for complex bunions seen in children with neuromuscular disorders [8].

Complications

Recurrence is common when bunions are corrected in late childhood. Bony remodeling reestablishes original deformity. **Overcorrection** may follow excessive soft tissue releases [9]. Metatarsal-phalangeal joint **subluxation**, may lead to arthritis. **Uneven** metatarsal head loading may occur if first metatarsal is excessively shortened or plantar flexed.

Consultant Ham Peterson, e-mail: peterson.hamlet@mayo.edu

References

1997 Mitchell osteotomy for adolescent hallux valgus. Weiner BK, Weiner DS, Mirkopulos N. JPO 17:781

1996 Modified Mitchell bunionectomy for management of adolescent hallux valgus. McDonald MG, Stevens DB. CO 332:163

1993 Adolescent bunion deformity treated with double osteotomy and longitudinal pin fixation of the first ray. Peterson HA, Newman SR. JPO 13:80

1990 Surgical treatment of adolescent hallux valgus. Geissele AE, Stanton RP. JPO 10:642

Tarsal Coalition Resection

Resection of tarsal coalitions is optimal management of refractory symptomatic coalitions. Resection of calcaneonavicular coalitions is much simpler and more consistently satisfactory than subtalar coalition resection. Subtalar coalitions often require secondary procedures due to continued pain, excessive valgus, or recurrence.

Calcaneonavicular Coalition Resection

This resection is based on technique of Cowell (1970) as described by Gonzalez and Kumar (1990). Under tourniquet hemostasis [1], make a 4 cm incision over the sinus tarsi. Avoid the sural nerve and peroneal tendons in the inferior aspect of the wound. Deepen the incision to expose the extensor digitorum brevis muscle [2]. Detach the origin of the muscle from the calcaneus and elevate it from the underlying coalition and reflect the muscle distally [3]. Identify the coalition with a Freer elevator. If location or extent of coalition is uncertain, identify with the aid of imaging. Resect the coalition with an osteotome as a single block [4]. The resected block should be rectangular, not triangular in shape. Remove any cartilagenous remnants of the coalition from both the calcaneal and navicular sides of the resection. Place a heavy absorbable suture in the origin of the extensor muscle. Thread this suture on a straight needle and pass the needle through the skin in the midportion of the longitudinal arch. Apply traction to the suture to pull the origin of the extensor muscle into the space previously occupied by the coalition. Secure the suture through a pad and the button [5]. Tie the suture with sufficient tension to maintain the position of the interposition but not so tight as to cause skin necrosis. The muscle interposed between the navicular and calcaneus prevents recurrence of the coalition [6]. Confirm the resection with an oblique radiograph of the foot [7]. Immobilize in a short-leg cast for about 3 weeks. Allow gradual return to full activity as comfort permits.

Talocalcaneal Coalition Resection

Based on Olney and Asher (1987) this is a description of resection of middle facet coalitions. Identify the coalition by CT scan [8]. Consider mapping the extent of the coalition as success is related to size. Make a 5–6 cm incision over the sustentaculum tali [9]. Reflect the abductor hallicus plantar-ward and divide the flexor retinaculum. Retract the flexor digitorum and the neurovascular bundle [10]. Between these structures, identify the coalition by elevating the periosteum and marking the anterior and posterior margins of the subtalar joint with Keith needles [11]. If uncertain about the location of the coalition, use imaging. Resect the coalition with a power burr, osteotomes, or rongeurs. Make the resection 5–7 mm wide. Be certain that the entire coalition is resected by visualizing joint cartilage around the resected area and demonstrating increased subtalar motion [12]. Place bone wax on the cut surfaces and harvest autogenous fat from the buttock crease. Place this graft into the defect [13]. Secure the graft under sutures in the overlying periosteal margins. Repair the flexor retinaculum, reattach the abductor origin, and close the skin in layers. Apply a short-leg non-weight-bearing cast. Remove the cast in the clinic in 2–3 weeks, maintain non-weight-bearing for an additional 4–6 weeks.

References

1998 Resection for symptomatic talocalcaneal coalition. Comfort TK, et al. JPO 18:283

1997 Results of the surgical treatment of calcaneo-navicular coalition. Jerosch J, Lindner N, Finnen DA. Arch Orthop Trauma Surg 116:379

1990 Calcaneonavicular coalition treated by resection and interposition of the extensor digitorum brevis muscle. Gonzalez P, Kumar SJ. JBJS 72A:71

1987 Excision of symptomatic coalition of the middle facet of the talocalcaneal joint. Olney BW, Asher MA. JBJS 69A:539

1970 Extensor brevis arthroplasty. Cowell HR. JBJS 52A:820

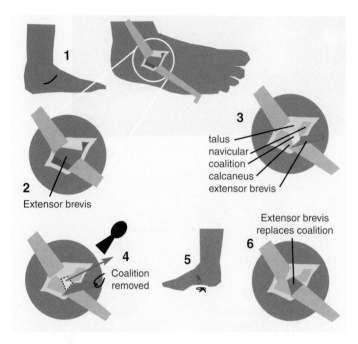

1

2 — Extensor brevis

3 — talus / navicular / coalition / calcaneus / extensor brevis

4 — Coalition removed

5

6 — Extensor brevis replaces coalition

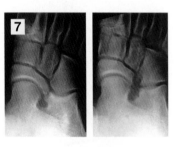
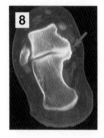

7

8

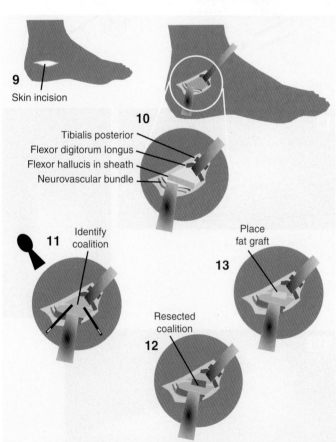

9 — Skin incision

10 — Tibialis posterior / Flexor digitorum longus / Flexor hallucis in sheath / Neurovascular bundle

11 — Identify coalition

12 — Resected coalition

13 — Place fat graft

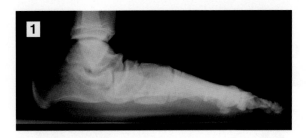

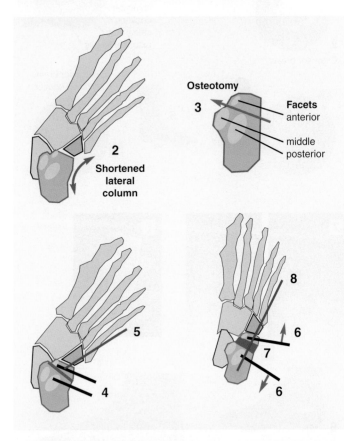

Calcaneal Lengthening

Calcaneal lengthening is the preferred method of correcting most pathologic flatfoot deformities. The procedure is joint preserving to avoid late degenerative change commonly associated with arthrodesing procedures. The procedure was originally described by Evan and more recently detailed by Mosca.

Indications

Severe symptomatic flatfeet are usually associated with cerebral palsy, myelodysplasia, skewfeet, or triceps contractures.

Preoperative Planning

Assess triceps for contracture. Obtain AP and lateral [1] standing radiographs of the foot (14-year-old with a flatfoot associated with heel-cord contracture). Shortening of the lateral column [2] and contracture of the heel-cord are typical features.

Technique (Mosca)

Position in the supine position with the operative side elevated. Make an oblique incision over the sinus tarsi. Expose the distal calcaneus dorsally, leaving the calcaneocuboid capsule intact. Lengthen the peroneus brevis, but not the longus. Select the site of osteotomy between the anterior and middle calcaneal facets [3]. Place Steinmann pins for traction [4]. Expose the plantar surface of the calcaneus and divide the periosteum. Using an osteotome or sagittal saw, divide the calcaneus. Apply distraction to the osteotomy site while observing the calcaneocuboid joint for evidence of subluxation. Place a smooth pin retrograde across the calcaneocuboid joint to maintain its normal relationship [5]. Prepare a trapezoid shaped graft. This may be an allograft or autogenous corticocancellous graft from the ilium. The graft should measure about 10–12 mm in lateral length and 4–6 mm in medial width. While distracting the osteotomy site with the Steinmann pins [6] place the graft [7]. Drive the pin across the osteotomy site well into the calcaneus to secure both the joint and the graft [8]. Remove the traction pins. Plicate the talonavicular joint and tibialis posterior tendon. Test for heel-cord tightness both with the knee flexed and extended. If the ankle cannot be dorsiflexed to neutral with the knee extended, perform a triceps lengthening procedure. Lengthen the heel-cord or the triceps aponeurosis, depending upon the site of contracture. In most cases, a gastrocnemius fascial lengthening is indicated. In most flatfeet, plantarflexion closing wedge osteotomy of the medial cuneiform is needed to correct the supination deformity of the forefoot. In skewfoot deformities, an opening wedge osteotomy of the medial cuneiform is indicated. Apply a short-leg cast and document with AP and lateral radiographs [9] in the cast. In these radiographs, the procedure was performed for a flatfoot deformity and a concurrent closing wedge osteotomy of the medial cuneiform was performed and fixed with a staple.

Postoperative Management

Maintain non-weight bearing for 8 weeks. Remove the original cast and pins in clinic [10] at 6 weeks. Replace the cast for an additional 2 weeks. Place over-the-counter arch supports in regular shoes thereafter.

Complications

The most common complication is subluxation of the calcaneocuboid joint. Avoid this by transfixing the joint with a percutaneous wire.

Consultation V. Mosca, e-mail: vmosca@chmc.org

References

2000 Technical details of calcaneal lengthening. Mosca VS. Personal communication.
1995 Calcaneal lengthening for valgus deformity of the hindfoot. Results in children who had severe, symptomatic flatfoot and skewfoot. Mosca VS. JBJS 77A:500
1993 Effect of calcaneal lengthening on relationships among the hindfoot, midfoot, and forefoot. Sangeorzan BJ, Mosca V, Hansen ST. Foot Ankle 14:136
1983 A review of elongation of os calcis for flat feet. Phillips GE. JBJS 65B:15

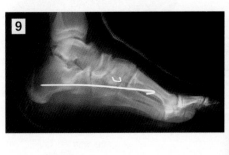

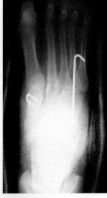

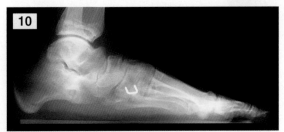

Subtalar Fusion and Arthroereisis Procedures

Procedures for arthrodesis, stiffening, or limiting motion of the subtalar joint are numerous and commonly performed. These procedures are often used to stabilize valgus feet secondary to cerebral palsy and to correct various types of flatfeet.

Types of Procedures

The procedures fall into several categories: arthrodesing procedures such as the interaarticular Dennyson–Fulford and bone dowel procedures [1]; extraarticular fusions such as the Grice–Green procedure [2]; subtalar procedures that stabilize the joint with a staple, plug of silastic, or bioabsorbable material [3]; and subtalar blocking procedures that limit eversion by implanting bone, metal, or plastic such as the STA-peg procedure [4]. These procedure are simple and commonly performed.

This simplicity of these procedures often leads to misuse by expanding the indications to include children with physiologic flexible flatfeet. Be aware that fusion of the subtalar joint increases stress on adjacent unfused joints and may lead to premature degenerative arthritis of the ankle and tarsal joints. Procedures that stiffen the subtalar joint may cause joint damage and eventual arthritis of the subtalar joint itself.

Indications

Subtalar stabilizing procedures have limited indications. These include feet with deformity, causing significant disability that cannot be corrected by joint preserving procedures such as calcaneal lengthening. Typical indications include feet with established osteoarthritis of the subtalar joint and deformity associated with stiffness of the midfoot eliminating the option of calcaneal lengthening.

Technique (Dennyson–Fulford)

Prep and drape the extremity free. Make a curved skin line incision (yellow line) over the sinus tarsi [5]. Expose the sinus tarsi by freeing the short extensor from the calcaneus and remove the soft tissues to expose the joint. With the foot in the neutral inversion–eversion position, decorticate the adjacent surfaces of the talus and calcaneus or use a dowel cutter to remove a segment of bone across the joint [6]. Obtain bone chips or a dowel graft from the ilium. Place the graft across the subtalar joint. While maintaining the neutral subtalar position, pass a drill vertically through the subtalar joint [7] and fix the joint with a cancellous screw to maintain the neutral position [8]. Confirm the position of the screw by radiography [9]. Lengthen triceps if contracted.

Postoperative Care

Immobilize in a short-leg nonwalking cast for 6 weeks. Place a walker on the cast to allow weight bearing for an additional 6 weeks.

Complications

1. Nonunion is best prevented by neutral positioning, autogenous grafting, and firm fixation.
2. Over- or undercorrection is avoided by careful positioning of the foot during grafting and fixation.

References

1998 Subtalar arthroereisis for the correction of planovalgus foot in children with neuromuscular disorders. Vedantam R, Capelli AM, Schoenecker PL. JPO 18:294

1998 Local bone-graft technique for subtalar extraarticular arthrodesis in cerebral palsy. Jeray KJ, Rentz J, Ferguson RL. JPO 18:75

1994 Dennyson-Fulford subtalar arthrodesis. Hadley N, Rahm M, Cain TE. JPO 14:363

1992 Totally absorbable screws in fixation of subtalar extra articular arthrodesis in children with spastic neuromuscular disease: preliminary report of a randomized prospective study of fourteen arthrodesis fixed with absorbable or metallic screws. Partio EK, et al. JPO 12:646

1990 Bilbo subtalar stabilization of the planovalgus foot by staple arthroereisis in young children who have neuromuscular problems. Crawford AH, Kucharzyk D, Roy DR. JBJS 72A:840

1990 Extraarticular subtalar arthrodesis: the dowel method. Pirani SP, Tredwell SJ, Beauchamp RD. JPO 10:244

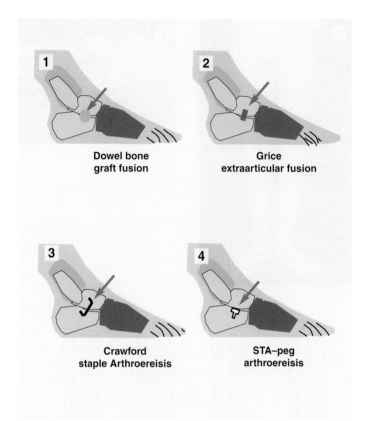

1 Dowel bone graft fusion

2 Grice extraarticular fusion

3 Crawford staple Arthroereisis

4 STA–peg arthroereisis

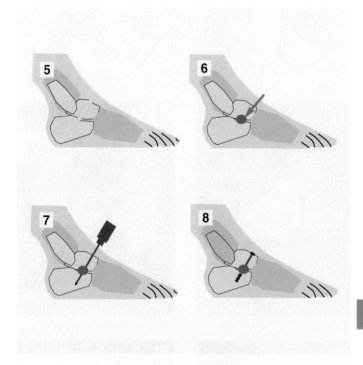

5

6

7

8

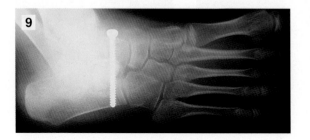

9

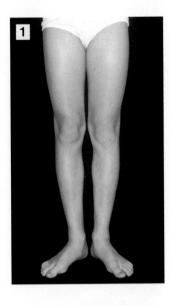

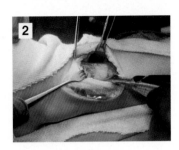

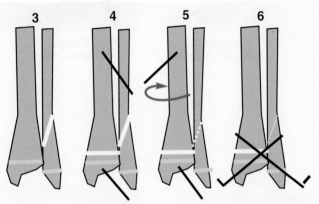

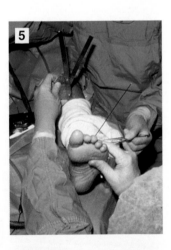

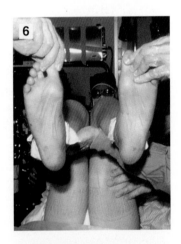

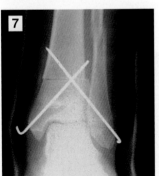

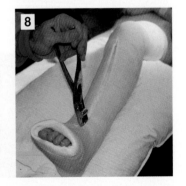

Distal Tibial Rotational Osteotomy

The distal tibia is the preferred level for rotational osteotomies of the tibia.

Indications

Rotational osteotomies may be performed for idiopathic tibial torsion, torsion associated with neuromuscular disorders, or occasionally torsion in clubfeet. Tibial torsion is rotation falling beyond the range of normal. Most rotational osteotomies are performed for lateral tibial torsion [1]. The thigh-foot angle usually exceeds 35°–40°. Because rotation changes with growth, delay rotation osteotomies until after 8–10 years. Bilateral procedures may be performed at one time. In the older child, performing one procedure at a time allows the child to crutch walk during recovery.

Technique

Using fluoroscopy, mark on the skin the sites of the growth plate and about 2–3 cm more proximal for the site of the tibial osteotomy. Make a 8 cm anterolateral longitudinal skin incision and expose the tibia proximal to the growth plate [2]. If deformity is severe, expose the shaft of the fibula more proximal and perform an oblique fibular osteotomy [3]. Place two smooth parallel K wires (black lines) proximal and distal to the osteotomy site to monitor the rotational correction [4]. Perform a transverse tibial osteotomy with a power saw. Rotate the distal segment while observing the relative position of the K wires [5]. Once the amount of correction is achieved, transfix the tibial osteotomy with two smooth percutaneous K wires [6]. Bend over the ends to prevent migration [7]. An alternative is to fix the osteotomy with a 4-hole plate. Apply a long-leg cast with the knee flexed about 20°. Split the cast to accommodate swelling [8].

Postoperative Care

Monitor neurovascular status during the early postoperative period. At 4 weeks apply a walker and allow weight bearing. Remove the cast and K wires in the clinic at 7–8 weeks.

Complications

Malrotation Avoid this complication by careful preoperative assessment, intraoperative monitoring of correction, and securing stable fixation.

Compartment syndrome This complication is avoided by operating distal to the compartment, splitting the cast, and monitoring clinical findings during the early postoperative period.

Nonunion This is most common in the fibula. Avoid this problem by avoiding any soft tissue interposition following the osteotomy. If the fragments are widely separated, they may be approximated by a heavy absorbable suture.

Consultant Lynn Staheli, e-mail: staheli@u.washington.edu

References

1998 Distal tibial/fibular derotation osteotomy for correction of tibial torsion: review of technique and results in 63 cases. Dodgin DA, et al. JPO 18:95

1998 Kinematic and kinetic analysis of distal derotational osteotomy of the leg in children with cerebral palsy. Stefko RM, et al. JPO 18:81

1994 The role of fibular osteotomy in rotational osteotomy of the distal tibia. Manouel M, Johnson LO. JPO 14:611

1994 Rotational osteotomies of the leg: tibia alone versus both tibia and fibula. Rattey T, Hyndman J. JPO 14:615

1992 Tibial rotational osteotomy for idiopathic torsion. A comparison of the proximal and distal osteotomy levels. Krengel WF 3d, Staheli LT. CO 283:285

1985 Rotational osteotomy of the distal tibia and fibula. Bennett JT, Bunnell WP, MacEwen GD. JPO 5:294

Proximal Tibial Osteotomy

Upper tibial osteotomy is appropriate for correcting angulatory deformity and combined deformities of angulation and rotation. Simple rotational deformity is best performed in the distal tibia as proximal osteotomies have a higher rate of complications.

Techniques

Select from the several techniques what seems like the best osteotomy and fixation for your patient.

Transverse osteotomy with external fixation [1]. This technique is ideal for management of tibia vara in the obese child. Cast supplementation is not necessary, correction can be gradually applied and easily modified, and monitoring compartment and nerve status simplified.

Transverse osteotomy with plate fixation [2] is useful when combining angular and rotational correction.

The oblique osteotomy provides correction both in rotation and angulation [3]. Calculate the angle for osteotomy before the procedure – (Rab 1988). The osteotomy is made from an anterior exposure with the entry point just inferior to the tibial tubercle. The osteotomy extends proximal and posterior at an angle necessary to correct both rotation and varus or valgus components of the deformity. Fixation is relative simple with a single AP screw. The large contact area increases the rate of union.

Dome osteotomy provides good contact with inherent stability, making fixation with crossed pins adequate [4].

Oblique closing wedge osteotomy provides a large contact area for rapid union and allows fixation with two transfixing screws [5].

Avoiding Complications

Complications of proximal tibial osteotomy are relative common. These include peroneal nerve injury, compartment syndromes, and physeal injury. Be aware of the anterior distal extension of the growth plate and make certain the osteotomy or fixation devices do not traverse the plate. In rare instances the peroneal nerve may be tethered, and mobilization may be necessary to avoid excessive stretch. For most osteotomies several steps are appropriate.

Prophylactic anterior compartment release Divide the fascia of the anterior compartment subcutaneously through the osteotomy incision [6]. Perform a fibular osteotomy [7], split the cast [8], and in the immediate postoperative period, follow carefully [9] for evidence of peroneal injury or compartment syndrome.

Clinical Examples

Bilateral tibial osteotomies in renal rickets [10].

Valgus osteotomy with external fixation [11 and 12] for tibia vara in obese adolescent.

Simple transverse osteotomy before plate fixation [13].

References

1997 Surgical correction of angular deformity of the knee in children with renal osteodystrophy. Oppenheim WL, Fischer SR, Salusky IB. JPO 17:41

1996 Treatment of adolescent Blount disease with the circular external fixation device and distraction osteogenesis. Coogan PG, Fox JA, Fitch RD. JPO 16:450

1996 Oblique proximal tibial osteotomy for the correction of tibia vara in the young. Laurencin CT, Ferriter PJ, Millis MB. CO 218

1995 Dynamic axial external fixation in the surgical treatment of tibia vara. Price CT, Scott DS, Greenberg DA. JPO 15:236

1994 Proximal tibial osteotomy with compression plate fixation for tibia vara. Martin SD, et al. JPO 14:619

1994 Peroneal nerve injury as a complication of pediatric tibial osteotomies: a review of 255 osteotomies. Slawski DP, et al. JPO 14:166

1992 Tibial rotational osteotomy for idiopathic torsion. A comparison of the proximal and distal osteotomy levels. Krengel WF, Staheli LT. CO 285

1988 Oblique tibial osteotomy for Blount's disease (tibia vara). Rab GT. JPO 8:715

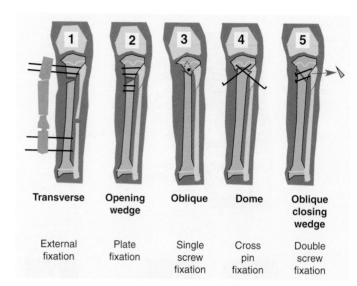

1	2	3	4	5
Transverse	Opening wedge	Oblique	Dome	Oblique closing wedge
External fixation	Plate fixation	Single screw fixation	Cross pin fixation	Double screw fixation

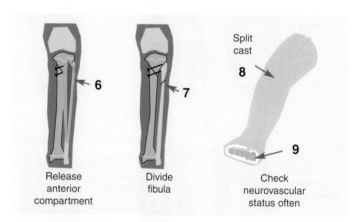

Release anterior compartment 6

Divide fibula 7

Split cast 8

Check neurovascular status often 9

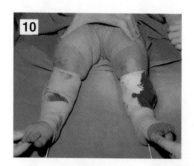

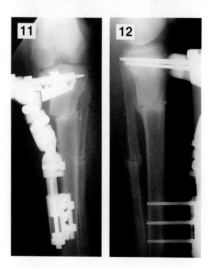

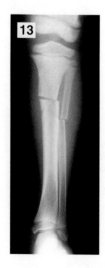

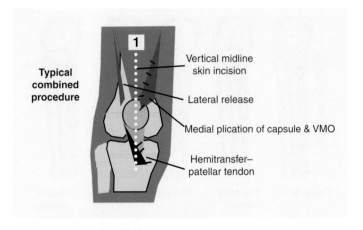

Typical combined procedure

Vertical midline skin incision

Lateral release

Medial plication of capsule & VMO

Hemitransfer–patellar tendon

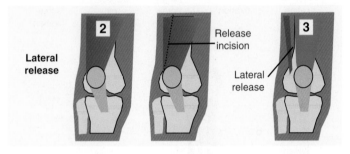

Lateral release

Release incision

Lateral release

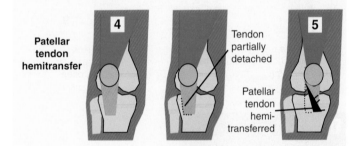

Patellar tendon hemitransfer

Tendon partially detached

Patellar tendon hemi-transferred

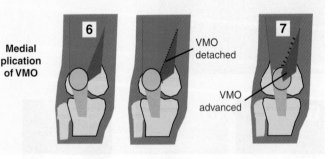

Medial plication of VMO

VMO detached

VMO advanced

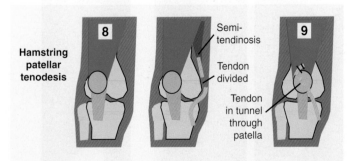

Hamstring patellar tenodesis

Semi-tendinosis

Tendon divided

Tendon in tunnel through patella

Patellar Realignment

Patellar realignment in childhood is complicated by the wide range of pathological elements. Lateral contracture, rotational and angular malalignment, condylar and patellar hypoplasia, muscle hypoplasia, and imbalance may be present alone or in various combinations. Often realignment requires a combination of procedures [1], which is often best accomplished through a direct anterior longitudinal incision. This allows intraoperative visualization of the pathology and tailoring of the repair to best correct the problems. Make certain at the end of the procedure that with passive flexion and extension of the knee the patella tracts vertically in the midline. Except for transfer of the tibial tubercle, these procedures may be performed in the growing child without the risk of growth arrest.

Lateral Release

Lateral contractures [2] are often present in congenital patellar dislocation or those that occur in infancy. In rare cases, very extensive, more proximal release is necessary. In others, a more limited release is adequate [3]. Be aware that lateral release is seldom indicated for most patellar instability cases. Excessive release may cause medial patellar dislocation from the loss of the normal lateral tether.

Patellar Tendon Hemitransfer

Patellar tendon hemitransfer [4] is often combined with other elements. It is rarely adequate alone. Detach the lateral side of the tendon from the tibia [5] and reflect it over itself and fix it medially with sutures. This provides the equivalent of medial transfer of the tibial tubercle without the risk of growth arrest.

Medial Plication

Attenuation of the medial capsule and the patello-femoral ligament follows acute patellar dislocation [6]. This may be corrected by first reefing the medical capsule, then advancing the VMO over the quadriceps and suturing to the anterior periosteum over the patella [7].

Hamstring Tenodesis

Tenodesis of the semitendinosis tendon into the patella creates a checkrein that is very effective in realignment [8 and 9]. Often this tenodesis is combined with a lateral release and medial capsular reconstruction.

Tibial Tubercle Transfer

This procedure is most commonly needed for the adolescent with malalignment that can be corrected by a distal procedure [10]. The tibial tubercle rotational transfer can be performed through a curved horizontal incision just below the tubercle. The scar from this incision is preferable to other knee incision [11].

Consultant Carl Stanitski, e-mail: stanitsc@musc.edu

References

1999 Soft-tissue realignment for adolescent patellar instability. McCall RE, Ratts V. JPO 19:549

1995 Operative realignment of patellar malalignment in children. Vahasarja V. JPO 15:281

1992 Congenital dislocation of the patella and its operative treatment. Langenskiold A, Ritsila V. JPO 12:315

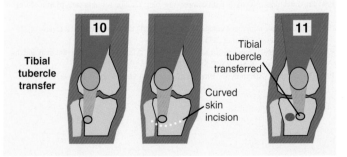

Tibial tubercle transfer

Curved skin incision

Tibial tubercle transferred

Hemiepiphyseal Procedures

Procedures that permanently or temporarily arrest half of the epiphysis are useful in correcting angulatory deformity in the growing child. Staples across the epiphysis provide temporary arrest and allow growth once removed. Hemiepiphysiodesis is permanent and requires careful timing to avoid over- or under-correction.

Hemiepiphysiodesis

Hemiepiphysiodesis requires careful timing and follow-up, as discussed in Chapter 4. The advantages are a small scar and a single procedure.

Technique Under imaging visualization use a K wire to identify the medial or lateral margin of the epiphyseal plate. Make a stab incision [1]. Place a 6 mm drill through the stab wound and just enter the growth plate [2]. Inspect the drilling for cartilage to confirm physeal entry. Through this drill hole place a small curette into the margin and perform a shallow curettage to remove the cortex and about a centimeter of underlying epiphysis [3].

Postoperative care Place compressive dressing and a knee immobilizer for comfort. Usually the patient is discharged the same day or the day after surgery. Follow clinically about every 3–4 months. If correction occurs before skeletal maturity, complete the epiphysis to avoid overcorrection.

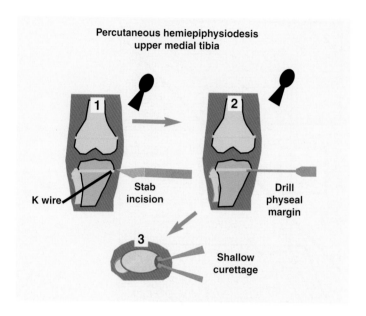

Percutaneous hemiepiphysiodesis upper medial tibia

1 K wire Stab incision
2 Drill physeal margin
3 Shallow curettage

Hemistapling

Stapling requires less accurate timing but a larger incision and a second procedure for staple removal.

Technique Under imaging using a K wire, mark the level of the physis [4]. Make a 3–4 cm longitudinal incision to expose the periosteum over the site of the physis [5]. Being careful not to damage or penetrate the periosteum, under imaging place a reinforced staple across the epiphysis at the midportion of the bone [6]. Leave the base of the staple extraperiostal. Place a second and possibly a third staple spaced about 2–3 cm apart across the plate, again avoiding a deep penetration [7]. Document the position of the staples with AP and lateral radiographs [8 and 9]. Close the wound with subcuticular skin sutures. Place a compressive dressing.

Postoperative care Follow the patient at 3–4 month intervals. When correction has occurred, remove the staples. Correction usually occurs at a rate of about 1° per month. Although staples rarely cause physeal closure, follow for this complication. If physeal arrest occurs, consider physeal bar resection and fat graft interposition or completion of the epiphysiodesis.

Complications

Hematoma Reduce risk by a compressive dressing following surgery.

Overcorrection Avoid by proper timing of staple removal or completing the epiphysiodesis in the hemiepiphysiodesis.

Undercorrection The procedure is performed too late.

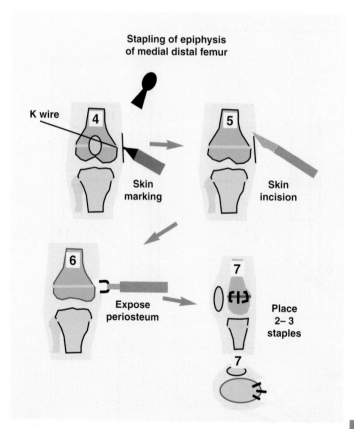

Stapling of epiphysis of medial distal femur

K wire 4 Skin marking
5 Skin incision
6 Expose periosteum
7 Place 2–3 staples
7

References

1999 Physeal stapling for idiopathic genu valgum. Stevens PM, et al. JPO 19:645

1997 Physeal surgery: indications and operative treatment. Guille JT, et al. Am J Orthop 26:323

1995 Medial physeal stapling for primary and secondary genu valgum in late childhood and adolescence. Fraser RK, et al. JBJS 77B:773

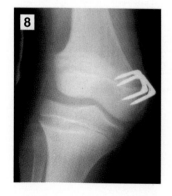

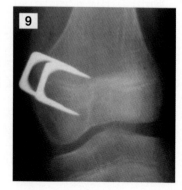

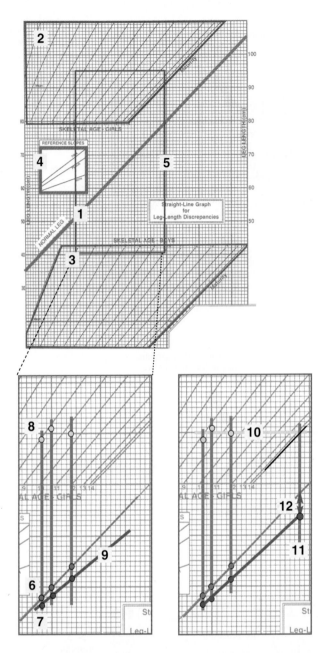

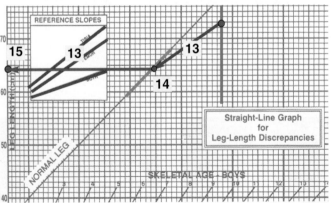

Timing for Epiphysiodesis (Moseley)

The straight-line graph method of Moseley is the most versatile but most difficult method of determining the timing for epiphysiodesis. This technique developed by Moseley is based on the Anderson and Green data and provides a system to graphically represent the data necessary to establish the appropriate time for epiphysiodesis. Plan to make radiographs with increasing frequency as the patient approaches the appropriate time for ephysiodesis. Be aware that the final timing is not based on the child's chronologic or skeletal age but when the long leg reaches the appropriate length for epiphysiodesis as determined by leg length radiographs.

The chart

The chart includes several elements: Normal leg growth [1] (green) and the skeletal ages for girls [2] (pink) and boys [3] (blue). The reference slopes [4] following epiphysiodesis are drawn for the femur, tibia, and combined level arrests (brown). Enlarged segments of the chart [5] (magenta) are shown to illustrate the details of assessment. Through a series of steps, the timing and epiphysiodesis level options can be established. The chart in full size in reproduced on page 412.

Assessment of Past Growth

Plot the point of length of the long leg [6] (sum of tibial and femoral lengths) on the green line (green dot) and draw vertical lines through the point (green line).

Plot the point representing the length of the short leg on the vertical green line [7] (red dot).

Plot the intersection (yellow dot) of the vertical green line and the bone age of the sloping nomogram line [8] (a girl in this example).

Plot the same points for each successive visit in the same fashion [9].

Prediction of Future Growth

Draw a horizontal straight line (yellow line) that best fits the points previously drawn representing skeletal age [10].

Draw a vertical line (blue line) from the intersection of the yellow line and the sloping line of maturity (black line) [11].

The points of intersection of the length at maturity (blue line) show the length of the normal and short leg at skeletal maturation [12]. The difference (red arrowed line) represents the leg length difference at the end of growth.

Prediction of Effect of Surgery

Based on the level and severity of the shortening, decide whether a tibial, femoral, or combined epiphysiodesis is best. From the point representing the length of the short leg at maturity, construct a line [13] with the appropriate slope back to the long leg growth line (green line). This point of interesection [14] represents the length of the long leg when the epiphsiodesis should be done. Determine the length in centimeters from the chart [15]. When the long leg is this length perform the procedure. In this example, a femoral epiphysiodesis should be performed when the normal leg length (combined femoral and tibial lengths) reaches 64 cm.

Full Size Chart

See page 412.

Consultant Colin Moseley, e-mail: cmoseley@ucla.edu

References

1992 The timing of epiphysiodesis. A comparative study between the use of the method of Anderson and Green and the Moseley chart. Dewaele J, Fabry G. Acta Orthop Belg 58:43

1991 Equalization of lower limbs by epiphysiodesis: results of treatment. Porat S, et al. JPO 11:442

1989 Assessment and prediction in leg-length discrepancy. Moseley CF. Instr Course Lect 38:3250

Epiphysiodesis

Epiphysiodesis is the safest procedure for correcting limb length inequality. The procedure is usually performed in the distal femur and or upper tibia, but the same principles apply for arresting the growth plate at other sites. Epiphysiodesis may be achieved by many techniques. Newer techniques are percutaneous and sometimes performed from only one entry site. The described techniques are suitable for both femoral and tibial level procedures.

Modified Phemister Epiphysiodesis

Technique Position the child supine with imaging available. Prepare the skin and drape. With imaging, mark the site of the medial and lateral sites of the physis [1]. The physis is usually at the mid-patella level. Under tourniquet hemostasis, make a 3 cm longitudinal incision centered over the physis [2]. Incise the periosteum and identify the cartilagenous physeal line. With a straight osteotome, remove a 2–2.5 cm square block of bone centered over the physis [3]. Curette about half of the physis [4]. Extend the curettage anterior and posteriorly, leaving the cortex intact. Rotate the block and replace it in the defect [5]. Repeat the procedure on the opposite side. Perform a subcuticular closure of both wounds. Inject marcaine in wound margins. Place a bulky compressive dressing and place in a knee immobilizer.

Postoperative care The day following surgery, replace the compressive bulky dressing with a conventional one, replace the knee immobilizer, and discharge the patient. Maintain non-weight-bearing status for 4–5 weeks with knee immobilizer in place. Physical therapy is not necessary. Allow full activity in 6–8 weeks. Evaluate at 6 months and yearly to assess effect of fusion. Check knee angle to identify asymmetrical fusion and limb lengths to assure complete physeal closure by a progressive reduction in length difference.

Percutaneous Epiphysiodesis

Technique Prepare and drape with the knee region exposed. Under tourniquet hemostasis, using a K wire marker, under image guidance with an 11 blade, make a 3–5 mm skin incision directly over the epiphysis [6]. Enter the epiphysis with a 6 mm (0.25 inch) drill [7]. Examine the drilling for cartilage fragments to confirm physeal penetration. Drill out the epiphysis by sweeping the drill from anterior to posterior. Leave the cortex intact. Make certain the entire central portion of the epiphysis has been removed (arrows) [8]. The epiphysiodesis may be performed from only the medial side. Some surgeons consider it prudent to perform the procedures on both sides of the epiphysis, as the growth plate is curved and sometimes difficult to access from only one side.

Postoperative care Discharge home the same day or the day after as with the modified Phemister technique.

Complications

Hematoma formation Reduce risk by placing a bulky compressive dressing following the procedure.

Compartment syndrome following tibial procedures is very rare. Identify early and release compartment.

Failure of fusion is rare and probably due to an inaccurate level of the procedure.

Asymmetrical fusion results in a progressive increase in varus or valgus deformity. Identify early and immediately refuse the open side.

References

1998 Percutaneous epiphysiodesis. Analysis of a series of 60 full-grown patients. Craviari T, et al. Rev Chir Orthop Reparatrice Appar Mot 84:172

1998 Percutaneous epiphysiodesis using transphyseal screws (PETS). Metaizeau JP, et al. JPO 18:363

1997 Epiphysiodesis using a cannulated tubesaw. Macnicol MF, Gupta MS. JBJS 79B:307

1996 Epiphysiodesis of the lower extremity: results of the percutaneous technique. Horton GA, Olney BW. JPO 16:180

1992 Fluoroscopic technique versus Phemister technique for epiphysiodesis. Liotta FJ, et al. JPO 12:248

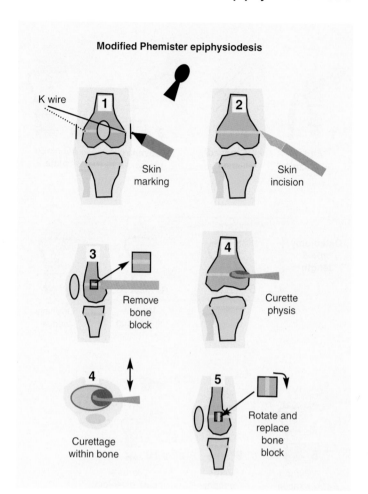

Modified Phemister epiphysiodesis

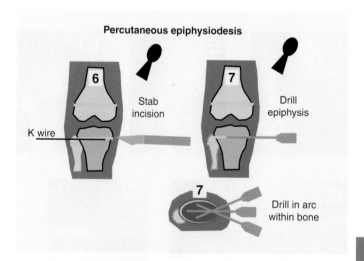

Percutaneous epiphysiodesis

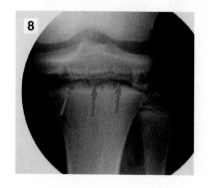

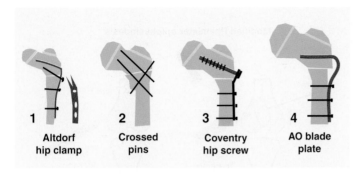

1 — Altdorf hip clamp
2 — Crossed pins
3 — Coventry hip screw
4 — AO blade plate

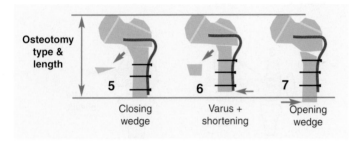

Osteotomy type & length

5 — Closing wedge
6 — Varus + shortening
7 — Opening wedge

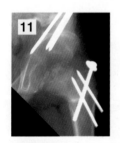 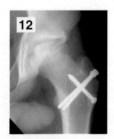 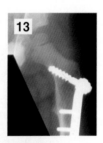

8 — Varus + rotation
9 — Varus + apophysiodesis
10 — Varus + pelvic osteotomy

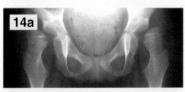

11

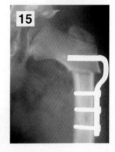

12

13

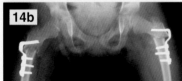

14a

15

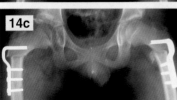

14b

14c

Varus Femoral Osteotomy

Proximal femoral osteotomy is useful in cerebral palsy, DDH, Perthes disease, and other conditions causing hip instability. To enhance stability and early union, perform the osteotomy at the intertrochanteric level and consider medial displacement of the distal fragment.

Fixation Methods

Select the method of fixation based on the procedure, age of patient, concurrent procedures, and available devices.

Altdorf hip clamp [1] is suitable for infants and young children. It is usually used in DDH. The clamp may be fabricated by cutting a notch in a standard fixation plate.

Cross pins or absorbable pins or screws [2, 11, and 12] require spica cast immobilization to supplement this fixation. The osteotomy must be high with a broad cancellous surface to provide stability. Multiple devices are necessary. Metallic fixation may be left in place.

Coventry hip screw [3 and 13] is suitable for children.

AO blade plate [4, 14, and 15] fixation is widely used. This fixation is very stable. Plan to place the fixation below the trochanteric apophysis.

Length Following Osteotomy

The osteotomy technique affects femoral length. Creating varus reduces femoral length. Intentional shortening may be appropriate when reducing a dislocated hip; maintaining length is an objective in Perthes disease.

Closing wedge osteotomy is often indicated as the shortening is minimal and a broad contact is created [5].

Intentional shortening [6, 14, and 15] is indicated when reducing a high-riding dislocation.

Opening wedge [7] design is useful when preserving length is desired, as in Perthes disease.

Combining Procedures

Creating varus to enhance hip stability is often combined with other procedures.

Varus, derotational osteotomy (VDRO) [8] is common in cerebral palsy. Use guide pins to monitor the amount of rotation.

Varus + greater trochanteric apophysiodesis [9 and 11] is used in managing Perthes disease. The apophysiodesis may be achieved by placing a screw with a washer across the apophysis, or by curetting out the apophysis.

Varus osteotomy + pelvic procedures [10, 11, and 14] is used to enhance stability. The bone from a closing wedge may be used in creating a shelf or to provide the opening wedge for the Salter or Pemberton procedures.

Examples

Some notable examples of varus osteotomy procedures are shown.

Perthes disease Double-level osteotomy with apophysiodesis [11].

Perthes disease Varus osteotomy fixed with AO screws [12].

Cerebral palsy sequence showing bilateral VDRO procedures combined with a limited periacetabular osteotomy on the right hip [14 and 15].

References

1999 Femoral varus osteotomy in Legg-Calvé-Perthes disease: points at operation to prevent residual problems. Kitakoji T, Hattori T, Iwata H. JPO 19:76

1998 Femoral varus derotation osteotomy with or without acetabuloplasty for unstable hips in cerebral palsy Song HR, Carroll NC. JPO 18:62

1997 Long-term effects of intertrochanteric varus-derotation osteotomy on femur and acetabulum in spastic cerebral palsy: an 11- to 18-year follow-up study. Brunner R, Baumann JU. JPO 17:585

1997 Outcome of Perthes' disease in unselected patients after femoral varus osteotomy and splintage. Lahdes-Vasama TT, et al. JPO-b 6:229

1995 The severely unstable hip in cerebral palsy. Treatment with open reduction, pelvic osteotomy, and femoral osteotomy with shortening. Root L, et al. JBJS 77A:703

1995 Varus derotation osteotomy for persistent dysplasia in congenital dislocation of the hip. Proximal femoral growth and alignment changes in the leg [see comments]. Suda H, et al. JBJS 77B:756

Rotational Intertrochanteric Osteotomy

This procedure is indicated for severe internal femoral torsion. Correction of femoral torsion may be done at any level of the femur but the intertrochanteric level offers several advantages. The osteotomy surfaces are broad to inhance stability and rapid union. Angular malunion is less obvious than osteotomies performed in the distal femur.

Preoperative Planning

Perform a rotational profile to document status of femur, tibia, and foot [1]. Review an AP radiograph of the pelvis to rule out other problems [2]. Consider the possible need for blood replacement and preop antibiotic prophylaxis. Access the amount of rotational correction needed. In most children, correct idiopathic internal femoral torsion by externally rotating the femur 45°.

Operative Setup

Make available interoperative imaging [3]. Prone positioning has several advantages: Interoperative measures of hip rotation are simplified. Gravity aids in exposure. Prep both legs. Drape allowing the limbs to be freely mobile [4].

Approach

Make a longitudinal lateral skin incision just distal to the greater trochanter. Incise the fascia and reflect the muscles anteriorly. Check position with the C arm to avoid injury to the trochanteric apophysis.

Guide Pins

Place two smooth parallel K wires to monitor rotation [5]. Place the pins far enough apart to avoid interfering with the fixation device. Access the alignment and record any differences in rotation between the pins. Place the nail guide pin and image to be certain that the position is appropriate [6]. Make the slot for the nail plate with a chisel.

Osteotomy

The level of the osteotomy is critical. The fixation device should be inserted just distal to the greater trochanteric apophysis. The osteotomy should be low enough to ensure adequate bone for the fixation of the nail but still be proximal enough to be intertrochanteric in location. Make certain the guide pin is preoperatively positioned. Check with an image to assure proper level. Complete the transverse osteotomy with a saw.

Rotation

Insert the blade plate into the slot and secure. Laterally rotate the leg until the pins show that the femur is 45° more laterally rotated than before the osteotomy. Screw the plate to the shaft, making certain not to lose the desired rotation [7]. Confirm position by assessing hip rotation [8] and imaging [9].

Postoperative Care

If fixation is secure, allow mobility in a wheelchair for the first 6 weeks. Allow crutch-walking for 2 additional weeks. Allow return to running at 16 weeks. Remove the plates in 6–12 months.

References

1999 Technique for illustrations. Dales M. surgeon.

1995 Surgical correction of idiopathic medical femoral torsion. Shim JS, Staheli LT, Holm BN. Int Orthop 19:220

1990 Osteotomy for femoral anteversion. A prospective 9-year study of 52 children. Svenningsen S, et al. Acta Orthop Scand 61:360

1989 Osteotomy for femoral anteversion. Complications in 95 children. Svenningsen S, et al. Acta Orthop Scand 60:401

1988 Valgus deformity following derotation osteotomy to correct medial femoral torsion. Fonseca AS, Bassett GS. JPO 8:295

1980 Medial femoral torsion: experience with operative treatment. Staheli LT, Clawson DK, Hubbard DD. CO 146:222

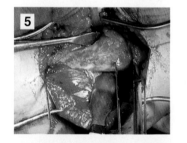
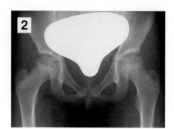
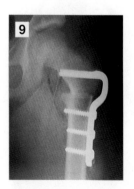
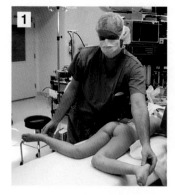
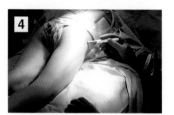
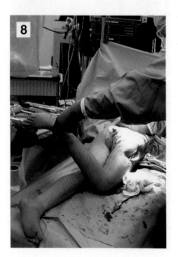
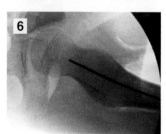
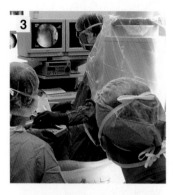
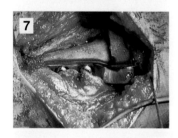

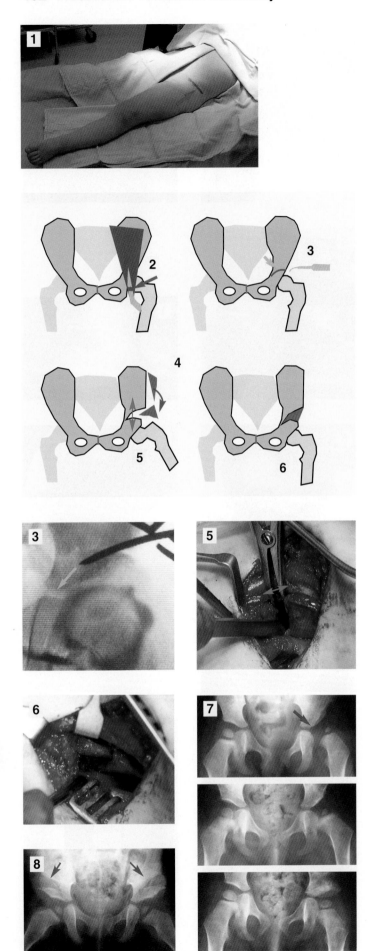

Pemberton Osteotomy

This pericapsular osteotomy was described by Pemberton in 1965. It has become more widely used with time for correction of dysplasia due to developmental hip dysplasia and neuromuscular disorders.

Indications

This osteotomy is indicated for correcting persisting acetabular dysplasia in the child less than 6–7 years with DDH and about 10–12 years with neurodysplasia. The procedure changes the shape of the acetabulum as the osteotomy hinges at the triradiate cartilage.

Pemberton and Salter osteotomies have similar indications. The advantages of the Pemberton procedure are the feasibility to perform bilateral procedures in one operative session, the lack of need for pin fixation, and a greater capacity for correction. The disadvantage is the alteration in shape of the acetabulum, which requires the procedure to be performed early in childhood to allow sufficient time for remodeling to create congruity with the femoral head.

Preoperative Planning

Make available curve osteotomes. Special Pemberton osteotomes with a 90° curve are available for the final portion of the osteotomy but are not essential. Determine in advance the need for an open reduction by abduction internal rotation radiographs and/or a preliminary arthrogram.

Technique

Prep and drape the leg free with the pelvis slightly elevated. Make a bikini incision parallel and slightly below the iliac crest [1]. Expose the inner and outer pelvis through a standard approach. Place a retractor in the sciatic notch. Perform a psoas release [2] and an open reduction if indicated. Perform the curved osteotomy that starts just above the insertion of the rectus and curves paralleling the acetabulum and into the triradiate cartilage just lateral to the sciatic notch [3]. If uncertain about the osteotomy, monitor with imaging. From the ilium, remove a triangular wedge of bone with the base about 2–3 cm [4]. Open the osteotomy with a lamina spreader and place the graft [5] in under compression. Create an acetabular index of about 10°–avoid overcorrection. Trim graft. The graft should be solidly impacted in the osteotomy and secure without fixation [6]. Close the wound and apply a spica cast with the hip in about 30° flexion, 30° abduction, and neutral rotation. Remove the cast in the clinic in 6 weeks. Hip stiffness may occur and will resolve spontaneously over a period of a few weeks or months.

Clinical examples

Unilateral dysplasia A 12-month-old infant with DDH following closed reduction is shown [7]. Persisting dysplasia was noted at 24 months. A Pemberton osteotomy was performed at 28 months.

Bilateral dysplasia A 30-month-old infant with DDH has persisting dysplasia corrected by concurrent bilateral Pemberton osteotomies [8].

Consultant Lynn Staheli, e-mail: staheli@u.washington.edu

References

1999 Injury to the growth plate after Pemberton osteotomy. Leet AI, Mackenzie WG, Szoke G, Harcke HT. JBJS 81A:169

1998 Pemberton osteotomy for the treatment of developmental dysplasia of the hip in older children. Vedantam R, Capelli AM. JPO 18:254

1997 Pemberton pericapsular osteotomy to treat a dysplastic hip in cerebral palsy. Shea KG, et al. JBJS 79A:1342

1996 Pemberton pelvic osteotomy and varus rotational osteotomy in the treatment of acetabular dysplasia in patients who have static encephalopathy. Gordon JE, et al. JBJS 78A:1863

1996 Pemberton's pericapsular osteotomy for the treatment of acetabular dysplasia. Szepesi K, et al. JPOB 5:252

1993 Pemberton osteotomy for residual acetabular dysplasia in children who have congenital dislocation of the hip. Faciszewski T, Kiefer GN, Coleman SS. JBJS 75A:643

1965 Pericapsular osteotomy of the ilium for treatment of congenital subluxation and dislocation of the hip. Pemberton PA. JBJS 47A:65

Salter Osteotomy

This single innominate osteotomy is useful to correct mild to moderate acetabular dysplasia from ages 18 months into adult life. The procedure is widely used and good to excellent outcomes are usually reported. Modifications include infrapelvic lengthening and performing the osteotomy with an osteotome, preserving the medial cortical periosteal attachments, enhancing stability, and eliminating the need for internal fixation.

Technique

Exposure Expose the hip through a bikini incision [1] and an iliofemoral approach splitting the iliac apophysis. Perform an open reduction as necessary. By subperiosteal dissection, expose the inner and outer surfaces of the ilium to expose the sciatic notch. Place retractors in the notch to protect the sciatic nerve.

Psoas tenotomy In most patients an intramuscular lengthening of the psoas is performed before the osteotomy. Identify the tendon within the muscle and divide only the tendon, leaving the muscle intact [2].

Osteotomy Perform the innominate osteotomy with a Gigli saw [3]. Passing the wire saw around the notch is the most difficult step in the procedure. This may be accomplished using the special saw passer, by placing a curved clamp around the notch, or by simply bending the saw blade and guiding it around with a curved clamp. Once the saw is passed, position the retractors to protect the soft tissues and perform the osteotomy. Make certain the osteotomy exits at the anterior inferior iliac spine.

Graft Place a towel clip in the anterior iliac spine to secure the graft. Remove a triangular graft that includes the anterior iliac spine using a bone cutter or osteotome. Reshape the graft into the desired triangular shape with the base about 2–3 cm in width [4].

Placing the graft Place a second towel clip through the ilium just above the acetabulum. Place the leg in a *figure 4 position* and with pressure on the flexed knee and traction on the towel clip, open and slightly laterally displace the acetabular segment. This should open the osteotomy laterally while keeping the medial cortical margins approximated [5]. Place the graft in the open defect.

Fixation Secure the fixation with two or three pins that penetrate the graft and both iliac surfaces [6]. These may be smooth or threaded. Make certain the pins do not penetrate the hip joint and are long enough for firm purchase on the lower fragment. Cut off the pins, allowing about 5–10 mm protruding above the cortical margin. It is important to cut the pins at a length that is long enough to facilitate removal but not so long as to cause skin irritation.

Closure is standard with a subcuticular skin closure. Immobilize in a spica cast for 6 weeks.

Differences Based on Disease

DDH Correct before age 4 years when possible. Immobilize in a spica cast for 6 weeks. In the older, cooperative child, with firm internal fixation non-weight bearing for 6 weeks is adequate. Make certain that the hip is concentrically reduced before performing the osteotomy.

Perthes disease When performed without a femoral osteotomy to decompress the joint, establish a good range of motion preoperatively and consider fixation with three larger pins to allow early mobilization following surgery.

Example

This 18-month-old female has a right DDH [7]. Open reduction was performed but acetabular dysplasia persisted [8]. At age 4 years a Salter osteotomy was performed [9]. Good correction was seen on radiographs taken at 8 [10] and 16 [11] years. The scar was linear and not noticeable [12].

Consultant John Wedge, e-mail: john.wedge@utoronto.ca

Reference
1961 Innominate osteotomy in the treatment of congenital dislocation and subluxation of the hip. Salter R. JBJS 43B:518

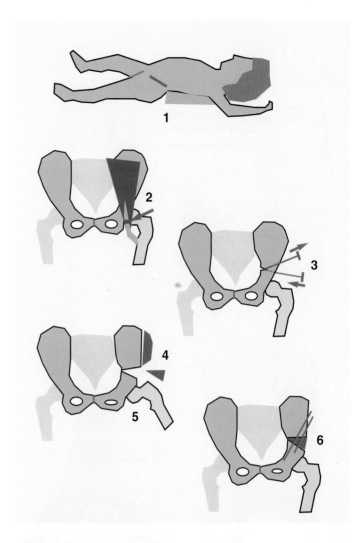

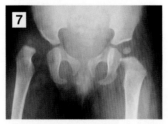

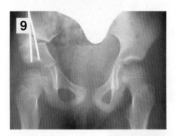

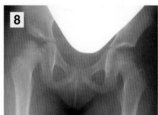

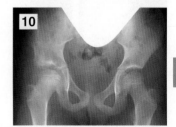

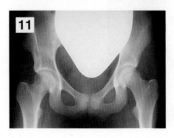

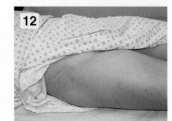

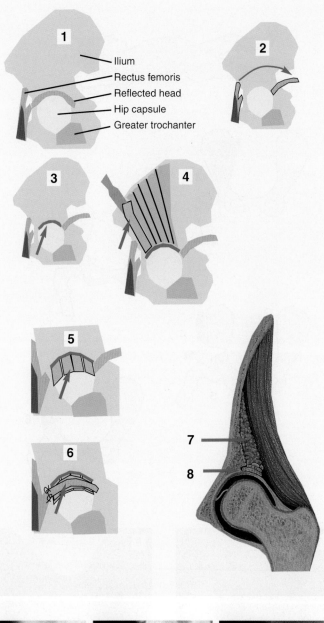

1

— Ilium
— Rectus femoris
— Reflected head
— Hip capsule
— Greater trochanter

2

3

4

5

6

7

8

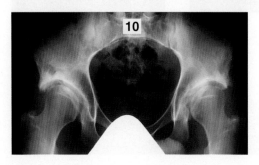

9

10

Slotted Acetabular Augmentation

This procedure is one of the many *shelf* operations. The shelf enlarges the acetabulum by grafting bone over the joint capsule. The joint capsule under the graft undergoes metaplasia to fibrocartilage. As the coverage is fibrocartilage, the shelf procedures are considered as salvage operations. Shelves are easily combined with other procedures. For example, if coverage or congruity is inadequate with a Chiari, Salter, or Pemberton procedure, consider adding shelf to improve coverage.

Indications

The procedure is indicated if the acetabular deficiency is severe, or non-spherical congruity is present. Other factors that make a shelf attractive include excessive scarring, bilateral augmentation as both sides can be corrected in one operative session, need for combined procedures, and to provide containment in Perthes disease.

Contraindications

When indicated, hyaline cartilage moving procedures such as the Salter or Pemberton osteotomy are preferred. Excessive laterization is best managed by Chiari procedure (unless bilateral).

Operative Planning

From a standing radiography of the pelvis, measure the CE angle and draw in a CE angle of 40°. Measure the needed width of the augmentation. Compare the standing radiograph with another taken in abduction in internal rotation. A difference in reduction indicates that the hip is unstable and a cast will be necessary.

Technique

   Anatomy Note that the reflected head of the rectus takes origin at the superior margin of the acetabulum [1].

   Approach Place a towel under the pelvis to elevate the hip. Prep and drape the leg free. Through a bikini incision expose the iliac crest. Identify the sartorius rectus interval. Incise the fascia over the sartorius and dissect through the interval to the hip joint without exposing the lateral femoral cutaneous nerve. Divide the apophysis or sharply divide the origin of the abductors from the iliac crest. Strip the abductor origin from the anterolateral side of the ilium to expose the hip capsule.

   Elevate tendon Identify the tendon of the reflected head of the rectus. Divide it anteriorly, sharply elevate it from the underlying joint capsule while preserving its posterior attachments [2].

   Create a slot in the ilium just at the lateral acetabular margin about 1 cm deep and 5 mm wide [3]. Extend it as far anterior and posterior as needed to provide required coverage.

   Graft Harvest abundant graft from the ilium [4].

   Place graft Place cancellous graft into the slot and over the capsule laterally as determined to create a CE angle of about 40° [5].

   Secure graft Secure the graft by resuturing the reflected head over the graft [6]. Reattach the abductors. Place the additional graft under the abductors to create a thick augmentation [7]. The graft should be congruous with the acetabulum [8]. Close the wound and apply a spica cast if the hip is unstable.

Postoperative Management

If the hip is unstable, immobilize in a cast for about 6 weeks. Crutch non-weight bearing is continued until the graft has consolidated– usually an additional 6 weeks. Full activity is allowed at 6 months.

Examples

   Unilateral augmentation Note the thick augmentation [9].

   Bilateral augmentation Bilateral procedures may be performed concurrently [10].

Consultant Lynn Staheli, e-mail: staheli@u.washington.edu

References
2000 Slotted acetabular augmentation: is a hip spica necessary? Walker KR, et al. JPO 20:124
1992 Slotted acetabular augmentation in childhood and adolescence. Staheli LT, Chew DE. JPO 12:569
1981 Slotted acetabular augmentation. Staheli LT. JPO 1: 321

Hip Releases in Cerebral Palsy

Hip contracture releases should be carefully tailored, taking into consideration the severity, location, child's age, and walking potential. Releasing of all contractures at one operative setting is usually best. Avoid overcorrection. The soft tissue releases may be combined with varus, rotational osteotomy, and if necessary a pelvic osteotomy.

This technique is based on Miller et al. (1997). Review the cross-sectional anatomy [1]. Plan to assess range of motion intraoperative with each step in the release. Releases may be performed through one medial incision.

Incision

Make a 5–6 cm oblique groin incision about 2 cm distal and parallel to the inguinal ligament and centered over the adductor longus tendon [2].

Adductor Release

Incise the fascia over the adductor longus and section the muscle [3]. Divide the gracilis muscle. If passive hip abduction <45°, progressively section adductors until 45° is obtained. Monitor muscle lengthening to assure both adequate correction and symmetry [4] are achieved. If the contracture is severe and hip subluxation is present, and it is unlikely the child will be ambulatory, section the obturator nerve.

Iliopsoas Release

Develop the interval between the pectineus and site of the divided adductor longus with finger dissection to palpate the lesser trochanter. Palpate the iliopsoas tendon attachment to the tubercle [5]. Place a right-angled clamp around the tendon and divide the tendon if the child is unlikely to walk [6]. If ambulatory, follow the tendon more proximally and perform an intramuscular lengthening of the tendon, leaving muscle bridging the tenotomy gap [7].

Proximal Hamstring Release

If the popliteal angle is <45° while under anesthesia and the child is likely to walk, lengthen the proximal hamstring tendons [8]. Extended the dissection by palpation medially under the adductor magnus muscle. With the knee extended, palpation will demonstrate the contracted proximal hamstring muscles. Differentiate the hamstring tendons–muscles from the sciatic nerve. The tendon and muscle take origin from bone, are somewhat more posterior in location, and the tendons are glistening white in color. Touch the tendon with the electrocautery tip before section to be absolutely certain the structure is not the sciatic nerve.

Asymmetrical Involvement

Asymmetry requires modifying the amount of release on each side to achieve symmetry [9]. Release more on the severe side. Try to achieve symmetrical passive abduction and popliteal angles releasing and assessing motion sequentially [10 and 11]. Passive motion should be symmetrical at the end of the procedure [12].

Postoperative Care

Miller recommends early intensive active and passive exercises provided by a physical therapist. An alternative is 2–3 weeks of immobilization in long-leg casts or knee immobilizer with a cross bar until the wounds are healed and the child is comfortable. Avoid prolonged immobilization, and mobilize the child as soon as possible to minimize postsurgical motor regression. Hospitalize 5–7 days. Follow at about 2 and 6 weeks, then every 6 months.

Consultant Freeman Miller, e-mail: miller@me.udel.edu

References

1998 Modified adductor muscle transfer in cerebral palsy. Beals TC, Thompson NE, Beals RK. JPO 18:522

1997 Soft-tissue release for spastic hip subluxation in cerebral palsy. Miller F, et al. JPO 17:571

1997 Psoas and adductor release in children with cerebral palsy. Spruit M, Fabry G. Acta Orthop Belg 63:91

1995 Adductor and psoas release for subluxation of the hip in children with spastic cerebral palsy. Moreau M, Cook PC, Ashton B. JPO 15:672

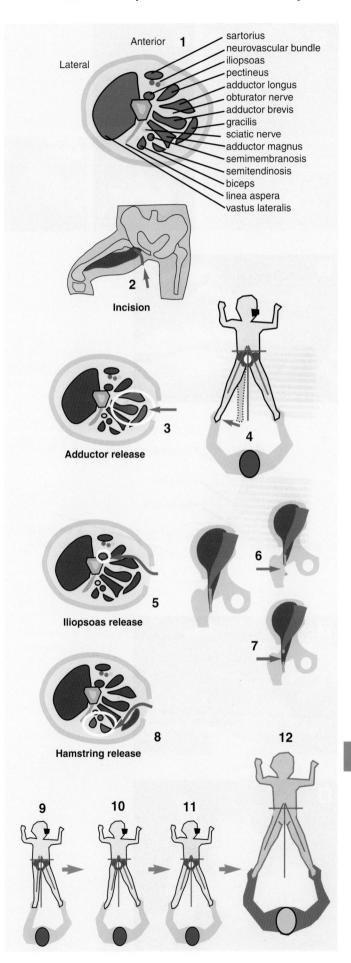

Anterior 1 — sartorius, neurovascular bundle, iliopsoas, pectineus, adductor longus, obturator nerve, adductor brevis, gracilis, sciatic nerve, adductor magnus, semimembranosis, semitendinosis, biceps, linea aspera, vastus lateralis
Lateral

2 — Incision

3 — Adductor release

4

5 — Iliopsoas release

6

7

8 — Hamstring release

9 10 11 12

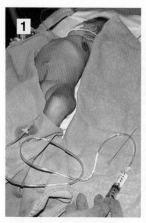

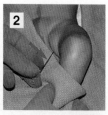

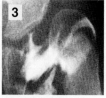

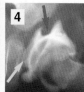

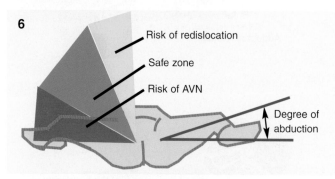

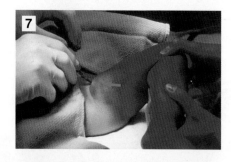

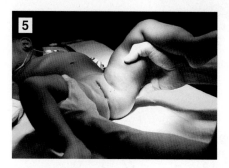

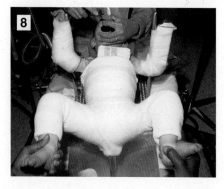

Closed Reduction of DDH

Closed reduction is appropriate management for most infants with DDH under about 18 months of age. Management involves four steps.

Arthrographic Evaluation

This step can be omitted if the hip easily reduces, is stable, and the conventional radiograph shows satisfactory reduction. If reduction or pathology is uncertain, perform an arthrogram. Fill a 20cc syringe with diluted dye [1]. Attach flexible tubing and fill the tubing with dye. Advance a 3 inch #20 needle through the adductor approach under fluoroscopic guidance into the empty acetabulum [2]. This step is facilitated by filling a second syringe with saline to be used to confirm joint entry. Once the joint is thought to be entered with the needle, inject a few cc of saline. Remove the syringe and medially rotate the leg. Joint entry is confirmed if saline drips from the needle hub. Repeat if necessary. Once entry is confirmed, attach the tubing and inject a few cc of dye while imaging the joint. Avoid excessive dye injection. Image in the position of dislocation [3] and reduction [4]. Note any obstacles to reduction. The labrum (red arrow) is interposed but the medial dye pool is not excessive (yellow arrow). Unless the hip is stiff, often an interposed limbus is accepted because the limbus will remodel with time.

Stability of Reduction

The second step is to determine the stability of reduction. Reduce the hip in flexion and determine the stability of reduction [5]. If an adductor contracture limits abduction, narrowing the arc of stability (green or safe zone), perform an percutaneous adductor tenotomy [6].

Percutaneous Adductor Tenotomy

This procedure is performed with a pointed blade through a stab incision just distal to the inguinal crease. Identify the palpable tendon of the adductor longus and divide the tendon by placing the blade first on the lateral side of the tendon and cutting in a medial direction away from the femoral artery [7].

Indications for an Open Reduction

If the limbus is interposed but the hip is stable, allow the interposition to be resolved by remodeling. If the interposition results in an unstable reduction or if the dislocation cannot be reduced or cannot be maintained without excessive abduction, perform an open reduction.

Immobilize in a Spica Cast

Most reductions may be safely maintained with the hip positioned in about 80° of flexion, 45° of abduction, and neutral rotation. While maintaining this position, position the infant on a spica frame and apply first the liner and padding [8] and then the cast. Be aware of the natural tendency for the person holding the position to allow the thighs to fall in greater abduction and less flexion during the cast application, making the reduction less stable and increasing the risk of AVN.

Post-Reduction Management

Document the reduction by an AP radiograph in the cast. If the quality of reduction is uncertain, confirm the reduction by a CT scan prior to discharge. Plan to change the cast under anesthesia in 4–6 weeks. If limbus interposition was present, repeat the arthrogram during the second cast change to firm a concentric reduction. Remove the second cast in the clinic. Follow with shielded AP pelvic radiographs at 3, 6, 12, 18, 24, 36, and 48 months following cast removal. Some advocate night splinting until age 3 years, but no data confirm the value of this splinting.

References

1994 The success of closed reduction in the treatment of complex developmental dislocation of the hip. Fleissner PR Jr, et al. JPO 14:631

1993 Acetabular development after closed reduction of congenital dislocation of the hip. Noritake K, et al. JBJS 75B:737

1992 Prognostic factors in congenital dislocation of the hip treated with closed reduction. The importance of arthrographic evaluation. Forlin E, et al. JBJS 74A:1140

Risk of redislocation

Safe zone

Risk of AVN

Degree of abduction

Medial Approach Open Reduction (Ludloff)

This procedure was described by Ludloff in 1908 to provide a direct approach for open reduction of the hip in DDH. This procedure is one of several approaches for open reduction [1].

Indications

The procedure is useful for management of dislocations of the hip due to DDH and arthrogryposis in infants under about 18 months of age.

Technique

Preparation Place a folded towel to elevate the pelvis [2]. If necessary both hips may be reduced at one operative setting. Perform an arthrogram if indicated [3]. Prepare the skin and drape with the limb(s) free [4]. Abduct the hip and identify the adductor longus tendon.

Approach Make a 3 cm skin incision 1 cm distal and parallel to the inguinal crease centered over the anterolateral margin of the adductor longus tendon. On the lateral aspect of the incision, identify and avoid the long saphenous vein. Identify the interval just lateral to the adductor longus muscle and tendon. Through this interval the lesser trochanter is identified. This is best done by palpation [5]. Bring the trochanter into profile by flexing and laterally rotating the thigh. Extend the finger dissection until the prominence of the trochanter is palpated. Place retractors to visualize the trochanter and free overlying soft tissue [6].

Psoas tenotomy Place a curve clamp around the psoas tendon just above its insertion [7]. Divide the tendon completely [8]. Free the hip capsule. Apply traction to approximate the femoral head within the capsule and rotate the thigh to feel the rotation of the femoral head.

Reduction Incise the capsule and extend the capsulotomy medially to include the transverse acetabular ligament. Perform a tendinotomy of the adductor longus tendon. Remove the ligamentum teres and pulvinar to allow a concentric reduction. To confirm that division of the ligament is complete, slide a curved clamp over the medial acetabular margin. Reduce the dislocation [9].

Stability Determine the arc of stability and the degree of flexion, abduction, and rotation that provides optimum stability while remaining within the safe zone. Obtain an AP radiograph with the hip reduced. The surgeon should maintain this position of stable reduction while an assistant performs the subcutaneous skin closure and applies the spica cast [10]. To ensure maintenance of the reduction, make a second comparable AP radiograph in the cast. If any loss of reduction is demonstrated, the cast is removed, the hip re-reduced, and a new cast applied.

Postoperative Care

Confirm the reduction with a CT scan. Expect considerable swelling about the perinenum. The patient may be discharged the next day. Reschedule for cast change in 6 weeks. Continue cast immobilization for 12 weeks. Maintain afterwards in a night splint [11]. About a third of the hips show persisting dysplasia and require a pelvic osteotomy.

Complications

Redislocation is best prevented by thorough release and careful positioning and follow-up in the cast. Avascular necrosis is the most common complication as with other methods of reduction. Try to avoid by careful dissection for exposure and positioning in the cast without excessive abduction.

Consultant Lynn Staheli, e-mail: staheli@u.washington.edu

References

1996 Ludloff's medial approach for open reduction of congenital dislocation of the hip. A 20-year follow-up [see comments]. Koizumi W, et al. JBJS 78B:924

1993 Open reduction through a medial approach for congenital dislocation of the hip. A critical review of the Ludloff approach in sixty-six hips. Mankey MG, Arntz GT, Staheli LT. JBJS 75A:1334

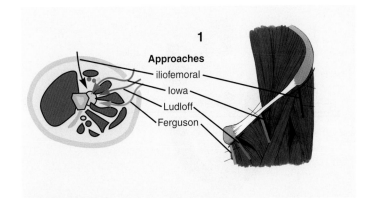

1

Approaches
iliofemoral
Iowa
Ludloff
Ferguson

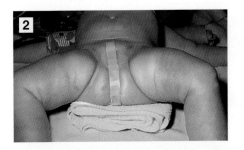

2

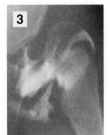

3

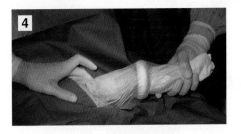

4

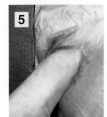

5

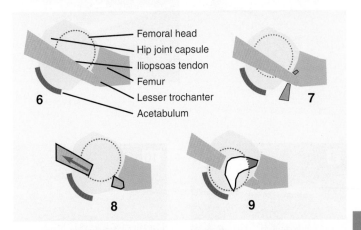

Femoral head
Hip joint capsule
Iliopsoas tendon
Femur
Lesser trochanter
Acetabulum

6   7

8   9

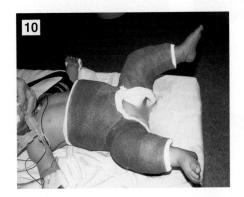

10

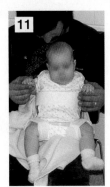

11

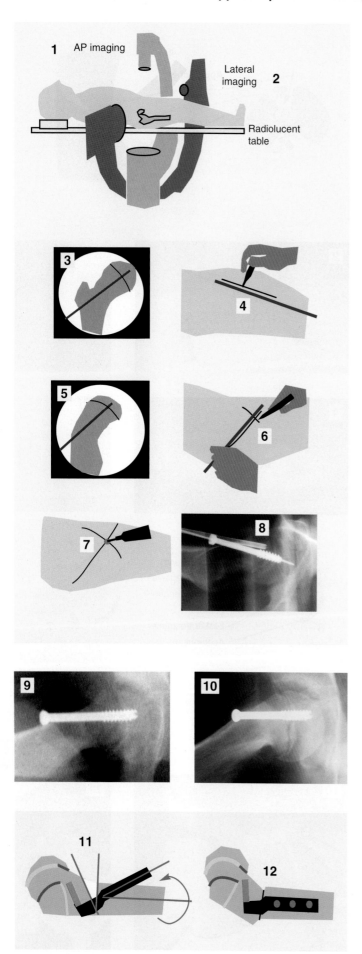

Fixation of Slipped Capital Femoral Epiphysis

Classify as stable or unstable. See page 153.

Percutaneous Pinning for Stable SCFE

Positioning Place the patient on a radiolucent table. Make certain that satisfactory imaging is possible for both AP [1] and lateral [2] views before starting the procedures. In the large, obese adolescent this may be difficult.

Determining position for pin entry Using guide wires, mark on the skin lines projecting optimal pin position for both the AP [3 and 4] and lateral [5 and 6] views. With greater degrees of slip, the entry point in the neck will become more proximal and anterior.

Fixation device Cannulated screws simplify fixation by allowing placement of a guide pin over which the fixation device may be placed.

Guide wire placement Prep the skin at the site the lines intersect, make a stab skin incision and place the guide wire in under imaging visualization [7]. Alternately monitor position by switching from the AP and lateral projections. Be certain to achieve accurate placement. Confirm accurate positioning by observing the position while imaging through an arc of motion that includes maximal profiling of the proximal femur.

Pin fixation Ream the femoral neck and head over the guide wire. Place the guide wire deep enough to avoid nonintentional removal when removing the reamer. Insert the cannulated screw at a depth that is short of joint penetration [8] but deep enough to provide 3–4 threads to engage the femoral head [9 and 10].

After treatment Walking is allowed as tolerated. Pin removal is usually not necessary. Follow to insure growth plate fusion and to monitor opposite side for possible slipping.

Unstable SCFE

Because the risk of avascular necrosis is great, open the joint to drain the hematoma and fix securely.

Joint decompression This is best achieved by opening the joint as soon as possible following the slip.

Reduction Adequate reduction is usually achieved by the act of positioning the leg in preparation for pinning. This positioning involves internal rotation and adduction of the limb. Avoid overreduction as this increases the risk of AVN.

Fixation Fixation is often adequate with one pin if good position and purchase is achieved. Add a second pin if fixation is tenuous.

After treatment Protect with bed rest for 3 weeks and non-weight bearing until callus is seen radiographically. Follow clinically for evidence of AVN by limited motion and radiographic changes.

Severe Deformity from SCFE

Slips >60° may cause persisting disability and be indications for corrective osteotomy. The simple flexion osteotomy has been shown to correct the deformity with little risk to femoral head vascularity.

Procedure Though a lateral approach, expose the intertrochanteric portion of the upper femur. From the measure of slip angle, determine the degree of correction. Place a right angle nail-plate in the upper fragment at an angle to the shaft equaling the slip angle. Perform an osteotomy just below the blade-plate entry site [11]. Flex the distal fragment to align the plate with the femoral shaft. Minimal rotational correction may be necessary. Fix with 3–4 cortical screws [12].

After treatment Protect with non-weight bearing until union is solid. Removal of the plate is usually not necessary.

Consultation Randy Loder, e-mail: rloder@shrinenet.org

References

1999 Intertrochanteric corrective osteotomy for moderate and severe chronic slipped capital femoral epiphysis. Parsch K, et al. JPO-b 8:223

1996 Treatment of the unstable (acute) slipped capital femoral epiphysis. Aronsson DD, Loder RT. CO page 99

Unicameral Bone Cyst Management

Select management based on the child's age, location, size, position in the bone, and previous treatment.

Selection of Treatment Method

Generally injection treatment is appropriate for cysts of non-weight-bearing bones. Cysts of the proximal femur and large cysts in other sites of the lower limb are best managed by curettage and grafting.

Diagnosis

Confirm the diagnosis by inserting a #18 spinal needle into the cyst through the thinnest wall [1]. Aspirate the cyst. Simple bone cysts are filled with clear yellow fluid. It may be slightly blood-tinged due to procedure. If blood is obtained, the cyst may be aneurysmal [2]. If no fluid is obtained, the lesion may be a solid tumor [3]. Consider biopsy [4].

Injection Treatment for Unicameral Cyst

If the cyst contains yellow fluid, perform a cystogram. Inject diluted contrast solution such as renografin to determine whether the cyst has single or multiple chambers [5]. For unilocular cysts, place a second needle and irrigate for several minutes [6]. Remove the second needle and inject the cyst [7]. The options for cyst treatment include:

Steroid Inject 50–100 mg of methyl prednicilone based on the cyst size.

Autogenous bone marrow Aspirate about 50 cc from the posterior iliac crest and inject the marrow into the cyst.

Treatment of Multilocular Cysts

If only part of the cyst fills during the arthrogram [8], modify the plan.

Injection. Inject each cavity with steroids or marrow [9] or break up the cyst.

Mechanical breakup of septa. Percutaneously introduce a trochar into the cyst and break up the septa [10]. Inject steroid or marrow as described before [11].

Radiographs

The arthrogram often shows a venogram (arrow) [12]. The cyst may fill completely [13], or incompletely [14].

Curettage Management

Manage cysts in weight-bearing bones, especially the upper femur [15] by curettage [16] and grafting. Following thorough curettage, fill cyst with autogenous or bank bone. Some recommend supplementing the curettage by freezing with liquid nitrogen, phenolization or burning with an aragon laser. The value of these supplemental measures has not been confirmed. Stabilize proximal femoral lesions with IM rods [17] or by nail-plate fixation [18].

Consultant George Rab, e-mail: george.rab@ucdmc.ucdavis.edu

References

1999 Percutaneous autologous bone marrow grafting for simple bone cysts. Kose N, et al. Bull Hosp Jt Dis 58:105

1998 Simple bone cysts treated with aspiration and a single bone marrow injection. A preliminary report. Delloye C, et al. Int Orthop 22:134

1997 Incomplete healing of simple bone cysts after steroid injections. Hashemi-Nejad A, Cole WG. JBJS 79B:727

1996 The choice of treatment for simple bone cysts of the upper third of the femur in children. Gennari JM, et al. Eur J Pediatr Surg 6:95

1996 Simple bone cysts treated by percutaneous autologous marrow grafting. A preliminary report. Lokiec F, et al. JBJS 78B:934

1995 Juvenile bone cysts. Relative value and therapy results of cortisone injections. Parsch K, et al. Orthopade 24:65

1994 Unicameral bone cyst of the calcaneus in children. Moreau G, Letts M. JPO 14:101

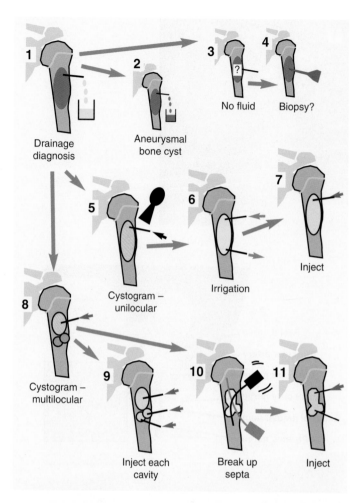

Drainage diagnosis — Aneurysmal bone cyst — No fluid — Biopsy?

Cystogram – unilocular — Irrigation — Inject

Cystogram – multilocular — Inject each cavity — Break up septa — Inject

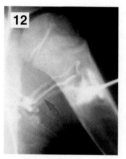
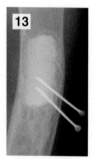
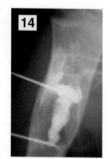

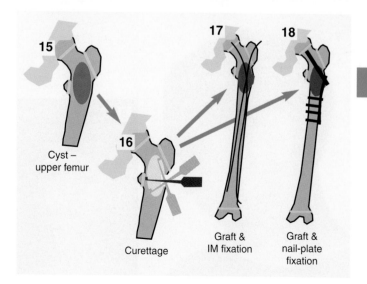

Cyst – upper femur — Curettage — Graft & IM fixation — Graft & nail-plate fixation

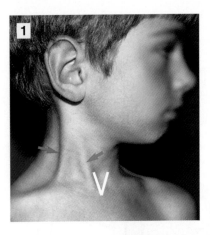

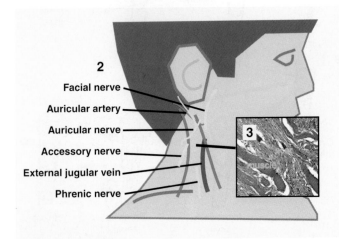

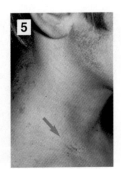

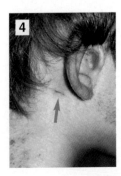

Facial nerve
Auricular artery
Auricular nerve
Accessory nerve
External jugular vein
Phrenic nerve

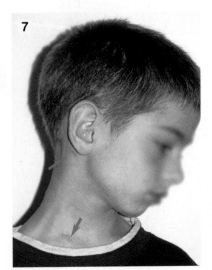

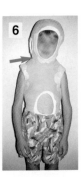

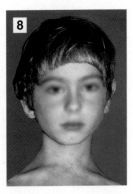

Bipolar Release for Muscular Torticollis

Most cases of muscular torticollis resolve during infancy. If the deformity persists into childhood and poses a cosmetic disability, release is indicated. Bipolar release of the contracted sternocleidomastoid muscle is usually appropriate, as double-level release provides better correction with less risk of recurrence. Endoscopic releases have been recommended; however, the open release can be performed through small skin line incisions that provides equivalent cosmetic results.

Preoperative Planning

Make certain the diagnosis is muscular torticollis (see page 188). Note the location of the contractures [1]. This boy shows the typical deformity with the clavicular head (red arrow) more contracted than the sternal head (blue arrow). If the deformity is severe, both distal heads should be released. If the deformity is moderate and if leaving the V contour is considered important, the sternal head may be left intact.

Technique

Position the child with a towel under the upper chest to allow extension of the head to make the contracture prominent during the release. Avoid nerves and vessels during the release procedure [2]. Although the array of these structures may seem worrisome, they can easily be avoided. The facial nerve lies well anterior, the auricular artery and nerve can be avoided by careful isolation of each segment of scar before excision. The accessory nerve lies distant, midway between the incisions. Distally, the vein and nerve lie deep to the fascia. The strands of fibrotic scar are distributed randomly within the muscle [3]. Perform the proximal release first [4]. Make a small transverse incision over the proximal portion of the muscle. With the muscle under tension, identify the fibrotic strands and divide each. Make certain that the release is complete. Make the second short transverse skin line incision in the skin crease well above the clavicle [5]. The mobile skin allows an extensive excision through a small incision. Release the muscle, fibrous tissue, and investing fascia. Close only the skin with subcuticular sutures. Reinforce the closure with paper tape. Apply a bulky dressing. Once the child is awake, a slightly compressive overdressing may be applied.

After Care

The child may be discharged the next day. Gentle stretching may be started within a few days. If the deformity is severe, apply a fiberglass jacket that includes the head (Minerva cast) [6]. Position the head in slight overcorrection in the cast. Cut windows for the face and ears. This cast may be applied in the clinic several days following discharge and worn for about 6 weeks. At 3 months after surgery, the scars [7] and the head tilt [8] are acceptable.

Complications

Residual head tilt is usually due to incomplete release or lack of postoperative range of motion or immobilization.

Bad scars may be due to excessive length, non-skin-line orientation, noncosmetic closure or keloid formation.

Neurovascular damage can be avoided by careful technique.

Recurrence is uncommon and cause may be uncertain.

References

1998 Endoscopic surgical treatment for congenital muscular torticollis. Burstein FD, Cohen SR. Plast Reconstr Surg 101:20

1992 Biterminal tenotomy for the treatment of congenital muscular torticollis. Long-term results. Wirth CJ, et al. JBJS 74A:427

1986 Surgical correction of muscular torticollis in the older child. Lee EH, Kang YK, Bose K. JPO 6:585

Spondylolisthesis Fusion

Fusion is indicated for slips of >50% and those that remain painful following nonoperative management. The need for reduction or instrumentional is controversial, but may be indicated for high-grade slips. Fusion of L5–S1 is often sufficient. Fuse from L4–sacrum when the transverse process of L5 are hypoplastic or displaced anteriorly, making a solid single-level fusion less certain.

Technique

Several approaches are effective. Consider tailoring the approach to the slip severity. With increasing slip severity and angle, increase the length of fusion and immobilization following surgery.

Positioning Place on rolls in the prone position. Prepare the skin and drape to allow visualization from L2–lower sacrum.

Skin incision Make a midline vertical skin incision. Alternatives include a curved transverse skin incision centered on the L1 spinous process or parallel paraspinal incisions [1]. Keep in mind the normal transverse anatomy [2].

Deep exposure may be made through the midline or through two paraspinal transfascial incisions. Make a midline incision through the lumbosacral fascia to expose the spinous process of each vertebral level to be fused. Expose the lamina, facet joints, and transverse processes [3]. As spina bifida is common, exercise caution in making this deep exposure to avoid accidental entry into the spinal canal.

An alternative is to make two paraspinal fascial incisions, leaving the transverse processes undisturbed and facilitating the lateral exposure [4].

In both approaches, extend the exposure to the tips of the transverse process. Avoid extending the exposure anterior or laterally beyond tips of the processes to avoid injury to the nerve roots and vessels.

Bone graft Retract the skin and subcutaneous tissues to expose the posterior ilium. Take a substantial bone graft of corticocancellous and cancellous bone.

Fusion Decorticate the transverse processes of each level to be fused. Create a notch in each sacral ala. Place cancellous bone from the sacral alar notch to L5 [5] or L4 [6] as planned. Place abundant graft in each lateral gutter [7] that extends laterally to the tips of the transverse process. Perform a facetectomy and graft the defect [8]. A posterior fusion is optional [9]. Some consider the posterior fusion increases the risk of spinal stenosis without improving the rate of fusion.

Postoperative care may include a pantaloon cast, TLSO, or no immobilization. The extremes include a cast and immobilization for 3–4 months or immediate mobilization with no external support. Most manage with a short period of immobilization and a TLSO for 3–4 months.

Illustration modified from Pizzutillo et al. (1986).

Consultation Kit Song, e-mail: ksong.chrmc.org

References

1997 Spondylolisthesis in childhood and adolescence. Schlenzka D. Orthopade 26:760

1988 Spondylolisthesis in children under 12 years of age: long-term results of 56 patients treated conservatively or operatively. Seitsalo S, et al. JPO 8:516

1986 Posterolateral fusion for spondylolisthesis in adolescence. Pizzutillo PD, Mirenda W, MacEwen GD. JPO 6:311

1985 Surgical fusion in childhood spondylolisthesis. Stanton RP, Meehan P, Lovell WW. JPO 5:411

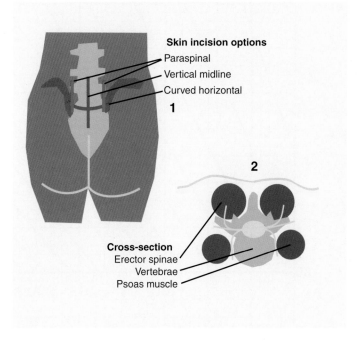

Skin incision options
- Paraspinal
- Vertical midline
- Curved horizontal

1

2

Cross-section
- Erector spinae
- Vertebrae
- Psoas muscle

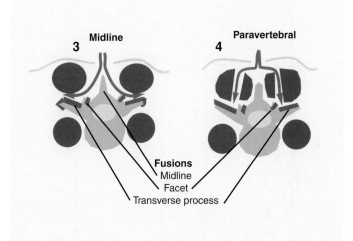

Midline

3

Paravertebral

4

Fusions
- Midline
- Facet
- Transverse process

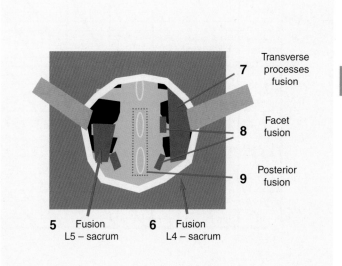

7 Transverse processes fusion

8 Facet fusion

9 Posterior fusion

5 Fusion L5 – sacrum

6 Fusion L4 – sacrum

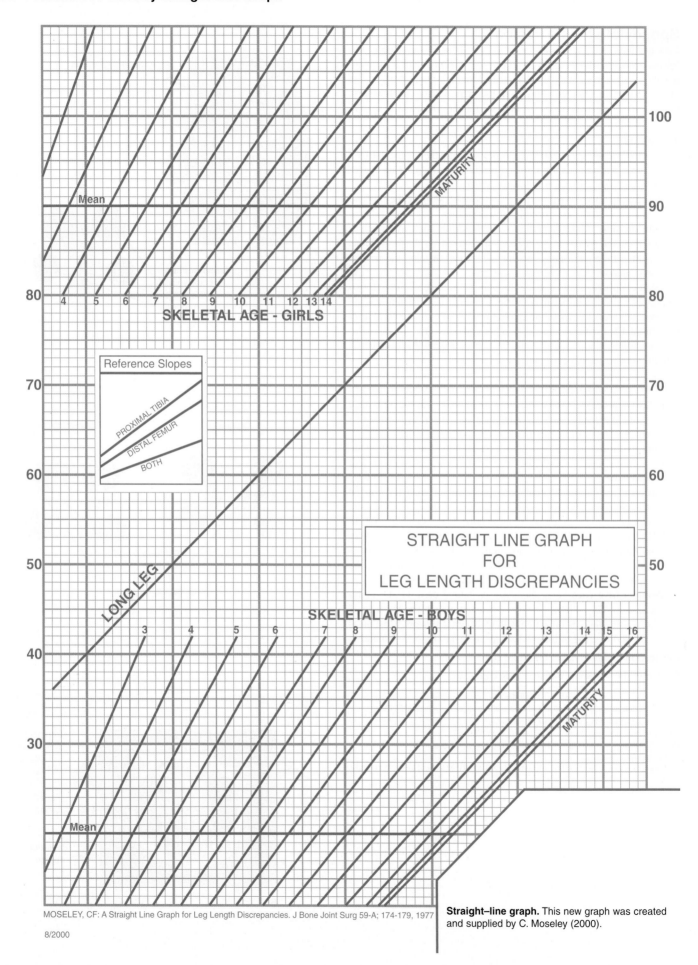

MATURITY

Mean

100

90

80   80

SKELETAL AGE - GIRLS

4   5   6   7   8   9   10 11 12 13 14

Reference Slopes

70   70

PROXIMAL TIBIA

DISTAL FEMUR

BOTH

60   60

STRAIGHT LINE GRAPH
FOR
LEG LENGTH DISCREPANCIES

50   50

LONG LEG

SKELETAL AGE - BOYS

3   4   5   6   7   8   9   10 11   12   13   14 15 16

40

MATURITY

30

Mean

MOSELEY, CF: A Straight Line Graph for Leg Length Discrepancies. J Bone Joint Surg 59-A; 174-179, 1977

8/2000

Straight–line graph. This new graph was created and supplied by C. Moseley (2000).

Chapter 17 – Reference Information

Questions Parents Frequently Ask

1. What are developmental variations?

These are common problems many infants and children develop during normal growth. These include flexible flatfeet, in-toeing and out-toeing, bowlegs, and knock-knees.

2. Why do infants and children develop these variations?

These variations are simply part of normal development that occurs in some children. It may be a pattern that is inherited or can occur for the first time in a family. Unfortunately, they may mimic deformities that are secondary to some underlying disease. Your physician will make certain the condition is not abnormal.

3. If I am concerned about the future, what should I do?

It is best to follow the advice of your physician. Your pediatrician or family physician will guide you. As they see many children with this problem, they are ideally qualified to advise you.

4. What are the features of these developmental variations?

They are very common. They occur in healthy infants and children. They resolve naturally over time.

5. How should these variations be managed?

It is best to allow the variation to resolve on its own.

6. Should we try to hasten the resolution by requiring my child to walk or sit in a corrected position?

No. This will not hasten the resolution and will simply frustrate your child.

7. Are corrective shoes or inserts useful?

No. Shoes and inserts do not hasten the resolution.

8. Is there any harm in such treatments?

Yes. Our studies have shown that adults who used these orthopedic devices as children remembered the experience as negative. Furthermore, the users had significantly lower self-esteem than adults who did not wear devices. This study suggests that the use of unnecessary treatment is not neutral but actually harmful.

9. Some doctors recommend shoe inserts, back manipulations, and other treatments. What should I do?

For a treatment to be imposed on your child, it should be both necessary and effective. We have not found any scientific evidence to support the use of these interventions.

10. My parents (grandparents) are insisting that we do something. What should we do?

If something must be done, do something that will clearly help your child. Follow the following recommendations:

  a. Do not focus attention on the variation because this may give your child a sense of being defective.

  b. Encourage your child to be physically active.

  c. Provide a healthy diet and avoid overeating to prevent obesity.

  d. Provide your child with flexible shoes that allow full mobility of the foot.

Handouts

The following pages may be photocopied and given to families to help them understand their child's condition.

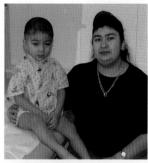
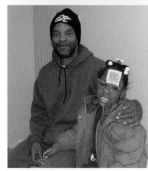
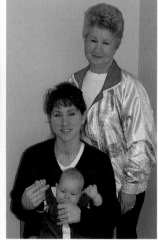

Fig. 17.1 Families. These are typical families that because of their concern often ask questions about their child's problem.

What Parents Should Know

about bent or twisted legs, flatfeet, and shoes for children.

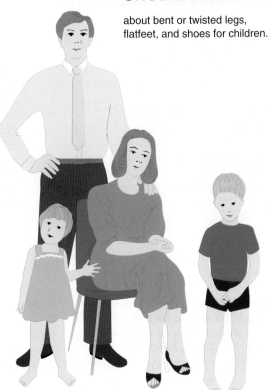

Most variations of normal childhood are outgrown.

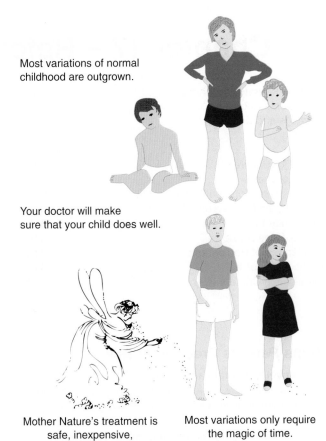

Your doctor will make sure that your child does well.

Mother Nature's treatment is safe, inexpensive, and effective!

Most variations only require the magic of time.

Bowlegs and Knock-knees

During normal development, children are bowlegged and then become knock-kneed. Special shoes or wedges make no difference.

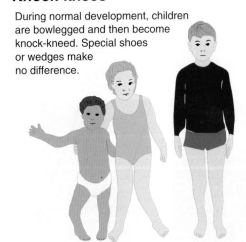

Your doctor will decide if your child's bowlegs or knock-knees are a normal form. If it is determined that the condition is normal, time is the best treatment.

Your doctor may be concerned if the condition is

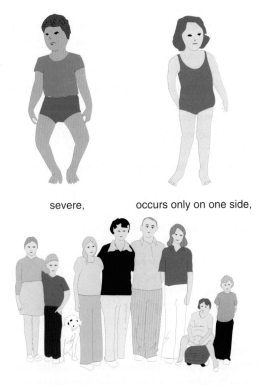

severe,   occurs only on one side,

or runs in the family (especially if the family tends to be unusually short in stature).

Intoeing

Intoeing is common in childhood and is usually outgrown.

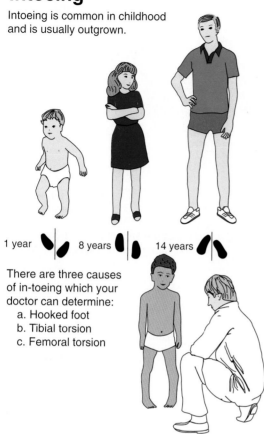

1 year   8 years   14 years

There are three causes of in-toeing which your doctor can determine:
a. Hooked foot
b. Tibial torsion
c. Femoral torsion

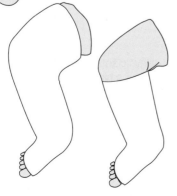

Hooked Foot

Hooked foot is caused by the position of the baby before birth.

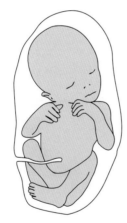

Most hooked feet get better without treatment during the baby's first month,

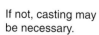

If not, casting may be necessary.

Tibial Torsion

Tibial torsion is a common cause of intoeing in toddlers.

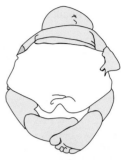

Most legs with tibial torsion get better without treatment.

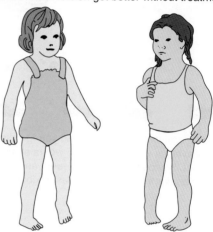

Femoral Torsion

The cause of femoral torsion is unknown. Femoral torsion is usually most severe when the child is about 5—6 years old. Most children outgrow this condition.

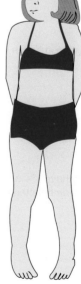

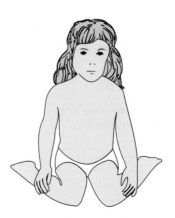

Shoe modifications and braces do not work for femoral torsion. They can make the child uncomfortable and self-conscious and can hamper play.

Flatfeet

Parents worry about flatfeet, but

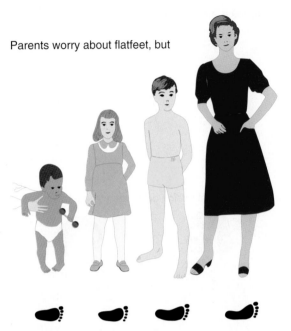

Flatfeet are normal in infants and young children. The arch develops whether the child wears shoes or goes barefoot. So special wedges, inserts, and heels are not necessary for the toddler who has flexible flatfeet.

Just as normal children are of different heights,

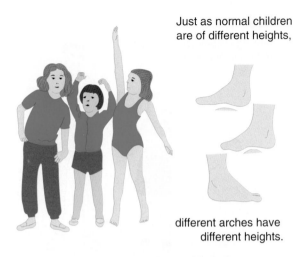

different arches have different heights.

Wearing a pad under the arch of a simple hypermobile flatfoot may make the child less comfortable,

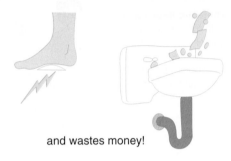

and wastes money!

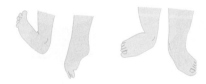

However, one in seven children never develops an arch.

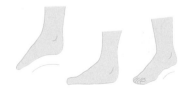

Children usually have low arches because they are loose-jointed. The arch flattens when they are standing.

The arch can be seen when these feet are hanging free or when the child stands on its toes.

The physician is concerned if the flatfoot is

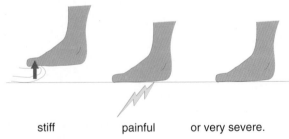

stiff   painful   or very severe.

Physicians are most concerned about a high arch.

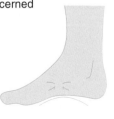

Shoes for Children

Barefoot people have the best feet!
Your child needs a flexible, soft shoe that allows
maximum freedom to develop normally.

1. Points in shoe selection
   Shoes are much better too large rather than too small.

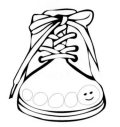
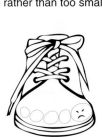

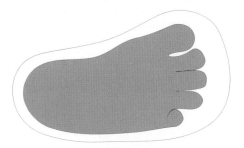

2. Flexible
   Stiff supportive shoes are not good for
   feet because they limit
   movement
   that is
   needed for
   developing
   strength and
   retaining foot
   mobility.

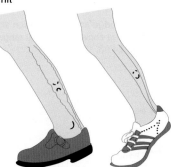

A child's foot needs protection from cold
and sharp objects, but it also needs
freedom of
movement.

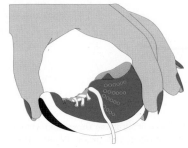

3. Flat sole
   Children's falls cause
   many injuries. A flat
   sole that is neither
   slippery nor sticky
   is best.

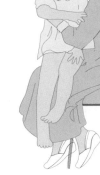

4. Soft porous upper
   A material that breathes is best,
   especially in
   for warm
   climates.

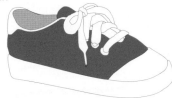

5. Avoid odd shapes.

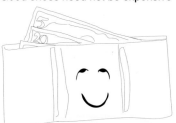

6. Good shoes need not be expensive

REMEMBER: The best shoe keeps the foot
warm and protected, but allows freedom of
motion and space to grow.

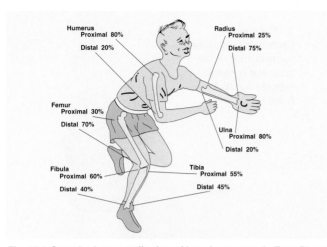

Fig. 17.2 Growth plate contribution of long bone growth. From Blount WB. Fig. 147, *Fractures in Children.* The Williams & Wilkins. Baltimore 1955.

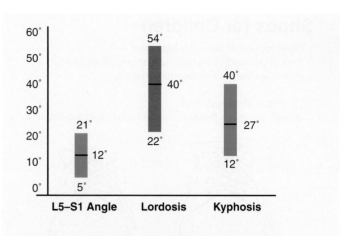

Fig. 17.3 Normal values of sagittal measures of spine in children. The range includes values from the 10th to the 90th percentiles. The **L5–S1 Angle** includes measures between the inferior surface of L5 and the superior surface of S1 (green). **Lordosis** is measured using the Cobb method between L1 and L5 (red). **Kyphosis** is measured using the Cobb method between T5 and T12 (blue). From Propst-Proctor & Bleck. JPO 3:344, 1983.

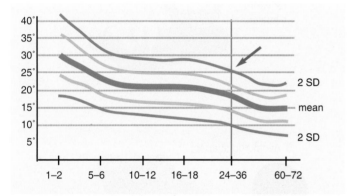

Fig. 17.4 Acetabular index. Illustration shows normal values by age group in months. Mean values (green line), 1 SD (orange) and 2 SD (red) are drawn. Note that at about 25 months the acetabular index should be below 25° (blue arrow). Redrawn from Tönnis D. Clin Orthop 119:39, 1976.

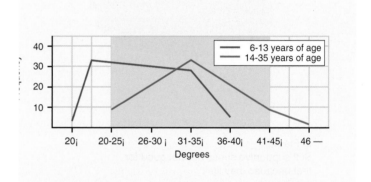

Fig. 17.5 Center-edge angle. Illustration shows mean values by age group. Green shaded area shows the normal range for adults. From Severin E. Acta Chir Scan 84:93, 1941.

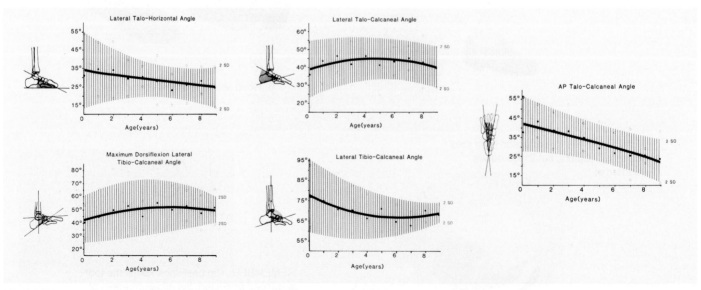

Fig. 17.6 Normal values for standing foot radiographs in infants and young children. These illustrations show mean values and normal range (plus or minus two standard deviations) in shaded areas. From Vanderwilde R, Staheli LT, Chew DE and Malagon V. JBJS 70A:407, 1988.

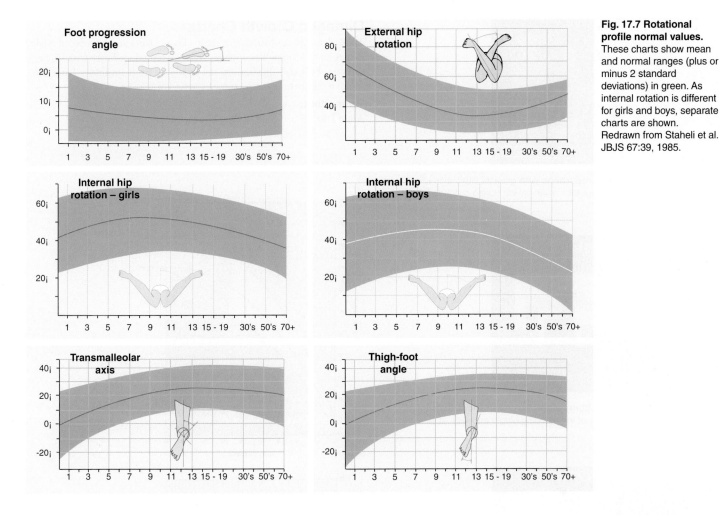

Fig. 17.7 Rotational profile normal values. These charts show mean and normal ranges (plus or minus 2 standard deviations) in green. As internal rotation is different for girls and boys, separate charts are shown. Redrawn from Staheli et al. JBJS 67:39, 1985.

Fig. 17.8 Ossification centers. Redrawn from Girdany BR and Golden R. AJR 68:922, 1952.

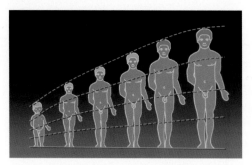

Fig. 17.9 Changes in body proportions with growth. Illustration shows that lower limb growth is greater than trunk growth during childhood.

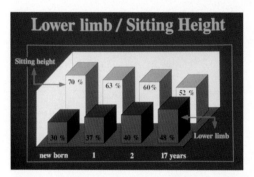

Fig. 17.10 Lower limb and sitting height. Illustration shows that at birth the lower limb represents 30% of the standing height and 48% at skeletal maturity.

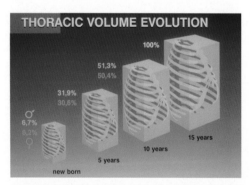

Fig. 17.11 Intrathoracic volume evolution. Illustrations shows that thorax volume increases more than tenfold from birth to maturity and doubles between age 10 years and the end of growth.

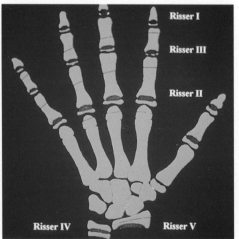

Dimeglio Growth Charts

These data and construction of these classic charts are the work of Alain Dimeglio of Montpellier, France. They are reproduced here with his permission. Full-size illustrations are available from Professor Dimeglio. Make requests by e-mail.

Consultant:

Alain Dimeglio, e-mail: a-dimeglio@chu-montpellier.fr

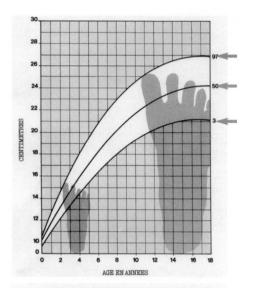

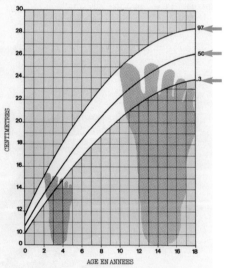

Fig. 17.12 Foot growth. These illustrations show foot growth of girls (upper) and boys (lower). Mean values (green arrows) and the two standard deviation levels above and below the mean values (red arrows) are shown.

Fig. 17.13 Hand and wrist radiographs, bone age, and Risser sign. The Risser sign is correlated with closure of the distal phalanx (Risser I), proximal phalanx (Risser II), middle phalanx (Risser III), distal ulna (Risser IV), and distal radius (Risser V).

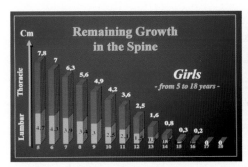

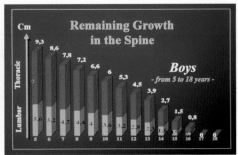

Fig. 17.14 Remaining growth in the spine. These illustrations show remaining growth in the thoracic (red) and lumbar (yellow) spine segments for girls (left) and boys (right).

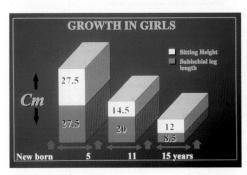

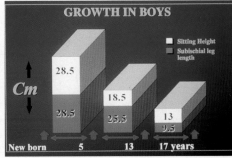

Fig. 17.15 Growth of the trunk and lower limbs. These illustrations show the proportions of the trunk and the lower limbs in infancy, childhood, and at the end of growth for girls (left) and boys (right).

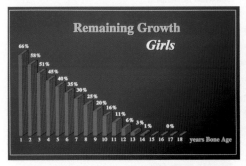

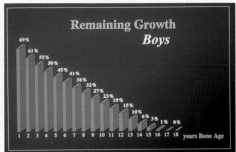

Fig. 17.16 Growth remaining. These illustrations show remaining growth (in percentages) for girls (left) and boys (right).

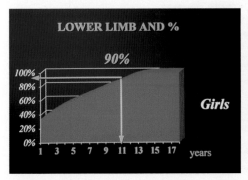

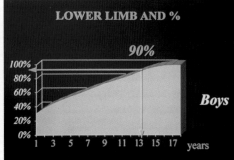

Fig. 17.17 Lower limb growth. These illustrations show the growth of the lower limb as expressed as a percentage of final length for girls (left) and boys (right).

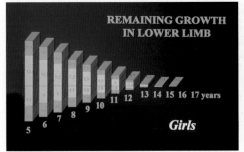

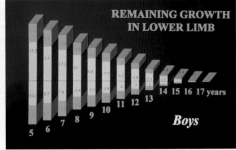

Fig. 17.18 Remaining growth of the lower limbs. These illustrations show remaining growth by age groups for girls (left) and boys (right). Growth contributions of each growth plate are shown from proximal to distal. These segments include the proximal femur, distal femur, proximal tibia, and distal tibia.

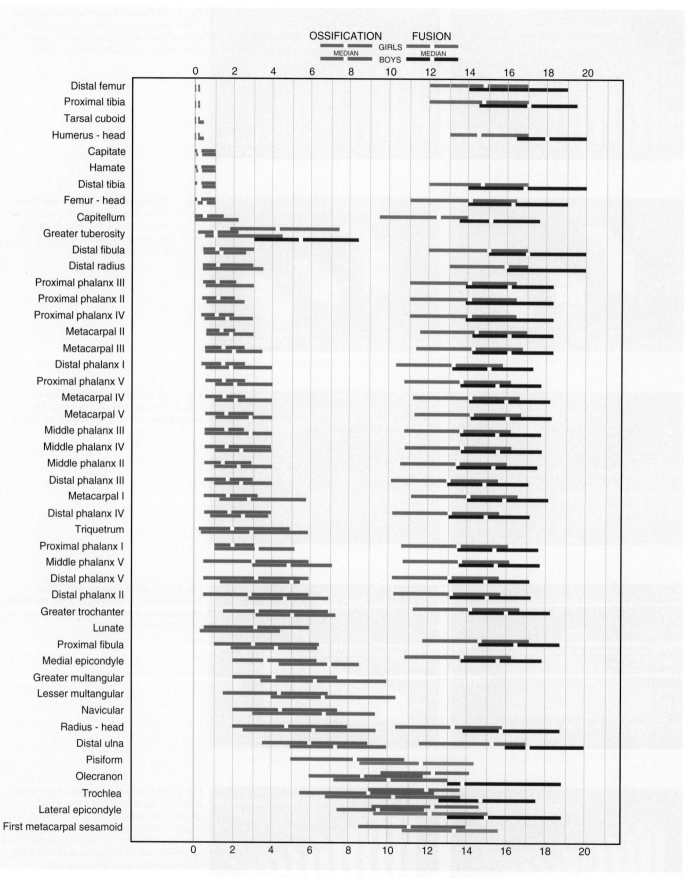

Fig. 17.19 Appearance and fusion of ossification centers. Redrawn from Hansman CF. AJR 88:476, 1962.

Chapter 18 – Index

Note: Page numbers in *italics* denote figures.